HISTOLOGY

SAUNDERS TEXT AND REVIEW SERIES

HISTOLOGY

RONALD A. BERGMAN, Ph.D.
Professor of Anatomy
The University of Iowa College of Medicine
Iowa City, Iowa

ADEL K. AFIFI, M.D.
Professor of Pediatrics, Anatomy, and Neurology
The University of Iowa College of Medicine
Iowa City, Iowa

PAUL M. HEIDGER, Jr., Ph.D.
Professor of Anatomy
The University of Iowa College of Medicine
Iowa City, Iowa

W.B. SAUNDERS COMPANY
A Division of Harcourt Brace & Company
Philadelphia   London   Toronto   Montreal   Sydney   Tokyo

W.B. SAUNDERS COMPANY
A Division of Harcourt Brace & Company

The Curtis Center
Independence Square West
Philadelphia, Pennsylvania 19106

Library of Congress Cataloging-in-Publication Data

Bergman, Ronald A. (Ronald Arly)

Histology / Ronald A. Bergman, Adel K. Afifi, Paul M. Heidger, Jr.

p.   cm.—(Saunders text and review series)

Includes bibliographical references.

ISBN 0-7216-3089-8

1. Histology.   I. Afifi, Adel K.   II. Heidger, Paul M.   III. Title.   IV. Series.
   [DNLM: 1. Histology.   2. Histological Techniques.   QS 504 B499h 1996]

QM551.B424 1996

611'.018—dc20

DNLM/DLC   95-33409

HISTOLOGY   ISBN 0-7216-3089-8

Copyright © 1996 by W.B. Saunders Company.

All rights reserved. No part of this publication may be reproduced or transmitted in any form or by any means, electronic or mechanical, including photocopy, recording, or any information storage and retrieval system, without permission in writing from the publisher.

Printed in the United States of America.

Last digit is the print number: 9   8   7   6   5   4   3   2   1

To our mentors,

through whom we learned;

and to our students,

through whom we learned what it means to teach

PREFACE

Biomedical research has been successfully directed in recent decades to probing the cellular and molecular bases of disease. Consequently, integration within the medical curriculum of molecular, cellular, tissue, and organ biology assumes paramount importance. This objective of integration has been a major motivating factor in our preparation of this text, which is thorough in its treatment of basic concepts at the various levels of biological structure while remaining of a size to be readable and useful to students. *Histology* is envisioned as a text that will be applicable in both newer integrated medical curricula as well as in more traditional presentations of microscopic anatomy. It is written for the student who has not had prior exposure to histology. We trust that the serious student will be directed to those more comprehensive treatments of topics, and to reviews of current concepts, referenced for each chapter.

Increasingly, the molecular and the microscopic are being melded into a more comprehensive understanding of structure-function relationships. The fabric and function of the human body cannot be understood solely in terms of the molecular—molecules function within the context of the cell. In turn, tissues and organs must be studied in terms of the functionally integrated cells and tissues that compose them. Within this unifying framework, we have organized this text in such a manner as to establish first the cellular basis for tissue structure; subsequently, organs and organ systems are considered in terms of the functional morphology of tissues. In no branch of biology does the maxim "the whole is greater than the sum of its parts" ring more true than in histology. The normal and abnormal functioning of organs must be studied at a far deeper level than that permitted by considering organs merely as aggregates of cells and tissues.

Where relevant, correlations are drawn between clinical syndromes and their underlying defects in morphology or alterations in cytophysiology and histophysiology. Such clinical correlations linking structure, function, and disease are included throughout the text in the anticipation that they will lead students in the health sciences to an appreciation of those mechanisms of disease that lie at the level of altered biostructure.

The illustrations within the text are computer-generated and have been prepared with the objective of presenting the beginning student with as clear and understandable depictions of biostructure as possible. The student desiring additional detail from original micrographic material is referred to the referenced comprehensive texts and atlases of histology, several of which contain superlative original light and electron micrographs. Many of the graphics within the text have been prepared from micrographs from our own collections and from illustrations in the literature.

The systematic arrangement of topics in *Histology* proceeds from cell to tissue, to organ and organ system. This organization was chosen on the premise, borne out in our professional experience, that only as students are first acquainted with the basis of biological structure, the cell, do the higher levels of biological organization at the tissue, organ, and systems levels appear intelligible. The organization of the present text parallels that of our

Atlas of Microscopic Anatomy, A Functional Approach: A Companion to Histology and Neuroanatomy. The *Atlas*, in addition to being an excellent guide to laboratory study, is therefore recommended as an excellent complement to the graphics presented in this text.

RONALD A. BERGMAN, PH.D.
ADEL K. AFIFI, M.D.
PAUL M. HEIDGER, JR., PH.D.

Acknowledgments

The editorial and publication staff at the W. B. Saunders Company deserves particular commendation for their empathetic and patient understanding during the preparation of the manuscript over a period in which trying personal circumstances and pressing professional obligations repeatedly beset us. Particularly, Mrs. Hazel Hacker, our developmental editor, deserves our highest praise and gratitude for her high professional standards, sincerity, and unfailing support and encouragement when needed most. We are indebted, as well, to Ms. Kim Kist, Senior Medical Editor, for encouraging us along the way.

The novel illustrations in this book have been prepared using computer graphics by JAK Graphics under the supervision of Joanna Koperski. We are indebted to Ms. Koperski and her staff for patience, good humor, high technical standards, and attention to detail in the preparation and revision of the graphic illustrations. The generous contributions of colleagues and of authors of other texts who have permitted modified and redrawn illustrations to be used in the present work are gratefully acknowledged; specific acknowledgements to authors are made within the figure legends of the text.

Finally, we acknowledge the support and sacrifice of our families, which permitted us to devote ourselves to the completion of an academic undertaking with the inevitable decrease in time available for family members and family responsibilities.

RONALD A. BERGMAN, PH.D.
ADEL K. AFIFI, M.D.
PAUL M. HEIDGER, JR., PH.D.

CONTENTS

CHAPTER ONE
The Cell 1

CHAPTER TWO
Epithelium 24

CHAPTER THREE
Connective Tissue 41

CHAPTER FOUR
Cartilage, Bone, and Joints 59

CHAPTER FIVE
Muscular Tissue 76

CHAPTER SIX
Blood Cells and Hematopoiesis 96

CHAPTER SEVEN
Neural Tissue 111

CHAPTER EIGHT
Cardiovascular System 133

CHAPTER NINE

LYMPHATIC SYSTEM AND IMMUNITY 142

CHAPTER TEN

INTEGUMENT 155

CHAPTER ELEVEN

THE DIGESTIVE SYSTEM 177

CHAPTER TWELVE

URINARY SYSTEM 213

CHAPTER THIRTEEN

RESPIRATORY SYSTEM 227

CHAPTER FOURTEEN

SPECIAL SENSES 240

CHAPTER FIFTEEN

ENDOCRINE SYSTEM 258

CHAPTER SIXTEEN

FEMALE REPRODUCTIVE SYSTEM 281

CHAPTER SEVENTEEN

MALE REPRODUCTIVE SYSTEM 303

BIBLIOGRAPHY 321

INDEX 325

ILLUSTRATION CREDITS 343

CHAPTER ONE

THE CELL

CELLS, TISSUES, AND ORGANS	2
SIZE DIMENSIONS IN THE STUDY OF BIOSTRUCTURE	2
PREPARATION OF TISSUES FOR HISTOLOGIC STUDY	2
Light Microscopy	2
Electron Microscopy	3
TECHNIQUES THAT PERMIT OBSERVATION OF LIVING CELLS AND TISSUES	4
PERSPECTIVES: THE QUICK AND THE DEAD	4
APPROACHES THAT FACILITATE ESTABLISHING FUNCTIONAL CORRELATES WITH HISTOLOGIC STRUCTURE	4
Histochemistry	4
Immunocytochemistry	5
Autoradiography	5
In Situ Hybridization	6
Cell Fractionation	6
CELL STRUCTURE AND FUNCTION	6
The Plasma Membrane	6
Cytoplasm	11
Organelles	12
Nucleus	19
Cell Division	21
CONCLUSION	23

CELLS, TISSUES, AND ORGANS

All living matter is organized into structural and functional units called *cells,* which are the smallest units of life capable of independent existence. In multicellular organisms, cells provide the building blocks for tissues, such as epithelium, connective tissue, muscle, and nerve. Organs are formed from these four primary tissues, and organs, in turn, function in the larger context of the major organ systems of the vertebrate body, such as the digestive, reproductive, and nervous systems.

Histology is the subdiscipline of anatomy that focuses upon the microscopic structure of normal tissues. The full appreciation of tissues is possible, however, only as they are studied in terms of both their fundamental units—cells—and their larger organizational and functional context—organs. For this reason, this text is organized in such a way that for each tissue, the specialized cells specific to that tissue are presented first, followed by the structural and functional roles played by the tissue within its organ and systemic context (Fig. 1–1). An accurate understanding of the structural and functional interrelationships of cells and tissues and organs relies increasingly upon the correlation of knowledge gained by means of traditional histologic techniques with the information contributed through powerful and sophisticated new techniques of molecular and cellular biology.

SIZE DIMENSIONS IN THE STUDY OF BIOSTRUCTURE

Students within the health sciences generally study human anatomy within several dimensional realms. Those structures that are studied with the unaided eye, as in the dissection room, fall within the province of gross anatomy—for example, the study of individual organs (organology), individual muscles, nerves, and the aggregate of connective tissue surrounding them. If two structures lie closer than 0.2 mm (the approximate *resolving power* of the human retina), however, they will be perceived as one structure, unless a supplemental lens system is employed to resolve them as separate entities. The study of such structures is necessarily relegated to microscopic anatomy. *Cytology,* the study of cells, and *histology,* the study of tissues, generally fall into this province.

The conventional unit of measurement in light-microscopic study, the *micrometer* (abbreviated μm, and formerly known as the micron, μ), is equal to one one-thousandth (10^{-3}) millimeter. No matter how great the magnification achieved by a light optical system, however, the practical limit of resolution of the average optical instrument (a good student laboratory microscope) is in the order of 0.2 μm. Resolving structures more closely placed than 0.2 μm, therefore, requires the use of electron optical instruments, such as the

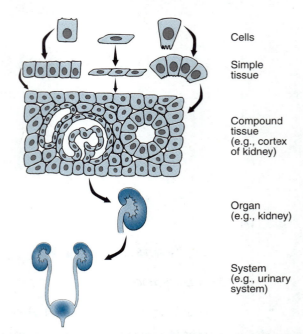

FIGURE 1–1. The interrelationship between cells, tissues, organs and organ systems. *Note that tissues are composed of cells, and organs of specialized tissues. Organs function together in an organ system.*

scanning and transmission electron microscopes. The current practical limit of resolution of most biologic electron microscopy is somewhat less than 0.5 nanometer (abbreviated nm; 1 nm equals 10^{-3} μm). Thus, biologic structure may be studied with electron microscopy close to the macromolecular level (the carbon-carbon interspace in a carbon lattice is approximately 0.2 nm). The recently introduced atomic force microscopes allow the cell biologist to probe the molecular and atomic dimensions of such structures as the cell membrane and cell junctions (Fig. 1–2). The subcellular detail resolved with electron microscopy is termed *fine structure* and includes, for example, those familiar cellular cytoplasmic organelles and inclusions as well as specializations of the plasma membrane not ordinarily resolvable with the light microscope.

PREPARATION OF TISSUES FOR HISTOLOGIC STUDY
Light Microscopy

Only as the student is aware of how tissues and cells are prepared for microscopic examination can he or she appreciate the validity, as well as the limitations, of histologic data. A knowledge of these procedures is essential if the student of histology is to be able to draw valid conclusions from the study of microscopic preparations and to distinguish genuine microscopic detail from those spurious features *(artifacts)* that are commonly introduced into microscopic preparations by tissue processing.

With few exceptions, students in most histology courses study only tissue specimens that have under-

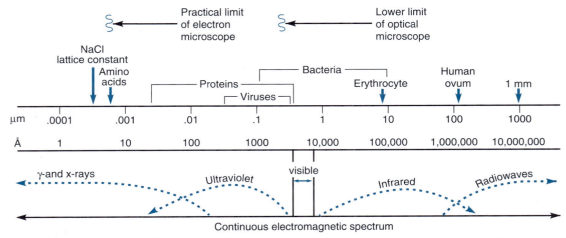

FIGURE 1–2. *This scale permits comparison of the overlapping realms of size dimensions in terms of the electromagnetic spectrum, dimensions of cells and organic molecules, and the resolution of light (optical) and electron microscopes.* Key: $\mu m = 10^{-3}$ mm; Å = Angstrom, $= 10^{-4}$ μm; 10 $\text{Å} = 1$ nm (nanometer).

gone extensive processing, and thus alteration, from the living state. Tissue specimens may be preserved *(fixed)* in a variety of fluids following their expeditious removal from the body and their blood and oxygen supply. The specific fluid, or *fixative*, chosen to preserve the tissue is selected on the basis of how well it maintains particular elements or constituents, usually by cross-linking or precipitating protein structures within the particular tissue under study. One of the most common fixatives used in the histology and pathology laboratory for the preparation of tissues for study by light microscopy is formaldehyde; for electron microscopy, glutaraldehyde is the primary fixative of choice. Other common fixatives for light microscopy contain picric and acetic acids and formalin (Bouin's fluid), and potassium bichromate, mercuric chloride, and formalin (Zenker-formol fixative and Helly's fluids).

The tissue, which is hardened during fixation, must be firmly *embedded* in a medium to facilitate the sectioning of the tissue into slices sufficiently thin to allow the passage of light through them (approximately 4 to 10 μm in routine practice). Such a medium has traditionally been paraffin or other waxes, although epoxy resin (plastic) embedment is frequently found to be superior for critical study of cells and tissues. Sectioning of appropriately embedded specimens is accomplished using a precision instrument, the *microtome*. When the thin tissue sections are mounted on glass slides and viewed in the light microscope, however, they do not exhibit an inherent contrast sufficient to permit differentiation of tissue components and cellular detail. Accordingly, tissues are routinely stained with various organic and inorganic compounds to enhance contrast. For example, selective staining of various cellular and tissue components allows nuclei to be distinguished from the cytoplasm, and various matrix and fiber components of the extracellular space to be differentiated from cells. A conventional combination of stains that allows such distinctions is hematoxylin and eosin (H&E); hematoxylin typically stains nuclei blue, and eosin stains cytoplasm pink.

Electron Microscopy

Three applications of electron optics to the study of tissues and cells are *transmission electron microscopy (TEM)*, *scanning electron microscopy (SEM)*, and *freeze-fracture microscopy*. In TEM, organs are usually fixed by the perfusion of glutaraldehyde-containing fixatives directly through the vascular system of the organ under study, and the organ thus is fixed in situ. Tissue specimens are then cut into very small cubes of tissue (1 to 2 mm on a side) to facilitate the penetration of fixing and embedding reagents into the interior of the specimen. Embedment is in epoxy resins, and sectioning is carried out using an ultramicrotome. The high resolution of TEM depends on the transmission of an electron beam through an extremely thin (50 to 80 nm) slice of tissue. "Staining" is accomplished by exposing the sections or tissue blocks to solutions of heavy metal salts (such as lead, uranium, and bismuth). These salts adhere selectively to various cellular and intercellular components and render them electron opaque under the electron beam. The thin sections are mounted on metal grids and viewed in the transmission electron microscope.

In SEM, fixed or rapidly frozen tissues (and in recent experimental advances, living specimens such as insects) are introduced into the electron beam, which scans the surface of the specimen, which has been coated with a microscopic layer of gold-palladium. Electrons that are reflected or are generated from hitting this metallic coating are electronically collected and focused, and a three-dimensional image is generated that faithfully depicts the microscopic details of cell and tissue surfaces.

In the freeze-fracture technique, biologic specimens are prepared for examination by snap-freezing them without fixation, dehydration, or embedment. This technique thus provides important confirmatory evidence of fine structural detail in cells that have not been exposed to the potentially deleterious procedures of fixation, shrinkage during dehydration, and organic solvent extraction of cellular and tissue components. The interior of such frozen specimens is revealed for study by fracturing the block and preparing a metal replica of the fractured surface for examination with TEM. The fracture face of such a preparation often runs within the interior of biologic membranes, and this technique thus has contributed much to our concept of the macromolecular structure of biologic membranes (see later discussion of membranes).

TECHNIQUES THAT PERMIT OBSERVATION OF LIVING CELLS AND TISSUES

Two optical techniques in routine use for the observation of living cells and tissues are *phase microscopy* and *differential interference (Nomarski) microscopy*. These techniques both employ special lens systems that render differences in refractive index within the specimen visible as differences in intensity and contrast. These differences are ordinarily undetected in routine light microscopy. The phase microscope accomplishes this by detecting the shift in phase imparted to light that is incident upon cells, in comparison with light that passes only through the surrounding medium in which the cells are suspended. These techniques permit direct observation of cells in culture, and although resolution is sacrificed for contrast, the correlations between microscopic observations of living specimens and of fixed specimens are crucial to interpretations of microscopic data. These techniques have found important application in the area of observation of cultured tissues and cells in cell biology and genetics. They are of value to the clinician as well, for examining cell samples *(biopsy specimens)* obtained from scraping cells from the skin, the lining of the oral cavity, or the female reproductive tract.

PERSPECTIVES: THE QUICK AND THE DEAD

Those students in the health sciences who have the opportunity and privilege of performing a dissection of the human body are encouraged to cross-reference their experiences in gross anatomy and microscopic anatomy in order to appreciate the full richness of the fabric of biostructure. It must be borne in mind, however, that the study of gross and microscopic anatomy from nonliving cells, tissues, and organs is fraught with the danger of conceptualizing structures (be they membrane systems, organelles, or even livers) as static entities, and not as the dynamic, interrelated and coordinated functioning systems that elegant phase-contrast and interference-contrast cinematographic analyses have revealed them to be. The electron-microscopist, particularly, must attempt whenever possible to correlate the static structural concepts generated from the high-resolution examination of fixed tissue with data derived from observations of living cells with various light-microscopic techniques. It is particularly in the areas of electron microscopy and molecular biology that the reductionist approach is so tempting and potentially so rewarding in terms of postulating cellular and molecular bases of structure and function. However, the integration of the multiplicity of detail concerning cell structure into a meaningful concept of the intact, functioning cell is perhaps the microscopist's and molecular biologist's greatest challenge and most common failing.

APPROACHES THAT FACILITATE ESTABLISHING FUNCTIONAL CORRELATES WITH HISTOLOGIC STRUCTURE

Histochemistry

The fields concerned with the identification and localization of chemical moieties within cells and tissues are *cytochemistry* and *histochemistry*, respectively. Histochemistry must be recognized as an imperfect marriage between histology and biochemistry, but one that has nonetheless contributed greatly to the understanding of structure-function relationships. The underlying principle of cytochemistry and histochemistry is that biochemical reactions that serve to identify organic and inorganic substances in homogenates and bulk samples may be applied validly to cells and to tissue sections. Within judicious limits, this assumption holds, provided that interpretations are made with the realization that the processing of tissues for histologic examination may extract partially or entirely the moiety in question or may (depending upon its water or lipid solubility) relocate the material within the tissue specimen.

Certain histochemical methods depend on a reasonably straightforward staining reaction of a dye for an organic molecule. For example, Sudan black and oil red O stains are widely used for revealing the presence and location of lipids within tissues.

Likewise, a recognized reaction for the detection of polysaccharides is the periodic acid–Schiff (PAS) reaction, in which 1,2 glycol groups exposed on glucose molecules in glycogen are first oxidized to aldehydes by the application of periodic acid to the tissue section. Subsequently, the Schiff reagent (containing the colorless, bleached form of the dye fuchsin) is applied to the tissue, with the result that purple fuchsin is generated and deposited in those areas in which it reacts with aldehydes. The PAS reaction is important to the pathologist in differentiating and diagnosing accumulations of ground substance (colloid), some varieties of which are PAS-positive and others are not.

The nucleic acids DNA and RNA are demonstrable histochemically (with the Feulgen reaction and with toluidine blue and hematoxylin staining, respectively). Proteins generally are not satisfactorily demonstrated histochemically except by means of immunocytochemistry, which is dealt with later in this chapter.

Enzyme histochemistry is used by both the histologist and the pathologist to localize enzymatic activity within tissue sections. Because of the lability of many enzymes and their sensitivity to routine procedures of fixation and embedment, frozen tissue sections are cut from blocks of tissue using a special microtome, the *cryostat*. The general principle of enzyme tissue chemistry involves incubation of the tissue slice or section in a medium containing (1) a substrate specific to the enzyme system under study, (2) a buffer chosen to maintain the pH optimum of the enzyme system, (3) any cofactors required by the enzyme, and (4) a visualizing molecule that will be precipitated within the tissue at the site of enzymatic activity. Many classes of enzymes are demonstrable in this manner, including the acid and alkaline phosphatases, esterases, and the dehydrogenases, oxidases, and ATPases of various metabolic cycles. When applied at the electron-microscopic level, these reactions are termed *electron cytochemistry*.

Immunocytochemistry

Immunocytochemistry is a powerful technique for the detection of tissue and cellular components, particularly protein molecules. It involves coupling, and subsequently visualizing, a labeled antibody to the component molecule of interest within a tissue section or cell population under study. The antibody may be a polyclonal antibody (raised in a species different from that under study) or a monoclonal antibody (generated in tissue culture by immortalized cell lines). The coupling site within the tissue is revealed microscopically by tagging the antibody either with a colored molecule visible in the light microscope or with a molecule of specific shape or electron opacity that can be recognized under the electron microscope. Fluorescent tags may also be used and the tissue examined under a fluorescence microscope. Pathologists are able to make selective diagnoses of disease through the use of immunocytochemistry. For example, certain tumors of connective tissues express antigens to intermediate-filament proteins, whereas prostatic tumors may express prostate-specific antigen, and other steroid-dependent tumors, such as breast tumors, express steroid receptor proteins that are detectable using this technique. Various strategies for labeling antibodies for use in immunocytochemistry are depicted in Figure 1–3.

Autoradiography

Investigations of the dynamics of cell turnover and of the metabolic synthesis of materials within tissues and cells have been made possible largely through the ability of researchers, using *autoradiography*, to detect and follow over time the incorporation of radiolabeled metabolic precursors within cells and tissues. For example, when tritium-labeled thymidine, a labeled precursor to DNA, is allowed to incorporate into a dividing cell population, the cells in S phase of the cell cycle incorporate the labeled thymidine. These cells are then visualized by means of autoradiography, the principles of which are diagrammed in Figure 1–4.

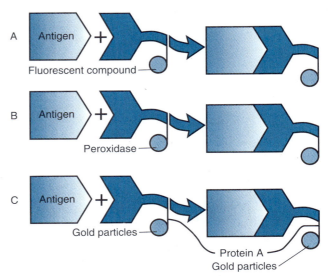

FIGURE 1–3. Three methods by which antibodies are labeled in immunocytochemical studies. A, Fluorescence labeling. A fluorescent marker (such as rhodamine or fluorescein isothiocyanate) is coupled to the antibody. Tissue sections are incubated with the label and are viewed using the fluorescence microscope. Tissue fluorescence indicates site of antibody localization. B, Peroxidase labeling. The protein horseradish peroxidase is coupled to the antibody. Tissue sections are reacted with the labeled antibody, and a histochemical reaction is run for peroxidase. With light microscopy, a brown deposition product is seen at the site of antibody-antigen coupling. With electron microscopy, an electron-opaque deposit marks the site of localization. C, Gold/protein A labeling. Gold particles of various dimensions may be coupled through protein A to antibody. Marker is detectable with both light and electron microscopy. It is a high-resolution marker, and "double labeling" of antibodies in single sections can be achieved using different-sized gold particles to label antibodies to one or more antigens.

Briefly, microscope slides prepared from an organ that has incorporated the radiolabeled material are dipped in photographic emulsion, such that a thin overlay of emulsion is deposited over each slide. The coated slides are stored in lightproof boxes for a period of time to allow for radioactive decay of the label. Beta particles (in the case of a tritium-labeled molecule) pass through the emulsion near their source in the underlying tissue. After an appropriate time, during which numerous beta particles travel through the emulsion, the slide and overlying emulsion are processed (developed) photographically, and the silver bromide molecules reduced by the passage of radiation are visualized as black grains of silver, theoretically over the source of the radiation in the tissue specimen. Dynamic processes, such as uptake and passage of precursor molecules through the endoplasmic reticulum and Golgi apparatus and secretory apparatus, for example, may be studied autoradiographically by injecting experimental animals with labeled precursor, sacrificing them at various intervals after the injection, and following the progression of incorporation.

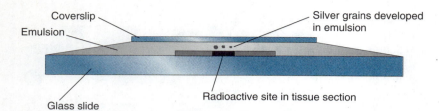

FIGURE 1–4. Diagram of a tissue section that has been processed for autoradiography. *Note the layer of photographic emulsion coating the tissue section. Reduction of silver bromide in the emulsion by radioactive decay from labeled elements within the tissue section deposits black silver grains over the site of radioactive emission.*

In Situ Hybridization

A powerful application of the principles of autoradiography involves the detection of radiolabeled DNA and RNA sequences within tissues. These radiolabeled, defined single-stranded nucleic acid sequences (probes) are prepared by molecular-biologic means in the laboratory. When they are exposed to tissue sections or slices, they bind to those complementary single-stranded segments within the tissue; following autoradiography, the site of binding is revealed. (Other labels are widely used, in addition to radiolabeled probes, e.g., *biotin*). This recent advance in technology, which provides a highly specific means of localizing genes or messenger RNA in tissue sections and chromosome squash preparations of mitotic cells, holds great promise for both research and clinical applications.

Cell Fractionation

The emphasis of the techniques previously described has been to localize biochemical and structural constituents within the context of the intact cell. However, a powerful adjunct tool to these techniques that allows for *quantitation* of cellular components and products is the biochemical tool of cell fractionation and differential centrifugation, to obtain pure fractions of cellular organelles or membranes, for example. Cells are disrupted by controlled homogenization, and the homogenate is centrifuged in a density gradient at high speed to separate and collect the various cellular fractions for study. The essentials of this technique are summarized in Fig. 1–5. One of the great advantages is that cell fractionation provides a means of quantifying cellular organelles and compartments under various physiologic and experimental conditions. As the biochemist and histologist pool the strengths of their respective approaches, a unified and satisfying concept of the cell will emerge.

CELL STRUCTURE AND FUNCTION

As noted earlier, cells in multicellular organisms are both structurally and functionally differentiated and specialized within tissues and organs. Accordingly, the universal, "typical" eukaryotic cell does not exist except as a construct in histology texts! Most cells of the mammalian body share certain hallmark features, however, and it is upon these common features that this section concentrates as a point of departure for the study of cells constituting specific tissues and organs.

Cells traditionally have been described as consisting of two separate compartments, the *cytoplasm* and the *nucleus*. A more functionally satisfying view of the cell is that of an intricately compartmentalized system of membranes encompassing both nucleus and cytoplasm.

As the noted cell biologist and physician Lewis Thomas has written, in the now classic work *Lives of a Cell,* "It takes a membrane to make sense out of disorder in biology." And so it does, particularly with regard to cell biology. The cell membrane (*plasma membrane,* or *plasmalemma*) serves as the interface of the cell both with the environment and with its companion cells within tissues. Internally, the fluid phase of the cell (*cytoplasm*) is compartmentalized by a membranous system, which includes the membrane-bounded organelles, the nucleus, and membranous vesicular system. It is these very membranes that are the enzyme systems essential to energy transduction and storage; it is at the level of the membrane that morphology and function are united (Fig. 1–6).

The Plasma Membrane

The outer limiting membrane of the eukaryotic cell is a dynamic structure, with morphologic and molecular variations from cell to cell that mirror the differentiated or physiologic state of the cell. In most cells, the plasmalemma exhibits a high protein content (50% to 60% dry weight) compared with its lipid content (20% to 30%). Carbohydrates, principally in the form of oligosaccharides covalently linked to lipid and protein, account for less than 10% of the weight of the plasma membrane.

Both the plasma membrane and those membranes that delimit the cytoplasmic organelles and nucleus exhibit a common macromolecular organization of these three components, namely a lipid bilayer into which specialized proteins are inserted and with which carbohydrates are associated. The lipid molecules of the membrane are asymmetric and *amphipathic;* one pole of the lipid molecule is hydrophilic, and the other hydrophobic. In aqueous solutions, such lipid molecules spontaneously aggregate into bimolecular sheets, with the hydrophobic ends directed inward, and the hydrophilic ends pointing outward (Fig. 1–7). Functionally, this arrangement of lipid and protein is highly significant: First, it allows for dynamic membrane re-

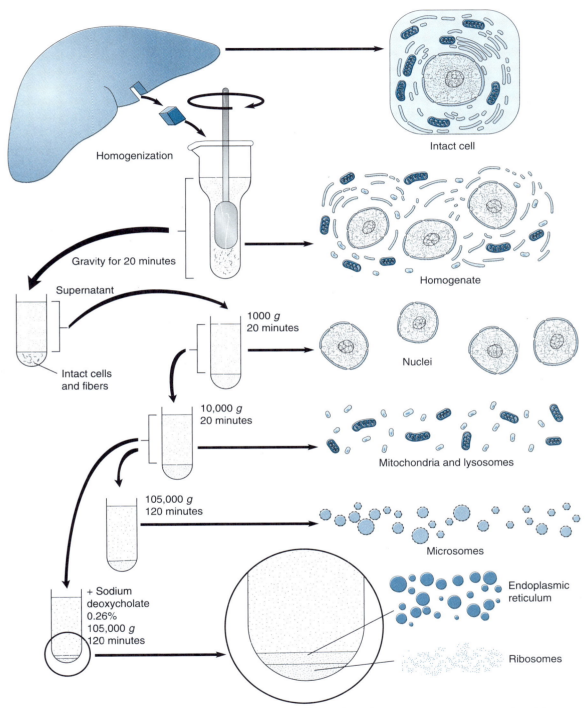

FIGURE 1–5. Subcellular components are isolated by means of homogenization and differential centrifugation. *Heavy components and particles are spun down as a pellet; the supernatant is re-centrifuged at progressively higher speeds, yielding pellets of less dense components. Number followed by g indicates number of times gravity achieved in centrifugation and necessary for separation of cellular constituents.*

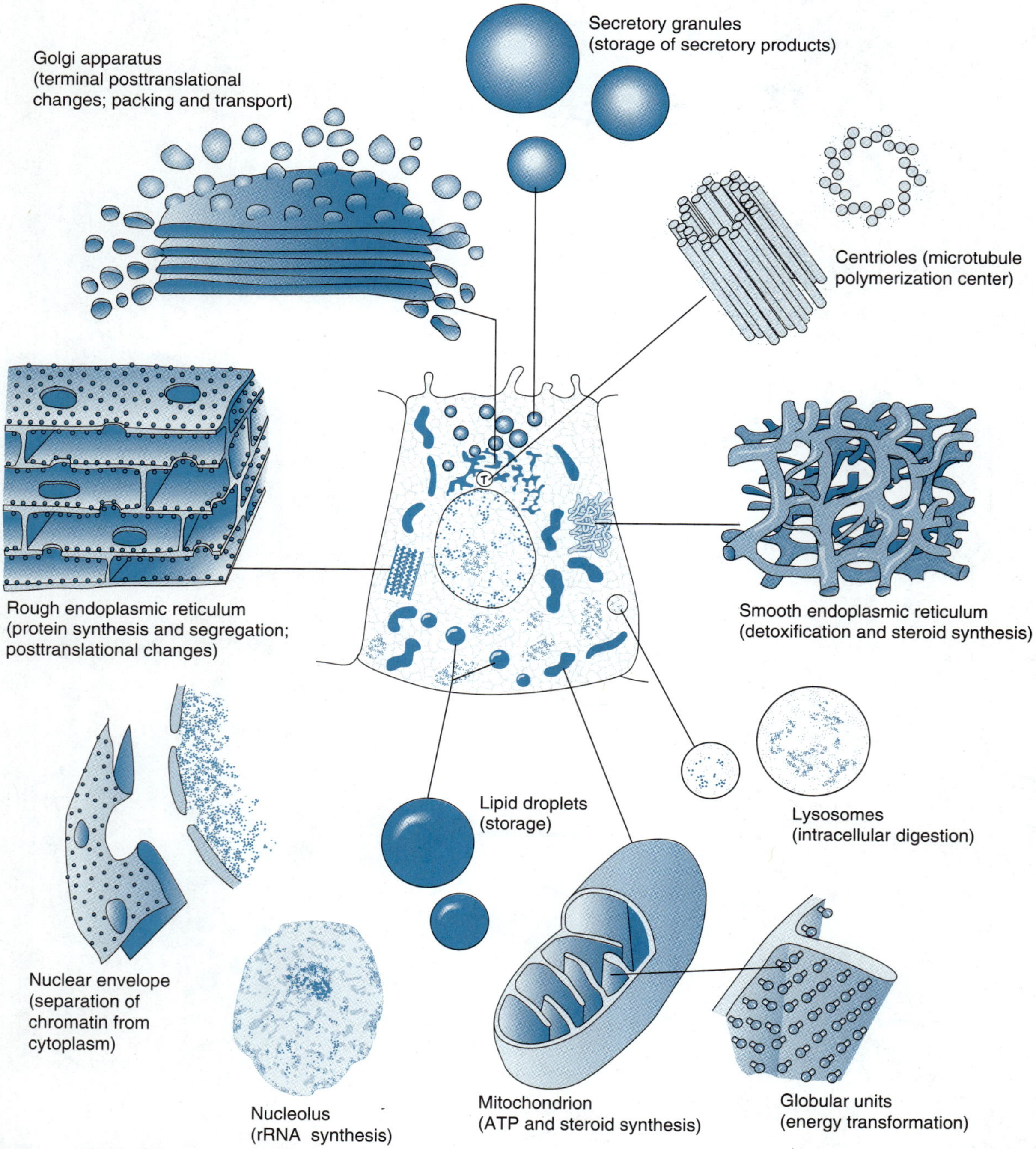

FIGURE 1–6. A schematic diagram of a "typical" mammalian cell, showing major membrane-bounded organelles as imaged with the transmission electron microscope.

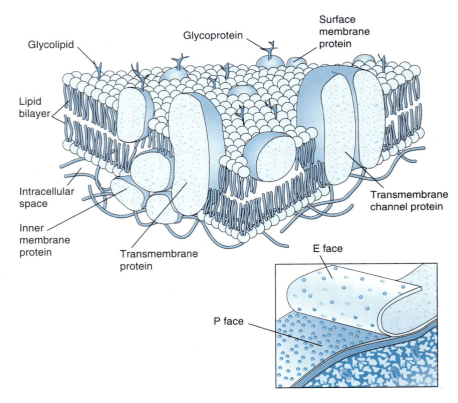

FIGURE 1-7. Macromolecular model of the mammalian cell membrane: fluid-mosaic model. Note the lipid bilayer, with hydrophilic (outward-facing) and hydrophobic (inward-facing) domains, into which are inserted protein and glycoprotein molecules. Inset, Diagram of freeze-fracture appearance of plasma membrane, with intramembranous particles (proteins) revealed by the fracture. The membrane leaflets are designated E and P, for extracellular and protoplasmic faces, respectively. The E face is generally particle poor, and the P face, particle rich. The E face exhibits depressions corresponding to particle placement in the P face.

modeling, or fluidity. The mosaic of inserted proteins and glycoproteins is capable of lateral displacement within the membrane, in their roles as transport, recognition, and attachment molecules. This feature of the model prompted its proposers (Singer and Nicholson) to name it the *fluid-mosaic model* of membrane structure. Second, this arrangement allows for differential permeability: lipid-soluble (hydrophobic) molecules pass readily through the membrane, but water and charged ions are thought to utilize protein-associated routes *(pores)* through the membrane. Third, it is self-sealing. Defects are naturally sealed if the hydrophobic groups are exposed to an aqueous environment.

Lipids of the Plasma Membrane

Three classes of lipid predominate in cell membranes: (1) phospholipids, (2) cholesterol, and (3) glycolipids. Of the phospholipids, four predominate—phosphatidylcholine (lecithin), phosphatidylethanolamine (cephalin), phosphatidylserine, and sphingomyelin. These phospholipids are not distributed uniformly throughout the membrane, but are selectively placed in the inner (cephalin and phosphatidylserine) and outer (lecithin and sphingomyelin) layers of the lipid bilayer. These molecules may serve to bind the transport proteins inserted into the bilayer (Fig. 1-8).

Cholesterol is an important component of cell membranes. It serves to stabilize them, perhaps by linking adjacent phospholipids.

Glycolipids are positioned only within the outer of the lipid bilayers of the membrane, with their carbohydrate moieties exposed on the cell surface. This arrangement facilitates their possible function in cell adhesion, intercellular communication and recognition, and other receptor-mediated interactions with the environment and other cells. Two glycolipids of particular note are galactocerebroside, a major component of the lipid-rich myelin sheath insulating nerve fibers, and

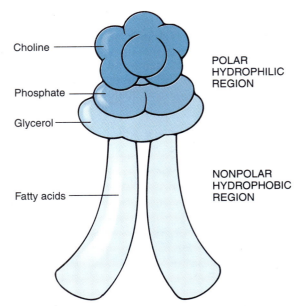

FIGURE 1-8. Phospholipid molecule of the plasma membrane. Note the molecular components of the molecule, which define its hydrophilic and hydrophobic domains.

gangliosides, which are abundant in nerve cell membranes.

Proteins of the Plasma Membrane

Two classes of membrane protein are recognized. The first is loosely associated with the cell surface and is easily extracted with salt solutions. Such proteins are termed *peripheral proteins*. More tightly incorporated proteins within the lipid bilayer are known as *integral proteins* and require detergent extraction for their removal. Furthermore, some of the integral proteins extend through the entire thickness of the plasma membrane. Termed *transmembrane proteins*, they are hypothesized to serve as pores or channels that facilitate the transport of water and charged ions across the membrane (see Fig. 1–7).

Carbohydrates of the Plasma Membrane

In addition to the carbohydrate moieties of glycolipids and glycoproteins that project to the cell surface, extrinsic carbohydrates, such as sialic acid, are commonly encountered attached to the cell surface. Together, these carbohydrates form what has been termed the "extrinsic coat" or *glycocalyx*. This "fuzzy coat," as it is also called, is particularly prominent over the microvillous lining of the small intestine.

Appearance of the Plasma Membrane with TEM

Cell membranes are resolved with transmission electron microscopy as trilaminar structures. Although the cell surface interface with the aqueous extracellular environment may be seen by light microscopy (LM), the bilayered plasma membrane, per se, lies below the limit of resolution of LM. It measures 7.5 to 10 nm in thickness, depending on the cell type and the preparative techniques used for microscopy. The "railroad track" configuration of membranes seen under TEM (Fig. 1–9) is thought to represent the deposition of osmium (a heavy metal fixative and stain used in TEM) within the lipid bilayer. This configuration, because it is common to most biologic membranes, has come to be termed the *unit membrane*. The asymmetry of inner and outer leaflets is apparent in critical preparations and reflects differences in macromolecular composition, as noted earlier.

Membrane Transport: Endocytosis and Exocytosis

Transport of fluids and particulates (apart from diffusion across the membrane, as discussed earlier) occurs across the plasma membrane via a system of transport vesicles. The uptake of material into the cell from the environment is termed *endocytosis*, and the analogous release of material from the cell to the environment is termed *exocytosis* (Fig. 1–10).

Endocytosis initially involves the formation of invaginations at the cell surface that subsequently seal off, forming a spherical vesicle called an *endocytosis vesicle*, or *endosome*. Essentially, the reverse of this process (see Fig. 1–10) occurs in the transport of cytoplasmic material via vesicles to the exterior of the cell.

Fluid transport into the cell via vesicles some 80 to 150 nm in diameter is called *pinocytosis*, whereas the term *phagocytosis* is reserved to describe the ingestion of particulates in larger (greater than 250 nm diameter) endosomes.

In contrast to the nonselective transport of fluid accomplished by the pinocytotic vesicle system, the cell membrane participates in highly selective transport processes, termed *receptor-mediated endocytosis*. The endocytotic invaginations form in relation to specialized regions of the cell surface, termed *coated pits*. These invaginations, unlike pinocytotic vesicles, exhibit a coating on the cytoplasmic surface of the pit consisting of several polypeptides, the primary one of which is *clathrin* (approximately 180,000 molecular weight). It is known that receptors for specific extracellular ligands, such as low-density lipoproteins and protein hormones, are aggregated within the clathrin-coated pits. After binding to their receptors, such ligands are endocytosed within coated vesicles, which form from the coated pits as depicted in Figure 1–11.

In the case of phagocytosis of particulates by macrophages or neutrophils, a larger endocytic vesicle forms, which engulfs the material to be endocytosed,

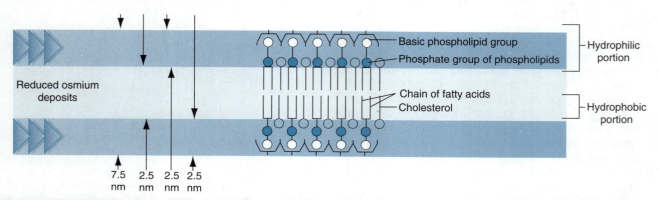

FIGURE 1–9. *Diagram of the appearance of the plasma membrane as viewed under the transmission electron microscope, correlated with the hypothesized molecular substructure of the membrane.* Osmium, which is electron opaque, is thought to be preferentially deposited during tissue fixation and staining in the hydrophilic domains of the phospholipid molecules of the membrane, imparting the typical "unit membrane" appearance visualized on electron microscopy.

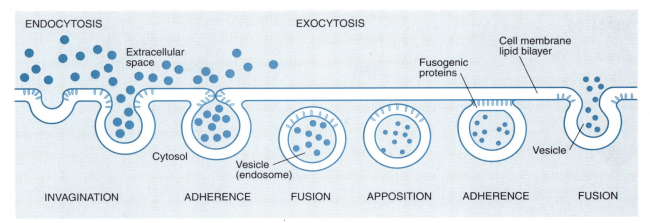

FIGURE 1-10. Diagrammatic representation of major features of endocytosis and exocytosis. *Note the formation of intracytoplasmic vesicles and their fusion in both endocytosis and exocytosis with the plasma membrane, a functional demonstration of their molecular compatibility in structure.*

and the phagocytic vacuole that forms facilitates the transport of the material to the lysosomal system of the cell (see later discussion of lysosomes).

Endocytosis and exocytosis are coordinated events—surface membrane incorporated into the endocytic vesicles is returned during exocytosis to the plasma membrane, resulting in conservation of surface membrane. This process of membrane recycling is termed *membrane trafficking*.

Cell-to-Cell Communication

The plasma membrane is integral to communication between cells within a given tissue, and between cells placed at a distance, in different tissue or body sites. It participates in the formation of specialized junctions (*gap junctions;* see Chapters 2 and 3) that are sites of altered ionic permeability and lowered electrical resistance. The membrane also has projecting from its surface specific receptor molecules that bind to and activate hydrophilic *signaling molecules* in the tissue fluids. These signaling molecules include nonsteroid hormones, neurotransmitters, and locally active *(paracrine)* chemical mediators. Circulating steroid hormones, owing to their hydrophobic nature, diffuse through the plasma membrane and couple with specific receptors within the cell. Thus, the plasma membrane facilitates the cell's responses to regulatory molecules from the endocrine and nervous systems and to local, paracrine chemical mediators of cell function.

Cytoplasm

The cytoplasmic compartment (cytosol) of the cell consists of a fluid matrix in which are suspended the membrane-bounded *organelles*, including the nucleus; filamentous elements of the *cytoskeleton;* and various cytoplasmic *inclusions*, such as free ribosomes, glycogen, pigment, and lipid stores in the form of droplets. Various cytosolic enzyme systems are present as well.

Until recent studies of the cytoplasm with high-voltage electron microscopy, it was assumed that the cytosol was essentially unstructured and that the various organelles and inclusions were suspended randomly within its fluid phase. It appears likely from recent evidence that such is not the case, but that there exists a *cytomatrix*, or *microtrabecular lattice*, that enfolds all formed elements of the cell. Confirmation of the presence of such a lattice, using other techniques, as well as biochemical characterization of the lattice is sorely needed, however.

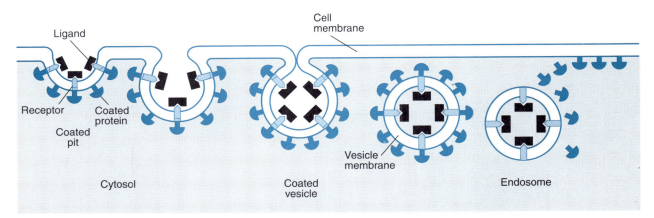

FIGURE 1-11. Receptor-mediated endocytosis occurs by means of clathrin-coated pits at the cell surface. *Note the binding of specific extracellular ligands with specific receptors in the cell membrane, and subsequent internalization of the ligand within a coated vesicle.*

Organelles

The Mitochondrion

Mitochondria are ubiquitous among eukaryotic cells. They were named for their threadlike appearance (*mitos* is Greek for "thread") by early microscopists, who resolved them with light microscopy. In terms of size, mitochondria generally appear as structures 0.5 to 1 μm in width but may reach several micrometers in length. They appear in numbers, sizes, and shapes characteristic of the cells in which they are found, and may be spherical, cylindrical, threadlike, or even of bizarre shape and size in certain pathologic conditions. Topographically within the cell, they are found in association with other organelles involved in synthetic activity, because they are the sites of oxidative phosphorylation and the sources of high-energy phosphate bonds (ATP), which fuel the cell's anabolic, active transport, and other cytophysiologic activities. Accordingly, mitochondria are often found at the base of cells synthesizing protein, in association with elements of the rough endoplasmic reticulum, and closely associated with the basal infoldings of the epithelial cells lining kidney tubules involved in active (energy-dependent) ion transport. The numbers of mitochondria within cells differ, but the number is relatively constant for cells within a particular tissue.

Despite their variation in size and shape, mitochondria present a characteristic structural profile under TEM. A double mitochondrial membrane (Fig. 1–12) bounds the organelle. The *outer membrane* defines the shape of the organelle and contains *porin*, a transport protein that facilitates the permeability of the outer membrane to molecules in the size range of 10 kD or less. The space between the inner and outer mitochondrial membranes is termed the *intermembranous space*. It is bounded internally by the *inner membrane*, which gives a pleated appearance caused by its folding into *cristae* (Latin for "ridges"). The core of the cristae (the *intracristal space*) is continuous with the intermembranous space. The remaining space in the mitochondrion, into which the cristae project, is the *intercristal* or *matrix space*.

The reduplicated cristae serve to increase the surface area of the inner mitochondrial membrane. The cristae contain the biochemical enzyme systems for oxidative phosphorylation and the electron transport chain. Phosphorylation occurs on specialized globular subunits of the cristae (see Fig. 1–12). It is significant that the inner mitochondrial membrane is impermeable to small ions, a reflection of its high content of cardiolipin. This facilitates the maintenance of electrochemical gradients as high-energy metabolites are produced. Other specific metabolic events and pathways are localized to specific compartments of the mitochondrion, as detailed in Figure 1–12.

A structural correlation exists between the energy requirements of a given cell population and its mitochondrial morphology. Cells of high oxidative metabolic activity (cardiac muscle, for example) exhibit numerous mitochondria with many cristae. Cells of low oxidative metabolic rate exhibit fewer mitochondria, bearing short, widely spaced cristae. Of note also is the observation that cristae of many steroid-synthesizing cells (of testes, for example) are tubular rather than shelflike.

Mitochondria reproduce their numbers by fission following cell division, in which approximately half the mitochondria are distributed randomly to each daughter cell. The matrix space contains mitochondrial DNA and the enzyme systems requisite for DNA transcription. This observation, together with the presence of systems within the mitochondrion for protein synthesis independent of direction from the cell nucleus, has led to the hypothesis that mitochondria may have evolved within eukaryotic cells from an ancestral symbiotic prokaryote.

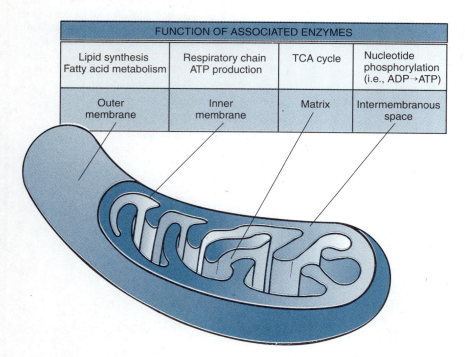

FIGURE 1–12. Schematic diagram of a mitochondrion. *The cytophysiologic compartmentation of the organelle by its system of double membranes is shown. Note the specific metabolic pathways associated with specific compartments.*

FUNCTION OF ASSOCIATED ENZYMES			
Lipid synthesis Fatty acid metabolism	Respiratory chain ATP production	TCA cycle	Nucleotide phosphorylation (i.e., ADP→ATP)
Outer membrane	Inner membrane	Matrix	Intermembranous space

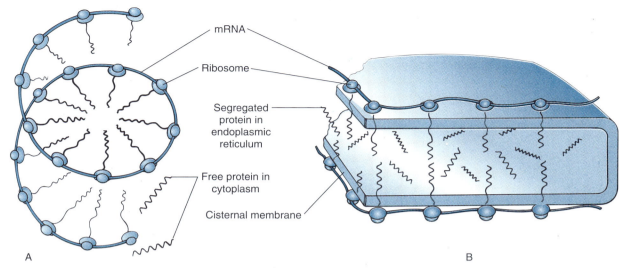

FIGURE 1–13. **Ribosomal arrangements.** A, Ribosomes attached to a strand of mRNA, synthesizing protein destined for release within the cytoplasm and for use within the cell. B, Ribosomes bound to the endoplasmic reticulum (ER) release synthesized protein into the cisterna of the ER, segregating it from the cytoplasm. This is typical of protein that is programmed for secretion from the cell as secretion product. The ER provides a means of transport to the Golgi complex for further molecular modification and packaging.

Ribosomes

Ribosomes are small (20 × 30 nm), electron-opaque particles of RNA and numerous proteins that lie free within the cytosol, are bound into clusters *(polysomes)* by means of a strand of mRNA, or are bound as polysomes to the rough endoplasmic reticulum (Fig. 1–13). Ribosomal RNA (rRNA) is synthesized in the nucleolus; ribosomal proteins are synthesized in the cytosol, are transported to the nucleus, and there associate with rRNA, which is organized into large and small ribosomal subunits. The subunits are transported out of the nucleus via the nuclear pore system. In the cytoplasm, the ribosomes function in the alignment of messenger RNA and transport RNA and the consequent formation of peptide chains in the biosynthesis of protein.

Ribosomes impart an intense basophilia to the cytoplasm of protein-synthesizing cells, owing to the numerous phosphate groups that react as polyanions with basic stains, such as toluidine blue, and with hematoxylin in routine H&E tissue staining. Regions of basophilia were noted in actively synthetic cells by early microscopists, but the resolution of ribosomes and endoplasmic reticulum as entities awaited the advent of TEM.

Cells that synthesize protein principally for their own use exhibit large numbers of free polyribosomes, whereas cells synthesizing protein for export (as in glandular epithelium of the salivary glands or pancreas) exhibit elaborate profiles of rough endoplasmic reticulum (see later).

Endoplasmic Reticulum

The endoplasmic reticulum *(ER)* is an interlacing network of membranous sheets that appose each other forming broad, interconnecting cisternae (in the case of the rough ER, RER) and tubular networks (in the case of smooth ER, or SER) (Figs. 1–14 and 1–15). The cytoplasmic surface of the RER is studded with

FIGURE 1–14. **Steps in the synthesis of protein on rough endoplasmic reticulum (RER).** A, Peptide synthesis is initiated within the cytosol. B, The ribosome becomes attached to the endoplasmic reticulum (ER) by means of a receptor. The peptide gains entry into the lumen of the ER via small pores thought to be protein lined. C, The signal sequence that permits peptide entry is cleaved, and protein is released into the ER lumen. D, The ribosome detaches from its ER receptor and returns free within the cytosol.

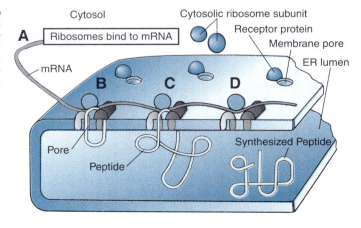

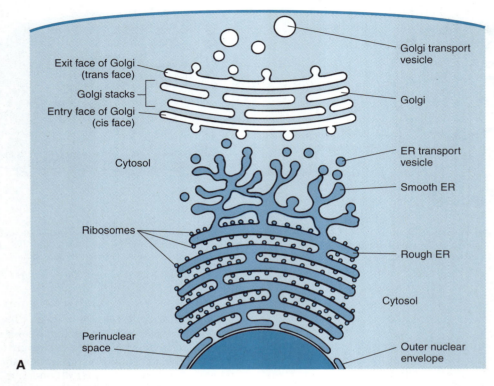
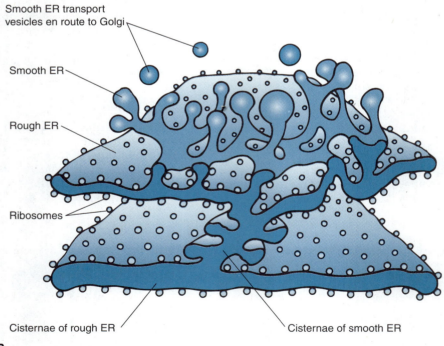

FIGURE 1-15. Three-dimensional representation of the rough endoplasmic reticulum (RER), as derived from transmission electron microscope (TEM) studies. A, *Diagrammatic representation of the membranous interrelationships of the outer nuclear envelope, the RER and SER, the Golgi, and the plasma membrane.* B, *Functional diagrammatic representation of the RER, and its association with the smooth endoplasmic reticulum (SER) and transport vesicles destined for the Golgi.*

polyribosomes and is intimately involved in secretory protein synthesis. Elements of SER (lacking ribosomes) are continuous with the RER, but the SER is specialized for other synthetic activities, such as steroid biosynthesis, as discussed later.

RER and Protein Synthesis

Protein synthesis is initiated in the cytoplasm with the attachment of mRNA to free polyribosomes. The translation step results in peptide synthesis. The initial portion of the peptide contains a *signal sequence*, which differs between peptides destined to remain in the cytosol and those programmed for export or for incorporation into membranes. Principal functions of the RER are segregation of these proteins, completion of the peptide synthesis initiated in the cytosol, and enzymatic removal of the signal sequence within the cisterna of RER, but include, as well, a wide range of posttranslational structural changes to the peptide, such as hydroxylation, sulfation, and phosphorylation. Importantly, the initial glycosylation of peptides destined for the Golgi complex and for exocytosis as secretory protein occurs in the RER; specifically, it is here that mannose oligosaccharides are incorporated into such peptides. Following this step, the nascent proteins are transported by elements of the SER toward the Golgi complex (Fig. 1–15). Smooth transport vesicles complete the delivery of those proteins segregated within the cisternae of the RER to the forming *(cis)* face of the Golgi apparatus, where the vesicles fuse with the membranous elements of the Golgi complex.

Functions of the SER

In addition to the coordinated role it plays with the RER in protein synthesis, the SER is the site of steroid biosynthesis; cells of the adrenal cortex and of the reproductive system (Leydig's cells, corpus luteum) exhibit extensive profiles of SER. The hepatocytes also contain abundant SER, where the organelle is involved in detoxification reactions and the breakdown of ingested alcohol, pesticide residues, and barbiturates. In the liver, also, this versatile organelle plays an important role in glycogen breakdown and mobilization, and in muscle, the SER (there termed the *sarcoplasmic reticulum*) functions in regulation of muscle contraction by sequestering and releasing calcium ion, upon which the contraction events are dependent. An additional important role of the SER is the synthesis of components of membranes, particularly phospholipid.

The Golgi Complex (Apparatus)

The Golgi apparatus represents another subcellular organelle that was discovered and named prior to the advent of electron microscopy, but whose function and full morphologic complexity were not appreciated until EM studies explored its crucial role in the secretion process. The Golgi complex lies within the apical portions of secretory cells; in favorable section, it is resolved as a series of parallel stacks of flattened saccules and associated vesicles (Fig. 1–16). A convex *forming face (cis)* is adjacent to profiles of RER, and a concave, *maturing face (trans)* is directed toward the cell apex. Transport vesicles from the smooth portion of the ER complex involved in protein synthesis convey material from the ER to the forming face of the Golgi. The Golgi complex is regionally specialized in terms of function. In the region of the forming face, transport vesicles from the ER are added to the Golgi membrane system, delivering their content to the cavities of the Golgi cisternae. It is in this *cis* region that phosphorylation of

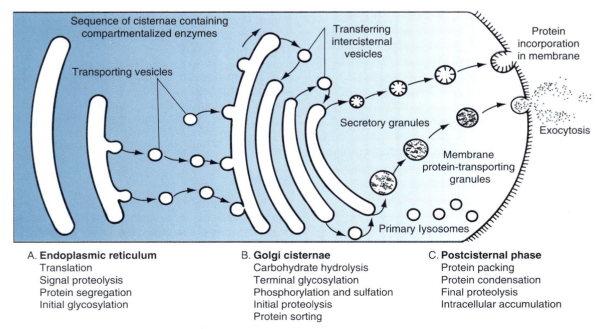

FIGURE 1–16. *Diagrammatic summary of events involving the endoplasmic reticulum (A), Golgi apparatus (B), and plasma membrane (C) in protein synthesis and exocytosis.*

protein occurs. In the mid-Golgi, sugar moieties are added to lipids and peptides in the formation of oligosaccharides. In the *trans* region, proteolysis and other final steps in the formation of secretory products occur, including the sorting of various macromolecules into appropriate vesicles, which are budded off the Golgi maturing face and contribute to the formation of lysosomes and secretory vesicles (Fig. 1–17).

Lysosomes

Lysosomes are membrane-bounded organelles formed from specialized vesicles from the Golgi, the *Golgi hydrolase vesicles*. Traditionally, lysosomes have been defined on the basis of their content of acid hydrolases and their function in the hydrolytic degradation of endocytosed materials. A more recent classification retains the benchmark of acid hydrolase content but includes lysosomes as only one element of the *acid vesicle system*. This system includes that group of cytoplasmic vesicles that contain within their limiting membranes a membrane H^+-ATPase, which serves as a hydrogen ion pump that can decrease the intravesicular pH to approximately pH 5. Those initial vesicles that bud from the Golgi (Golgi hydrolase vesicles) lack this enzyme system and thus the capacity to lower pH and to activate the acid hydrolases sequestered within them. These hydrolases typically include acid phosphatase, cathepsin B, and β-glucuronidase. Fusion with an endosome containing this enzyme system, however, sets the stage for activation and hydrolysis of the ingested material within what is termed an *endolysosome*. Endolysosomes can recruit other endosomes to form large *phagolysosomes*. Likewise, *autophagolysosomes* may form and clear damaged or nonfunctional organelles from the cytosol through the acid vesicle system. The digested residue material from this process is called a *residual body*. Large accumulations of such material are recognized by pathologists as *lipofuscin,* or age pigment. The dynamics of the acid vesicle system are summarized in Figure 1–18. Clinically, important syndromes are recognized to be results of hereditary deficiencies in the ability of the body to produce specific acid hydrolases. Lysosomal glycogen storage disease (acid maltase deficiency) results in the accumulation of large stores of glycogen, which cannot be broken down because of the enzyme deficiency. Likewise, Tay-Sachs disease involves a lysosomal deficiency in which the lysosomes of neurons accumulate inordinate stores of lipid, owing to a hexosaminidase A deficiency, which does not permit degradation of sphingolipids.

Peroxisomes (Microbodies)

Peroxisomes are membrane-bounded organelles, typically smaller in diameter than mitochondria in the same cell, that contain enzyme systems for the β-oxidation of long-chain fatty acids; D- and L-amino acid oxidases; and catalase, which degrades peroxide to oxygen and water. The action of catalase is important in that it protects the cell against the deleterious intracellular accumulation of the oxidizing agent hydrogen peroxide. A serious clinical condition, adrenoleukodystrophy, arises from the impaired ability of cells in the brain, spinal cord, and adrenal gland to accomplish β-oxidation of fatty acids, with resultant lipid accumulation in these organs accompanied by dementia and failure of adrenal function.

The Cytoskeleton

The cytoplasm contains, in addition to the membranous organelles considered previously, other formed elements: the *microtubules, microfilaments,* and *intermediate filaments.* Collectively, these tubular and filamentous structures contribute to the internal support and scaffolding of the cell, termed the *cytoskeleton*.

Microtubules

Microtubules, approximately 25 nm in diameter, exhibit a hollow core that differentiates them (aside from their larger size) from cytoplasmic microfilaments. Microtubules are constructed of subunits, the alpha and beta *tubulin* molecules, arranged in a helical profile of 13 subunits (Fig. 1–19). Polymerization of tubulins into microtubules occurs in relation to organizing centers, such as centrioles and basal bodies. The microtubules are in a constant state of flux of polymerization-depolymerization, their structure being stabilized by other proteins with which they are associated—microtubule-

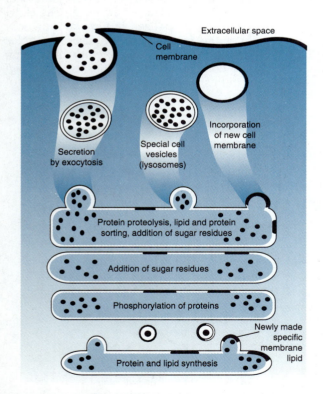

FIGURE 1–17. A diagrammatic representation of the functional specialization of the Golgi apparatus. *The Golgi is regionally specialized for the addition of specific moieties to proteins synthesized within the endoplasmic reticulum and delivered to the Golgi for further processing and packaging.*

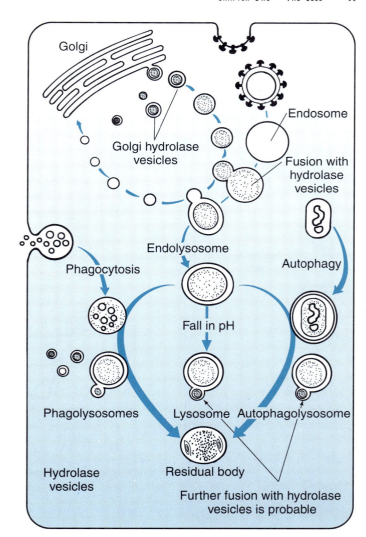

FIGURE 1–18. The acid vesicle system and its relationship to the formation and function of lysosomes. Note the formation of lysosomes from the fusion of endocytic vesicles and Golgi hydrolase vesicles. Phagolysosomes, lysosomes, and autophagolysosomes are functional in acid hydrolysis of the material within them, segregated from the cytoplasm by the lysosomal membrane. Residual bodies result from intracellular digestive processes in these three lysosomal components.

associated proteins (MAPs). Microtubules may be found randomly arranged within the cytosol or organized into more discrete, straight arrays.

Because they seldom are observed to bend, they are considered cytoskeletal elements that function in the maintenance of cell shape. Microtubules are, however, considered to have an important role (in concert with the *attachment proteins,* dynein and kinesin) in the movement of cytoplasmic organelles within the cell. Disruption of microtubular arrays halts such translocation of organelles, and treatment of cells with antimitotic alkaloids, such as colchicine and vinblastine, disrupts the mitotic tubular spindle and arrests mitosis. This capacity has found clinical application in cancer chemotherapy.

Microtubules also form the backbone for other cellular structures, namely, centrioles, basal bodies, flagella, and cilia. Centrioles and basal bodies have the same cross-sectional profile under TEM: Nine microtubular triplets set at the angle of a pinwheel and bound together with linking proteins (see Fig. 1–19). Centrioles are usually found as a single pair of structures in the interphase cell. During S phase of the cell cycle, they duplicate themselves, move to opposite poles of the cell, and serve as the organizing centers for the mitotic spindle.

Cilia and flagella both exhibit a central microtubular array of nine peripheral doublets arranged around one central pair of microtubules. This is the so-called *axoneme* (9 + 2) arrangement basic to motile cilia in both vertebrates and invertebrates. Critical TEM studies of cross-sections of the axoneme confirm that each of the peripheral pairs of doublets utilizes a shared wall of several heterodimers, and that there is an asymmetry between the two members of the doublets; subfiber A consists of the expected 13 heterodimers, but subfiber B has only 10, by virtue of sharing heterodimers with subfiber A. Extending from subfiber A are two arms of *dynein,* a protein exhibiting ATPase activity. These structural details, derived from careful TEM studies, have led to hypotheses of ciliary and flagellar motility. Such hypotheses posit that the bending of the cilium may arise as the result of coordinated sliding of adjacent doublets in relation to each other and to the axis of the cilium. The dynein arms of subfiber A of one doublet are conceived as binding the surface of

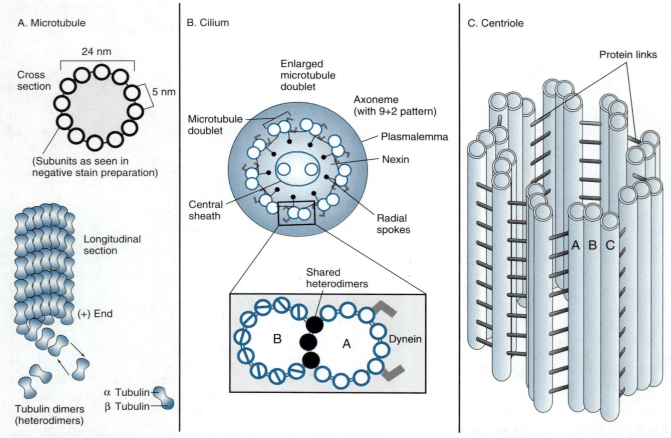

FIGURE 1–19. Diagrammatic representation, based on electron-microscopic studies, of a microtubule, the axoneme of a cilium, and a centriole. A, *Note the formation of microtubules from tubulin subunits.* B, *Microtubular doublets are shown in the "9 + 2" axonemal complex of a cilium (see text).* C, *The triplet microtubular organization of a centriole.*

subfiber B of the adjacent doublet. Such binding is postulated to be ATP-dependent. Adjacent doublets are bound to each other by protein bridges termed *nexins*. This binding is thought to constrain the movement of the microtubular pairs relative to each other, and to contribute to the bending and complex movement of cilia observed in living specimens. Such models of ciliary motility gain credence in the clinical observation that in patients with Kartagener's immotile cilia syndrome, the dynein arms are absent from subfiber A in the peripheral doublets. The beauty of the biologic symmetry of the system is further illustrated in that the dynein arms always are directed clockwise when viewed up the cilium from the vantage point of the basal body.

Microfilaments

Fine filaments measuring 5 nm in diameter are routinely found coursing throughout the cytoplasm and commonly occur also as a thin sheet of filaments in the region immediately subjacent to the plasmalemma, *the cell cortex*. These filaments have been biochemically characterized as *actin filaments*, and they are widely accepted as playing both a cytoskeletal role as well as a role in endocytosis, exocytosis, the movement of subcellular organelles within the cytoplasm, the stricturing of cytoplasm between daughter cells in mitotic telophase, and stabilizing the cell surface during adhesion and cell movement.

Unlike the stable actin filaments in muscle, the actin filaments in other cells appear to dissociate and repolymerize readily, a process under control of calcium ion and cyclic AMP. This property holds advantages for a biologic system, which must accommodate to changes in size and shape related to growth or physiologic requirements. Actin-severing proteins contribute to the dynamic remodeling of the cytoskeleton; one of the better-characterized of these is *gelsolin*, which is stimulated by high cytosolic calcium levels. The network of cortical actin fibers is thought to attach to the plasma membrane via anchoring proteins, similar to *spectrin* and *ankyrin* found in the erythrocyte. Also, actin may attach to transmembrane proteins in specialized junctional regions of the plasmalemma. With respect to lending stability to membrane specializations, such as microvilli, the actin core of microfilaments is linked together with the linker proteins, *fimbrin* and *fascin*. In addition, *myosin* and *minimyosin* may be present in the cytoplasm in unpolymerized form and can polymerize into filaments attached to organelles during translocation.

Intermediate Filaments

A population of filamentous cytoskeletal elements commonly observed in most cells lies intermediate in diameter between the thin microfilaments of actin and the thick filaments of myosin. These *intermediate filaments* exhibit an average diameter of 10 to 12 nm and represent several different proteins. The distribution of these filaments across cell and tissue types is quite narrowly restricted, as determined by immunocytochemical studies. Table 1–1 summarizes six major classes of intermediate filaments and their tissue distribution. In terms of functional significance, they insert into transmembrane proteins at the site of cell junctions (desmosomes and hemidesmosomes; see Chapter 2). *Keratin intermediate filaments,* by serving as linker proteins between the outer layers of the skin of the body surface, contribute to the permeability barrier of the skin. In neurons, the *neurofilaments* exhibit particularly long side-arms, which are thought to support nerve cell processes. Furthermore, in the event of cell trauma, the intermediate filament network serves to isolate the damage and to support physically the necessary rebuilding phase. This is evidenced clinically in chronic alcohol excess, when keratin intermediate filaments collapse within the liver cells, accumulating in a pattern known as *Mallory's hyaline.* Finally, in the nucleus, the *nuclear lamins* elaborate a lattice immediately deep to the nuclear envelope, which probably interacts with link proteins to lend structural stability to the nucleus.

Nucleus

The nucleus may be considered the cell's largest discrete organelle. It is bounded by a concentric double membrane, *the nuclear envelope,* and contains the cellular DNA in the form of *chromatin* and one or more *nucleoli.* The size, shape, and staining characteristics of nuclei vary considerably from tissue to tissue, but the morphology of the nucleus within cells of the same tissue is remarkably uniform. The nucleus moves within limits within the cytoplasm and may assume a basal or more central position, depending on physiologic state. A remarkable feature of nuclei is that they are capable of rotating within the cytoplasm, as demonstrated by phase-microscopic cinematography. Thus, they cannot adequately be described as uninteresting safe-deposit boxes for the cell's genetic code! Alterations in the size, uniformity, and staining characteristics of nuclei within a tissue may indicate early signs of neoplastic transformation. Cancer cells often exhibit bizarrely shaped nuclei, with deep invaginations and chromatin concentrated around the periphery of the nucleus (marginated chromatin). As noted previously, the *nuclear matrix* of lamin filaments is instrumental in the maintenance of nuclear shape.

Nuclear Envelope

A double-trilaminar membrane, the nuclear envelope enfolds the entire nucleus and forms a uniform space (40 to 70 nm) between the two membranes termed the *perinuclear cisterna.* The membranes of the envelope are individually specialized: the inner membrane is closely applied to the nuclear matrix and the marginated chromatin, whereas the outer leaflet is continuous with the RER and frequently exhibits polysomes bound to its surface. *Nuclear pores* are present in the envelope, at sites where the inner and outer membranes have fused (Fig. 1–20). They have an approximate diameter of 70 nm. Nuclear pores are critical to the transport of materials to and from the nucleus. They have a complex fine structure, with eight subunits and a thin membrane covering the aperture of each pore. This fine structural configuration suggests that they may be selectively permeable in the case of some macromolecules, allowing small molecules free access and restricting larger molecules. Nuclear pores are permeable to mRNA and certain cytoplasmic proteins.

Chromatin

Chromatin derives its name, not from any inherent coloration, but from its avid affinity for basic histologic stains. On the basis of relative staining characteristics, early microscopists distinguished two morphologic varieties of chromatin. The first consisted of clumps of densely stained material, which frequently was present near the nucleolus and at the margins of the nucleus. This *heterochromatin,* under the electron microscope, is very electron opaque and coarsely granular. More lightly stained areas running throughout the regions of heterochromatin, and characterizing large portions of some nuclei, particularly secretory cells, were called *euchromatin.* These regions, under the electron microscope, appear finely granular Both light-microscopists and electron-microscopists hypothesized that euchromatin, denatured and amorphous as it is as a result of the preparative techniques employed, represents a relatively loose coiling of DNA-histone complexes. This

TABLE 1-1. Six Classes of Intermediate Filaments and Their Distribution in Tissues

Filament Type	Cell Type	Examples
Keratins Variable kDs, depending upon 40- to 70-kD polypeptide subunits incorporated	Epithelial cells; not cells of mesenchymal origin	Particularly keratinizing, but also nonkeratinizing epithelia; e.g., "tonofilaments"
Vimentin (58-kD protein)	Mesenchymal cells	Fibroblasts, macrophages, and other mesenchymal derivatives
Desmin (53-kD acidic protein)	Muscle	Striated muscle; smooth muscle, with the exception of vascular smooth muscle
Glial filaments (51-kD fibrillary acidic protein)	Glial cells	Astrocytes, oligodenodrocytes, and microglia
Neurofilaments (210-kD, 160-kD, and 68-kD polypeptide subunits)	Neurons	Neuronal perikarya, axons, and dendrites
Filaments of nuclear lamina, composed of lamins, polypeptides, 60–75 kD	Form the nuclear lamina of most cells (30–100 nm in thickness), associated with the inner aspect of the nuclear envelope	

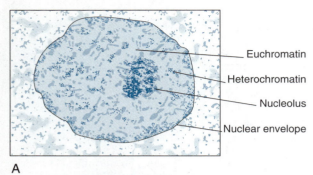

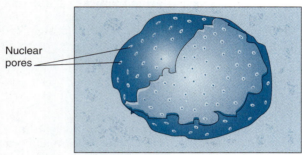

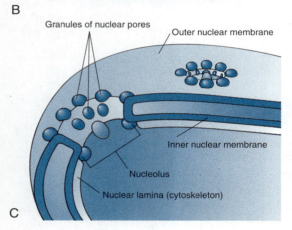

FIGURE 1–20. Diagram of the nucleus and nuclear pore system. A, The nucleus as imaged in the transmission electron microscope, showing the heterochromatin, euchromatin, nucleolus, and the nuclear envelope. B, Freeze-fracture electron micrograph reveals that the nuclear envelope is perforated by pores—the nuclear pores—revealed here by the cryofracture that passed through the nuclear envelope. C, Diagrammatic representation of the molecular arrangement of the nuclear pore complex. The pores are complex in terms of both structure and function. They are not merely passive openings in the nuclear envelope, as their name might imply.

interpretation is consistent with the extensive regions of euchromatin that typify the nuclei of cells actively synthesizing protein, in that the uncoiling of the nucleoprotein complex (and its consequent light-staining reaction) correlates with active genetic transcription. The precursors of messenger, ribosomal, and transfer RNAs are synthesized within chromatin DNA.

Molecular-biologic techniques have permitted the nature of the coiling of the DNA-histone complex to be probed. The fundamental unit of chromatin structure is recognized as the *nucleosome*. Within the nucleosome, dimers of four histones (H2A, H2B, H3, and H4) form an octomer that is wrapped by a segment of DNA double helix consisting of 166 base pairs. It is recognized that nonhistone proteins also are associated with chromatin, but their molecular architecture and significance are not yet clear. Nucleosomes (Fig. 1–21) form the building blocks for the next-higher order of chromatin organization, a 30-nm fiber referred to as a *solenoid*. Six nucleosomes participate in each turn around the coiled axis of the solenoid structure. Less detail is known of the yet still-higher order coiling and packing of chromatin material that must occur to account for the appearance of the dense, thick mitotic chromosomes.

It is of both biologic and clinical interest that female X chromosomes do not both uncoil in interphase: one remains intensely heterochromatic and is routinely detectable in cells from buccal smears and in leukocytes of mammalian females of the species. This chromatin, referred to as the *sex chromatin*, is readily visible as a small "drumstick" appendage to the nuclei of the neutrophils of peripheral blood. Clinically, this feature permits identification of the genotype of individuals whose external genitalia do not readily permit gender determination. Careful analysis of the chromosomal pattern of a patient requires the preparation of a *karyotype*, utilizing special staining techniques of metaphase chromosomes to study the complex banding patterns peculiar to each chromosome. Alterations in the banding patterns of suspect chromosomes are used to diagnose certain genetic disorders (Fig. 1–22).

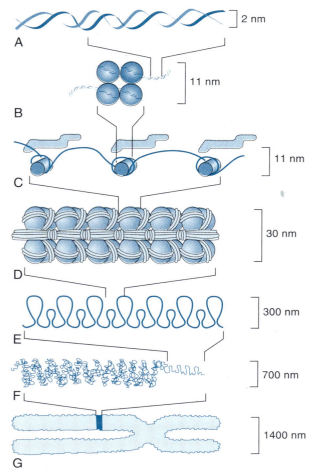

FIGURE 1–21. Diagram representing the different orders of packing that DNA and protein are thought to undergo in chromatin and the metaphase chromosome. The DNA double helix (A) is associated with histones in the formation of nucleosomes (B). Nucleosomes linked to histones (C) form fibers (D). Fiber loops (E), in association with protein cores, form chromosomal regions, which, when condensed (F), are visible under the light microscope, after appropriate staining, as bands (G) (see Fig. 1–22).

Nucleolus

The nucleolus, or "little nucleus," its literal Latin descriptor, was recognized and named by early light-microscopists, who remarked upon its size and prominence within nuclei of synthesizing cells. Nucleoli are also prominent in the actively synthetic cells of the embryo and of many neurons, and in tumors. Although in some cells the nucleolus is of irregular and complex shape, it typically is identified in sections as a round structure, closely associated with clumps of nuclear heterochromatin, the *nucleolus-associated chromatin.* The nucleolus stains basophilically (blue) with hematoxylin. Examination of nucleoli under the electron microscope reveals three components of the nucleolus. The first is usually a number of pale-staining regions within the nucleolus, the *nucleolar organizer DNA;* these have been determined to represent bases that code for ribosomal RNA. Nucleoprotein fibers, some 5 to 10 nm in diameter, constitute the *pars fibrosa* of the nucleolus,

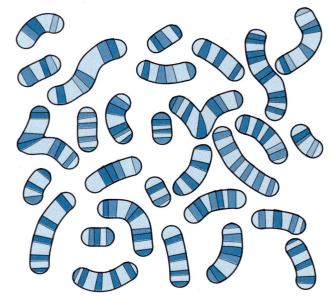

FIGURE 1–22. Karyotype. *Special stains of metaphase chromosomes allow segregation of the chromosome pairs and identification of the banding patterns of individual chromosomes; such a preparation is called a* karyotype.

representing primary transcripts of the rRNA genes. The third component, the *pars granulosa,* is composed of granules some 20 nm in diameter, which are maturing ribosomes (Fig. 1–23).

Cell Division

On the basis of the demonstrated uptake of radiolabeled DNA precursors, cell populations within the body have been classified as static, stable, or renewing.

Static cell populations are those incapable of mitosis in the adult. Examples are neurons of the central nervous system, and cardiac muscle cells. Stable populations are those that although they ordinarily do not divide, would respond to loss of cells from an organ

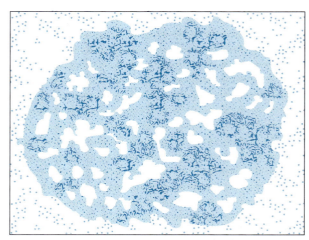

FIGURE 1–23. Diagram of the nucleolus. *Amorphous, granular, and fibrous components, as revealed in transmission electron microscopic studies.*

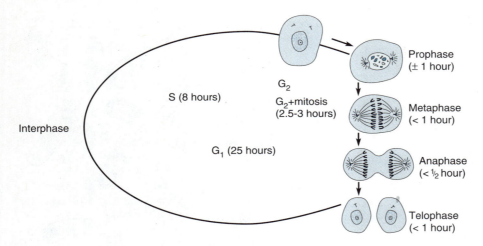

FIGURE 1–24. *Diagram of a typical mammalian cell cycle.* Note that the pre-DNA synthesis phase (G_1) is variable among tissues, depending upon its cellular turnover rate. A postsynthesis phase (G_2) follows the S or synthesis phase of DNA. Mitosis, visible with the light microscope, lasts a comparatively short time in relation to the other, morphologically indistinguishable phases of the cycle. Times given are for bone tissue. (From R. W. Young, J. Cell Biol. *14:*357, 1962).

with an attempt to replace them by division. An example within the human body is the liver.

Renewing cell populations, on the other hand, are characteristic of those organs that regularly lose cells from trauma and cell death (for example, the skin and the epithelial lining of the gastrointestinal tract) and that must replace them continuously to retain structural integrity. Observations of cell populations that have such differing potential for cell division, or *mitosis,* have led to the development of the concept of the *cell cycle.* Even though the events of mitosis are the most visible signs of cell division, other phases of the proliferative dynamics of a dividing cell population must be appreciated. Figure 1–24 summarizes the concepts of the cell cycle.

Briefly stated, cells that are not dividing do not cycle in and out of the two major phases of a cell's natural history, *interphase* and *mitosis.* Rather, they remain in interphase, in G_0. Figure 1–24 helps place the events of cell division into these two phases. *Mitosis* is that visible expression of the proliferative cycle; the named, time-honored "steps" of mitosis are summarized here and shown in Figure 1–25.

INTERPHASE. *Interphase* is that interval between the final telophase event of mitosis, and the visible reappearance of prophase. Interphase consists of the G_1, S, and G_2 phases; cells remain in interphase (either arrested in a phase designated G_0) or in other phases preparatory to undergoing mitosis for the majority of their lives. The G_1 *phase* is the most variable in length from one dividing tissue to another and depends on a variety of tissue-specific factors. In this phase, cells are engaged in anabolic metabolic activity and exhibit growth following the previously completed mitotic phase. In the *S phase* of the cycle, which follows the G_1 phase, DNA is synthesized, and the centrioles replicate. Following the S phase, the dividing cell enters the G_2 phase, during which energy is generated and stored by metabolic means for the events of mitosis, and tubulin is synthesized to be used in the elaboration of the mitotic spindle.

PROPHASE. Mitotic prophase is the first morphologic

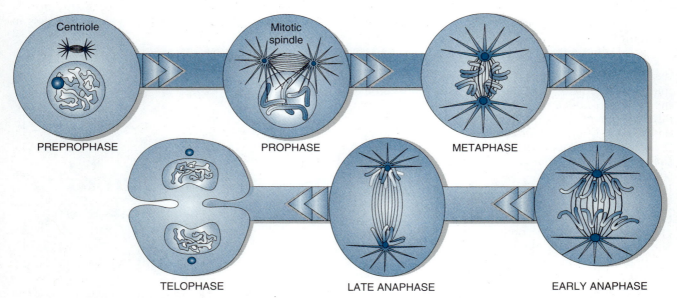

FIGURE 1–25. *Diagram of the various phases of mitosis.* Hallmark events in the process of mitosis are noted (see text).

manifestation that division will occur in a given cell. Chromosomes condense but the nuclear envelope is retained. Separation of centrioles (duplicated in the S phase of interphase) begins, and microtubular assembly occurs.

METAPHASE. Both the nucleolus and nuclear envelope disappear. Chromosomes migrate to the equatorial plate, with division of each chromosome into two chromatids. Chromatids attach to centromeres.

ANAPHASE. Sister chromatids separate and migrate toward centrioles at opposite poles of the cell.

TELOPHASE. Nuclei reappear, chromosomes redisperse, and nucleoli reappear, together with chromatin and the nuclear envelope. Actin and myosin belt–like constriction of the daughter cell cytoplasm appears preparatory to *cytokinesis*, the divison of cytoplasmic components.

CONCLUSION

As emphasized earlier, it must be realized that the cell cycle and mitotic stages are part of a continuum and must be appreciated and studied as such. As the student gains an understanding of how cells regulate their growth and cell cycles, so will he or she begin to appreciate how tumors and other abnormal growth and developmental patterns arise. The process of **meiosis** is examined in relation to the study of the reproductive systems and gametogenesis in Chapters 16 and 17.

CHAPTER TWO

EPITHELIUM

A STRUCTURAL-FUNCTIONAL CLASSIFICATION OF THE EPITHELIUM	25
Simple (Single-Layer) Epithelia	28
Stratified Epithelium	34
GLANDS	35
Classification of Glands	35
Exocrine Glands	37
Endocrine Glands	38

Epithelial cells cover the body surfaces. They may be single or multilayered. Although a highly specific term (*epi*, upon; *thelos*, nipple), *epithelium* has been redefined through usage to comprise the specialized cellular surfaces of all cavities and vessels as well as the exterior of the body. The epithelia vary in form and are derived from all three embryologic cell layers. The cells covering the skin or integument, alimentary tract, and the most distal parts of the urogenital tracts arise from both ectoderm and endoderm. Those epithelia lining internal cavities and the proximal parts of the urogenital system arise from mesoderm. The linings of the pericardial, peritoneal, and pleural cavities are termed *mesothelia*, and those lining blood vessels and the chambers of the heart are *endothelia*; they also arise from mesoderm.

In general, many epithelial cells have a free surface, which is actually or potentially exposed to the external environment (skin and respiratory tract) or to a moist environment continuous with the external environment (digestive, reproductive, and urinary tracts). Other epithelial cells, constituting glands found in underlying connective tissue, are in continuity with the surface epithelium by means of epithelial duct cells. The glandular epithelium secretes diverse products, which are carried to the external surface. The products of these glands include sweat, bile, urine, reproductive cells and associated glandular secretions, mucus, milk, digestive enzymes and hydrochloric acid. Some epithelial cells have migrated away and have lost contact with the free surface. These cells form distinctive cellular masses, termed *endocrine glands*. The secretory products of these cellular masses are delivered into the vascular system, to be carried to their specific sites of activity. The endocrine glands are discussed in detail in Chapter 15.

It is important to remember that everything that enters or leaves the body is either modified or synthesized by epithelial cells or has diffused or has been transported through this tissue. The various functions of epithelium are protection, secretion, excretion, digestion, absorption, lubrication, sensory reception, and reproduction. Such a diversity of functional activity depends upon structurally diverse cell types and cell groupings classified as epithelium.

In some classifications, the epithelia are separated from the mesothelia and endothelia. Because the latter two types are derived from mesenchyme rather than from ectodermal or endodermal elements, they have characteristic mesenchymal features. For example, their cytoskeletal intermediate filaments are composed of vimentin rather than the keratin filaments found in epithelia. The functions of epithelia include their being selective-permeability interfaces. They may facilitate or prevent the passage of substances across the surfaces they cover. They protect underlying tissues from desiccation and from chemical and mechanical damage. The epithelia synthesize and secrete materials into the spaces they bound. Also, they may function as sensory surfaces.

The epithelial cells rest upon a basement membrane composed of glycoproteins, which are discussed in Chapter 3. In addition, a 20-nm intercellular gap typically exists between adjacent cells, which is also filled with glycoproteins. Intercellular junctions are also numerous in epithelia; these junctions have already been discussed in Chapter 1 but are also considered briefly in this chapter. Cell shape is variable, from cuboidal or polygonal to flask-shaped to columnar. The shapes of these cells are partially determined by surrounding tissues or cells, by their cytoplasmic contents, and by other considerations, such as physiologic state.

The epithelia are continuously replaced and some have an exceptional capacity for regeneration; this quality can be seen in the skin and liver, as examples. Replacement is an essential factor for the maintenance of epithelial integrity and for survival of the organism, since fragile single or even multiple cell layers are vulnerable to abrasion or other trauma.

An epithelium is a thin layer of cells, so even where it is thickest (e.g., the skin), nutrients and waste products are provided and removed by the immediate proximity of the underlying vascular system. There is a limit, however, to the number of layers of viable cells that this type of vascular relationship can sustain.

A STRUCTURAL-FUNCTIONAL CLASSIFICATION OF THE EPITHELIUM

This basic tissue can be divided or grouped into simple epithelia (single cell layer) and multilayered epithelia (more than one cell thick). Additional structural details permit further refinement of this classification (Fig. 2–1).

Accordingly, epithelia are classified by histologists on the basis of cell layering and cell shape. Two distinct types of epithelium are recognized: (1) *simple*, which is a single cell layer, and *pseudostratified*, a single cell layer that appears to have two or more layers, and (2) stratified, which is composed of several to many cell layers. Only the simple and stratified epithelia have important subgroupings, which are classified according to the shapes of the cells that are exposed to the free surface. The simple epithelia are described as *squamous* (sheets of flattened cells), *cuboidal* (in which the cells are roughly equal in height and width when seen in sections—they are actually five- or six-sided when seen in cross-section as in Figures 2–1 and 2–6, and *columnar* (in which the cells are greater in height than width when seen in most sections—these, too, are actually five- or six-sided in cross-section). The stratified epithelia are *stratified squamous*, in which the superficial cells on the free surface are flattened; *stratified cuboidal*, in which the superficial cells on the free surface are cuboidal; and *stratified columnar*, in which the superficial cells on the free surface are columnar.

From a functional point of view, the simple epithelia carry out the most diverse activities, i.e., absorption, excretion, synthesis, secretion, and sensory reception, whereas the stratified epithelia have protective functions, serve as conduits or ducts, and produce repro-

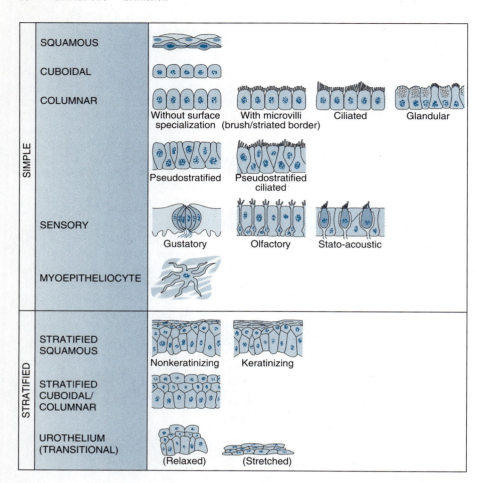

FIGURE 2–1. Epithelial variety. *Diagrammatic representation of epithelial types, both simple (A) and stratified (B).*

TABLE 2–1. Classification of Epithelial Cells

Cell Type	Some Locations in Body	Cell Type	Some Locations in Body
Simple epithelium		Simple Epithelium *(Continued)*	
Squamous (Fig. 2–2)	Innermost lining of blood and lymph vessels and heart (endothelium)	Pigmented (Fig. 2–7)	Epithelium of retina
	Lining of pleural, cardiac, and abdominal cavities	Neuroepithelium (Fig. 2–8)	Receptors of cells of taste, hearing, and balance
	Initial segments of ducts of glands		
	Air sacs or alveoli	Myoepithelium (Fig. 2–18)	Specialized contractile cell associated with glands
	Renal glomeruli and corpuscles		
	Kidney tubules (thin segment of loop of Henle of nephron)	Stratified epithelium	
Cuboidal (Fig. 2–3)	"Germinal" epithelium covering ovaries	Stratified squamous (Fig. 2–9)	Keratinized and nonkeratinized epithelium of skin, palpebral conjunctivum, oral cavity, esophagus, and anus
	Ducts of many glands and kidney tubules		Urethra near external orifice
	Ciliary body of eye		Vagina
	Secretory cells of many glands (endocrine and exocrine) vary from cuboidal to columnar; size and shape may vary with the functional state (e.g., thyroid gland)	Stratified cuboidal (Fig. 2–10)	Ducts of sweat and sebaceous glands
			Graafian follicles
Columnar (Fig. 2–4)	Stomach, intestines, and gallbladder	Stratified columnar (Fig. 2–11)	Portions of pharynx, larynx, and urethra
	Small bronchi		Portions of excretory ducts of salivary and mammary glands
	Uterine tubes		
Pseudostratified (Fig. 2–5)	Pharynx, trachea, and large bronchi	Transitional (uroepithelium) (Fig. 2–12)	Renal calyces and pelvis
	Male secretory ducts (epididymis and vas deferens)		Ureter
	Parts of male and female urethra		Urinary bladder
Specialized (unicellular glands) (Fig. 2–6)	Glands of intestinal tract		
	Nasal cavity and bronchi		
	Uterine tubes		
	Accessory sex glands		

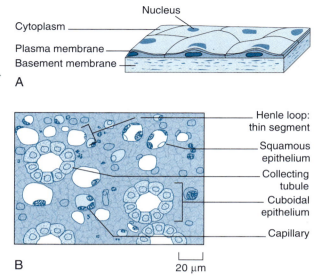

FIGURE 2–2. Squamous epithelium. *Note the distribution of this type in capillary blood vessels and certain kidney tubules. Compare with cuboidal type seen in the same illustration. See also Figure 2–3.*

ductive cells. In order to serve their distinctive functional roles, epithelial cells often display distinctive cell membrane or surface modifications and appendages.

The epithelial types shown in Figure 2–1 represent the morphologic varieties of simple and stratified epithelia. The structural features of many other epithelial cell types and groupings are found in other sections of this text, where their functional roles are considered in the context of organ function. The morphologic characteristics have important functional considerations.

A classification of epithelial cell types and some of their locations in the body are given in Table 2–1. The various types are shown in Figures 2–2 through 2–12.

Several specializations of epithelial cells found on

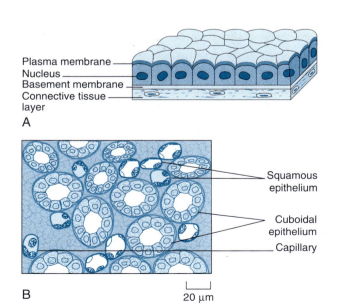

FIGURE 2–3. Simple cuboidal epithelium in kidney tubules. *Compare with squamous type seen in the same illustration. See also Figure 2–2.*

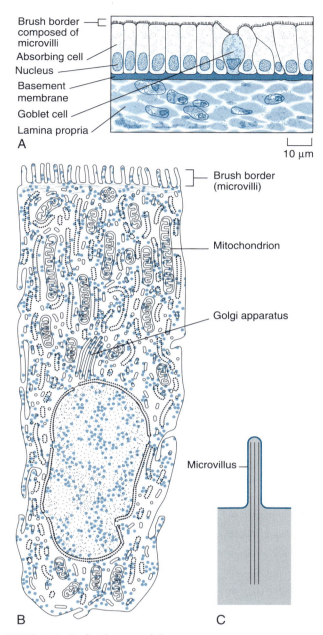

FIGURE 2–4. Simple columnar epithelium. *This epithelium is found in the digestive tract. Its free surface has microvilli, which vastly increase the cell surface area and absorptive capacity. A, Light microscopic appearance. B, Diagram of electron micrograph of a columnar epithelial cell. C, Fine structure of a microvillus.*

their free or exposed surface are the brush or striated border of the absorbing cells of the intestine and kidney (Fig. 2–4), motile cilia of the pseudostratified epithelium of the respiratory system (Fig. 2–5), and nonmotile stereocilia of the pseudostratified epithelium lining the epididymis (Fig. 2–13). Specializations that structurally and functionally link adjacent cells together include the *terminal bars* or adhesion belts and the *intercellular bridges* or desmosomes associated with prickle cells found in stratified squamous epithelium (Fig. 2–14). Marked infoldings of the basal cell membrane, termed *basal striations*, are seen in certain active transport cells,

28 CHAPTER TWO EPITHELIUM

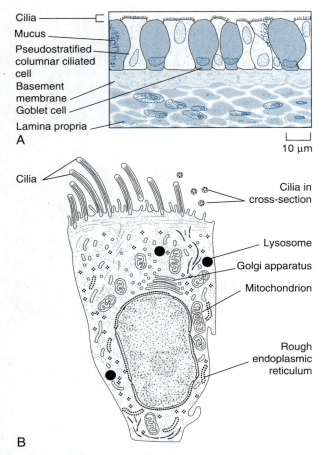

FIGURE 2–5. Simple, pseudostratified epithelium. This type of epithelium, found in the respiratory system, has cells with nuclei at various levels, producing the illusion that it is stratified. All cells rest on the basement membrane, but all cells do not reach the free surface. Note the unicellular glands (goblet cells) and the typical, very thick basement membrane. A, Light microscopic appearance. B, Diagram of an electron micrograph of the principal cell type in this epithelium.

such as the proximal convoluted tubule cells of the kidney and ducts of certain glands (Fig. 2–15). Between the basal surface of epithelial cells and the underlying connective tissue is the *basement membrane*, which varies markedly from place to place and in certain disease states. This extracellular structure has been shown, by electron microscopy, to have several components (among them, the basal lamina) that are produced by both epithelial cells and the underlying connective tissue fibroblasts (Fig. 2–15).

Simple (Single-Layer) Epithelia

A classification of epithelium based on cell shape would comprise squamous, cuboidal, and columnar forms. In general, epithelial cells with little cytoplasm, few organelles, and low metabolic rates tend to be squamous and cuboidal types, and epithelial cells that are absorbing or primarily transporting, ciliated, or secretory tend to appear columnar (Figs. 2–4 to 2–6). Highly active cells have abundant mitochondria, endo-

plasmic reticula, and in the case of secretory cells, a well-developed Golgi apparatus (Figs. 2–13 and 2–18).

The simple epithelia (unilaminar) have also been divided according to their structural-functional characteristics, such as cilia, microvilli, secretory activity, and sensory receptor characteristics. Myoepithelial cells are included in this type of epithelium but are discussed elsewhere.

Squamous Epithelium

Squamous epithelial cells are flat, polygonal cells that frequently have interlocking surfaces (Fig. 2–2). The thickness of the cell may be only 0.1 μm; as a result, the nucleus may produce a surface bulge on the cell. Cells of this type are found lining the alveoli of lungs, parts of the urinary system, the pericardial, pleural, and peritoneal cavities, and the vascular and lymphatic systems. In the pericardium, pleura, and peritoneum, the lining cells are known as the *mesothelium;* in the vascular system, the *endothelium*. The mesothelia and endothelia differ from other forms of squamous cells because they possess vimentin filaments rather than epithelial keratin filaments.

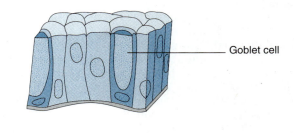

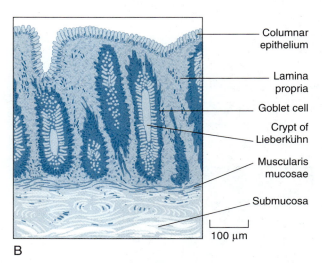

FIGURE 2–6. Unicellular glands (goblet cells). These structures are found in abundance in the digestive, respiratory, and genitourinary tracts. Note the five- and six-sided shapes due to tight packing, which are characteristic of so-called cuboidal and columnar cells. The columnar cells of the large intestine possess a thin microvillous surface (not shown). A, Diagram of columnar cells in longitudinal and cross-section. Note the polygonal shape seen in cross-section. A single complete goblet cell is also seen. B, Numerous unicellular goblet cells are seen.

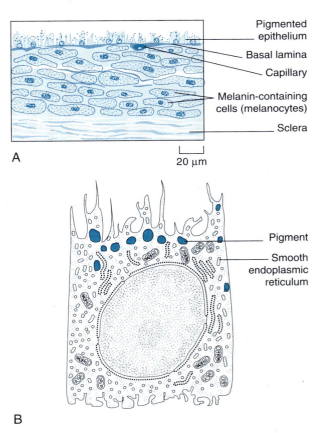

FIGURE 2-7. Simple pigmented (cuboidal) epithelium. *Cuboidal cells that synthesize melanin line the eye and absorb light. A, Light microscopic magnification of the pigment epithelium of the eye. B, Diagram of an electron micrograph of a pigment epithelial cell.*

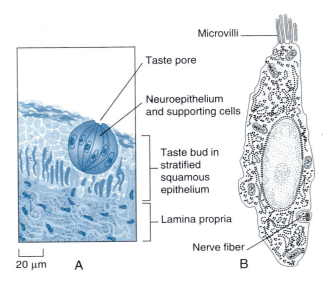

FIGURE 2-8. Simple gustatory neuroepithelium. *Sensory receptor cells with supporting cells are shown. The receptor cells for taste have an elongated nucleus, whereas supporting cell nuclei tend to be round. A, Light micrograph magnification of a taste bud containing taste cells. B, Diagram of an electron micrograph of a taste receptor cell.*

30 CHAPTER TWO EPITHELIUM

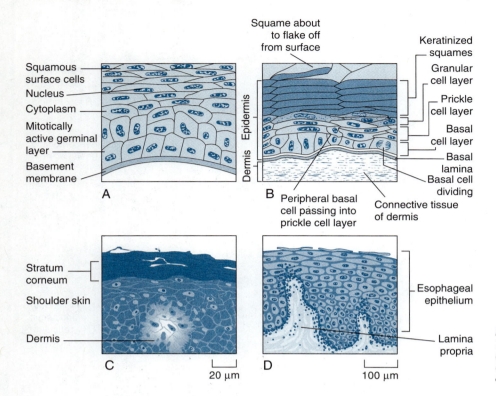

FIGURE 2–9. Stratified squamous epithelium. *Two types are shown, the nonkeratinizing (esophageal) (A and B) and keratinizing (skin) (C and D). Note that the stratum corneum is absent in A and B.*

FIGURE 2–10. Stratified cuboidal epithelium. *The follicular cells surrounding the ovum constitute a stratified cuboidal epithelium. A, Light micrograph appearance of the stratified cuboidal epithelium in a follicle. B, Higher magnification of the stratified cuboidal (follicular) epithelium.*

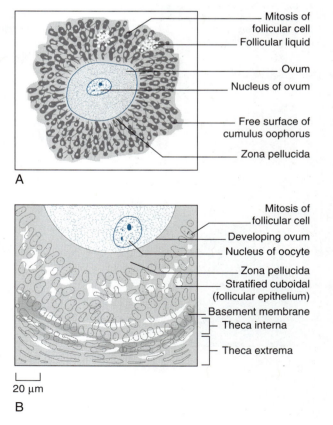

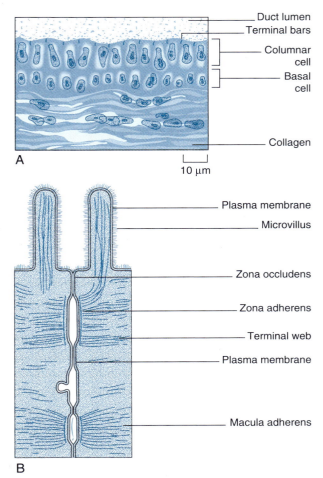

FIGURE 2-11. Stratified columnar epithelium. This type and a stratified cuboidal type form the large ducts of glands. A, The so-called terminal bars are well seen. B, The special junctional complex revealed by electron microscopy represents the terminal bar seen by light microscopy. Other features of junctional complexes are described in the text. This illustration, however, is typical of columnar epithelial cells that possess microvilli.

Functionally, the thin squamous epithelia are designed to allow rapid diffusion or transport of gases, water, and other substances. In some locations, the endothelium is not firmly attached by occluding junctions, thus permitting materials to pass between cells; in other places, the endothelium has numerous "pores" that selectively permit certain substances to pass; in still other locations, active transport via endocytic vesicles appears to be the mechanism by which materials pass across squamous cells (see Chapter 8).

Cuboidal and Columnar Epithelium

In vertical section, cuboidal and columnar epithelial cells appear square or rectangular (Figs. 2–3 and 2–6). In cross-section, however, the cells are seen to be polygonal. Although misnomers *cuboidal* and *columnar* are used with the understanding that this terminology is based on their appearance (height) in longitudinal section. Cuboidal epithelium is found in urinary, reproductive, and glandular systems, whereas columnar cells are seen in the respiratory and digestive systems. There are important additions to the location of both cell types, but these are mentioned in the appropriate places in subsequent chapters. It must also be remembered that although cuboidal and columnar epithelia usually retain their shapes, some epithelia may appear cuboidal in one physiologic state and columnar in another (e.g., thyroid follicles).

Variation in height is only one aspect of these cell types. Another variation is cell surface specializations, which serve very important functional roles. In some cuboidal and columnar cells, the free surface may be composed of microvilli. The microvilli enormously increase the surface area of the cell, thereby facilitating absorption and transport of substances into the body, e.g., in the digestive system, urinary system, and certain glands (Fig. 2–15). Details of these cell types are considered in later chapters. Ciliated epithelium, responsible for the removal of mucus and particulate matter from the respiratory tract, is commonly called respiratory epithelium, although columnar and cuboidal cells are found in addition to the squamous cells (alveolar cell type I) where respiratory exchange actually takes place in the alveoli (see Chapter 13). Ciliated cells in the uterine tube assist in moving the ova from the peritoneal cavity to the uterus for implantation (see Chapter 17).

Certain columnar cells are actually unicellular glands. These cells usually reside among nonsecretory cells, as in the respiratory epithelium. Here, the secreted mucus traps "dust" and it is swept along for removal at

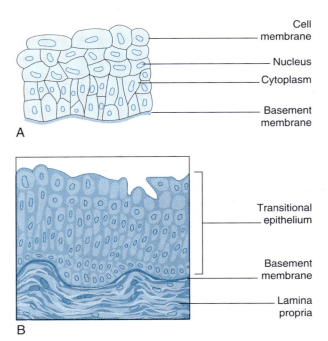

FIGURE 2-12. Stratified transitional epithelium. Transitional epithelium (uroepithelium) is characterized by "cuboidal" cells rather than squamous cells on its free surface. As the epithelium is stretched physiologically (e.g., bladder filling), the cells flatten. They return to their "cuboidal" shape upon relaxation. A, Diagram of stratified transitional epithelium. B, Diagram of a light micrograph of transitional epithelium.

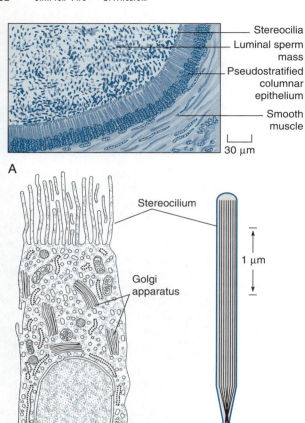

of a bottle brush (see Chapter 3). These huge molecules have a molecular weight of 2 million or more. The carbohydrate residues include glucose, fructose, galactose, and sialic acid (negatively charged N-acetylglucosamine). The terminals of some of the carbohydrate chains are similar to blood group antigens of the ABO group found in 80% of the population. They may therefore have an antigenic function. The long carbohydrate chains bind water and thereby protect epithelial surfaces from dehydration. Mucus also provides surfaces with reduced friction; this lubricating property protects underlying tissues from abrasion and trauma.

Mucus is synthesized in the granular endoplasmic reticulum and moved to the Golgi apparatus, where it is conjugated with sulfated carbohydrates to form a glycoprotein, which is carried away from the synthetic apparatus in small dense vesicles that swell as they approach and fuse with the cell membrane at the apex of the cell, where it is released (Fig. 2–16).

Pseudostratified Epithelium

Pseudostratified epithelium is a simple columnar epithelium, because each cell actually lies on the basement membrane (Fig. 2–13). In addition, not all cells reach the free surface, and the nuclei are found at different levels. Cells that do not reach to the free

FIGURE 2–13. Simple pseudostratified columnar epithelium with stereocilia. This epithelium has its nuclei at several levels, giving it a stratified appearance. Actually, all cells of this epithelium contact the basement membrane, except for wandering cells of the immune system. Stereocilia are immobile but are a functionally significant part of this epithelium in that they facilitate resorption. A, Diagram of a light micrograph of pseudostratified columnar epithelium with stereocillia. B, Diagram of an electron micrograph of the principal cell type. C, Diagram of a stereocilium at the electron microscopic level.

the pharynx by swallowing. The mucus is synthesized as small globules that fill the upper end (apex) of the cell, giving the cell a distinctive wine goblet–like appearance. The columnar cells that produce mucus are known therefore, as *goblet cells* (Figs. 2–4 and 2–5). They are found in the respiratory and digestive systems. In both cases, their function—the production of mucus—is thought to be protective in nature. These cells are often located between "nonsecretory" cell types (see Chapters 11 and 17).

Mucus is a viscid suspension of various very complex glycoproteins and many other products from non–mucus-producing cells that are added inadvertently to the suspension. The mucus glycoproteins consist of core proteins to which carbohydrate chains are added, which stand out from the core protein like the bristles

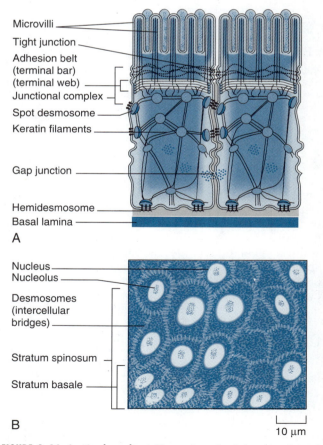

FIGURE 2–14. Junctional complexes. The variety of cell junctions formed by epithelial cells of the small intestine (A) and skin (B).

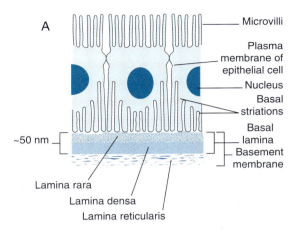

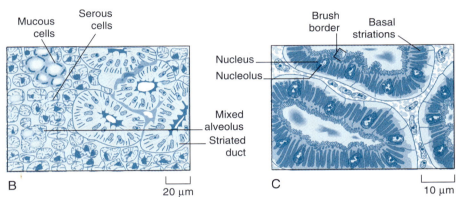

FIGURE 2-15. **Epithelial apical and basal surfaces.** *Microvilli and basal cell membrane invaginations are commonly observed in specialized epithelia. They increase the cell surface area and facilitate absorption or the excretion process. A, Diagram showing microvilli and basal striations (invaginations) and the basal lamina. B, Striated ducts with basal striations (invaginations) in salivary glands. C, Microvilli (brush border) and basal striations (invaginations) in kidney tubules.*

surface of the epithelium often constitute a basal cell layer. These cells are mitotic and provide replacement cells when the mature cells either die or are damaged.

Lymphocytes, which are migratory, are typically found within this type of columnar epithelium, and their nuclei are found at different levels and contribute to the pseudostratified appearance.

Neuroepithelium (Sensory Cells)

The sensory receptor cells of the gustatory, olfactory, and statoacoustic systems contain receptor cells surrounded by supporting epithelial cells. Olfactory receptor cells are modified neurons, whereas the others are regarded as modified or specialized epithelial cells. The neurons of olfactory receptors pass directly through the cribriform plate of the skull to the brain itself; the others synapse with nerve fibers peripherally (Fig. 2–17).

Myoepithelial Cells

Sometimes referred to as "basket cells," myoepithelial cells are actually stellate or fusiform. Because they contain significant numbers of actin and myosin filaments, they are able to contract when stimulated by nervous or neurohormonal activity. These cells surround the secretory elements and ducts of lacrimal, mammary, salivary, and sweat glands. They lie within the basal lamina (basement membrane) located at the basal surface of these secretory cells. Because they lie on the epithelial cell side of the basement membrane, they are classified as epithelial cells. The contraction of myoepithelial cells results in the flow of secretion into larger channels, thereby facilitating the expulsion of the secretory product.

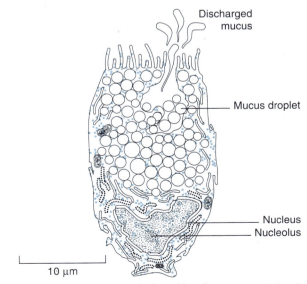

FIGURE 2-16. **Simple unicellular gland or goblet cell.** *These unicellular glands provide a protective mucous coating to cell surfaces of the respiratory and digestive tracts.*

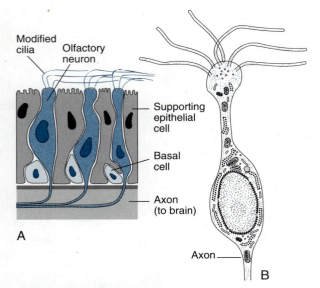

FIGURE 2–17. Specialized neuroepithelium: olfactory. *This specialized nerve cell has modified cilia, which have receptors that respond to odors of various types. These cells may be replaced, if damaged, by the maturation of basal (stem) cells. The supporting cells are true epithelial cells. A, Diagram at the light microscopic level of the olfactory epithelium. B, Diagram of an electron micrograph of an olfactory receptor neuron.*

ing constant formation, maturation, and loss. These cells are formed mitotically in the deepest or basal layer of the epithelium. The cells are pushed more superficially, changing their shape from columnar or cuboidal to squamous (Fig. 2–9). The squamous cells are normally removed from the surface by abrasion. This tough epithelium, when exposed to other stresses, provides continuous protection for the underlying tissues from chemical, microbial, mechanical trauma, and sunlight.

The viable cells of the stratified squamous epithelium are held together by innumerable desmosomes ("intercellular bridges") that form a stratified layer of significant strength (Fig. 2–14).

Two varieties of this kind of epithelium are found, namely, keratinized and nonkeratinized stratified squamous epithelium.

KERATINIZED STRATIFIED SQUAMOUS EPITHELIUM. The keratinized variety of stratified squamous epithelium is found over the entire external body surface—the mucocutaneous junctions such as the lips, nostrils, distal anal canal, and the outer surface of the tympanic membrane. The cells of this epithelium, keratinocytes, are formed by mitosis of basal stem cells located in the deepest layer,

Myoepithelial cells are similar in ultrastructure to smooth muscle cells, in their complement and arrangement of actin and myosin proteins. Myoepithelial cells arise, however, from both ectoderm and endoderm, unlike smooth muscle cells (Fig. 2–18).

Pigmented Epithelial Cells

Pigmented epithelial cells are widely distributed, and all have a light barrier function. They are found in the eye as the external layer of the retina and in the posterior layer of the iris. In these locations, the melanin-containing cells are densely filled with pigment granules. In the skin, melanocytes produce and transfer pigment granules to other cells but do not store them within their cytoplasm. The melanocytes of stratified squamous epithelium are derived from the neural crest. These cells migrate into the epithelium during development (Fig. 2–7).

Stratified Epithelium

Although all epithelial surfaces are subjected to wear and tear, those in some locations are at greater risk for damage and trauma. Multilayered epithelia may be replaced continuously (stratified squamous epithelium of skin), or they may be replaced only when damaged or traumatized.

Stratified Squamous Epithelia

As its name suggests, *stratified squamous epithelium* is a multilayered, stratified collection of cells undergo-

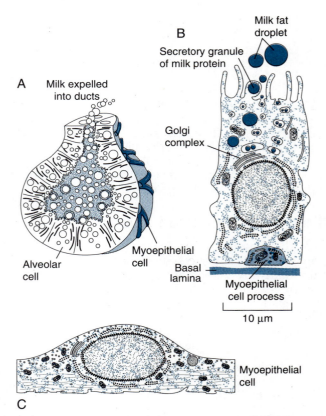

FIGURE 2–18. Specialized myoepithelial cell. *Myoepithelial cells are modified muscle cells associated with glands. Note the abundant cytoplasmic myofilaments. These cells are thought to facilitate secretion by contraction, as in the mammary gland, the example used here. A, Myoepithelial cells associated with an alveolus. B, Diagram of an electron micrograph showing the myoepithelial cell adjacent to the secretory cell. Note the myoepithelial cell is contained between the basal lamina and the secretory cell. C, Diagram of an electron micrograph of a portion of a myoepithelial cell containing myofilaments.*

the *stratum basale*. The deepest basal layer is attached to the basal lamina by *hemidesmosomes*. These basal cells move toward the free surface, changing their ultrastructure during their progression. After the basal cells divide, they synthesize many ribosomes, mitochondria, and other metabolically active organelles. The cells are also rich in cytoskeletal keratin filament bundles known as *tonofibrils*, which are securely fastened into the plasma (cell) membrane at desmosomal contacts with other cells (so-called prickle cells with intercellular bridges, because of their appearance by light microscopy). These cells, having a spiny appearance, compose the *stratum spinosum*. As these cells continue to divide and move, they begin to flatten and synthesize a dense, basophilic protein known as *keratohylin*, which fills the cells along with keratin filaments. The stainable granules give this layer a granular appearance; hence it is called *stratum granulosum*. An additional feature of the cells in this state of differentiation is the synthesis and secretion of a "waterproofing" glycolipid. This glycolipid not only "waterproofs" the cell surface but also is a thick lipidic, water-resistant cement between the adjacent squamous cells. Also at this stage, the cells lose their nuclei, and keratin filaments become embedded in the matrix protein; the cells are dense and form the upper, outer, final layer, the *stratum corneum*. The nonliving cells are squamous, tough, and hornlike and are continuously shed from the free surface (Fig. 2–9).

NONKERATINIZED STRATIFIED SQUAMOUS EPITHELIUM. Nonkeratinized stratified squamous epithelium can be found where it may be subject to abrasion but is protected from drying. It is located in the buccal cavity, oropharynx, laryngopharynx, esophagus, a part of the anal canal, the vagina, distal cervix of the uterus, distal urethra, conjunctiva of the eye, cornea, and vestibule of the nasal cavities. The cells of the nonkeratinizing epithelium undergo the same stages of differentiation, but these appear to be incomplete. They produce keratin, but the keratin does not fill the cell; they secrete glycolipid to a lesser extent; and the nucleus is not lost until an entire cell desquamates at the free surface of the epithelium. Where there is potential trauma or significant abrasion, the epithelium becomes thicker, with many more cell layers, and the superficial cells may respond with additional keratin synthesis and accumulation within cells. Such places can be found on the hard palate, the gingivae, and the dorsum of the tongue.

It is of interest that cells of this type of epithelium can be collected by abrasion of the reproductive tract or cheek with a swab and studied for pathologic manifestations or for sexing of individuals in questionable cases (Fig. 2–9).

Stratified Cuboidal and Columnar Epithelium

Stratified cuboidal and columnar epithelium is characteristic of larger ducts of some exocrine glands. They can be found in the pancreatic, salivary gland, and sweat gland ducts. The function of this type of epithelium is not fully understood, but it may provide the duct with greater strength than other combinations of stratified cell types (Fig. 2–11).

Uroepithelium

As its name implies, *uroepithelium* lines the free surfaces of the urinary tract, from the large collecting ducts of the kidneys, through the ureters and bladder, to the initial or proximal part of the urethra. This epithelium is also known as *transitional epithelium*.

In the female urethra, uroepithelium extends as far as the urogenital diaphragm. This type of epithelium is believed to be derived from all three germ layers in development. In males, it lines the urethra as far as the ejaculatory ducts. After this point, the epithelium becomes irregular and is replaced by pseudostratified epithelium in the membranous urethra.

Uroepithelium appears to be about six cells thick and lines some organs capable of considerable distention and contraction. When stratified, the cells flatten, but their relative position in regard to adjacent cells is maintained by the presence of numerous desmosomes. When relaxed, the cells located deep (basally) are cuboidal and uninucleate and contain numerous ribosomes; hence, the cells are somewhat basophilic. Those cells located nearer the free surface appear large and binucleate. This trend continues as the cells fuse to form still larger cells. The cell surface of this epithelium possesses glycoprotein plates embedded in the lipid bilayer. These plates apparently stiffen the membrane to such an extent that in the relaxed state (when the surface area of the cell is reduced), the glycoprotein plates are folded into the cell, only to reemerge when the epithelium is once again stretched.

Uroepithelium forms an effective barrier, preventing urine from crossing it, because urine contains toxic substances that may be harmful to surrounding cells and tissues (Fig. 2–12).

GLANDS

Glands are epithelial and are specialized for secretory activity. In many cases, the secretory epithelium may be located below the surface cell layer but is connected with the surface by a duct system. These exocrine glands secrete onto the free surface of the epithelial cell and the secretion is carried by a duct to the surface of the skin, buccal cavity, or elsewhere. More is said of such glands in the chapters on skin and digestive, respiratory, and urogenital systems. Some glands lose their connection with the free surface, and the secretion of endocrine glands is directed into the blood stream and lymphatic vessels, with which they are richly supplied (Fig. 2–19).

Classification of Glands

Glands may thus be classified as shown in Table 2–2.

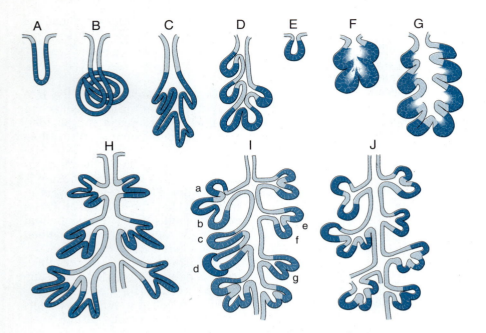

FIGURE 2-19. Diagrammatic representation of various types of exocrine glands. A and G show simple glands; H to J show compound glands. A, *Simple, nonbranched tubular.* B, *Simple coiled tubular.* C, *Branched tubular.* D, *Branched tubuloacinar (tubuloalveolar).* E, *Simple nonbranched alveolar.* F and G, *Branched alveolar as in sebaceous glands.* H, *Compound tubular.* I, *Compound tubuloacinar,* showing some of the various types of terminations. a, serous acinus with simple, nonbranched canal; b and c, variations in size of lumen of mucous terminations, as in sublingual; d, tubuloalveolus of mucous tubule and serous demilune; e, f, and g, serous terminations with branched canals, or intercellular secretory canaliculi, as in parotid gland. J, Compound alveolar gland.

Simple Glands

The simple glands of the human are classified as tubular, coiled tubular, branched tubular, and acinous or alveolar (see Fig. 2-19).

SIMPLE TUBULAR GLANDS. There is no excretory duct in a simple tubular gland, and the terminal portion is a straight tubule that opens directly on the epithelial surface. Such are the intestinal glands (crypts) of Lieberkuhn.

SIMPLE COILED TUBULAR GLANDS. The terminal of a simple coiled tubular gland portion is a long coiled tubule that passes into a long excretory duct. The sweat glands belong to this category. In the large axillary sweat glands of apocrine type, the terminal portions branch.

SIMPLE BRANCHED TUBULAR GLANDS. The tubules of the terminal portions in simple branched tubular glands are split forklike into two or more branches that sometimes are coiled near their ends. An excretory duct may be absent, as in the glands of the stomach and uterus, or there may be but a simple short excretory duct, as in some of the small glands of the oral cavity, the tongue, and the esophagus, and in some of the glands of Brunner (duodenal glands).

SIMPLE BRANCHED ACINOUS GLAND. If the terminal portion of a gland has the form of a spherical or elongated sac, the gland is called *acinous* or *alveolar*. If only one acinus is present with one excretory duct, it is a simple acinous gland; this type does not occur in mammals. If the acinus is subdivided by partitions into several smaller bodies, or if several acini are arranged along a duct, it is called a simple branched acinous gland (sebaceous glands of the skin, meibomian glands in the eyelids).

Compound Glands

A compound gland may consist of larger subdivisions called *lobes*, which are further subdivided by connective tissue into smaller parts. The smallest that can be observed easily with the naked eye is called a macrolobule. This, in turn consists of smaller, often incompletely separated, microscopic lobules that contain the glandular units. Glands of each order of complexity may be found in the body. A compound gland consists, then, of a varying number of simple glands whose small excretory ducts join to form ducts of a higher order, which in turn combine with other ducts of the same caliber to form larger ducts of a still higher order (see Fig. 2-19).

The compound exocrine glands are sometimes classified according to the secretion they furnish. Thus, mucous, serous, and mixed glands are distinguished. This classification can be applied with partial success chiefly to the glands of the oral cavity. Another classification is based on the form of the terminal portions.

COMPOUND TUBULAR GLANDS. In compound tubular glands, the terminal portions of the smallest lobules are more-or-less coiled, usually branching tubules. To this category belong the pure mucous glands of the oral cavity, glands of the gastric cardia, some of the glands of Brunner, the bulbourethral glands, and the renal tubules. In special cases, as, for instance, in the testis, the terminal coils anastomose with one another.

TABLE 2-2. Classification of Glands

Duct glands (glands of external secretion; exocrine glands)	
Simple	Tubular—straight, coiled, or branched
	Tubuloalveolar (tubuloacinous)
	Alveolar (acinous, saccular)
Compound	Tubular
	Tubuloalveolar (tubuloacinous)
Ductless glands (glands of internal secretion; endocrine glands)	

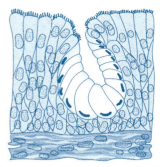

FIGURE 2–20. Intraepithelial gland. *These glands are found in pseudostratified ciliated epithelium of the laryngeal surface of the epiglottis in humans.*

COMPOUND ACINOUS (ALVEOLAR) GLANDS. In the compound acinous or alveolar glands, the terminal portions are supposed to have the form of oval or spherical sacs. As a rule, however, they are irregularly branched tubules with numerous saccular outgrowths on the wall and on the blind ends. These glands can be designated *compound tubuloacinous*. To this group belong most of the larger exocrine glands—the mixed glands of the oral cavity and respiratory passages, and the pancreas.

In some cases, the excretory ducts do not all join into a single main duct, but open independently on a restricted area of a free epithelial surface (lacrimal, mammary, and prostatic glands).

Exocrine Glands

Exocrine glands may be unicellular or multicellular. Unicellular glands are a part of the epithelium with which they are associated. Their function is to coat the surface of the epithelium with a protective covering. These glands, known as *goblet cells* because of their occasional similarity to a wine goblet, are found in the digestive and respiratory systems (see Figs. 2–4, 2–5, and 2–16); additional details can be found in Chapters 11 and 13. Intraepithelial glands may also be found in the urethra, nasal cavity, and epiglottis (Fig. 2–20).

Multicellular glands have ducts to carry their secretions from outlying areas to the free surface. In these cases, we describe a duct and secretory parts of the gland. *Simple glands*, which have a single duct as just described, can be found, for example, in the sweat glands of the skin and the tubular glands of the digestive system. *Compound glands* have branched ducts accommodating a greater number of secretory units; these glands can be found in the digestive system, e.g., the salivary glands and pancreas. The ducts are therefore either unbranched or branched.

The secretory part of the gland may be straight or coiled and is essentially tubular, flask-like or acinous, and rounded or alveolar. Intermediate forms are also known, such as tubuloacinous and tubuloalveolar; these are usually enlarged, distended, or saccular. Large glands are supported by a strong connective tissue framework composed in large measure of reticular fibers and collagen (see Chapter 3). Lobules and lobes may be differentiated by their connective tissues. The connective tissues also support the essential vascular system, nerve bundles, and ducts. Ducts may be classified as *intralobular* or *interlobular* if they lie within or between lobules of glands, respectively. The largest duct, usually composed of several layers, is the final common path of the secretory product via this so-called excretory duct.

The secretory process varies from place to place. In so-called *holocrine glands*, such as the sebaceous gland associated with hair follicles, the apex and much of the cell disintegrates to free the thick, oily secretion of the gland. In *apocrine glands* of the mammary gland, a small amount of the cell surface may be discharged with the secretory vesicles. Finally, in *merocrine glands*, the most common form of secretory gland, the secretion is discharged by having the membrane surrounding the secretory product fuse with the plasma membrane and, in doing so, releasing only the contents of the secretory vesicle. Membrane added to the cell surface in this kind of secretory process can be recombined with the cytoplasmic membranes by endocytosis and reutilized in the formation of new secretory vesicles (Fig. 2–21).

The stimulus for secretion may be nervous or hormonal, but the process itself varies from gland to gland. In the case of mucous cells, a so-called second messenger system involving cyclic AMP pathway, which causes internal calcium release in the cytoplasm, is involved.

Glands may be classified according to their secretory products. The three primary salivary glands can be used as examples; the parotid gland has primarily a *serous* (watery) product; the submandibular gland has

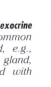
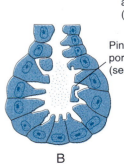
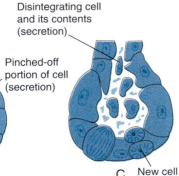

FIGURE 2–21. Types of secretion in exocrine glands. A, *Merocrine gland, e.g., common sweat glands.* B, *Apocrine gland, e.g., axillary sweat glands.* C, *Holocrine gland, e.g., sebaceous glands associated with hair follicles.*

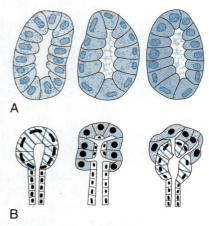

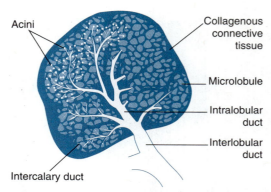

FIGURE 2-22. Characteristics of glandular cells. A, Note the position of the nuclei, and their shape in serous glands (left), mucous glands (middle), and mixed acini in human salivary glands (right). B, The diagram shows the proximal part of the intercalary duct system and its relationship to the various secretory cells. Mucus-secreting cells are cross-hatched, and serous-secreting cells are stippled.

FIGURE 2-23. Glandular duct system. This diagram shows the branches of the duct system and its relationships to secretory parts of a lobule of a gland. Collagenous stroma may completely or incompletely separate the microscopic lobules. The main duct shown is a branch of the interlobular duct. The interlobular duct branches into intralobular ducts, which divide several times. The intralobular ducts are ultimately joined to the secretory cells unit by intercalary ducts.

a *mixed serous and mucous* secretion; and the sublingual gland is entirely *mucus secreting*.

In general, mucous glands have a vesicular cytoplasm with nuclei flattened out against the basal cell membrane. These cells stain with mucus stains, are metachromatic, and are also stained by the periodic acid–Schiff (PAS) method. On the other hand serous cells tend to have rounded, centrally positioned nuclei (Fig. 2-22). These cells have a granular cytoplasm containing numerous mitochondria, ribosomes, and Golgi membrane, and they secrete proteinaceous products, such as digestive enzymes. The duct system in exocrine glands is seen in Figure 2-23. A greater understanding of epithelial cell structure and function can be gained from subsequent chapters specifically considering each type of epithelium.

Endocrine Glands

Cells belonging to these types of glands have an extraordinary blood supply. They occur in clusters or cords of cells supported by a framework of reticular connective tissue. The thyroid gland is composed of cells that form hollow balls of cells known as *follicles*. The secretory product is stored in follicles. In some places, endocrine cells may occur singly and are scattered among epithelial cells of another kind (e.g., in

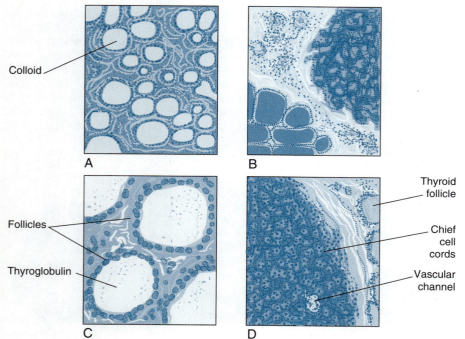

FIGURE 2-24. Endocrine glandular units as follicles or cords. A and B, the cuboidal cells constituting the thyroid follicle are seen. The secretory product of the cuboidal cells is delivered into the follicle. When needed, the stored secretion is mobilized from the follicle to the blood supply for global distribution. C and D, the cords of cells secrete their product directly into the extracellular space and then enter the capillaries, whereby the hormone is delivered to its target sites.

the digestive system) (Fig. 2–24). The rich capillary network surrounding endocrine gland cells is usually of the fenestrated type.

The endocrine glands secrete their specific products, called hormones, directly into the blood stream. The endocrine glands are all circumscribed, with minor exceptions. They are thus set aside from numerous other structures believed to produce internal secretions and also important in coordination and integration within the organism. The circumscribed endocrine glands of the human are the adrenal, hypophysis, thyroid, parathyroid, islets of Langerhans, and portions of the testis and ovary. Other glands that resemble them morphologically in some respects, but do not produce a known secretion, are the pineal body and the paraganglia.

CHAPTER THREE

Connective Tissue

THE CELLS OF THE CONNECTIVE TISSUE 42
    Fibroblasts and Fibrocytes 43
    Macrophages 43
    Mast Cells 44
    Lymphocytes 45
    Plasma Cells 46
    Eosinophils 46
    Adipocytes 46
    Pigment Cells 48

CONNECTIVE TISSUE MATRIX 48
    Collagen Fibers 49
    Tropocollagen 49
    Types of Collagen 50
    Molecular Structure of Banded Collagen 52
    Synthesis of Collagen 52
    Reticulum Fibers 52
    Elastin Fibers 52
    Ground Substance or Extracellular Hydrated Gel 54
    Structural Glycoproteins 55
    Basement Membrane 55
    Microscopic Appearance of Connective Tissue 57
    Mucoid Tissue 58
    Pigmented Connective Tissue 58

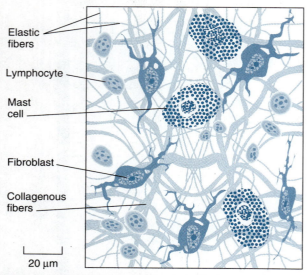

FIGURE 3–1. Aveolar or loose connective tissue. *This most widely encountered connective tissue contains many cellular and fibrous elements found in connective tissues.*

Connective tissue is concerned with maintaining the structural integrity of the body. It does this by first contributing the essential structure upon which minerals form the skeleton. The skeleton is a specialized connective tissue. The parts of the skeleton are held together by aggregations of connective tissue fibers known as ligaments. The muscular attachments to the skeleton are in the form of bundles of collagenous fibers, which form tendons. The force developed by a muscle is transmitted to the skeleton via tendons, resulting in movement. Connective tissue forms the framework on which specialized cells form organs, and these organs may be encapsulated or supported by connective tissue.

Connective tissue is also the supporting tissue, which may be loosely formed (nontendinous or nonligamentous type), permitting the migration of innumerable cells of various types. Some of these migratory cells are concerned with the inflammatory response to pathogens, others are immunocompetent, still others are phagocytic (Fig. 3–1). Foreign bodies and hostile organisms are usually recognized and combated within the connective tissues; it should be remembered that in many places, the septic external environment and the sterile internal environment may be separated by the width of only one cell.

The connective tissues, in general, are composed of three parts–cells, fibers, and matrix (or ground substance)–and the proportions of each component are variable, depending on structural considerations. For example, connective tissues include such highly specialized forms as bone, cartilage, blood, and adipose tissue; these subjects are, because of their complexity, discussed in separate chapters.

Connective tissues generally develop from embryonic mesoderm, although not exclusively. The mesodermal cells are migratory, and they penetrate and surround, and thus contribute to the organization of, developing organs.

THE CELLS OF THE CONNECTIVE TISSUE

The cells of the connective tissue are generally of two varieties: the resident types, such as the fibroblasts and fibrocytes, and the transient types, including lymphocytes, macrophages, plasma cells, and mast cells. Neutrophils, eosinophils, and basophils may also be found. The structure and function of these cells are considered in Chapter 6.

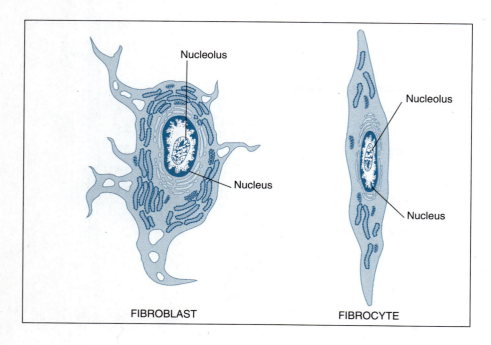

FIGURE 3–2. Fibroblast and fibrocyte. *The structure of one cell type in two functional states is shown. The fibroblast actively synthesizes and secretes connective tissue components. The fibrocyte is the inactive form of the same cell; it can be stimulated to revert to the fibroblast form.*

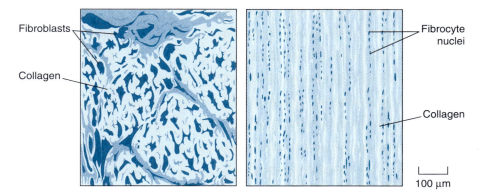

FIGURE 3–3. Collagenous connective tissue. *This dense, regular connective tissue is composed primarily of collagenous fibers. Left, Fibroblasts are secreting collagen fibers organized in bundles, seen in cross-section. Right, At low-power magnification is a longitudinal section of a tendon, showing bundles of fibers, regularly aligned, and "strings" of fibrocytes.*

Fibroblasts and Fibrocytes

Fibroblasts and fibrocytes are the same cell with a functional difference. *Fibroblast* is the name of the cell that produces the fibrous component and the amorphous ground substance. The *fibrocyte* is the inactive form of the fibroblast, which retains its capacity to revert to the intensely synthetic "blast" form. The two forms of the same cell are morphologically distinctive and reflect their different metabolic activity (Figs. 3–2 and 3–3).

The fibroblast is large and irregularly shaped with abundant cytoplasm and an ovoid nucleus. The cytoplasm contains a highly developed rough endoplasmic reticulum, a Golgi complex, as well as numerous mitochondria. The nucleus is large and is pale or weakly stained except for a prominent nucleolus. The nucleus therefore reflects that of a functionally active cell type.

Fibrocytes are smaller and thinner than fibroblasts. This is shown in the rough endoplasmic reticulum, Golgi complex, and mitochondria, which are reduced in size and number and perform only maintenance levels of activity. In wound healing, fibrocytes revert to the active fibroblastic appearance and function.

The fibroblasts are functionally versatile, producing collagen, elastin, and reticular fibers as well as glycosaminoglycans and glycoproteins, which form the amorphous ground substance in which the fibers are embedded. The fibrocyte is capable of cell division, which occurs when the organism needs to repair connective tissue that is damaged.

Other cells are commonly found in the connective tissue but are unrelated to the formation of connective tissue; they are transient.

Macrophages

Macrophages arise from precursor cells that are found in the bone marrow and that form monocytes, which are ameboid phagocytic cells. Mature monocytes enter the blood stream and then leave the vascular system to enter the connective tissue spaces. When these monocytes (mononuclear cells) begin this phase of their existence, they are called macrophages. Tissue macrophages can also proliferate within the connective tissue, producing more of these voracious scavenging cells (Figs. 3–4 and 3–5).

Most of the organs of the body have macrophages, because they migrate freely throughout most of the connective tissue–filled spaces. Macrophages may differ

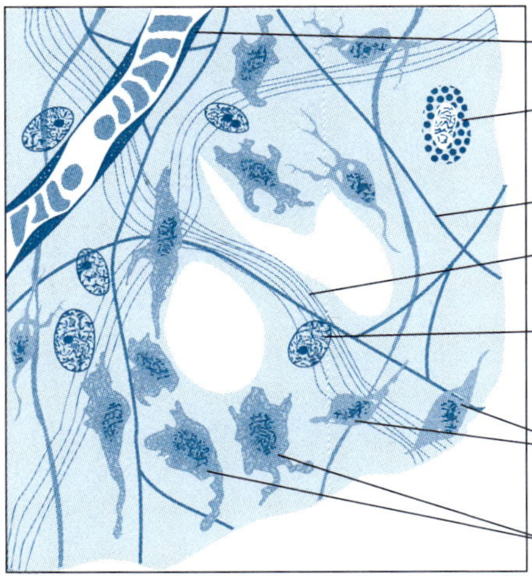

FIGURE 3–4. Preparation of human omentum. *Note the cellular and fibrous composition of the mesentery, a form of loose connective tissue found in the abdomen.*

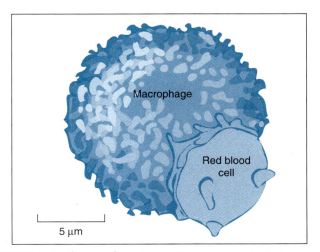

FIGURE 3–5. The macrophage. *One cellular component of the loose connective tissue is the macrophage. In this illustration, the macrophage is ingesting a red blood cell.*

slightly in appearance, but they all possess the phagocytic capability. These cells are part of a group of macrophages known as the mononuclear phagocytic system. The following cells are parts of this system: alveolar macrophages of the lung; Kupffer's cells of the liver; macrophages of the loose connective tissue, lymph nodes, spleen, pleura, and peritoneum; microglia of the central nervous system; and osteoclasts of bone (Fig. 3–6).

In general, these cells can be characterized structurally as having a highly irregular surface, characteristic of cells actively engaged in pinocytolic and phagocytic activity. They have numerous lysosomes, a well-developed Golgi complex, rough endoplasmic reticulum, and numerous vesicles of both Golgi and pinocytic origin, reflecting two-way traffic into and out of the cell.

Macrophages are generally larger than their rounded, monocytic precursors. The apparent growth takes place during their foraging, extravascular period. The active phagocytic period results in an increase in all of the cellular organelles and cytoplasm. Usually, macrophages vary in size between 10 and 35 μm and have an eccentrically placed nucleus. These cells have relatively long lives, 1 or more months, within the connective tissue.

Mast Cells

Mast cells can be readily characterized by numerous, uniformly round granules that frequently obscure the nucleus of the cell. Each cell is about 20 μm in diameter.

Electron microscopy of mast cells reveals them to have a well-developed Golgi complex, few rounded mitochondria, and few short segments of the rough endoplasmic reticulum. This secretory cell synthesizes heterogeneous granules about 0.3 to 0.5 mm in diameter that are membrane bound.

It was discovered many years ago that the granules stained in a remarkable way with certain aniline dyes. For example, with toluidine blue, the granules appeared purple rather than the color of the dye, which is blue. This example of metachromatic staining occurs because glycosaminoglycans (heparin or chondroitin sulfate) are components of the granules. Other components of the granule are histamine, proteolytic enzymes, and an eosinophil chemotactic factor (ECF-A) (Fig. 3–7). In routine hematoxylin and eosin stained sections, the granules take the dye eosin and appear red.

Some investigators distinguish two varieties of mast cells. One, most commonly found in areolar or loose connective tissue, has heparin as the primary granular proteoglycan, whereas the second variety, located in the mucosa of the digestive tract, has granules that contain chondroitin sulfate. Heparin is an anticoagulant, and chondroitin sulfate is a mucopolysaccharide composed of alternating residues of β-D-glucuronic acid and N-acetylgalactosamine in a β(1–4) linkage (Fig. 3–8). Mast cells also produce leukotrienes, which are not stored but rather are thought to be synthesized from the phospholipids of membrane. Mast cells arise from

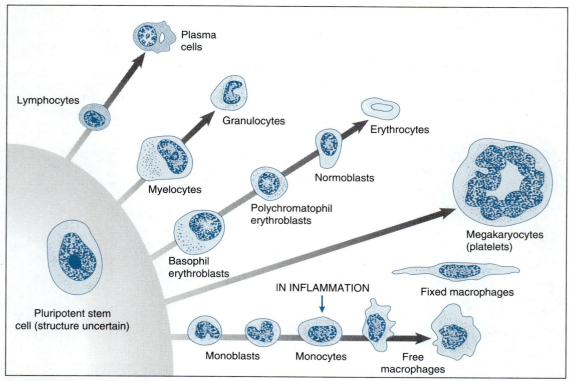

FIGURE 3–6. Cell lineage of mononuclear cells. See index to find discussions of the varied functions of the mature cell types. Note that in an inflammatory condition, monocytes are readily converted to active macrophages.

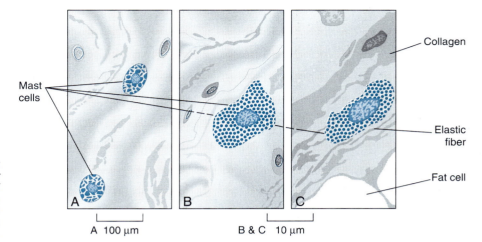

FIGURE 3-7. Mast cells. *Mast cells at different magnifications. Found in loose or alveolar connective tissue and around blood vessels, these cells produce heparin and histamine in humans. The coarse granules stain metachromatically with toluidine blue and other basic aniline dyes.*

stem cells located in the bone marrow. They share some structural and functional characteristics of basophilic leukocytes, but they have a separate stem cell and are therefore unrelated. The surface of mast cells possesses receptors for immunoglobulins IgE and IgG4, antibodies produced by plasma cells.

Lymphocytes

Lymphocytes are found in great numbers in loose connective tissue only during pathologic conditions. They migrate into affected areas from nearby lymphoid tissue or from the general circulation.

The majority of tissue lymphocytes are small cells, about 6 to 8 mm in diameter. Their nuclei are generally round and deeply heterochromatic, although some may be deeply indented. The nucleolus is not recognized by light microscopy. These cells are a heterogeneous group with variable life spans, which may be only a week or less or as long as several months to years. Two major functional groups are present, B and T lympho-

cytes. The B groups originate in the bone marrow and migrate to lymphoid tissues, where they reside and proliferate. When antigenically stimulated, B lymphocytes undergo additional mitotic divisions, then enlarge and mature into plasma cells, which synthesize and secrete antibodies (immunoglobulins) (Figs. 3–9 and 3–10).

T lymphocytes arise from cells originally formed by bone marrow, but during late stages of development, they migrate into the thymus (before seeding peripheral lymphoid tissues), where they continue to proliferate. When antigenically stimulated, T lymphocytes enlarge and their cytoplasms become filled with free polyribosome clusters. The functions of T lymphocytes are numerous but still incompletely understood. Those functions that are recognized include the identification and destruction of virus-infected cells, tumor cells, fungi, tissue and organ grafts; modulation of B lymphocytes; and other cell-to-cell interactions. It is known that functional subsets of T lymphocytes have specific roles in regard to these activities.

Further details of lymphocytic activity are dis-

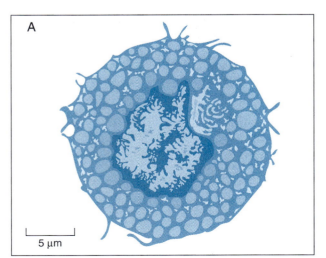 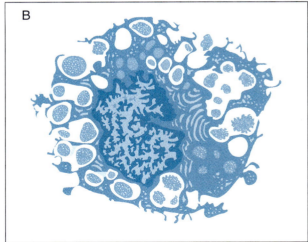

FIGURE 3-8. Mast cells. *Mast cells degranulate when they are traumatized or, more commonly when they are exposed to IgE antibodies or to antigens. Degranulation releases histamine and other associative agents, such as interleukins and prostaglandins. The mast cell plays an important role in defense against the invasion of pathogens.*

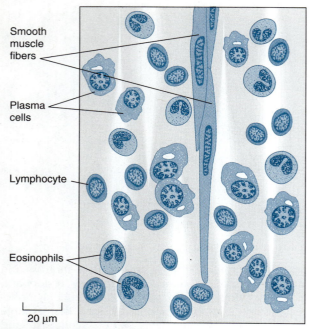

FIGURE 3–9. Lamina propria. The lamina propria located beneath the epithelium is primarily a reticular fiber network containing eosinophils, lymphocytes, and plasma cells. These cells actively deter the invasion of the organism by pathogenic organisms.

cussed along with the lymphatic system (see Chapter 9).

Plasma Cells

Plasma cells are most numerous in areas of the body where penetration of the epithelial surface of the body by microbes and toxins can be most readily accomplished. The lamina propria of the digestive tract is the outstanding example (Figs. 3–9 and 3–11).

Plasma cells are large. They have a distinctive nucleus described as similar in appearance to a cartwheel or a clockface, with clumps of chromatin equally disposed around the nuclear membrane, as well as a well-defined nucleolus, a basophilic cytoplasm filled with a granular (RNA) endoplasmic reticulum, and a highly developed Golgi apparatus. This cell is a classic example of a protein-secretory cell, and its products are specific globulin antibodies. Circulating antibodies are synthesized by the enormous numbers of plasma cells located in sites of infection or potential infection.

Plasma cells arise from B lymphocytes. They generally do not divide, and their turnover rate is about 15 days.

Eosinophils

Eosinophils and other granulocytes are discussed in Chapter 6; it is useful to point out here, however, that granulocytes are often found in the loose connective tissue and in the lamina propria of the skin, digestive system, and respiratory tracts. In particular, the number of eosinophils is enormously increased in the connective tissue of individuals who have parasitic infestations, allergic reactions, and other diseases. Eosinophils are phagocytic in regard to antigen-antibody complexes but they do not phagocytose microorganisms or foreign materials.

Eosinophils are attracted to sites of allergic reactions by eosinophil chemotactic factors that are liberated by mast cells and basophils. Basophils are not commonly found in the connective tissues. Mast cells are an abundant connective tissue cell type capable of reacting to allergens.

Adipocytes

Also known as lipocytes or fat cells, adipocytes appear oval or round when they occur in small numbers. When they are found in large numbers, they assume a polygonal appearance. Adipocytes vary in size but usually average about 50 mm in diameter.

Each cell has a thin rim of cytoplasm in which the nucleus is located, giving an adipocyte the appearance of a "signet ring." The cell usually contains a large single droplet of fat, which is liquid at body temperature (Fig. 3–12).

The nucleus of the cell is oval and is compressed against the cell membrane. A slight accumulation of cytoplasm occurs around the nucleus. In this cytoplasm is a Golgi complex. Elements of rough endoplasmic reticulum and mitochondria and microfilaments are also found throughout the scanty cytoplasm surrounding the lipid-filled vacuole.

If sections are not specifically prepared for the preservation of fat, the fat is usually dissolved out, because both xylol and similar solvents are used in preparing slides of tissue sections. In this case, only the peripheral rim of cytoplasm, with its slightly thickened rim where the nucleus resides, will remain. This appearance reminded early histologists of a signet ring; hence the name signet ring cells.

Fat may be fixed and stained (black) with osmium tetroxide. Other dyes may also be used with frozen (cryostat) sections, including oil red O, Sudan III, Sudan black, and Sharlach R. These dyes are successful because they are more soluble in oil or fat than they are in water.

The stored fat is composed of glycerol esters of oleic, palmitic, and stearic acids.

Fat cells are probably not exclusively concerned with fat storage. They are also involved in the synthesis of specific kinds of fatty substances.

Fat cells deprived of lipid are stellate and appear similar to fibroblasts. As lipid accumulates within the cell, it initially appears as isolated droplets; these later coalesce to form a single large droplet. As lipid is depleted from these cells, the large droplet decreases in size and breaks into smaller, isolated droplets. The depleted fat cell again becomes fibroblastic in appearance. Fat cells have defined as well as generalized

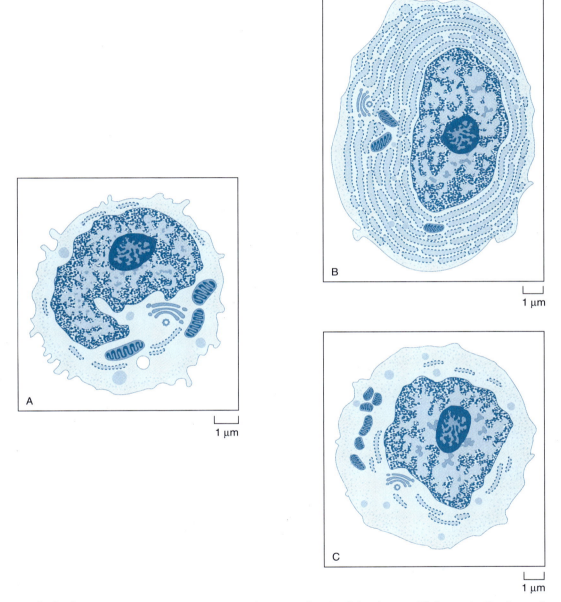

FIGURE 3-10. T and B lymphocytes. *In this figure, the structural transformation of resting B lymphocytes (A) into active B cells, or plasma cells (B), capable of producing circulating antibodies is seen. Structural transformation of resting T cells (A) produces several activated forms (C) capable of evoking a variety of cell-mediated defense responses known as* **cellular immunity.**

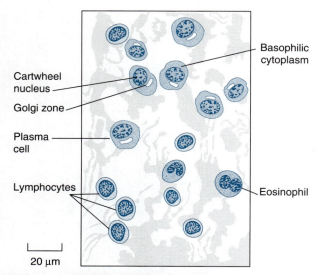

FIGURE 3-11. Transformed B lymphocytes (plasma cells). *Shown here in the jejunum, but found throughout the body in loose connective tissue, plasma cells, or activated B cells, produce circulating antibodies.*

locations within the body, but they are all a single definitive cell type.

A second interesting adipose cell type found in most mammals, including humans but especially animals that hibernate, is called *brown fat* (Fig. 3–13). The fat droplets are located in numerous separate droplets that do not coalesce. In these cells, mitochondria are large and elongate with numerous cristae. These fat deposits are concerned with heat production mediated by the mitochondrial activity. In human neonates, brown fat is located mainly in the intrascapular region and elsewhere in lesser amounts. Although its importance in later years is uncertain, brown fat is particularly sensitive to, and proliferates in the presence of, cortisone. The mobilization of fat is believed to be under sympathetic nervous or adrenal and endocrine system control. Other factors may also be involved.

Pigment Cells

Pigment cells are found in the dermis of the skin, particularly in darker races, and in the iris and choroid

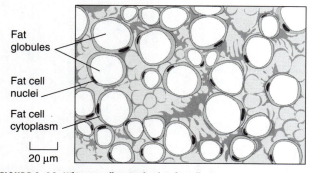

FIGURE 3-12. White or yellow (unilocular) fat cells. *The most common lipid-containing cells are characterized by a single lipid droplet. Such a cell is often called a signet ring cell, because the cell nucleus bulges from one point of the cytoplasm, which is reduced to only a thin rim owing to the large lipid droplet.*

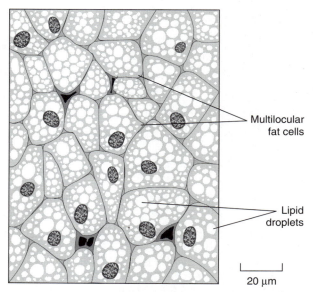

FIGURE 3-13. Brown (multilocular) fat cells. *These cells are found in the interscapular region of the upper back in adult humans. This form of fat cell is more widespread in embryonic and early postnatal life. Note that the lipid is in the form of many small droplets, rather than the one large droplet characteristic of white or yellow fat cells.*

of the eye. Most of these cells are unable to synthesize melanin or related pigments and are named chromophores or melanophores. These cells contain pigment, which they have ingested after their release from the melanocytes that synthesize the melanin. Melanocytes are derived embryologically from the neural crest. These cells are stellate with long processes containing dark brown or black granules thought to be melanin. The function of melanocytes is to prevent light from reaching more deeply placed cells (Fig. 3–14).

CONNECTIVE TISSUE MATRIX

The matrix of connective tissue contains all the extracellular components, including fibers and ground substance. The fibers can be divided into two major

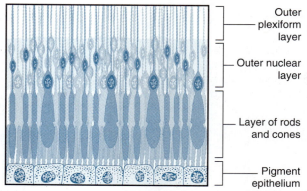

FIGURE 3-14. Pigment epithelial cells in outer portion of retina of eye. *The pigment epithelium consists of cells that possess large numbers of melanin granules. The granules ultimately absorb light that has entered the eye and has stimulated the receptor segments of the rods and cones.*

classes, collagen (including reticular) and elastin. The ground substance is composed of hydrated networks of proteins known as glycoproteins and proteoglycans. In the space between the fibers and the ground substance networks, water, salt, and other diffusible substances, as well as migrating nonconnective tissue cells in certain types of connective tissue, are found.

The matrix of connective tissue has complex mechanical properties that vary from stiffness and strength to elasticity and pliability, depending on the location and function. It is through the matrix that food and waste, gas, and hormones pass. The matrix contains the molecular environment, which permits cells to survive and carry out their specific functions. The matrix of skeletal tissues is hard and is the framework by which the soft tissues are supported. In other places, certain arteries have a matrix that is elastic and permits volume changes to occur as required. These aspects are discussed throughout the book as well as on the following pages.

Collagen Fibers

Collagen fibers make up most of the fibrous component of connective tissues. Collagen is a major component of cartilage and bone, tendons, aponeuroses, ligaments, muscle and nerve sheaths, meninges, dermis, cornea, sclera, and other structures.

Collagen is tough, with high tensile strength (equal to that of steel), and has the very desirable quality of being freely flexible with very little elasticity. This connective tissue is vital to the performance of mechanical functions of the body.

Collagen fibers generally appear in bundles. Although smaller bundles may leave a larger one to join an adjacent bundle, the collagen fibers themselves do not branch. In tissue sections, they may appear limp, coiled, or as taut cables.

Microscopic Appearance

Histologically, collagen may be stained pink with eosin (although not specifically) with the standard hematoxylin and eosin method, or blue with aniline blue (with greater specificity), as in Mallory's connective tissue stain, as well as by other methods familiar to the special histologist or pathologist (Fig. 3–15). Because of their usually regular arrangement, collagen fibrils forming bundles show birefringence when examined microscopically with cross-polarized light. On electron microscopy, collagen fibers are seen to be composed of thin, 20 to 200 nm collagen fibrils. The fibrils consist of even smaller (3.5-nm) microfibrils, and finally, the microfibrils are aggregates of tropocollagen molecules.

Although different types of collagen have somewhat different structural details (Table 3–1), those forms that aggregate into fibers are primarily cross-banded in a characteristic and quantitative way (see Fig. 3–11). X-ray diffraction measurements reveal that the regularly repeating pattern occurs every 67 nm, although the dehydrated collagen prepared for electron microscopy

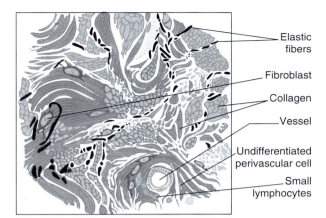

FIGURE 3–15. Human dermis. *Dense, irregularly arranged connective tissue consists primarily of collagen fibers interspersed with short, thick sections of elastic fibers.*

yields a value of 64 nm between major bandings. The structural organization of a collagen fibril is seen in Figure 3–16.

The ability of collagen assemblies to cross-link adjacent collagenous elements at every level of structural organization accounts for the great tensile strength and mechanical stability of collagen fiber already mentioned. This ability is enhanced by proteoglycans, which form regular connections between microfibrils, fibrils, and fibers. Further, individual tropocollagen molecules cross-link by various chemical bonds between specific amino acids as well as between the polypeptide subunits of which tropocollagen is composed (Fig. 3–16).

Tropocollagen

Collagen fibers swell and disintegrate if they are treated with acid or alkali. The byproduct of this treatment is the production of filamentous molecules of tropocollagen, which are about 300 nm long (or 200 nm when dried) and 1.4 nm thick.

Gelatin, which is formed when collagen is boiled, is composed of disorganized networks of tropocollagen molecules.

The tropocollagen molecule is composed of three polypeptide chains, known as procollagen, in the form

TABLE 3-1. Four Major Types of Collagen and Their Distributions

Type	Molecular Formula	Polymerized Form	Tissue Distribution
I	$[\alpha 1(I)]_2 \alpha 2(I)$	Fibril	Skin, tendon, bone, ligaments, cornea, internal organs (almost 90% of body collagen)
II	$[\alpha 1(II)]_3$	Fibril	Cartilage, intervertebral disc, notochord, vitreous body of eye
III	$[\alpha 1(III)]_3$	Fibril	Skin, blood vessels, internal organs
IV	$[\alpha 1(IV)]_2 \alpha 2(IV)$	Basal lamina	Basal laminae

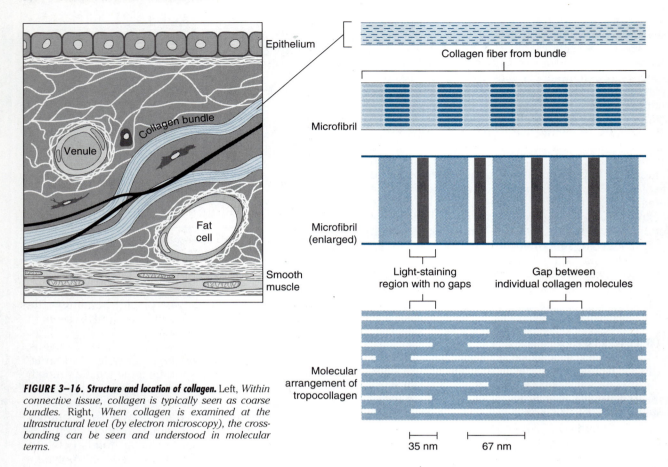

FIGURE 3–16. Structure and location of collagen. Left, *Within connective tissue, collagen is typically seen as coarse bundles.* Right, *When collagen is examined at the ultrastructural level (by electron microscopy), the cross-banding can be seen and understood in molecular terms.*

of a triple helix. Procollagen can be further divided and consists of 100 repeating amino acid triplets characterized by a glycine molecule at the third position. The other two amino acids that form the triplet may differ in type but are usually hydroxyproline and hydroxylysine. It is of interest that these latter two amino acids are not commonly found except in collagen.

The triple helix of procollagen is maintained by covalent bonds between the polypeptide chains. Of special interest are the hydroxyproline bonding sites for specific carbohydrates, because these sites have an essential role in the assembly of tropocollagen molecules when they are released from the cell into the extracellular space (Fig. 3–17).

Types of Collagen

Variations in amino acid sequence of procollagen chains have been found in different parts of the body; at least 11 types of collagen are recognized, although most are not fully understood (Table 3–2). Only relatively recently has immunohistochemistry detected this rather large group of related molecular types of collagen. The variety of types are not uniformly distributed, but rather, they are located in different tissues or joined in different stages of development, or they appear during tissue repair as characteristic structural and functional collagen types. The variety of types and their structural features are due to specific combinations of their component polypeptide chains. As Table 3–1 shows, types I through V are the most common and best known.

As indicated earlier, molecular tropocollagen is composed of three polypeptide chains with an α-helical chemical structure, so-called α-chains, with each major type of tropocollagen having its own specific varieties. For example, note that type I collagen has two α1 polypeptides. The notation for type I collagen would then read $[\alpha 1\ (I)]_2\ \alpha 2(I)$, and its subclass $[\alpha 1(I)]_3$.

Type I collagen is the most abundant kind found in tendons, ligaments, skin, and bone. It is, in fact, the

TABLE 3–2. Glycosaminoglycans

Glycosaminoglycan	Molecular Weight (daltons)	Tissue Distribution
Hyaluronic acid	4000 to 8×10^6	Various connective tissues, skin, vitreous body, cartilage, synovial fluid
Chondroitin sulfate	5000 to 50,000	Cartilage, cornea, bone, skin, arteries
Dermatan sulfate	15,000 to 40,000	Skin, blood vessels, heart, heart valves
Heparan sulfate	5000 to 12,000	Lung, arteries, cell surfaces, basal laminae
Heparin	6000 to 25,000	Lung, liver, skin, mast cells
Keratan sulfate	4000 to 19,000	Cartilage, cornea, intervertebral disk

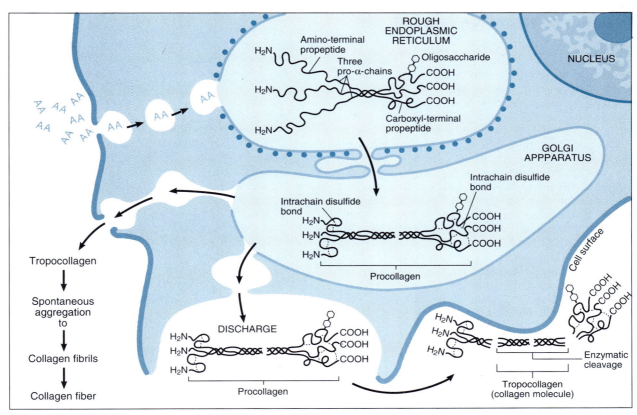

FIGURE 3-17. Collagen synthesis. *Within and outside the fibroblast, the development of the collagen molecule can be followed. AA, amino acids.*

most abundant protein of any kind from any source. Its fibers are usually flexible and of high tensile strength, and electron-microscopically, they are markedly cross-banded. The staggered gaps between tropocollagen molecules (see Fig. 3-16) may provide sites for calcium salt deposition in developing bone; hence, they play an important role in the overall calcification process.

Type II collagen is found in cartilage and only a few other places, including cornea, vitreous humor, and notochord, and the nucleus pulposus of the intervertebral disk. Type II collagen is composed of a mixture of some fibrils about 100 nm in diameter and others 20 nm in diameter. The smaller variety is shorter and does not have distinct cross-bands characteristic of the larger fibrils. The larger, type II fibrils predominate in articular or hyaline cartilage, where mechanical strength is important.

In fibrocartilage, a mixture of type I and type II collagen can be found. The smaller, thinner type II collagen fibrils are usually transparent, because they bind large amounts of carbohydrates and, therefore, water, and as a consequence, they form stiff gels of short, separated fibrils. They are not cross-banded and do not form fibers. As one might expect, collagen in this form is found in the eye vitreous body as well as in hyaline cartilage.

Type III collagen is reticulin, a fibrous structure rich in carbohydrate. The fibers are thinner than those of type I collagen. Reticulum forms an extensive open network that supports the cells of glands, lymphoid tissue, and bone marrow. It is also a component of basement membranes and the papillary layer of the skin. Type III collagen is revealed by certain stains containing silver salts and by the periodic acid–Schiff (PAS) method; these stains do not stain other types of collagens.

Type IV collagen, found in the lamina densa of basal laminae, is formed of short units aggregated to form complex feltworks. It is believed that this type of collagen forms the primary skeleton of the basal lamina, to which other of its components are attached.

Type V collagen also does not form fibrils. Although very widely distributed, it is a minor component of the connective tissues. It is also known to be highly glycosylated and is located primarily in the pericellular parts of organs. Its function is not known.

Type VI collagen forms tetramers like type IV. Type VI collagen does, however, assemble into microfibrils, and it is often associated with elastin.

Type VII collagen is a very small component of the entire complement of placental membrane collagen. Its function is not known.

Type VIII collagen is a product of endothelial cells. Its function is also not known.

Collagen *types IX, X,* and *K* are synthesized by chondrocytes, but their function is also unknown. Types IX and X are located in the perilacunar region of cartilage. Type X has been found in regions of hypertrophying cartilage cells.

Molecular Structure of Banded Collagen

Banded collagen has been found to have a highly ordered arrangement of tropocollagen molecules.

The microfibril is composed of tropocollagen molecules 300 nm in length. They are aligned longitudinally in five rows, with a gap of 40 nm between the end of each molecule and the beginning of the next in each longitudinal array of microfilaments. Grossly, the major band repeat is 67 nm, and each tropocollagen molecule spans four 67-nm intervals and overlaps a fifth by about 32 nm. Each row is staggered by 67 nm in relation to the adjacent molecule; this arrangement is maintained by covalent cross-links by amino acid residues. This arrangement also provides the basis for the appearance of the cross-banding, which is due to variable densities of the collagen and its staining propensities. Within the fibril, the microfibrillar units are maintained and aligned by glycoproteins, resulting in the banded appearance of the collagen fiber.

Synthesis of Collagen

The synthesis by collagen of fibroblasts has been studied in detail by autoradiographic electron microscopy as well as biochemically. Amino acids are taken up by fibroblasts and synthesized on ribosomes of the rough endoplasmic reticulum, forming long polypeptides or procollagen α-chains (pro-α-chains). It is of some interest that these polypeptides are longer than the final α-chains of tropocollagen, because extra polypeptides, which apparently function in the assembly of the tropocollagen molecule, are subsequently removed from both ends of the procollagen chain.

The polypeptide chains, once synthesized, move into the cysternae of the endoplasmic reticulum, where various enzymes hydroxylate some proline and lysine residues to form hydroxyproline and hydroxylysine. Completion of this step requires ascorbic acid (vitamin C), molecular oxygen, iron, and other factors. Hence, deficiencies in any of these factors reduce or stop collagen synthesis.

As the hydroxylation proceeds, carbohydrate is linked to some hydroxylysine residues, followed by the association of the three pro-α-chains by their extension peptides and their twining together as cross-links are formed. This results in the formation of the triple helix of the procollagen molecule. This molecule is then transferred by the Golgi apparatus to the exterior of the cell in secretary vacuoles. Outside the cell, the extension polypeptides are removed by enzymes, procollagen peptidases, at the cell surface. The newly formed tropocollagen molecules then aggregate spontaneously to form collagen fibrils. These fibrils are cross-linked at the lysine and hydroxylysine residues by the action of an enzyme, lysol oxidase, which is also released by the fibroblast.

Collagen fibrils can be laid down in precise and regular patterns, as is the case in ligaments and tendons and organ connective tissue capsules (so-called regular connective tissues). The most remarkable pattern is found in the cornea, where successive layers of collagen fibrils are formed at right angles to each other.

Genetic mutation may lead to molecular defects in collagen. The defects can be recognized through the inheritance pattern, clinical signs, and the defective product itself. Ehlers-Danlos syndromes are manifest in patients with inherited defects in the synthesis and chemical stability of collagen. Such patients exhibit hyperextensible skin, unstable joints, poor wound healing, defective blood vessels, as well as other serious skeletal deformities related to defective collagen. The defective collagen is type III.

Scurvy, due to a dietary deficiency of vitamin C, results in the stoppage of collagen synthesis. Vitamin C is needed for the enzymatic hydroxylation of prolyl and lysyl residues of normal collagen. Bone growth and dentition are abnormal in the young individual deficient in vitamin C. Wound healing is poor, and blood vessels rupture when placed under normal increases in pressure.

Reticulum Fibers

Reticulum fibers are fine and branching, and reticulum forms the supporting network in cells of many organs, including the kidney, lymph nodes, spleen, and liver. Reticulum is an important component of basement membranes. These fibers are specifically stained black with silver salts and red by the periodic acid–Schiff method, as mentioned previously (Fig. 3–18).

Reticulum fibers have the same periodic band pattern as collagen, the same x-ray diffraction pattern, and a similar chemical composition. Reticulum is now classified as collagen type III and is known to be highly glycosylated, accounting for its affinity for silver salts. Reticulum is synthesized by fibroblasts, which are called reticular cells in places where reticulin is the primary connective tissue or is found in high concentration.

Elastin Fibers

Elastin fibers are branched and usually thinner (0.1 to 0.2 μm) than bundles of collagen. Frequently, they occur as thicker fibers, as in the ligamentum flavum, or in sheets, as in the fenestrated elastic lamellae of the aortic wall (Fig. 3–19). Elastic fibers are easily stretched and have the capacity to recoil with a very high degree of reproducibility. In older individuals, however, the elasticity may decrease in number or the fibers may calcify. In the genetic disease pseudoxanthoma elasticum, elastin fibers calcify throughout the body in relatively young individuals, who ultimately perish from the disorder.

Elastin fibers are very resistant to acid and alkali, to boiling, and to organic solvents. Elastin fibers can be digested by elastase, an enzyme found to be associated with crude extracts of trypsin and produced by bacteria.

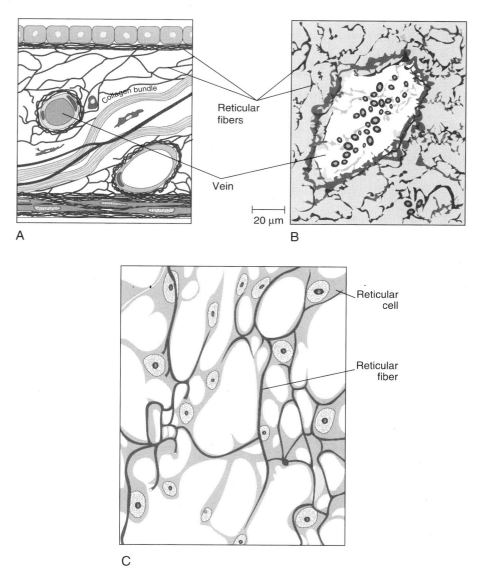

FIGURE 3-18. Reticular fibers. In a section of lymph node after removal of lymphocytes, the network of reticular fibers and their intimate relationship with reticular cells can be seen. A, The low magnification shows general distribution of reticular fibers. B, At higher magnification, the distribution of reticular fibers and their relationship to a blood vessel are seen. C, At highest magnification, stellate reticular cells and fibers are shown.

Elastin is stained red with orcein, black with Verhoeff's hematoxylin, violet with Wright's resorcinfuchsin, and blue with toluidine blue used for light-microscopic studies.

Elastin fibers contain molecules in a relatively disordered or coiled configuration; they are not birefringent in the unstretched condition. The birefringence of elastin fibers becomes intense, however, when the fibers are stretched, indicating that the molecules become aligned in parallel arrays, fulfilling the conditions necessary for polarization.

At the level of magnification of the electron microscope, elastin is seen as an amorphous mass surrounded by microfibrils about 10 nm thick. The microfibrils are known as the elastic tissue microfibrillar component. Two additional thin filaments 10 to 12 nm in diameter are related to and associated with elastin, known as oxytalan and elaunin. These filaments have elastic properties but do not share staining reactions with the larger elastin fiber.

Elastin is formed of subunits of tropoelastin. The subunits consist of unfolded, irregularly coiled polypeptide chains (random coils). The chains are strongly cross-linked, forming a three-dimensional network capable of mechanical deformation and recoil (Fig. 3-20).

Elastin has a high content of the amino acids alanine and valine plus another, probably unique to elastin, named desmosine.

In connective tissues, fibroblasts synthesize elastin fibers, but in organs where elastin occurs in the form of sheets (aorta and arteries in general) and in other organs, elastin is synthesized by smooth muscle cells. During elastin formation, the microfibrillar part is secreted first, and then the amorphous part is added.

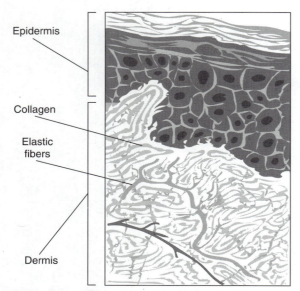

FIGURE 3–19. Elastic fibers. *In this simulated tissue section, note the elastic fibers and other tissue components in their typical locations. The fibers intermingle with collagen bundles in the skin and elsewhere, and elastic tissue forms a membranous ring or rings in blood vessels.*

Ground Substance or Extracellular Hydrated Gel

Ground substance is the material in which connective tissue cells and fibers are embedded and supported, with the exception of mineralized tissue (bone). It is a viscous gel containing large amounts of water bound to long-chain carbohydrate molecules and protein-carbohydrate complexes (Fig. 3–21). The outstanding biologic features of these molecules are that they form hydrated gels and fill an extraordinary amount of tissue space. The ground substance constitutes only about 10% of the total weight of "connective tissue," but it occupies most of the tissue space. Two major classes of protein carbohydrate molecules are known: the proteoglycans and the so-called structural glycoproteins.

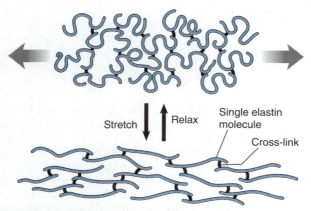

FIGURE 3–20. Elastin molecules. *Each elastin molecule is capable of expansion when stretched but recoils to its original coiled form when the force deforming the molecule is eliminated.*

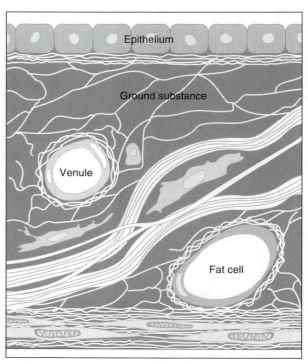

FIGURE 3–21. Ground substance. *The fibrous and cellular components beneath the epithelium are within a viscous gel containing water, bound largely to long-chain carbohydrate molecules and protein-carbohydrate complexes known as* proteoglycans *and* structural glycoproteins.

In proteoglycans, the carbohydrate is mainly in the form of glycosaminoglycan (GAG) molecules. These are long, unbranched polymers of repeating disaccharides, each unit being a hexamine residue bearing an acetyl group and a hexuronate or galactosyl residue. The disaccharide may also bear either a carboxyl or a sulfuric ester group. The resulting polymer has a very strong negative charge, permitting it to be stained with acidophilic or cationic dyes, such as alcian blue, and metachromatic dyes such as toluidine blue. Because of its carbohydrate content, the polymer can also be stained red with the PAS method.

Molecules of this type range in molecular weight from 6000 to several million daltons. Wide variations in chemistry are possible because of their complex nature, and various combinations of these molecules can be found together in close association. Within tissues and organs, they are usually associated with long filamentous proteins, and these complexes are termed *glycoproteins* or *proteoglycans,* depending upon the ratio of the two compounds that make up the molecule. The most common glycosaminoglycans are chondroitin 4-sulfate and chondroitin 6-sulfate (or chondroitin sulfate A and C, respectively), hyaluronate, dermatan sulfate (or chondroitin sulfate B), keratan sulfate, and heparin sulfate. With the exception of hyaluronate, which is an enormous coiled molecule several million daltons in molecular weight, glycosaminoglycans are normally attached to a core protein. They extend from the core protein like the bristles on a test tube brush, because they are negatively charged and because they actually

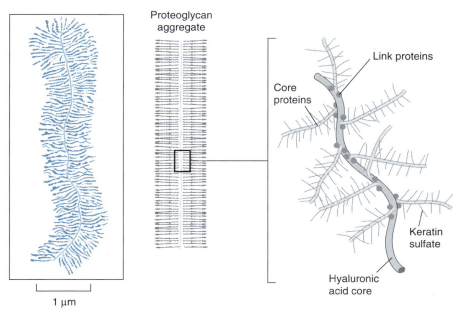

FIGURE 3-22. Proteoglycan aggregate. *Electron-microscopic and schematic appearance of a proteoglycan aggregate. The giant molecule is composed of proteoglycan molecules bound by link proteins to a hyaluronic acid core. The molecular weight of proteoglycan aggregate can be as much as 10^8 daltons.*

repel one another, resulting in the extended ("test tube brush") form (Figs. 3-22 and 3-23). The glycosaminoglycan-protein units (GAG-proteins) can also be grouped as even larger complexes when they are joined by hyaluronated molecules through a linking protein. When this occurs, the ground substance becomes very viscous, because of the formation of huge three-dimensional networks capable of binding water. The water of the ground substance is the medium through which metabolites, electrolytes, and gases diffuse between capillaries and the cells embedded within the ground substance. The negatively charged GAG-proteins not only bind ions but also act as selective barriers to the movement of inorganic ions and other charged molecules.

Structural Glycoproteins

These fibrous proteins, along with their associated carbohydrated side groups, play a role in cell adhesion to other matrix components and apparently to other cell-matrix interactions as well. The structural glycoproteins include laminin, which is present in the lamina lucida of the basal lamina of many cell types, and fibronectin, which is found in both blood plasma and the connective tissue matrix and which acts as an adhesive between various matrix components and between these components and fibroblasts. In a similar manner, chondronectin and osteonectin are specific adhesives between chondroblasts and type II collagen and between osteoblasts and type I collagen (Figs. 3-24 and 3-25).

The ground substance is synthesized by fibroblasts, osteoblasts, chondroblasts, and, under some circumstances, smooth muscle cells. The site of synthesis is within the granular endoplasmic reticulum and the Golgi complex.

In hypothyroidism, the production of ground substance is increased, resulting in a condition termed *myxedema*. The high viscosity of ground substance is a barrier to rapid deployment of microbial invaders, although many of these organisms can secrete hyaluronidase to reduce the viscosity of the ground substance and thereby facilitate their invasion.

The ground substance is difficult to demonstrate structurally because of its water solubility. Although proteoglycans are demonstrable by electron microscopy as small dense granules in tissue sections, it is thought that the proteoglycan's extended or bristly or feathering structure collapses when fixed and dehydrated. The more natural extended condition can be seen in preparations of isolated molecules that are negatively stained and examined on electron microscopy (see Fig. 3-22).

Basement Membrane

The basement membranes are laminae of dense amorphous substances of varying kinds and locations throughout the body. These membranes are found primarily with epithelial and endothelial cells and are intimately associated with connective tissue. In some cases, the basement membrane is unusually thick, and these areas have been intensively investigated. In particular, the basement membrane is usually thick beneath the ciliated epithelium of the trachea, in the glomerulus and lens capsule, and in the anterior limiting membrane in the cornea (Fig. 3-26). Also, in diabetes and myasthenia gravis, the capillary basement membranes may be markedly thickened. This is also true of the glomerular capillaries in glomerular nephritis. The stimulus for and consequences of these changes in the thickness of the basement membrane are unknown.

The structure of this "membrane" is complex, ap-

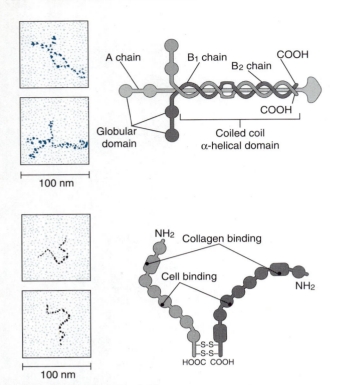

FIGURE 3–23. Laminin and fibronectin. *Diagrams of electron micrographs and a schematic model of laminin* (top) *and fibronectin* (bottom). *Laminin is a glycoprotein made up of three polypeptides composed of more than 4500 amino acid residues. The polypeptides are disulfide bonded in a crosslike configuration. Fibronectin is a dimer composed of two different polypeptide chains, which are joined together by two disulfide bonds near their dicarboxyl ends. Note three of the many possible binding sites, which are specialized for molecular, tissue, and cellular components of living organisms.*

pearing as two distinctive parts or zones. The basal lamina lies adjacent to the plasma or cell membrane of adjacent cells, and the reticular lamina lies next to the subjacent connective tissue. The reticular lamina becomes continuous with the so-called reticular layer of the dermis of the skin.

The *basal lamina* can be characterized ultrastructurally as being about 80 nm thick. It can be subdivided into a fibrillary layer called the lamina densa (about 35 nm wide) and an electron-lucent zone, the lamina lucida, which is located between the cell or plasma membrane and the lamina densa. The lumina lucida is composed of regularly spaced particulate and fibrillar material and contains laminin fibronectin and a variety of proteoglycans. The lamina densa is primarily composed of type IV collagen fibrils and heparin sulfate proteoglycan.

It is thought that laminin, fibronectin, and proteoglycans have an important role in the adhesion of cells to the basal lamina and of the basal lamina to the adjacent connective tissue matrix.

These molecules may, in some as yet unknown way, carry "information" that guides morphogenesis and subsequent development. There is evidence that the basal lamina plays a role in the regeneration of injured axons by guiding their outgrowth. A similar role

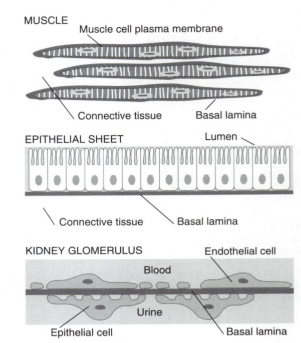

FIGURE 3–24. Basal lamina. *Characteristically, the basal lamina completely surrounds muscle fibers (smooth, cardial and skeletal)* (top), *underlies epithelial cells* (middle), *and separates epithelial and endothelial cells* (bottom).

has been suggested for the regeneration in angiogenesis of capillary beds.

The basal laminae all have similar components, but their ultrastructural organization varies from place to place. The various specializations of the basal laminae are considered in later chapters, where their functional role can be properly understood.

The *reticular lamina* is important because it is composed of a matrix containing a network of reticulum fibers. This lamina varies in thickness and is a major component of the total basement membrane. At the light-microscopic level, the membrane is stained by the PAS method.

The basal lamina is usually synthesized by the

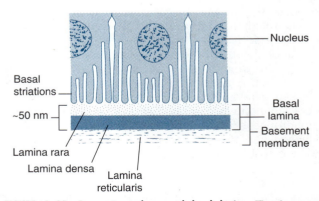

FIGURE 3–25. Basement membrane and basal lamina. *The basement membrane includes several component parts visible under the electron microscope: lamina rara, lamina densa, and lamina reticularis. The basal lamina is composed of the lamina rara and lamina densa alone.*

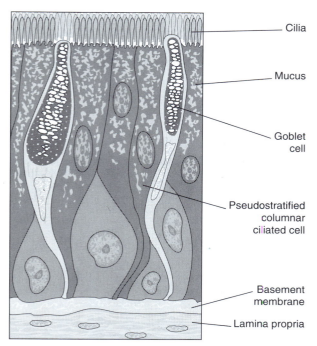

FIGURE 3–26. Basement membrane. *The basement membrane is shown here beneath the pseudostratified ciliated columnar epithelium, where it is characteristically much thicker than when underlying most epithelia.*

adjacent epithelium or endothelium, and the reticular lamina is thought to be produced by fibroblasts and by smooth muscle cells; hence, the two distinctive layers or zones.

Microscopic Appearance of Connective Tissue

The connective tissues vary from place to place in their appearance, consistency, and composition, according to their functional requirements. The structural variation depends on cellular constituents, the amount and arrangement of the fibrillar components, and the ground substance or matrix. With these considerations as a basis, the most common connective tissues are divided into irregular and regular types.

Irregular Connective Tissues

Irregular connective tissue has been subdivided for convenience into the so-called loose, dense, and adipose forms.

Loose connective tissue, also known as areolar connective tissue, is the most common type, and its primary function is to join various parts of the body together in places where significant amounts of movement take place (see Fig. 3–1). Such places are the connective tissue between muscles and investing nerves and blood vessels, between skin and underlying tissues except in specialized areas, and around skeletal joints (but not the joint capsules). This type of connective tissue occurs in the submucosa of the digestive tract as well as within organs and glands.

Loose connective tissue is characterized structurally as being composed of a meshwork of small collagen bundles intermixed with elastic fibers. The arrangement provides both strength and extensibility. The meshwork is embedded in a soft, pliable, gel-like ground substance, in which a variety of cells characteristic of this type of connective tissue are found: macrophages, mast cells, lymphocytes, and the ubiquitous source of connective tissue, the fibroblast or fibrocyte.

Dense connective tissue is found where strength is essential. The ground substance matrix is filled with collagen fibers in thick bundles that course in three dimensions. The principal fiber type is the fibrocyte, and very few other cell types are found in very small numbers. Dense connective tissue is found in organ sheaths and coverings such as occur in the penis, testis, sclera of the eye, and periostea (Fig. 3–27). It is the reticular layer of the skin, the deep fascia of muscles, and also the nerve sheaths. The metabolic activity of dense connective tissue is low; hence, its blood supply is not extensive.

Fat cells are found in the loose connective tissue in most parts of the body but do not constitute the major part of the connective tissue. In adipose connective tissue, however, fat cells are the most abundant component. *Adipose tissue* normally occurs in specific, genetically determined regions. The subcutaneous connective tissue or superficial fascia is rich in fat cells, as is that in the female breast, as well as around the kidneys, the mesenteries and omenta, the orbits, the marrow of bone, and the synovial pads in many joints. Fat distribution in the subcutaneous connective tissue shows both age and sex differences.

Adipose tissue is composed primarily of adipocytes contained within an areolar (or loose) connective tissue. The areolar tissue contains other cell types common to all loose connective tissue. The tissue is highly vascularized as well as being divided into loculi by

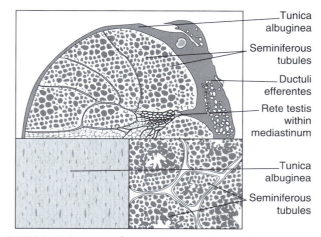

FIGURE 3–27. Dense irregular connective tissue. *Note the dense outer layer of the testis, the tunica albuginea. It is classified as dense irregular connective tissue, because the connective tissue fibers do not course in any specific direction. This arrangement of collagenous fibers makes the outer layer of the testis very strong.*

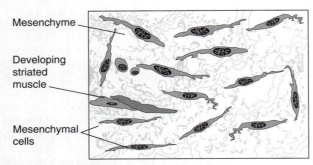

FIGURE 3-28. Mesenchymal tissue. *Mesenchymal tissue is composed of mesenchymal cells, fine fibers, and copious ground substance. It serves as a precursor of definitive connective tissue cells and tissues.*

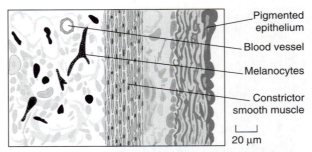

FIGURE 3-29. Melanocytes and pigmented epithelium. *In this diagram of a section through the iris of a rhesus monkey, spindle-shaped melanocytes can be found containing the yellow-brown pigment known as melanin. The pigmented cells vary considerably in their concentration of melanin granules.*

fibrous bands or septa containing blood vessels. Adipocytes are round (see Fig. 3-12), but when compressed, they assume a polygonal shape. Fat cells are the energy storehouse in times of abundant nutrition. They are the source of metabolic lipids, serve as insulation against a cold external environment, are a resilient shock absorber, and fill all otherwise empty extracellular spaces. In times of nutritional deficits, the fat cells release their storage fat. In certain societies, adipose tissue has a cosmetic function.

In the newborn infant, as discussed earlier, there are areas of specialized adipose tissue, so-called brown fat, which generates heat through the metabolic breakdown of fat by specialized and structurally unusual mitochondria.

Regular Connective Tissue

Regular connective tissue, as its name implies, is formed of fibrous bands that are all oriented in a similar direction. The fiber bundles may be flat sheets, known as aponeuroses, or may be thickened to form bundles known as ligaments and tendons (see Fig. 3-3). The direction of the collagen fibers that make up regular connective tissue appears to be determined by the lines of force exerted on the fibers. In the case of the cornea, collagen is arranged in a very precise manner, with layers of collagenous fibers stacked at right angles to each other.

Fibroblasts secrete the collagen that forms the aponeuroses, ligaments, and tendons. When this function ends, the cells remain in the connective tissue in their inactive form, fibrocytes. Fibrocytes can be reconverted into fibroblasts if the collagenous bands are damaged and need repair or replacement.

Regular connective tissue is primarily collagenous, but some ligaments are composed primarily of elastic fibers. Elastic ligaments of this type are associated with the vertebral column (the ligamenta flava) and also the vocal folds of the larynx.

Mucoid Tissue

Mucoid tissue is the fetal or embryonic form of connective tissue. It is found primarily where the connective tissue is developing from mesenchyme. It is also located in the umbilical cord, where it is known as Wharton's jelly. Mucoid connective tissue consists of an extensive matrix composed of hydrated mucoid substances (proteoglycans) and a fine meshwork of type II collagen fibers. Fibroblasts are present and highly branched but are characteristically few in number. In the adult, the vitreous body of the eye and nucleus pulposus of the intervertebral disk are generally considered to be similar to mucoid connective tissue (Fig. 3-28).

Pigmented Connective Tissue

Pigmented connective tissue occurs in the choroid, iris, and lamina fusca of the sclera of the eye. The lamina fusca contains a benzodipyran derivative, which is the melanin-like pigment of the retinal epithelium (Fig. 3-29).

CHAPTER FOUR

Cartilage, Bone, and Joints

CARTILAGE 60
    Hyaline Cartilage 60
    Elastic Cartilage 62
    Fibrocartilage 63

BONE 64
    Methods of Studying Bone 64
    Bone Cells 65
    Histogenesis 66
    Haversian Systems 70
    Bone Matrix 72
    Collagen 73
    Ground Substance 73
    Ectopic Ossification 73

JOINTS 73
    Synarthroses 73
    Amphiarthroses 74
    Diarthroses 75

The skeleton consists of cartilage, bone, and joints.

Cartilage is a tough, resilient connective tissue composed of cells and fibers embedded in a firm gel-like matrix. The physical characteristics of matrix permit effective responses by the tissue to mechanical deformation, weight-bearing, and other stresses.

Three histologic types of cartilage are recognized: hyaline cartilage, elastic cartilage, and fibrocartilage. Hyaline cartilage is the most abundant. It provides a smooth, "Teflon-like" surface for the bones of a joint to move against each other. Hyaline cartilage is also the precursor or model on which most bone development takes place. Elastic cartilage provides maximum flexibility while retaining the capacity to return to its undistorted or original shape. Fibrocartilage provides strength and direction to ligaments at some joints and a matrix for the connective tissue of the anulus fibrosus of intervertebral disks. Elastic cartilage and fibrocartilage may be considered modifications of hyaline cartilage.

Bones have a complex architecture and are composed of several tissues. The most abundant, however, is the specialized, mineralized matrix known as bone. Both bone and (to a lesser extent) cartilage support, and are acted upon by, the soft tissues of the body.

Joints may be defined as the connections between any rigid component parts existing in the skeleton, whether they are cartilaginous or bony. On the basis of their most characteristic structural features, joints may be classified into three main types: fibrous, cartilaginous, and synovial.

CARTILAGE

Cartilage is composed of cells, or chondrocytes, embedded in an extensive matrix of fibers and ground substance. The chondroblasts are responsible for the synthesis and secretion of the matrix, which they secrete until they are completely immersed (Fig. 4–1). The spaces in which chondroblasts are located are known as *lacunae*.

The principal macromolecules in the matrix of all cartilage are collagen, hyaluronic acid, proteoglycans, and glycoproteins. Elastic fibers are present in elastic cartilage, giving it its springlike capacity to return to its original shape when it is deformed. Fibrocartilage is characterized by an abundance of fibrous connective tissue, a small amount of matrix, and few characteristic cartilage cells in small clusters of isogenous groups. Hence, three types of cartilage are distinguished on the basis of the amount of matrix and the collagenous and elastic fibers embedded in it.

Cartilage is avascular, and cartilage cells receive their nutrients and dispose of their waste by diffusion from and to capillaries outside the tissue or from the synovial fluid of the joint cavity. Cartilage has, as might be expected, a low metabolic rate. It has no nerve supply or sensory receptors.

Hyaline Cartilage

The most abundant type of cartilage is hyaline cartilage, which in the adult is found on the articular

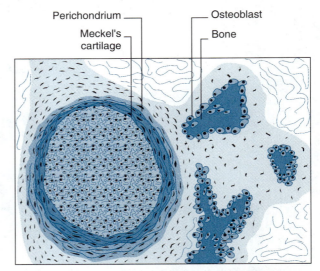

FIGURE 4–1. Meckel's cartilage and bone developing from mesenchyme. *Hyaline mandibular (Meckel's) cartilage developing in the embryonic mesenchyme. Isolated islands of so-called membranous bone can also be seen. Membranous bone is discussed later.*

surfaces of joints, at the ventral ends of ribs of the thorax, and as the tracheal rings and laryngeal cartilages. Hyaline cartilage is firm but permits some deformation of its tough gel-like matrix. It has an opalescent, bluish white hue (Fig. 4–2).

Developmental Aspects

At sites of cartilage development, mesenchymal cells aggregate to form "centers of chondrogenesis." These protochondrial cells are small and tightly packed. As they enlarge, they begin to secrete a metachromatic*

---

*Metachromatic staining by certain dyes occurs when the components of cells and tissues contain, for example, a significant amount of strongly acidic sulfated proteoglycans. The dye toluidine blue will demonstrate metachromasia by staining structures purple or red if they contain sulfated proteoglycans.

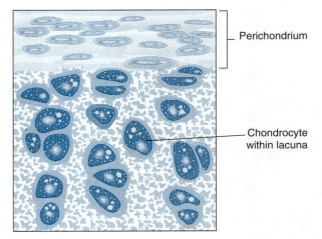

FIGURE 4–2. Hyaline cartilage. *Hyaline cartilage develops from the cells of the perichondrium. These cells migrate, divide, and produce a tough resistant ground substance in which they are embedded. The spaces the cartilage cells are housed in are called* lacunae.

extracellular matrix, which increases the distance between cells, resulting in so-called interstitial growth. The secreted matrix also contains tropocollagen fibers. The tropocollagen molecule, about 280 nm in length and 1.4 nm in diameter, consists of three polypeptide chains, designated α_1-chains. Each chain has a molecular weight of 100,000 and a left-handed helical configuration; the three polypeptide chains are entwined and cross-linked in a triple helix. The tropocollagen fibers that form extracellularly are masked by the matrix that contains them.

The secretion of interstitial matrix results in the growth and separation of chondrocytes. This is one mechanism by which cartilage grows. The second is cell division or mitosis. As soon as a chondroblast divides and starts synthesizing and secreting matrix and tropocollagen, the cells become separated from one another and are housed in separate lacunae. A second cell division results in a cluster of four cells, and a third in a cluster of eight cells. These clusters of two, four, or eight cells are called an *isogenous* (of common origin) grouping of cells (Fig. 4–3).

The outermost cells of developing cartilage form a layer of cells called perichondrium, a specialized connective tissue covering. The cells of the inner surface of the perichondrium differentiate into chondroblasts, which can secrete matrix and tropocollagen, thereby increasing the overall size of the cartilage. This growth mechanism is called appositional growth (Fig. 4–4). After birth, the perichondrium ceases producing chondroblasts; nevertheless, the potential for such growth remains in postnatal life.

Chondrocytes

When cartilage is examined under the microscope, the most peripheral lacunae appear oval and somewhat

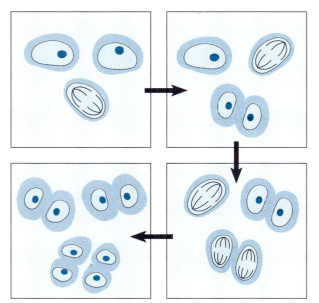

FIGURE 4–3. Cartilage growth. *Cartilage enlarges as chondroblasts divide and synthesize matrix. The shaded area around the chondroblasts signifies newly formed matrix. Once synthetic activity of chondroblasts ceases, they become inactive and are renamed* chondrocytes.

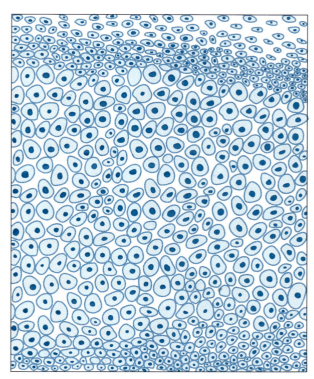

FIGURE 4–4. Mature hyaline cartilage. *A low-power view of hyaline cartilage reveals an outer layer of small cells and fibrous material known as the* perichondrium. *The larger cartilage cells are located within lacunae, and these are surrounded by a bluish white matrix. Hyaline cartilage plays an important role in skeletal formation.*

flattened. This appearance is well seen in articular cartilage. Lacunae are stacked with their ovoid long axes parallel to the free surface. Deeper in the cartilage, the lacunae are more round or square, and they are roughly 15 to 30 μm in diameter. The cells have the typical appearance of all protein-secretory cells and contain one or two nuclei. Adjacent to the nuclei, the cytoplasm contains centrioles and a typical and well-developed Golgi complex. Around this cell center are elongated mitochondria, lipid droplets, and glycogen. When matrix is being synthesized and secreted, as in developing and growing cartilage or cartilage under repair, the cells become basophilic, and the Golgi complex enlarges. The increased basophilia seen by light microscopy can be translated on electron microscopy into increases in cytoplasmic RNA attached to endoplasmic reticulum. Associated with the dilated sacs of the Golgi complex are vacuoles containing filaments and granules that extend to the surface of the cell and discharge their products into the surrounding matrix. When growth or repair ceases, the Golgi complex and the rough endoplasmic reticulum decrease in size and complexity, and the cytoplasm loses its basophilia.

Cartilage Matrix

The secretory product of the chondroblast is the matrix in which the cells become embedded. Superficially, newly synthesized cartilage appears homogenous in texture. It is composed of both tropocollagen fibers and a gel-like ground substance with similar refractive indices.

Light microscopy has shown that the matrix is deeply stained by the periodic acid–Schiff (PAS) method, indicating the presence of the disaccharides of glycosaminoglycans. Intense basophilia is due to the presence of strongly acidic proteoglycans composed of chondroitin 4-sulfate, chondroitin 6-sulfate, and keratin sulfate covalently linked to a core protein. These same compounds also account for the metachromasia that occurs when cartilage is stained by toluidine blue. The intensity of these staining reactions is especially prominent in the cartilage immediately adjacent to each chondrocyte, thereby outlining its lacuna. The deeply staining rim is called *capsular* or *territorial matrix*, whereas the less basophilic area between cell groups is called *intercapsular* or *interterritorial matrix*.

Molecular Aspects of Matrix

The extracellular matrix of cartilage is composed primarily of collagen type II and proteoglycans. The collagen fibrils are quite small, 10 to 20 nm in diameter. They usually lack distinct cross-banding typical of type I collagen. The collagen is an assemblage of molecules of a single kind–$\alpha 1(II)$–and is distributed in the matrix as a loose network rather than bundles of fibrils. The core protein to which the proteoglycans are attached is composed of 2000 amino acids and is about 300 nm long, with a molecular weight of about 250,000. The remainder of the molecule is composed of complex glycosaminoglycans, which radiate from the core protein like the bristles of a test tube brush. Approximately 80 chondroitin sulfate chains and 100 keratin sulfate chains radiate from each core protein. One end of the core protein is bound to a hyaluronic acid molecule. Keratin sulfate–chondroitin sulfate, the major proteoglycans of cartilage, has been shown to form large aggregates that are bound covalently to a single hyaluronic acid molecule. As many as 200 proteoglycan monomer aggregates are bound to a single hyaluronic acid chain by a linking protein, forming a huge complex with a molecular weight of about 1 million. In the in vivo, hydrated state, these giant molecules occupy a very large volume relative to their molecular weight. The high content of bound water (60%) gives the cartilage matrix its gel-like and resilient characteristics. This is particularly important in weight-bearing joints. The consistency of cartilage matrix depends upon (1) electrostatic bonds that exist between collagen and glycosaminoglycan side chains of matrix proteoglycans and (2) binding of water to negatively charged glycosaminoglycan chains extending from the proteoglycan core proteins.

Synthesis and Secretion of Hyaline Cartilage

The chondrocytes synthesize and secrete the collagen and proteoglycans of their surrounding matrix. The amino acid precursors of collagen have been traced in their course from the site of synthesis through the rough endoplasmic reticulum, Golgi complex, and secretory vacuoles at the cell periphery, with an intercellular time of about 3 hours. A similar sequence of events takes place for the production of matrix proteoglycans. The core protein is synthesized on the ribosomes of the rough endoplasmic reticulum, and the initial oligosaccharide is added at the same time within the cisternae of the endoplasmic reticulum. The initial product is collected in the cisternae of the reticulum and transported to the Golgi complex, where synthesis and sulfonation of glycosaminoglycans take place. The core proteins are synthesized and secreted into the Golgi complex, which adds additional glycosaminoglycans to the core protein to form the proteoglycans. It has been suggested that proteoglycans and type II collagen are synthesized at the same time and that they are packaged by the Golgi complex and secreted together. Proteoglycans are secreted as monomers; their assembly into aggregates occurs extracellularly.

Functional Aspects of Hyaline Cartilage

Hyaline cartilage covers the articular surfaces of bone and the junctions between ribs and sternum and provides support for the airway (preventing collapse) and several small cartilages of the larynx. It is also the model from which the bone is formed by a process called *endochondral calcification* of cartilage matrix; this process is discussed in detail later. The cartilage of adults does not repair as well as that of young children. When regeneration does take place, it is due to the action of perichondral cells, which secrete the "healing" matrix. In older people with osteoarthritic conditions, it is believed, cartilage cells have lost the ability to replace proteoglycans at a rate equal to the erosion of the matrix.

Elastic Cartilage

Elastic cartilage has a limited distribution. It is found in the pinna of the external ear, part of the external auditory canal, auditory tube, epiglottis, and the small cartilages of the larynx, the corniculate and cuneiform cartilages (Fig. 4–5). All of these structures have the capacity to be temporarily deformed without being structurally damaged.

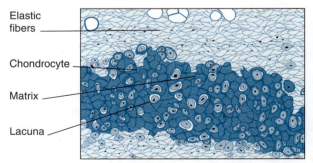

FIGURE 4–5. Mature elastic cartilage. *Elastic fibers are found in the matrix surrounding cartilage cells located in lacunae. This cartilage is flexible and less brittle than hyaline cartilage.*

Elastic cartilage, when unstained, is yellow, opaque, and more elastic than hyaline cartilage.

The cells of elastic cartilage are similar in appearance to those of hyaline cartilage. They occupy lacunae, are rounded, and occur singly or in isogenous groupings of two or four cells.

Unlike hyaline cartilage, the intercellular matrix or ground substance is often obscured by a meshwork of fibers or sheets of elastin. Special stains have been developed that are specific for elastin, such as Verhoeff's elastic tissue stain.

Growth of elastic cartilage is appositional owing to the presence of a perichondrium not unlike that associated with hyaline cartilage.

Molecular Aspects

The main component of elastic fibers is elastin, which is a highly hydrophobic, nonglycosylated protein of 830 amino acids. It is rich in proline and glycine like collagen, but differs in having little hydroxyproline and no hydroxylysine.

Like collagen molecules, elastin molecules are secreted from the Golgi complex in vesicles into the extracellular space. Here, filaments and sheets are formed in which the elastin molecules are highly cross-linked to one another, thereby forming an extensive network.

Elastin molecules differ from most other proteins in that their specialized function requires their polypeptide backbones to remain unfolded as random coils, i.e., the molecule does not have a unique or specific configuration. It is the random-coil, cross-linked structure that allows the molecules to be stretched and to recoil like rubber bands. Elastin is about five times as extensible as rubber of the same cross-sectional area. Interwoven with the elastic tissue are inelastic collagen fibrils, which limit the extension of elastin, preventing its rupture. Elastic fibers are not composed exclusively of elastin. They contain a glycoprotein in the form of microfibrils on their surface. Elastic fibers are assembled, along with other components of the elastic cartilage matrix, near the surface of the plasma membrane that secreted the matrix.

Fibrocartilage

Fibrocartilage has a very limited distribution in the body. It is found closely associated with the dense connective tissue of joint capsules and ligaments, in the ligamentum teres femoris, intervertebral disks, and symphysis pubis (Fig. 4–6). It is regarded as a transitional form of dense connective tissue and is always associated with it.

Fibrocartilage contains widely scattered chondrocytes, which occur singly or in isogenous groupings of two or four. They are arranged in rows, in the line of stress on the matrix, in the long axis between dense rows of collagenous (type I) connective tissue bundles. The matrix of fibrocartilage is not abundant and contains equal amounts of chondroitin sulfate and derma-

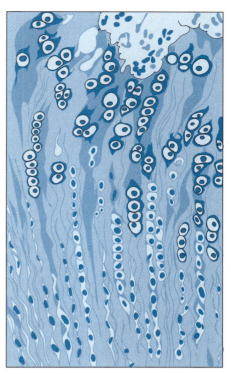

FIGURE 4–6. Mature fibrocartilage. *This drawing of a low-power view emphasizes the alignment of cartilage cells in their lacunae at the insertion of a tendon into bone. The alignment of both cells and fibers is determined by the direction of stress placed on the tendon. This cartilage is very strong and inelastic.*

tan sulfate, which stain metachromatically with certain basic dyes because of the strongly acidic sulfated protein polysaccharides that constitute the glycosaminoglycans.

Fibrocartilage develops like ordinary collagenous connective tissue, from fibroblasts that produce large amounts of type I collagen. Some fibroblasts apparently differentiate into chondrocytes and begin to secrete matrix. Only those collagen bundles in the immediate neighborhood of cartilage cells become embedded in matrix, which is never very extensive.

Functional Aspects

In young animals, cartilage is subject to many alterations resulting from dietary deficiency and hormonal imbalance. Deficiencies of proteins, vitamins, and minerals have severe effects on cartilage.

Protein deficiency results in a pronounced reduction in size of the epiphyseal plate of cartilage in growing bones, leading to an early cessation of growth.

Vitamin deficiencies affect cartilage in several ways. Vitamin A deficiency has an effect similar to that of protein deficiency. Vitamin C affects the synthesis of collagen and matrix formation. Vitamin D deficiency reduces uptake of calcium and phosphorus, leading to improperly calcified cartilage, defective bone growth, and bowing of the legs characteristic of rickets.

Hormones also influence the growth of cartilage. In excess, growth hormone stimulates the growth of cartilage, which under normal circumstances would have stopped growing. Growth hormone deficiency results in cessation of mitotic activity, reduction in size, and cessation in growth of cartilage cells; these changes can be readily reversed by the provision of growth hormone.

Molecular Considerations

Vitamin C deficiency in humans causes scurvy. The vitamin prevents proline hydroxylation and inhibits procollagen helix formation. Although normal collagen is slowly degraded by collagenase, this process is greatly enhanced in scurvy when defective pro-α-chains fail to form a triple helix. The progressive loss of normal collagen without replacement results in loss of teeth and in collagen-deficient organs and blood vessels.

BONE

Bone constitutes most of the human skeleton. Because of its strength, bone is the framework on which soft tissues are attached and act against to produce movement. It houses and protects vital organs in the skull, thorax, abdomen, and pelvis and contains the blood-forming tissue. Bones of varying length are associated with one another, forming joints for movement of body parts and other objects. Bone stores and releases calcium, phosphorus, and other ions when demands are made on it by hormones to control and balance the ionic content in body fluids (homeostasis).

Bone is a calcified connective tissue. The synthesis, maintenance, and resorption of the calcified matrix are performed by three cell types: osteoblasts, osteocytes, and osteoclasts (Figs. 4–7 and 4–8). Unlike cartilage, bone does not permit diffusion of nutrients through it; hence, osteocytes reach their blood supply through

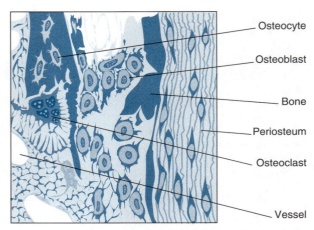

FIGURE 4–8. Osteoblast, osteocyte, and osteoclast. *Key criteria used to identify these cells are as follows: Osteocytes are surrounded by bone and located in their lacunae. Osteoblasts are located near or on bony spicules, where they line up; they are cuboidal or rounded in shape. Osteoclasts are multinuclear and situated on bony spicules or within depressions in spicules called Howship's lacunae.*

canaliculi. Minute osteocytic filopodia reach nearby capillary beds and contact other osteocytes, with which they form *gap junctions*.

Bone is covered on its external surface by a specialized osteogenic connective tissue, the *periosteum*, which is similar to the perichondrium that covers cartilage. It contains cells capable of differentiating into osteoblasts and producing bone. The periosteum is absent from surfaces that are normally covered by articular (hyaline) cartilage and from the area covered by articular capsules. The internal surfaces of bone are also covered by a thin cellular layer, the *endosteum*, which also possesses osteogenic capabilities.

Bone combines great tensile strength with relative lightness. It is very responsive to changes in individual weight. With increased body weight, bone thickens, and with weight loss and weightlessness (absence of gravity), bone becomes thin. Weightlifters have greater bone mass than nonweightlifters. Because of bone's physiologic responsiveness and its ability to repair itself, several medical specialists (otolaryngologists, orthopedic and plastic surgeons, orthodontists, and others) can perform many desirable alterations in bony imperfections or damage.

Methods of Studying Bone

Bone, being very hard, can be studied most easily by two techniques. First, pieces of bone may be ground by abrasives until they are extremely thin, so that the calcified framework may be examined. Although most of the cells, connective tissue, and blood vessels are no longer present, their former locations are readily examined by light microscopy. Second, bone may be fixed and then decalcified in dilute acid (5% formic or nitric acid) or by a calcium-binding chelating agent. Following decalcification, the bone is readily embedded, sectioned, and stained with many routine histologic methods.

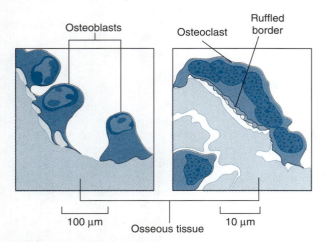

FIGURE 4–7. Bone Cells: osteoblasts and osteoclasts. *The cells that produce bone are known as osteoblasts. They are mononuclear cuboidal cells that line cartilage or newly formed bone. The cells that reorganize or remodel or reshape bone are known as osteoclasts. They are multinuclear, appear rather foamy, and have a ruffled border, particularly at the surface of the bone; they are very large and can be identified in tissue sections by means of these criteria.*

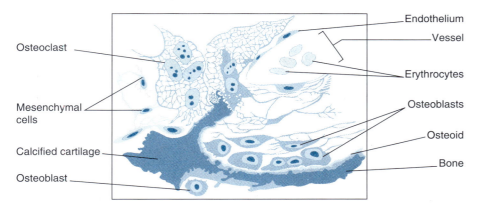

FIGURE 4–9. Bone development: remodeling of calcified cartilage. This illustration shows a pair of osteoclasts eroding away a piece of calcified cartilage in the marrow cavity near the zone of endochondrial ossification.

Additional details may be obtained with high-resolution electron microscopy, by sectioning undecalcified bone with a diamond knife and viewing the sections.

Bone Cells

Four cell "types" are recognizable in actively growing bone, although three of these are merely functional stages of the same cell type. The first three are the osteoprogenitor cell, osteoblast, and osteocyte, and the fourth type is the osteoclast. It is thought that the first three arise from mesenchyme and the fourth from monocytes that are formed in the bone marrow and found in the circulating blood.

Osteoprogenitor Cells

Osteogenic or progenitor osteoblastic (*osteoprogenitor*) cells are found on the inner layer of the periosteum adjacent to the external surface of the bone, in the endosteum lining haversian canals, and on the trabeculae of cartilage matrix at the metaphysis of growing bone. These cells are elongate, with oval nuclei, and have an acidophilic or slightly basophilic cytoplasm. They proliferate during the period of rapid bone growth but become less active during adult life. When a bone is broken or is being reorganized for any reason, these cells will again begin to proliferate. The cells undergo cell division and become indistinguishable from osteoblasts. When the bone has been repaired or reorganized and the functional activity of these cells is complete, they may revert structurally and functionally to the resting progenitor state. In many instances, they may be incorporated into the repaired bone and become functional osteocytes. Osteoprogenitor cells are not multipotential mesenchymal cells, because they have a very limited capacity to differentiate into other cell types, unlike mesenchyme.

Osteoblasts and Osteocytes

Osteoblasts synthesize bone matrix, which includes type I collagen, proteoglycans, and glycoproteins. This uncalcified matrix is known as *osteoid* (Fig. 4–9). Calcium phosphate is then added to the matrix to form bone; this process requires the presence of osteoblasts, perhaps indicating certain essential enzymatic activity (discussed later) or additional unknown functions for these cells.

Osteoblasts line the free surfaces of bone in a continuous layer, interrupted only by osteoclasts (Figs. 4–10 and 4–11). These cells are polarized: They usually have a flattened face adjacent to the bony surface and a rounded distal free surface.

Osteoblasts are typical protein-secretory cells; hence, they have the typical cytoplasmic organelle profile. The cytoplasm contains abundant, rough (RNA-studded) endoplasmic reticulum, a large Golgi complex, and numerous mitochondria. Typical of cells with abundant cytoplasmic RNA, osteoblasts are basophilic when stained with basic dyes and examined by light microscopy. In thin sections, the cell center containing the Golgi complex can be seen as an area of diminished staining capacity but acidophilic in character. Special stains are needed to stain the Golgi complex. Histochemical evaluation reveals significant alkaline phosphatase activity in active osteoblasts. This enzyme decreases when synthetic activity decreases. The enzyme probably plays a role in calcification of newly synthesized matrix. It is possible that localized increases in phosphate ions would facilitate the precipitation of minerals and their subsequent crystallization. The serum levels of alkaline phosphatase reflect the level of new bone formation, regardless of the stimulus initiating the process.

When the synthetic activity of the osteoblast decreases, the cells flatten, their basophilia disappears,

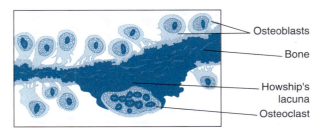

FIGURE 4–10. Bone development: the development of a trabecula. Note the relationship of the osteoblasts to the developing trabecula. A single multicellular giant cell, an osteoclast, is shown in a depression known as a Howship's lacuna.

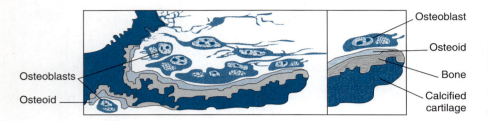

FIGURE 4-11. Osteoid. *Bone is laid down first as osteoid, or uncalcified bone, and then is subsequently calcified. Hence, two layers usually can be identified when bone is formed. Bone formation is shown at a very early stage on the left side, and after 4 months on the right.*

and their enzymatic activity decreases. As osteoblasts become embedded in the matrix they are producing, they develop long, thin processes or filopodia, which allow them to maintain contact through gap junctions with the filopodia of neighboring osteoblasts, which will also become osteocytes. In the course of their embedment, the processes become enclosed, forming canaliculi in which they will reside until they are uncovered by erosion of the calcified matrix during bone remodeling or repair.

Once osteoblasts are embedded in matrix, they are renamed *osteocytes*. The embedded osteocytes are stellate with many thin processes. As indicated earlier, these cells cannot synthesize matrix in their present state, but the potential remains; they are potential osteoblasts. Calcification greatly reduces the diffusion of fluids, gases, and nutrients; hence, osteocytes must be nourished and sustained via the minute canaliculi and their enclosed osteocytic filopodia. The filopodia are surrounded by a thin layer of uncalcified matrix. Uncalcified matrix is known as *osteoid*.

Osteoclasts

Osteoclasts have an interesting and distinct origin from that of osteoprogenitor cells. It has been demonstrated that osteoclasts originate from bone marrow cells, most probably from the fusion of monocytes (see Figs. 4–9 to 4–11).

Osteoclasts are giant cells as large as 100 μm in diameter and may contain as many as 50 nuclei. These giant cells are always located in regions of bone resorption, frequently in shallow depressions known as Howship's lacunae. These cells are polarized, with their free surface rounded. The acidophilic cytoplasm contains the numerous nuclei mentioned previously. The part of the cell adjacent to the bone is composed of many cell processes, not unlike the surface of a brush in appearance. The processes are not, however, of uniform diameter and are always seen actively moving; this surface of the cell is called the *ruffled border*. Deep infoldings of the cell membrane vastly increase the cell's surface area and its capacity to degrade bone. The narrow extracellular spaces between the processes often contain small pieces of bone matrix undergoing dissolution.

The nuclei of osteoclasts are not unusual in appearance, being similar to those of osteoblasts. The cytoplasm is strongly acidophilic, although a ribosome-studded endoplasmic reticulum is present in these giant cells. An analysis of the function of these cells indicates that they are involved in protein secretion in the form of collagenase and other hydrolytic enzymes. The rough endoplasmic reticulum is small and does not influence staining, because this organelle is overshadowed by the abundant agranular endoplasmic reticulum and several Golgi complexes. It is of interest that the number of centriole pairs corresponds to the number of nuclei. Cytoplasmic vacuoles, lysosomes, and free ribosomes complete the organelle profile for osteoclasts.

Hormones have a profound effect on bone. It has been shown that normal blood levels of calcium depend on the action of two hormones that act antagonistically on bone. Parathyroid hormone causes bone resorption and the release of calcium ions into the blood. Calcitonin acts to decrease mobilization of calcium from bone. In this regard, it causes the disappearance of the ruffled border of osteoclasts, suggesting that bone resorption is directly related to osteoclastic function.

In hyperparathyroidism, bone is greatly resorbed and is replaced with fibrous tissue containing numerous osteoclasts. These changes are similar to those seen in osteitis fibrosa or von Recklinghausen's disease.

Histogenesis

Bone formation occurs by two mechanisms. The first occurs in embryonic connective tissue and is known as intramembranous ossification. The second mechanism involves the replacement of preexisting cartilage and is called endochondral ossification. In endochondral ossification, cartilage is gradually replaced before bone is laid down.

Although these two modes of bone formation have different starting points, the cellular deposition of bone is identical.

Intramembranous Ossification

The skeleton is composed of several bones that develop by intramembranous ossification. These so-called membrane bones include the frontal and parietal, parts of the occipital and temporal, and the mandible and maxilla of the skull (Fig. 4–12).

Intramembranous bone formation begins when the embryonic mesenchyme becomes a dense aggregation of cells in contact with one another by numerous long, tapering processes. These cells produce randomly placed, delicate collagen fibrils and a gel-like matrix that fills the intercellular space. This is followed by a thickening of the matrix, which is eosinophilic (acidophilic), with a decreased number of cells within the

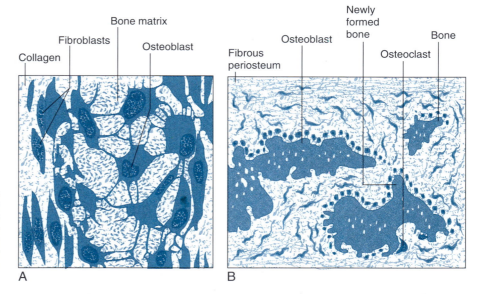

FIGURE 4–12. Membrane bone. Bone formation without a cartilaginous model is termed membranous bone formation. It starts in the mesenchyme with the differentiation of osteoblasts possessing numerous processes that contact adjacent osteoblasts. The osteoblasts lay down bone matrix, which subsequently calcifies.

matrix. The cells within and adjacent to the matrix line up and become cuboidal but retain their contact with one another via their now foreshortened processes. Those within the matrix become osteocytes but also retain, through their extensive processes, their contact with peripheral cells via gap junctions. This region is called a *primary ossification center*.

The cells outside this region are primarily spindle-shaped or fusiform and fibroblastic. They form an outer covering for the developing bone of the primary ossification center.

The cuboidal cells become increasingly basophilic and are now designated osteoblasts. These osteoblasts secrete osteoid or bone matrix, and through appositional growth, bony trabeculae develop, becoming larger and longer.

Osteoblasts secrete both collagen molecules and proteoglycans. The collagen molecules polymerize extracellularly to form large numbers of randomly oriented collagen fibrils throughout the osseous matrix. Because this early, immature, primary bone matrix is composed of a feltlike distribution of collagen, it is sometimes referred to as *woven bone*. Shortly after secretion of the matrix, calcium phosphate is deposited to complete the ossification process. During remodeling of this immature bone, the newly synthesized collagen is arranged in aligned bundles.

Immature bone has randomly distributed osteocytes and large, irregular channels occupied by blood vessels. These irregular channels also contain mesenchyme that differentiates into blood cell–forming tissue or bone marrow cells (hematopoietic tissue).

Replacement of the woven bone results in a highly ordered distribution of osteocytes arranged in concentric rings (or lamellae) around relatively straight blood vessels (so-called haversian canals).

Numerous primary centers undergoing growth eventually fuse with adjacent bony spicules, forming a series of trabeculae and having a microscopic appearance that resembles a sponge, so-called spongy bone or primary spongiosa.

As the osteoblast is incorporated into the newly formed bone and becomes an osteocyte, additional osteoblasts appear from the surrounding mesenchyme, where they undergo cell division. Once the cells differentiate into osteoblasts, they lose their capacity to divide.

At birth, bone development is not complete, and the bones of the skull are as yet not united. Fontanelles, the spaces between the bones, are filled with osteogenic connective tissue.

Bone has characteristic patterns of development. A specific bone may develop from two or more sites. These sites, called ossification centers, grow in size and ultimately fuse to complete the proper shape or form of the bone. Should the ossification centers fail to fuse, a single bone may appear as two or more parts. The bones of the skull grow faster at their periosteal surfaces than at their endosteal surfaces, resulting in two layers of compact bone separated by a layer of spongy bone, the diploë. In those areas where the primary spongiosa ultimately becomes compact bone, the trabeculae diminish and are obliterated. Although the compact bone here appears superficially to be lamellar bone, it is not so designated, because the collagen fibrils are randomly distributed in the feltlike pattern. Where membrane bone is destined to remain spongy bone, e.g., diploë, trabeculae thicken to a certain size, and bone formation ceases. The mechanism for this is unknown. The spaces between trabeculae contain vascular and connective tissues, which differentiate into hematopoietic, or blood cell–forming, tissue.

As a final stage of membrane bone formation, the peripheral connective tissue forms a true fibrous covering, the periosteum. The osteoblasts facing the bone lose their bone-forming organelle profile and revert to fusiform cells resembling fibroblasts. The same events take place on the endosteal surface, and the osteopro-

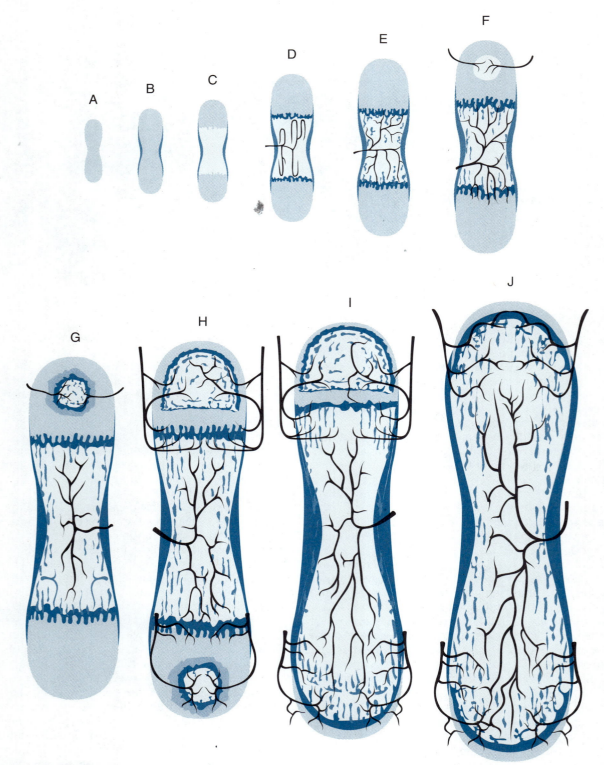

FIGURE 4-13. Bone development. *Cartilaginous bone model and progressive changes that occur in the ossification process.* A, *The cartilage "model" of a long bone.* B, *Appearance of periosteal bone before the development of calcified cartilage.* C, D, *and* E, *The "breakdown" of the cartilage model and the invasion of vascular mesenchyme.* F *and* G, *Vascular mesenchyme enters the model at two points, dividing the ossification process into two parts.* H, *The* epiphysis *(upper, smaller part) develops and grows larger.* I *and* J, *Bone growth in the region of the* diaphysis *takes place at the ends of diaphysis, known as the* metaphyses. *At this point, cartilage can divide and grow. The advancing growth of the bony collar distally defines the inferior border of the metaphysis in long bone development. The upper and lower epiphyseal cavities join the shaft (diaphysis) of the bone when the bone stops growing. The marrow cavity is continuous throughout the length of the bone. After the disappearance of the cartilaginous plates at the zones of ossification, the blood vessels of the diaphysis, metaphysis, and epiphysis anastomose.*

genitor cells appear fibroblastic. In bone fractures, these cells become reactivated to repair the break.

Endochondral Ossification

The vertebral column, pelvis, and limbs are initially formed of hyaline cartilage. The cartilage resembles, on a small scale, the bone to be formed from the cartilaginous model. This type of bone formation is called *endochondral ossification*.

The process is best understood by studying a model of a series of developing long bones of the limbs (Fig. 4–13). The first indication that the hyaline cartilage model is to undergo ossification is the appearance of a thickening of the perichondrium and the deposition of a thin layer of bone around the middle of the cartilage model, which is known as the *diaphysis*. The initiation of bone formation is intramembranous, as discussed previously. The bony collar greatly decreases diffusion of nutrients for the cartilage cells, which undergo atrophy and death. As a result, the hyaline cartilage surrounding the cells is broken down, leading to the enlargement of lacunae. The dying cartilage cells are unable to maintain the cartilage, and by some unknown mechanism, the cartilage is calcified.

At this stage, blood vessels from the periosteum penetrate the bony collar and invade the degenerating cartilage and lacunae. The blood vessels bring osteogenic progenitor and bone marrow stem cells into the decaying cartilage, which differentiate into osteoblasts, osteoclasts, and blood cells. The osteoblasts assume their positions on the spicules and remnants of lacunar cartilage and begin to lay down osseous tissue, or osteoid, which will subsequently become calcified. The osteoclasts begin the task of resorbing the bone as growth continues on both the external and internal surfaces of the decaying cartilage. Hyaline cartilage extends and grows from either end of the bony collar. As the bony collar grows distally, toward each end of the developing bone, additional cartilage becomes part of the ossification process. Lacunae break down, the space is invaded by blood vessels, calcification of cartilage spicules occurs, and osteoblasts line the calcified cartilage spicules and lay down osteoid. Subsequently, these bony spicules are resorbed by osteoclasts, and the marrow cavity is filled with blood cell–forming stem cells.

As bone formation advances toward the ends of the cartilaginous model, the rows of cartilage cells adjacent to the degenerating cartilage cells are known as the *epiphyseal plate*.

Secondary centers of ossification begin at the ends of the cartilaginous model. The secondary centers are found in that part of the bone known as the *epiphysis*. Ossification occurs in the epiphysis when invading blood vessels bring in chondroclasts (Figs. 4–14 and 4–15). It should be noted that the epiphysis does not have a perichondrium. The epiphyses become the articular surfaces of joints. No perichondrium, bony collar, or any other cover forms over the epiphysis; hence, it remains hyaline cartilage.

Growth of the developing bone depends on growth

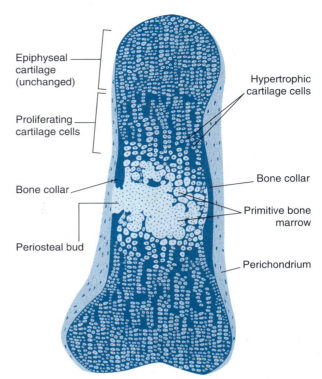

FIGURE 4–14. Penetration of vessels into the diaphysis. *The presence of a bony collar around the shaft of the cartilage model initiates the breakdown of adjacent cartilage and the penetration of blood vessels, which carry osteogenic and osteolytic cells.*

of the cartilage of the epiphyseal plate by proliferation of chondroblasts, with the bony collar (diaphysis) growing toward the ends of the cartilaginous model. The most mature chondrocytes begin to die, the lacunae break down, lacunar spicules begin to calcify, osseous tissue is laid down by osteoblasts, and new bone formation continues until the cells of the epiphyseal plate are depleted. When this happens, bone growth ceases permanently.

A fracture of a long bone in a child may have serious consequences if it damages the mitotically active epiphyseal plate. Growth may be retarded or arrested, resulting in a permanent shortening of the bone.

The process of growth involves both the secretion and the reabsorption of bone, which occur at the same rate. Until bone growth ceases, the epiphyseal plate remains uniform in thickness. Bone growth is usually complete in young adults (about 26 years). Ossification is not complete until after the 32nd year (Table 4–1).

Using a developing long bone as an example, one can summarize the events or stages in bone formation by endochondral ossification; five critical histologic zones can be recognized.

1. Zone of resting chondrocytes: Hyaline cartilage contains resting chondrocytes at the distal ends of the structural model.

2. Zone of proliferating chondrocytes: Cells undergoing division form isogenous cell groupings, arranged in columns perpendicular to the epiphyseal

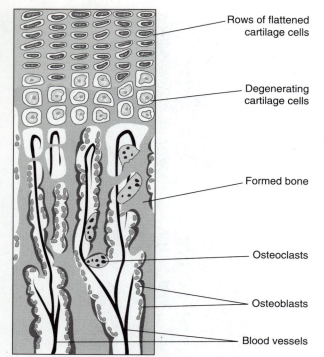

FIGURE 4–15. Developing bone: vascular penetration. *Hypertrophic and degenerating cartilage cells lead to the breakdown of lacunae walls, allowing penetration of lacunae by blood vessels carrying osteogenic mesenchyme. Elements of cartilage present are calcified; they are covered by osseous tissue deposited by osteoblasts. These ossified cartilage trabeculae or spicules are subsequently resorbed, and the developing bone is remodeled.*

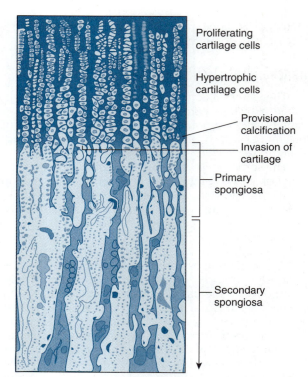

FIGURE 4–16. Endochondrial ossification: zone of epiphyseal growth. *The cartilage of the future bone is rapidly removed except for longitudinal remnants that were calcified, ossified by osteoblasts, and vigorously remodeled by osteoclasts. The peripheral growth of the bony collar and the proliferation of cartilage beyond (distal to) the bony collar results in growth of the shaft of the bone. Primary spongiosa is immature bone formed of cartilaginous spicules. The secondary spongiosa becomes compact bone with osteocytes lodged within lacunae.*

plate and parallel with the long axis of the developing bone.

3. Zone of hypertrophic chondrocytes: These large cells have pyknotic nuclei and glycogen accumulations. Matrix is resorbed, with thinned septae between cells. A thin bony collar surrounds the cartilage starting at this point and centrally.

4. Zone of chondrocyte degeneration and death: Cell death and breakdown of cartilaginous transverse septae occur, forming cartilaginous spicules that undergo provisional calcification with hydroxyapatite crystals. Blood vessels invade the degenerating cartilage (Fig. 4–16).

5. Zone of matrix calcification: Osteoblasts cover the spicules of calcified cartilage and lay down osseous tissue, which is subsequently calcified.

Haversian Systems

Parts of spongy bone formed during development become converted into compact bone (Figs. 4–17 and 4–18). Bony spicules located in the highly irregular, marrow-filled cavity of spongy bone increase in size through osteoblastic synthesis of new bone. The numerous bony spicules enlarge layer by layer, forming concentric bony lamellae. This process continues until the former marrow cavity becomes a rather narrow channel containing blood vessels and marrow cells. This system of concentric bone lamellae is referred to as the *primitive haversian system*.

The next step in the complicated process involves places where bone resorption is taking place through the action of osteoclasts. This process may include parts or all of the newly formed primitive haversian system. In this process, wide cylindrical cavities are formed and are filled with blood vessels and embryonic bone marrow. The bone destruction ceases, osteoblast activity begins, and concentric systems are laid down on the walls of the newly formed cavities. These are known as *second-generation haversian systems*. Bone dissolution

TABLE 4–1. Average Age at Which Bony Ossification Is Complete

Bone	Chronological Age of Fusion (yr)
Scapula	19 ± 1
Clavicle	27 ± 4
Bones of upper limb (arm, forearm, hand)	19 ± 2
Os coxa	21 ± 3
Bones of lower limb (thigh, leg, foot)	20 ± 2
Vertebra	~25
Sacrum	24 ± 1
Sternum (body)	~23
Sternum (manubrium, xiphoid)	30+

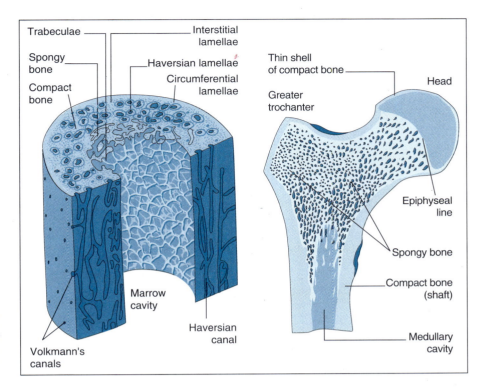

FIGURE 4-17. Shaft of the femur: definitive bone. Various parts of a bone are located and named. Left, A portion of the shaft of the bone. Right, The parts known as the head and trochanter are identified. See also Figure 4-18.

may be initiated, followed by the formation of the *third-generation haversian systems* (Figs. 4-18 and 4-19).

Haversian systems are formed by appositional growth of bone on the inner surfaces of lamellae of bone surrounding blood vessels, which results in a developmental decrease in the size of haversian canals and an increase in the compactness of the bone.

Three types of bony lamellae are recognized and result from the activity just described. As the bone thickness increases, the periosteum and the endosteum provide the osteoblasts that lay down successive layers, into which they are incorporated. These lamellae are known as *inner basic lamellae*. Reconstruction or modeling of bone results in the destruction and replacement

FIGURE 4-18. Bone: lamellae. Note the types of lamellae—interstitial and outer circumferential (periosteal circumferential)—formed by remodeling of the bone during growth. Haversian and Volkmann's canals are identified. Haversian canals run longitudinally (in the long axis of the bone), and Volkmann's canals extend transversely from the periphery and join haversian canals. These canals contain neurovascular bundles.

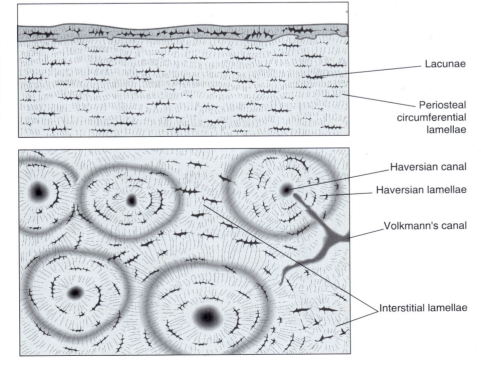

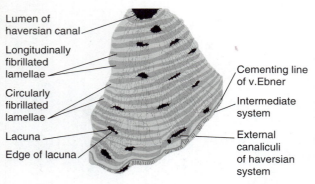
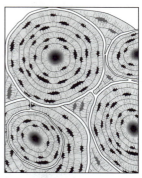

FIGURE 4–19. Haversian system: canaliculi link osteocytes with blood supply. *The canaliculi contain extracellular fluid, which carries nutrients and provides for gaseous exchange.*

of haversian systems. This results in the formation of incomplete (incompletely destroyed) haversian systems known as *interstitial lamellae* or the interstitial system. These lamellae do not have a blood vessel core (Fig. 4–20).

Cells of the periosteum form first a thin and later a thick periosteal bony band (or collar), which surrounds the diaphysis or shaft of the developing bone. The outer layer or band is the *circumferential* or *outer basic lamellae*. These lamellae also do not have a blood vessel core. The outer basic lamellar system is covered by periosteum, and the inner basic lamellar system contains blood vessels, bone marrow, variable amounts of fat, and nerve fibers.

Excessive amounts of vitamin A accelerate remodeling of bone. A deficiency of vitamin A results in a slowing of the rate of growth of bones, and of the overall growth of the skeleton. Because the growing central nervous system is not affected by vitamin A, the spinal cord may be damaged owing to the discrepancy in size between the spinal cord and the neural foramina of the vertebra.

Bone Matrix

Bone is formed of two primary components, an organic matrix and inorganic salts, in a ratio of 1:1. The

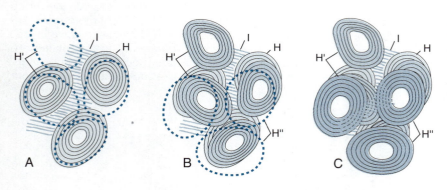

FIGURE 4–20. Bone development: haversian systems remodeled. *Haversian systems undergo remodeling on a continuing basis, even in the mature form of compact bone. A, B, and C, Three generations of haversian systems are seen (H, H', H''). Interstitial lamellae are also modified (I). Incomplete portions of haversian systems are therefore found in sections of mature compact bone.*

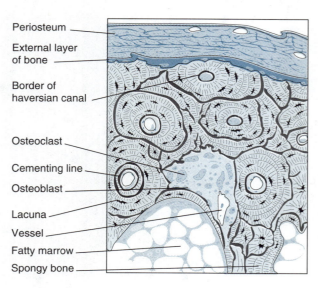

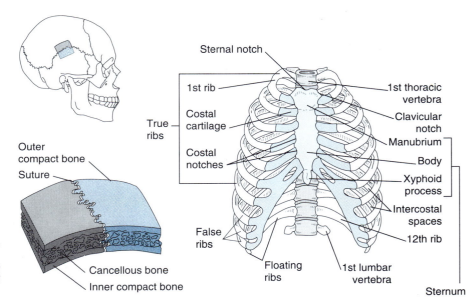

FIGURE 4–21. Synarthroses. *These joints are stable, strong, and relatively immobile. They are typically found in the skull and at the junctions between the ribs and costal cartilages.*

organic matrix is about 95% collagen and 5% ground substance. The inorganic salts are primarily calcium phosphate, with small amounts of bicarbonate, citrate, magnesium, potassium, and sodium.

Collagen

The collagen of bone is type I and occurs as fibrils that are cross-striated. The fibrils are 50 to 70 nm in diameter. The cross-striations have a repeat period of 67 nm.

Type I collagen is resistant to dilute acid and relatively insoluble to solvents used to extract other collagen types.

Ground Substance

Histochemical evidence suggests that the ground substance contains glycosaminoglycans. Three have been identified: chondroitin sulfate, keratin sulfate, and hyaluronic acid. Among the important glycoproteins in ground substance are sialoprotein and osteocalcin, both of which strongly bind calcium.

Ectopic Ossification

Ectopic ossification has been described in such diverse locations as the pelvis of the kidney, the walls of arteries, the eyes, the dura mater, muscles, and tendons. Many types of connective tissue have latent osteogenic potencies, which are only rarely seen away from the skeletal system. There is evidence that excessive use of alcohol alone induces ectopic bone formation and that it shares this ability with other irritating substances. Older individuals may also be subject to ectopic bone formation.

JOINTS

There are three principal types of joints: synarthroses (immovable), amphiarthroses (slightly movable), and diarthroses (freely movable).

Synarthroses

There are three subtypes of synarthroses (Fig. 4–21): syndesmoses, synchondroses, and synostoses.

Syndesmoses

Syndesmoses permit little or no movement between adjacent bones. The bones are united by fibrous connective tissue with osteogenic capabilities. The sutures of the skull are examples of this type of joint. The bones of the skull are joined by layers of connective tissue, both fibers and cells. The osteogenic cells of the joint can produce bone by appositional growth at the free ends of the bone joined by connective tissue. When an individual matures, the skull stops growing, and the connective tissue is gradually replaced by bone. The joint then becomes a synostosis. Another example of syndesmosis is the tibiofibular joint.

Synchondroses

In synchondroses, bones are joined by hyaline cartilage. An example of this type of joint is found where the ribs join the sternum.

Synostoses

Synostoses, found in adults, stabilize parts of the skeleton once growth has stopped. As indicated previously, the skull provides examples of this type of joint.

Fractures of the skull are common in adults but

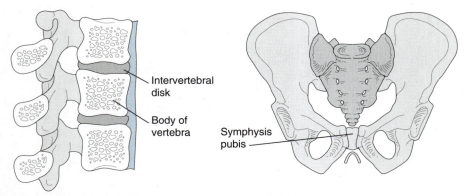

FIGURE 4–22. Amphiarthroses. *The intervertebral disks and pubic symphysis are examples of slightly movable joints.*

are much less so in children. The skull of the child is more resilient because of the immature nature of the developing membranous bone and because of the connective tissue within the sutures. The skull of an adult is brittle, like an eggshell, and it will frequently splinter on impact.

Amphiarthroses

Two examples of amphiarthroses are intervertebral disks and the symphysis pubis (Fig. 4–22).

The vertebral bodies are joined together by intervertebral disks and ligaments. The intervertebral disk is composed of a soft gelatinous inner core and an outer rim of fibrous concentric rings, the *anulus fibrosus*. The fibers of the anulus are securely attached to the vertebral bodies. The fibers forming the fibrous lamellae are layered and run at various angles to adjacent lamellae.

The anulus fibrosus is composed of fibrocartilage within a sheath of dense connective tissue derived from mesenchyme. The *nucleus pulposus* arises from the notochord and is composed of a mucoid semisolid gel. The nucleus absorbs and dissipates forces on the spine. In older individuals, the nucleus pulposus becomes brittle and inelastic. The anulus also becomes less resil-

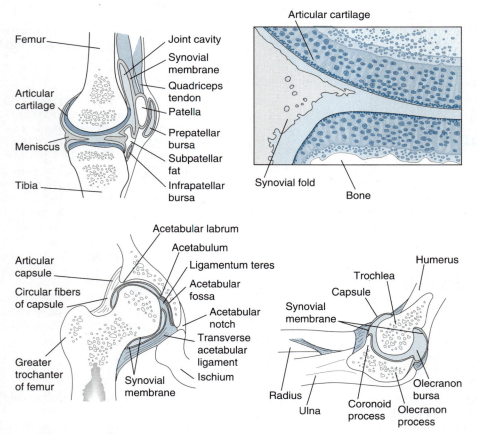

FIGURE 4–23. Diarthroses. *The knee, hip, and elbow joints are examples of freely movable joints.*

ient, owing to an increase in collagen and a decrease in glycosaminoglycans.

Hormonal action in a pregnant woman causes the symphysis pubis and the sacroiliac and sacrococcygeal joints to soften and become flexible. Relaxation of pelvic joints reduces the potential for trauma during childbirth by increasing the diameter of the pelvic outlet. After childbirth, the joints stiffen, but the diameter of the pelvis remains slightly wider than it was initially.

Diarthroses

In freely movable joints, the ends of adjacent bones are joined by a capsule of connective tissue (Fig. 4–23). The capsule is lined by a synovial membrane and encloses a fluid-filled cavity, which greatly reduces friction between the articular cartilages of opposing bones.

Two types of cells line the synovial membrane. One is macrophage-like and is called a *histiocyte type A or M* (macrophage-like) *cell*. The second cell resembles a fibroblast and is characterized by greater eléctron density; it is called a type *B or F* (fibroblast-like) *cell*.

Synovial fluid is an ultrafiltrate from synovial membrane capillaries. The fluid differs from blood serum by having less protein. The viscosity of synovial fluid is due primarily to mucin secreted by the type B lining cells. Mucin consists of hyaluronic acid covalently bound to protein. The lubricating qualities of synovial fluid are due to a glycoprotein. The microscopic examination of synovial fluid is used in the diagnosis of joint disorders.

Osteoarthritis is a degenerative disease of the articular cartilage of diarthrotic joints accompanied by the formation of bony spurs in the joint cavities. Immobility may occur if, for example, the hip joint is affected by this disease. In such cases, the entire hip joint can be replaced by orthopedic surgeons in a procedure known as *hip arthroplasty*.

CHAPTER FIVE

MUSCULAR TISSUE

BASIC CONCEPTS 77

STRIATED SKELETAL MUSCLE 77
    Histologic Organization of Skeletal Muscle 77
    Molecular Basis of Striations 79
    Band Patterns in Contraction 81
    Structural-Functional Orientation 82
    Fiber Type Heterogeneity (Red, White, and Intermediate) 83
    Ultrastructure of Skeletal Muscle 83
    Molecular Basis of Striated Muscle Fiber 84
    Molecular Basis of Contraction 86

STRIATED CARDIAC MUSCLE 88
    Functional Architecture of Fibers 89
    Excitation-Contraction Coupling: The T System and Sarcoplasmic Reticulum 89
    Intercalated Disks 90
    Fiber Heterogeneity 90
    Myocardial Pacemakers and Stimuli-Conducting Fibers 91

SMOOTH MUSCLE 92
    Molecular Basis of Smooth Muscle Function 94
    Nerve Supply 94

MYOEPITHELIAL CELLS 95

Movement is carried out by cells that are specialized to contract (shorten); these cells are normally controlled by the central nervous system. One cannot overestimate the role of the brain and spinal cord in the programming, initiation, and control of movement through muscular contraction. Every overt manifestation of central nervous system function and life is expressed as some movement or mechanical work, carried out by muscle or other contractile cell types, all of which use similar "contractile proteins." There is no life without movement.

BASIC CONCEPTS

Histologists generally recognize three kinds of muscle cells or fibers, although almost all cells have the capacity to change shape: (1) *striated skeletal muscle,* which contracts at will (so-called voluntary) and requires the participation of the somatic nervous system, (2) *striated cardiac muscle,* which contracts spontaneously (so-called involuntary), although the autonomic nervous system controls its rate of contractile activity, and (3) *smooth* or *plain* muscle, which also contracts spontaneously (involuntary) through the overall control of the autonomic nervous system.

The basic organization of each muscle type is considered first in this discussion, followed by light- and electron-microscopic structure, function, and molecular basis of contraction.

STRIATED SKELETAL MUSCLE

The study of muscle has had a long history. It began (from the histologic point of view) when Anton van Leeuwenhoek studied the muscle from fat and lean cows with his single-lens microscope in 1683. He was able to see *cross-striations,* which are characteristic of both skeletal and cardiac muscle (Fig. 5–1). It was not until 1840, however, that Bowman, a British physician, reported his microscopic studies of the structure and function of muscle. This early work is relevant today and is still the basis on which all structural-functional correlations have been developed.

Most striated muscle is associated with the skeleton, hence the term *skeletal muscle,* and it is concerned primarily with the movement of bony levers for skeletal movement. Striated muscle is also found in the tongue, upper pharynx, and esophagus, hence the term *visceral striated muscle.*

A muscle is composed of muscle cells or fibers that are variable in diameter, length, number of fibers, and internal structure, depending on the specific function for which the muscle was designed. Muscles designated as striated skeletal are associated, for the most part, with movement of skeletal parts or stabilization of the articulated skeleton. Muscle function may be highly refined and controlled (e.g., playing a violin, painting a picture, writing) or rather coarse (e.g., lifting heavy weights, running) (Fig. 5–2). These functions are a matter of muscle fiber internal architecture, number of fibers, and degree of control exercised by the nervous system. Although controlled by nerves activated by the will of the individual, some movements are involuntary or reflex in nature (e.g., the sudden withdrawal of one's hand when it touches a hot item, or the knee jerk when the patellar tendon is struck). Nerves carrying muscle-activating nerve impulses determine what kind of contraction will take place; a train of many impulses may result in a sustained (tetanic) contraction of variable force, whereas a single nerve impulse produces a brief (twitch) contraction of small force (Fig. 5–3).

Muscle fibers, surrounded by connective tissue and acting as a functional unit, are given specific names, such as latissimus dorsi and biceps. Their proper or specific name is usually descriptive. The examples just cited, when translated, are the broad flat muscle of the back and the two-headed muscle.

Histologic Organization of Skeletal Muscle

A skeletal muscle is a structurally definable unit composed of muscle fibers surrounded by connective tissue. A muscle has a blood supply and a nerve supply. The blood vessels enter and leave the organ after forming a profuse capillary network around individual muscle fibers (Fig. 5–4).

Striated skeletal muscle fibers do not function unless they have a nerve supply; if deprived of their nerve supply, they atrophy *(denervation atrophy).* Nerve fibers contact muscle fibers in specialized regions called motor end-plates (Fig. 5–5).

In addition, muscles that are prevented from shortening or contracting undergo *disuse atrophy.* This is readily seen in people who have recovered from broken bones. To allow broken bones to repair themselves, muscle activity is restricted, usually by a cast. Upon removal of the cast, the inactive muscle will be seen to be smaller by comparison with the active muscle on the normal side.

Sensory nerves in skeletal muscles emanate from muscle spindles and Golgi tendon organs. Muscle spindles sense muscle stretch or lengthening and control muscle length and the force that a muscle generates. The Golgi tendon organs measure tension development in the tendon, where force is transmitted by muscle fibers to cartilage, bone, or skin (Fig. 5–6).

Muscle fibers are longer than they are wide (i.e., asymmetric). The fibers are collected into fascicles

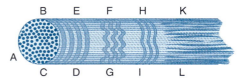

FIGURE 5–1. Muscle: early observation. *This drawing shows both cross and longitudinal striations (long axis) and solid rods in cross-section. These observations and this diagram by Leeuwenhoek were among the earliest histologic observations.*

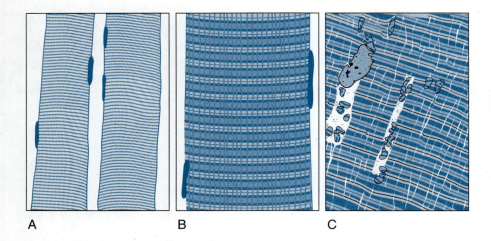

FIGURE 5–2. Muscle striations as seen with modern microscopes. A, Alternating dark and light bands can be seen. These are the A and I bands, respectively. B, Higher-magnification view on light microscopy shows the darker A band to be divided by a lighter band, or H zone, and the lighter I band to be divided by a thin dark line, the Z line. C, When seen with the electron microscope, the H zone is divided by a thin dark line, the M line. The other zone, bands, and lines remain the same as those in the middle frame. See also Figures 5–7 and 5–10.

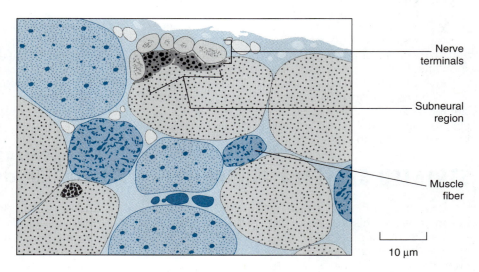

FIGURE 5–3. Muscle fiber types as seen with light microscopy at low magnification. Note that the largest fibers have the fewest and smallest dark spots, which are mitochondria revealed by a histochemical method. The so-called white muscle fibers, they are the fast-contracting fibers. Muscle fibers of middle size and with a greater number of mitochondria are intermediate muscle fibers; they contract more slowly than the larger white fibers. The smaller fibers with large spots are red muscle fibers, which they contract even more slowly than the intermediate fibers. Many muscles are composed of these three fiber types. Note the nerve terminals of a motor end-plate.

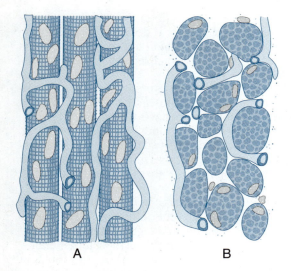

FIGURE 5–4. Muscle blood supply. Note the numerous blood capillaries, which lie in the interfiber connective tissue (endomysium). The capillaries supply muscle fibers with nutrients and oxygen and remove lactic acid and carbon dioxide and other waste products. A, Longitudinal section. B, Cross-section.

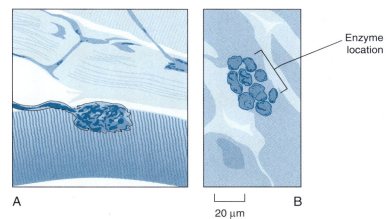

FIGURE 5–5. Muscle motor end-plate and subneural apparatus. A, A motor (excitatory) nerve arborizes and nerve terminals lie over a limited area of the muscle sarcolemma. B, As revealed by this histochemical reaction, acetylcholinesterase lies in the sarcolemma of the muscle fiber. The muscle fiber is activated when acetylcholine is released from the nerve terminals activating the muscle. The acetylcholine must be enzymatically broken down to prevent it from acting on the muscle.

(bundles), all of which have the same orientation or direction. When a fascicle of muscle fibers contracts (shortens), it exerts a force in one direction. A muscle is usually made up of many fascicles, and some of the fascicles may be oriented in more than one direction (like a fan); hence, a single muscle may be able to develop force in more than one direction (e.g., pectoralis major).

If a small piece is taken from a muscle fascicle and properly preserved and prepared for microscopic examination, the long and short axes of the constituent muscle fibers can be examined, and one can begin to appreciate how muscle structure defines function (contraction) (Fig. 5–7).

Light microscopy of thin slices (about 5 μm) of muscle fibers in their long (longitudinal) axis reveals numerous coarse fibrillar elements, the myofibrils that are banded or striated. Muscle fibers are multinucleated. In addition, connective tissue, blood vessels, nerve fibers, and muscle spindle sensory receptors can usually be recognized between the bundles (fascicles) of muscle fibers.

Three histologic arrangements of connective tissue are associated with striated skeletal muscle. The outermost covering is called the *epimysium;* it is this connective tissue that defines the functional unit called a muscle. Within the epimysium, the *perimysium* gathers together a number of muscle fibers, forming fascicles. Blood vessels and nerves that have passed through the epimysium are distributed to the fascicles in the perimysium (Fig. 5–8). The *endomysium* surrounds and is intimately associated with individual muscle fibers. It should be remembered that all three connective tissue elements or coverings are similar and are in continuity with one another, and that the force generated by the muscle must pass through all three.

Molecular Basis of Striations

The striations or bands result from the relative density (mass) of specific parts of the fibrillar structures called *myofibrils* (see Fig. 5–7). In noncontracted or relaxed muscle, the basic band pattern is alternating light and dark. This pattern was demonstrated by Bowman in 1840. Brucke, in 1858, demonstrated that the dark band was anisotropic and named it the *A band*. He also showed that the light-appearing, less dense band was isotropic and named it the *I band*. *Anisotropic* and *isotropic* refer to the internal molecular organization of the components of these specific regions of the myofibril. The A band is anisotropic because the

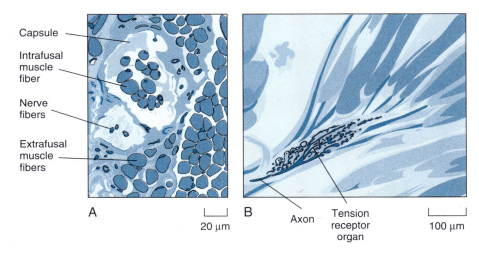

FIGURE 5–6. Muscle sensory receptors. A, Cross-section of a muscle spindle. The encapsulated receptors monitor muscle stretch and can react to this stimulus by inhibiting or reducing the extension of the muscle. B, A Golgi tendon organ monitors contraction or force development but does not have the ability to reduce excessive force.

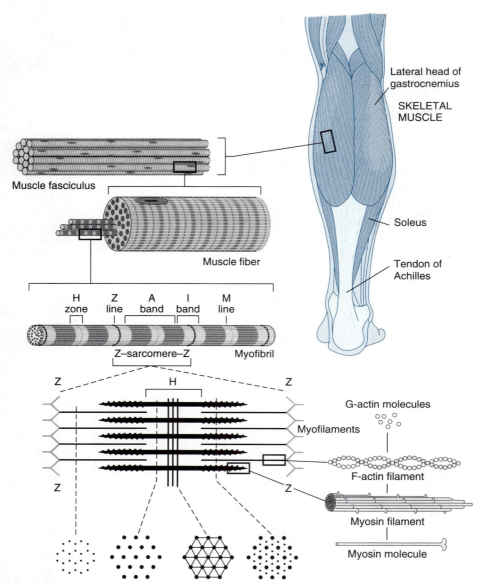

FIGURE 5–7. From muscle to molecules. *This diagram traces the component parts of a muscle to its molecular components and their topographical relationships. Muscle tissue is composed of muscle cells (termed* fibers*) collected into bundles, or fasciculi. Muscle fibers contain myofibrils within their cytoplasm, which in turn are composed of myofilaments of actin and myosin.*

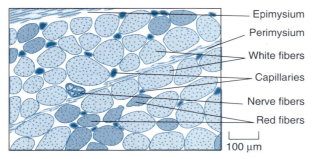

FIGURE 5–8. Muscle connective tissue and fiber types. *A small fascicle of striated muscle fibers in cross-section reveals a mixed composition of fiber types, both white and red. The outermost connective tissue investment of the muscle is termed the* epimysium. *Groups of muscle fibers are bounded by perimysium; the endomysium (not labeled) surrounds individual muscle fibers.*

molecular substructure of the region contains filaments that are asymmetric (they are longer than they are wide), arranged in an orderly pattern, and spaced closer together than the wavelength of light. Such molecular architecture restricts the passage of light rays except where they are oriented parallel to the elongated molecules within the A band. Because ordinary light rays radiate in all planes, most are restricted and cannot pass through the A bands, which thus appear dark. On the other hand, the I band regions are much less restrictive and appear light or bright under the same conditions of illumination (Fig. 5–9). The light-and-dark band pattern is enhanced by histologic staining methods (Fig. 5–10).

Closer inspection of the A band in noncontracted muscle reveals a zone of variable width in the middle, which is not as dark as the remainder of the band. Because it is relatively lightly stained and appears bright, it is known as the *H zone* (H from the German word *heller*, meaning "bright"). The H zone is also an area of reduced density of filamentous material within the A band. Similar inspection of the I band reveals a thin dark band across its middle known as the *Z line* (Z from the German word *Zwischenscheibe*, meaning "middle line"). This pattern of lines and bands—Z line, I band, A band, I band, Z line—occurs repetitively in the myofibril and is called the *sarcomere* (see Figs. 5–2 and 5–10).

Band Patterns in Contraction

If a muscle sample is permitted to shorten and is then fixed or preserved, the basic band pattern just described changes. The A bands remain constant in length but move toward the Z line, and the usually bright H zones narrow and may disappear, after which they become dark (reversal) and increase in length (Fig. 5–11). At the same time, the I bands become progressively narrower in length as the A bands approach each other, and, finally, the I bands completely disappear into the A bands. Contraction ends when the A bands strike the Z line barrier. The A bands now possess a dark central H zone, the I bands are entirely contained within the A bands, and the Z lines, a barrier to further shortening, appear to increase in density when maximum shortening has taken place. This appearance was seen by Bowman in 1840, and both the contracted and relaxed band patterns can usually be seen at the light-microscopic level when muscle is sectioned in the longitudinal axis of the muscle sample (Fig. 5–12).

It has been shown in some muscles that electrical stimulation at the level of the Z line causes two adjacent

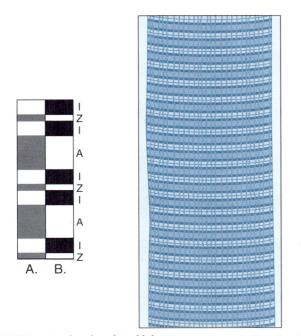

FIGURE 5–9. Muscle under polarized light. *Compare* A *and* B. *Note that the A band, which appears dark on conventional light microscopy* (A), *appears bright in cross-polarized light* (B); *the A band exhibits anisotrophy, and hence is called the A band. The I band appears bright on conventional light microscopy* (A) *but dark in cross-polarized light* (B); *the I band exhibits isotrophy, and hence is called the I band. The Z line also exhibits anisotrophy. Structures that can refract light have certain structural characteristics that provide clues to their internal or molecular structure.*

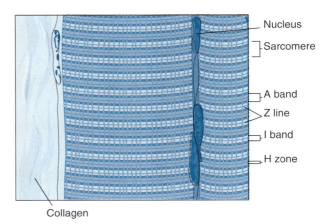

FIGURE 5–10. Definitive cross-bands of skeletal muscle. *Note the A and I bands, H zone, and Z lines. Two adjacent Z lines define a single sarcomere, with an identical band pattern being repeated more than 4545 times per cm. See also Fig. 5–7.*

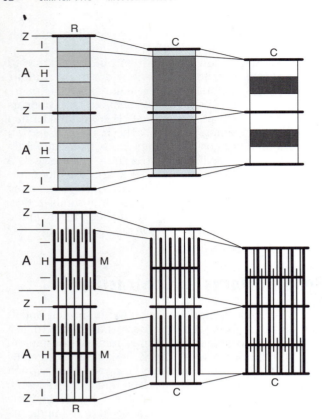

FIGURE 5-11. Muscle band patterns. *The appearance of band patterns and their density in skeletal muscle in relaxation and contraction. Top, The light-microscopic appearance of resting and contracting myofibrils. R, resting; C, contracted. Bottom, The corresponding arrangements of myofilaments within a sarcomere. In each case, the volume of the sarcomeres remains constant.*

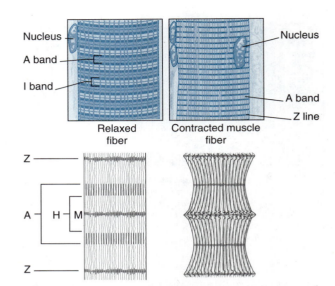

FIGURE 5-12. Relaxed and contracted muscle fibers. *The configuration of sarcomeres in relaxed and contracted myofibrils. Note that the Z line and M line are of equal width in relaxed fibers and that the Z line is wider than the M line in fully contracted myofibrils.*

A bands to move toward the Z line. No other position of the stimulating electrodes causes the bands to move or local contraction to occur. In other muscles, the only sensitive points are located at the level of the A band–I band junction, and here, only one A band moves to abut the Z line. Thus, there appear to be two fundamental (functional) units of contraction: (1) the symmetric movement of two A bands toward a Z line, which involves two half-sarcomeres, and (2) the movement of a single A band toward a Z line, which involves one half-sarcomere. For pragmatic reasons, the sarcomere is commonly, but incorrectly, called the functional unit of contraction.

Contracted muscle fibers and myofibrils are known to increase in width; the shortening is isovolumetric (no change in volume).

The molecular basis of contraction is discussed with the ultrastructure of striated muscle.

Structural-Functional Orientation

If a muscle is cut transversely (to the long axis), a so-called cross-section, the constituent muscle fibers appear as irregular polygons of variable size and number arranged in bundles or fascicles (see Figs. 5–3 and 5–8). Only immature or diseased muscle fibers are round in cross-section. These closely packed polygons are enclosed by a cell membrane, the *sarcolemma*, which defines the outside perimeter of the fiber (also recognized by Bowman in 1840). Within the polygons, numerous small, rounded subunits, the myofibrils, represent the cut ends of the elongated and banded structures seen in longitudinal section. They vary in size and number depending on the type of muscle fiber (Fig. 5–13).

Muscle nuclei, normally found beneath the sarcolemma (so-called subsarcolemmal or peripheral nuclei), are a diagnostic feature of healthy striated skeletal

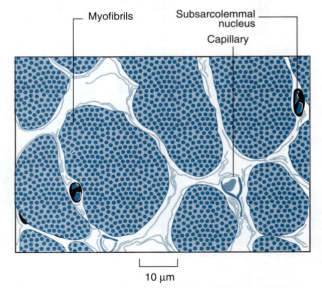

FIGURE 5-13. Skeletal muscle fibers in cross-section. *Muscle fibers in cross-section reveal myofilaments that constitute myofibrils. Note a key characteristic of skeletal muscle: the nuclei are subsarcolemmal in normal muscle fibers. In disease states, they may become central.*

muscle seen in cross-section and longitudinal section (also recognized by Bowman in 1840). In diseased muscle, for example, long rows of 20 to 100 subsarcolemmal nuclei or centrally located nuclei may be found.

In addition to the myofibrils, mitochondria, lipid droplets, glycogen, and a highly organized membranous system can be found. In order to see these structures, special fixatives (preservatives), stains, and histochemical procedures are employed (Figs. 5–14 to 5–16). These organelles are discussed later.

Fiber Type Heterogeneity (Red, White, and Intermediate)

Muscle fibers are not uniform in size, structure, or functional characteristics. There are two major muscle fiber types: one with a relatively large diameter (~ 100 μm) and the other consistently smaller (~ 20 μm). The large muscle fibers appear white (e.g., chicken breast muscle) because they have little *myoglobin,* an iron-containing protein structurally and functionally related to the hemoglobin of red blood cells. The *white muscle fibers* have small-diameter myofibrils and relatively few mitochondria, and they store glycogen (a polymer of glucose), which is used as the primary energy source by mitochondria. They contract and fatigue quickly and are designed for fast but brief bursts of muscular activity.

Small muscle fibers, on the other hand, are red because of the presence of myoglobin. They have large myofibrils and numerous mitochondria, and they store lipid droplets for use as their energy source. They contract slowly and are resistant to fatigue. Examples of *red muscle fibers* are the postural muscles (e.g., the soleus), which support the body in the upright position, and the breast muscles of birds, such as the pigeon and hawk, that excel in prolonged flight, unlike the chicken with its rapidly fatiguable white breast muscle.

Subtypes of red and white muscle fibers are

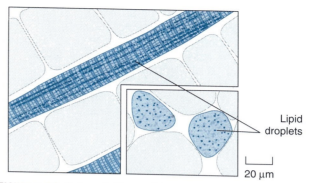

FIGURE 5–15. Red muscle fibers and high lipid content. *Red muscle fibers usually contain greater numbers of lipid droplets, which can be seen in these sections. White fibers store glycogen preferentially.*

known. The *intermediate* type has certain characteristics of the two main fiber types. Most muscles are a variable mixture of two or three fiber types (see Figs. 5–3, 5–8, 5–14, and 5–15). In the human, the red muscle fibers are known as *type I* and the white fibers as *type II,* terminology used in classifying muscle diseases.

Ultrastructure of Skeletal Muscle

By the late 1800s, the light-microscopic structure of muscle was well established, and some well-founded hypotheses concerning muscle ultrastructure had been proposed, particularly the fibrillar nature of the A bands. It was not until the middle 1900s, however, that muscle biochemistry and electron microscopy identi-

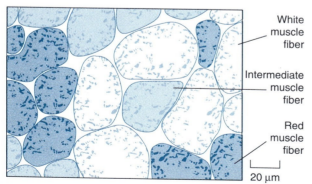

FIGURE 5–14. Red and white muscle fibers. *Red muscle fibers are darker than white muscle fibers, owing in part to the presence of myoglobin, which imparts a red color. Myoglobin is related to the hemoglobin of red blood cells and has the capacity to carry oxygen used in the cells' metabolic function. Red fibers have the capacity for sustained, slow contraction, whereas white fibers are designed for short-term, fast contractions. Intermediate types are also seen.*

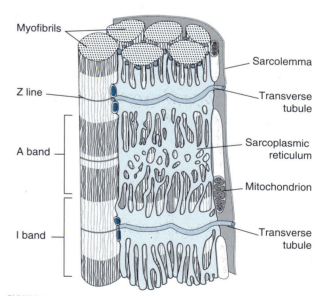

FIGURE 5–16. Muscle fibers: sarcoplasmic reticulum and transverse tubules. *The sarcoplasmic reticulum ensheaths each myofibril. The transverse tubules bring the sarcolemma into the muscle fiber, here, at the level of the Z line. In other skeletal muscles, the transverse tubules may be located at the A band–I band junction. The sarcoplasmic reticulum stores and releases calcium ions, and the transverse tubules carry excitatory impulses into the depth of the muscle fiber.*

fied the basic proteins and confirmed the filamentous nature of myofibrils. Subsequently, additional studies extended our understanding of the molecular nature of the contractile process.

The advent of electron microscopy permitted in-depth study of muscle structure. The myofibrils were found to contain two types of microfilaments: a "thick" (12 nm × 1.6 μm) type composed primarily of myosin and a "thin" (9 nm × 1.0 μm) type composed primarily of actin (see Fig. 5–7).

Molecular Basis of Striated Muscle Fiber

Thick filaments are composed of many myosin molecules, each with a molecular weight of about 480,000 daltons (Fig. 5–17). The myosin molecule is composed of six polypeptide chains, two so-called heavy chains (each with a molecular weight of about 200,000 daltons) and four light chains (each with a molecular weight of 20,000 daltons). The two heavy chains form a double helix. At one end of each of these chains, the molecule has a globular mass called the *myosin head*. There are two heads for each myosin molecule. The remainder of the molecule is called the *tail*. Two additional light chains are also considered part of the myosin head; hence, each myosin molecule has two globular heads and two light chains for each head. The light chains are thought to control the function of the head during the process of muscular contraction.

Composition of the Myosin Molecule and Thick Filament

Each myosin filament is composed of about 200 individual myosin molecules (see Fig. 5–17). The central molecules are joined by their tails at the middle of the filament, and the other molecules aggregate and extend outward in both directions for a distance of 0.8 μm. The total length of a single "thick" filament is 1.6 μm. The tails form the body of the myosin filament, with the heads and part of the tail (arms) extending outward from the sides of the body. The protruding arms and heads are called *cross-bridges*, and each of these is thought to be flexible at two places called *hinges*. The hinges are located at the point where the two heads are joined to the arms and where the arms join that part of the molecule forming the body of the filament. The hinged heads participate in the contractile process, and the hinged arms allow the cross-bridges to move outward from the body of the filament.

Although the total length of the myosin filament is

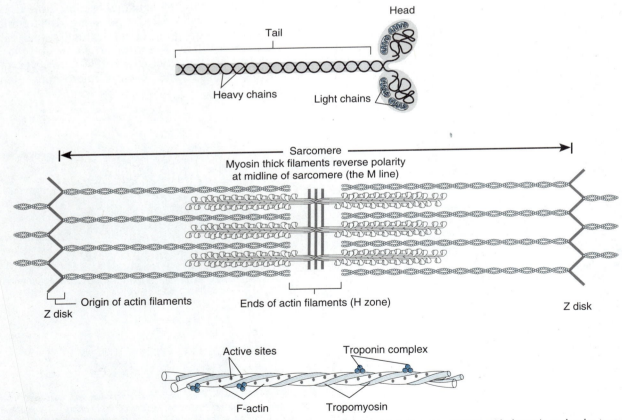

FIGURE 5–17. Muscle sarcomere. Top, *Myosin is composed of a head and a tail. The head is believed to interact with the actin molecules to produce movement.* Middle, *The myosin molecule composes the thick filaments found in the A band.* Bottom, *Actin is found extending from the Z line (or disk) through the so-called I band into the A band. The F-actin and the troponin and tropomyosin components may be seen. A sarcomere extends from Z line to Z line, as indicated on the middle illustration.*

1.6 μm, there are no cross-bridges in the center of the filament for a distance of about 0.2 μm, because the hinged arms extend from the body of the filament toward the two ends. The center, therefore, has only tails but no heads. The myosin molecules aggregate so that each successive set of cross-bridges is displaced axially from the previous set at an angle of 120 degrees. Hence, cross-bridges are placed strategically around the filament.

The head of the myosin molecule has another feature essential to the contractile process; the enzyme ATPase, which cleaves the terminal phosphate of ATP. This allows the energy derived from ATP's high-energy phosphate bond to be utilized for the contractile process.

Composition of the Thin Filament and Actin, Tropomyosin, and Troponin Molecules

The thin filament is slightly more than 1 μm long. Its base is attached to the Z line, and the other end protrudes into the A band, between the thick filaments, in a highly ordered manner (Figs. 5–17 and 5–18).

Thin filaments are composed of a double-stranded F-actin protein molecule, tropomyosin, and troponin. The backbone of these filaments is the double-stranded F-actin protein molecule wound in a helix with a complete revolution every 70 nm.

Each strand of the double F-actin helix is composed of polymerized G-actin molecules, which have a molecular weight of 42,000 daltons. There are about 13 molecules in each revolution of each strand of the helix. Attached to each one of the G-actin molecules is one molecule of ADP. It has been suggested that each of the ADP molecules is the active site on the actin (thin) filaments with which the cross-bridges of the myosin (thick) filaments interact to cause shortening. The active sites on the two F-actin strands of the double helix are staggered, with one active site on the overall actin filament about every 2.7 nm (see Fig. 5–17).

The thin filament contains two additional protein strands that are polymers of tropomyosin (see Fig. 5–17). Each has a molecular weight of 70,000 daltons and a length of 40 nm. It is thought that each tropomyosin strand is attached loosely to an F-actin strand and that, in the resting state, the tropomyosin strand physically covers the active sites of the actin strands so that no interaction between the thick and thin filaments may occur to cause contraction.

Attached approximately two thirds of the distance along each tropomyosin molecule is a complex of three globular protein molecules called *troponin*. One of the proteins (troponin I) has an affinity for actin, another (troponin T) for tropomyosin, and a third (troponin C) for calcium ions. This complex of three globular molecules is thought to attach tropomyosin to actin. The strong affinity of troponin for calcium ions is thought to initiate contraction.

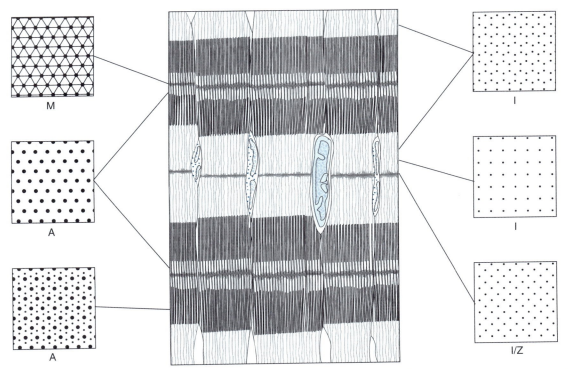

FIGURE 5–18. Molecular arrangement of muscle. Note how the configuration of the myosin (larger filaments) molecules, cut in cross-section, are arranged in the A band. Upper left, The M line, formed of three sets of bridging proteins, links the myosin filaments, which are in a hexagonal array. Middle left, This arrangement is clearly seen in the H zone, where at rest, only thick filaments can be found. Lower left, In the region of thick filament–thin filament overlap in the A band, the two sets of filaments are in a double hexagonal array. Upper right, Only thin (actin) filaments are seen in the I band in a hexagonal array. Middle right, The filaments are approaching the Z line, where they conform to a quadrilateral array. Lower right, Finally, at the Z line, the filaments form a double quadrilateral array.

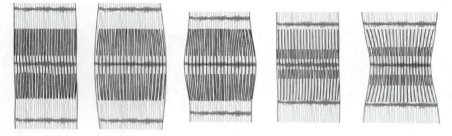

FIGURE 5–19. **Muscle contraction.** *Muscular contraction involves the symmetrical reduction of the I band, as the thin filaments are drawn into the A band and the Z lines strike the ends of the thick filaments. There is also an overall configurational change in the shape of the sarcomere. Stages seen from left to right, relaxed to fully contracted.*

Thin filaments are joined at the Z line, where each thin filament is joined to four thin filaments that emanate from the opposite side of the Z line. The Z line also is composed of the protein *desmin*. Desmin is found in all three types of muscle. It provides a cytoskeleton for the attachment and structural integration of contractile proteins at the Z line and the attachment of the Z line to the sarcolemma. In smooth muscle, desmin links together the dense bodies that are the structural equivalent of Z lines in striated muscles.

Interaction of Thick and Thin Filaments

In the presence of ATP and magnesium ions, a pure solution of myosin and actin binds to form actomyosin. When troponin and tropomyosin are added, actin and myosin do not bind. For contraction to occur (i.e., the interaction of actin and myosin), the influence of troponin and tropomyosin on this process must be negated.

Calcium ions negate the influence of troponin and tropomyosin by a mechanism that is not understood. It is known, however, that four calcium ions bind to troponin C, resulting in the "uncovering" of active sites on actin. This event allows the contraction process to begin.

Molecular Basis of Contraction

Contraction begins when calcium ions uncover active sites on the actin thin filaments, thus allowing the heads of cross-bridges of thick myosin filaments to interact with the active sites. The mechanism of the movement of the cross-bridge heads is not understood, but some movement of these heads must occur if there is to be relative movement between the thick and thin filaments.

It has been postulated that the cross-bridge heads alternately attach to and detach from the uncovered active sites on actin thin filaments. The heads probably move (tilt), resulting in what is known as the *power stroke*. After the movement, the heads detach from the active site after moving the site and the filaments forward. The detached head returns to its original position before re-attaching to a new site, where it will again move (tilt), and this process is repeated for as long as the muscle is excited to contract. The movement draws the thin filaments (I band) into the spaces between the thick filaments (A band) (Fig. 5–19).

Energetics for Contraction

When a muscle contracts against a load, work is performed. Energy is required for this process, and ATP is the energy source. During the contractile process, ATP molecules are cleaved enzymatically, resulting in the formation of ADP and inorganic phosphate (P_i).

Before contraction begins, it is thought, the heads of the myosin cross-bridges bind ATP, which is degraded enzymatically to ADP and P_i, and these degraded products remain bound to the head. In this state, the cross-bridge is prepared but does not become attached to actin because of the inhibitory effects of the troponin-tropomyosin complex. The inhibitory influence is abolished when calcium ions, released from the sarcoplasmic reticulum, flood into the interstices between the filaments (raising the concentration to a critical level), expose the "active sites" on the actin filament, and bind to the myosin heads (see Fig. 5–9).

The binding of the cross-bridge head to the "active site" and the subsequent tilting of the head unidirectionally toward the arm of the cross-bridge or the middle of the myosin filament (or *M line*) is called the power stroke. It moves the actin filament toward the middle of the A band (Fig. 5–20). The energy for this movement is supplied by the breakdown of ATP.

After the power stroke, ADP and P_i are released and reconverted to ATP, and another molecule of ATP is bound, resulting in the detachment of the cross-bridge from the actin filament. In the absence of ATP (e.g., after death), the cross-bridges remain bound to the actin filament, and the condition known as *rigor mortis* occurs (Fig. 5–21).

Calcium is actively returned to the sarcoplasmic reticulum, lowering its concentration in the cytosol, and

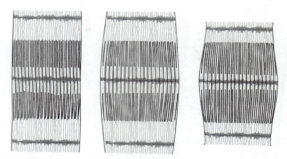

FIGURE 5–20. **Isometric muscle contraction.** *In isometric contraction the muscle length is held constant, but the shape of the contracting sarcomeres (middle and right) appears barrel-shaped compared with the cylindrical appearance of the resting sarcomere (left).*

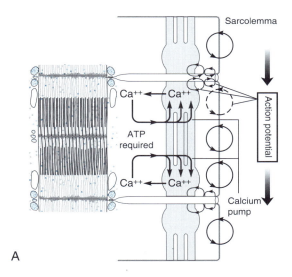
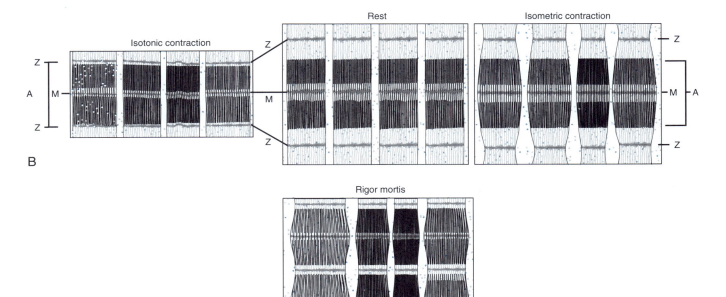

*FIGURE 5-21. **Muscular contraction and rigor mortis.** A, An activating stimulus (action potential) is carried into a muscle fiber by means of the transverse tubules. At the level of the sarcoplasmic reticulum, the stimulus causes release of stored calcium ions. The released calcium ions catalyze the breakdown of ATP by myosin-ATPase, thus releasing the energy to move the two sets of filaments in relation to each other. When the stimulus ceases, calcium is re-sequestered, and relaxation (withdrawal of actin filaments from the A band) takes place. B, Note the configurational changes that occur in sarcomeres during isotonic and isometric contractions. C, Note the configuration of sarcomeres in rigor mortis, in which it is believed thick and thin filaments are "locked" in their fully interactive state; all cross-bridges from the myosin molecules are linked to adjacent actin filaments. Rigor mortis occurs in the absence of ATP.*

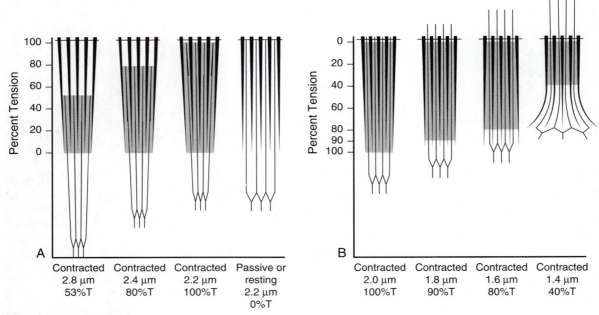

FIGURE 5–22. Contraction of half-sarcomere. *Myosin/actin filaments overlap, and the force development (Tension) at various sarcomere lengths, together with the configurational changes (shown here in half-sarcomeres) that accompany the force development, are shown. A, Isotonic contraction. B, Isometric contraction.*

the "active sites" are again covered (Fig. 5–21). Once the head has detached, its newly bound molecule of ATP is split. The head binds to another "active site" made available by the release of calcium ions from the sarcoplasmic reticulum, tilts, and, as before, draws the actin filament forward. This process continues as long as the fiber is activated to contract, or until the A band strikes the Z line and contraction stops. This type of activity is called *isotonic contraction* (Figs. 5–19 to 5–22).

If the load the muscle is to support equals the force generated by the cross-bridges, the muscle does not shorten, but the load is supported; this is called *isometric contraction* (Figs. 5–20 and 5–22). When this load is to be released, a decrease in the number of active sites occurs, and the load is lowered slowly. The number of active sites decreases as a result of the decrease in the frequency of the excitatory stimuli delivered to the muscle fiber.

STRIATED CARDIAC MUSCLE

Striated cardiac muscle differs from striated skeletal muscle in four important ways, although the contractile proteins and striations are similar (Fig. 5–23):

- Cardiac muscle fibers are shorter than skeletal muscle fibers, and they branch and join each other end-to-end, end-to-side, or side-to-side, forming sheets rather than bundles or fascicles of fibers.
- The junctions between successive muscle fibers are uniquely cardiac and are called *intercalated disks*. They run transversely across the fiber and are complex specializations of the sarcolemma that join adjacent fibers and form a complex network of interconnected muscle fibers.

The nuclei are always centrally located in cardiac muscle fibers, rather than peripherally located beneath the sarcolemma as in skeletal muscle fibers (Fig. 5–24).

- Cardiac muscle fibers contract spontaneously but are under the control of the autonomic nervous system, not individual will. The sympathetic com-

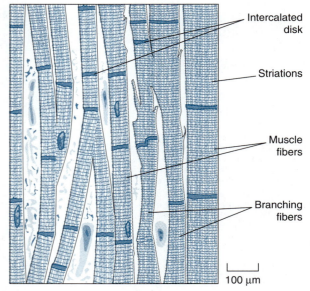

FIGURE 5–23. Cardiac muscle. *Note the characteristic branching muscle fibers with centrally located nuclei. An additional characteristic of cardiac muscle is the presence of intercalated disks.*

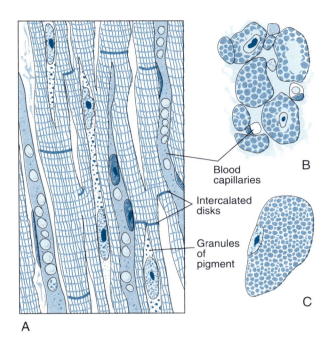

FIGURE 5–24. Cardiac muscle. A, Note the blood vessels between branching cardiac muscle fibers. B, Note the centrally located nuclei in cardiac muscle. C, By contrast, in a skeletal muscle, the muscle nuclei are always found beneath the sarcolemma (peripherally), except when the muscle is diseased.

ponent of the autonomic nervous system increases the rate of the contraction-relaxation cycle, whereas the parasympathetic component slows the heart rate. In addition, norepinephrine secreted by the adrenal medulla increases the rate of cardiac muscle contraction.

Functional Architecture of Fibers

Cardiac muscle fibers have a cell membrane or sarcolemma similar to that of skeletal muscle, with certain exceptions. Cardiac fibers have more mitochondria than skeletal muscle fibers (40% versus 2% of cell volume, respectively), a less elaborate sarcoplasmic reticulum, more lipid, and less glycogen. They also have more myoglobin than most skeletal muscle fibers. Heart muscle contracts more slowly than skeletal muscle. These differences are functionally important, because cardiac fibers have a lifetime of sustained rhythmic contractile activity, unlike other muscle fibers. The A and I bands, H zone, and M and Z lines are identical with those of skeletal muscle. One or two euchromatic nuclei are found in cardiac fibers, whereas many times that number are found in skeletal muscle fibers. Because cardiac fiber nuclei are centrally located, myofibrils diverge around the nuclear region and form a conical area on either pole of the nucleus or nuclei. Several important organelles are found in this area, including a small Golgi complex, ribosomes, and vesicles of the agranular reticulum. In older individuals, lipofuscin pigment granules also may be found within the conical area.

The myofibrils outlining the nuclear region in cardiac muscle are poorly delineated compared with those in skeletal muscle, because they are unusually large and the sarcoplasmic reticulum is not as highly developed. As a result, mitochondria, elements of the sarcoplasmic reticulum, lipid droplets, and glycogen appear embedded within the myofilaments of the contractile apparatus when cross-sections of cardiac muscle are examined by electron microscopy.

The mitochondria are large and long and are located throughout the myofibrillar mass in the long axis of the cardiac muscle fiber. They commonly are intimately associated with lipid droplets at their distal ends. Mitochondria constitute 30% to 40% of the cell volume. Because of their size and linear arrangement, they provide an illusion of units, similar to myofibrils, when thin sections of cardiac muscle are studied. This type of organization of the contractile apparatus is seen in some skeletal muscles, for example, the soleus muscle, a postural muscle that is continuously active when one is in the upright position. Like cardiac muscle, the soleus muscle is deep red and contracts slowly. Soleus muscle fibers contain myoglobin in significant quantity; one should remember here that myoglobin is related to hemoglobin and stores oxygen for use in metabolic activity.

Glycogen is seen in electron micrographs as 40-nm granules; its more general distribution is best demonstrated when cardiac muscle is stained with the periodic acid–Schiff (PAS) stain. Although glycogen granules are not abundant, they fill the interstices between the mitochondria, sarcoplasmic reticulum, and other spaces and the myofilaments of the contractile apparatus. Glycogen granules may also be seen between myofilaments in the I band, H zone, and M line (Fig. 5–25).

Excitation-Contraction Coupling: The T System and Sarcoplasmic Reticulum

The sarcolemma or cell membrane invaginates to form tubular structures, so-called *T tubules*, at the level of the Z line, similar to some skeletal muscle fibers. These T tubules (transverse tubules) contain extracellular fluid and are generally larger than those seen in skeletal muscle fibers. The invaginations also possess an external glycoprotein layer, which covers the entire sarcolemma. The T tubules bring the sarcolemma and the extracellular "space" to the interior of the fiber, so that no part of the fiber is more than a few microns from the extracellular space. The T tubules carry the excitatory impulses (propagated depolarizations) into the interior of the cardiac fiber, where they effect the release of calcium ion from the sarcoplasmic reticulum.

Although the sarcoplasmic reticulum in cardiac muscle fibers is not as highly organized as that found in most skeletal muscle fibers, it carries out the same function and is suited to the activity of the heart. The reticulum is plexiform and lies in narrow clefts within the mass of the contractile apparatus. Each functional

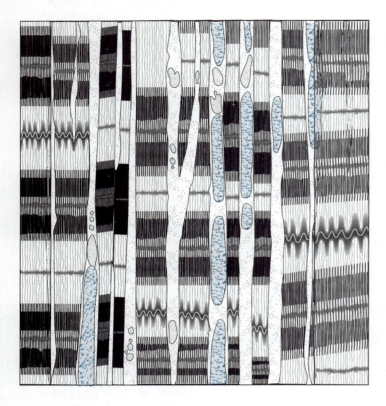

FIGURE 5–25. Cardiac muscle as seen by electron microscopy. *Except for branching and the presence of intercalated disks, the striations look like those in skeletal muscle. Intercalated disks incorporate variations of the sarcolemma: typical sarcolemma anchors Z line elements (ends of the myofibrils); gap junctions carry the excitation of one cardiac muscle fiber to its neighbor; and desmosomal contacts provide adhesion between fibers.*

unit of sarcoplasmic reticulum is located between Z lines and terminates distally as small dilated sacs on the T tubules located at the Z line. The terminal cysternae are not aligned opposite other cysternae as they are in skeletal muscle; hence, they are called *diads* (a terminal expansion of the sarcoplasmic reticulum opposite a T tubule) rather than the triads found in skeletal muscle. Although the intrafiber membrane system is less extensive than that found in most skeletal muscle fibers, it is scaled to fit the needs of the cardiac muscle fiber. It is the function of the sarcoplasmic reticulum to release calcium ion when the reticulum is depolarized via its T tubules and to resequester calcium ion when the excitation ceases.

Unlike skeletal muscle fibers, which extend from tendon to tendon over relatively long distances, cardiac muscle fibers are small and branched; they are joined at their distal ends and side branches to form sheets or layers of fibers. They are 80 to 110 µm in length and about 15 to 20 µm in diameter.

Intercalated Disks

A distinguishing feature of cardiac muscle relates to how adjacent fibers are structurally and functionally linked together. On light microscopy, the interfiber junctions stain more heavily than other parts of the fiber. These so-called intercalated disks are not straight but appear to cross cardiac fibers stepwise; however, they are always located at the level of the Z line. At the macromolecular level, the opposing ends of adjacent muscle fibers are composed of corresponding projections, pits, grooves, and ridges forming complex junctions between muscle fibers that stain densely by light-microscopic techniques. At the electron-microscopic level, however, several important components of the fiber-to-fiber interface can be identified (see Figs. 5–23 to 5–25).

The first is the *desmosome* (zonula adherens of epithelial junctions), which keeps adjacent fibers joined together. The second specialization is the *fascia adherens*, one half of a Z line, from which thin or actin filaments of the sarcomere emanate. It is the distal end of the contractile apparatus of a cardiac fiber. The third component is the *gap junction*, which functionally links adjacent fibers by providing areas of low electrical resistance (Fig. 5–26). Gap junctions allow the rapid and systematic spread of excitatory impulses from cell to cell, throughout the entire myocardium as though it were one large cellular syncytium.

Fiber Heterogeneity

Although the muscle fibers of the heart are generally similar in structure, some very important regional differences have been detected by both light and electron microscopy. The cardiac fibers forming the atria are generally smaller in diameter than those of the ventricles and appear to require or to have fewer T tubules and sarcoplasmic reticulum elements. A noteworthy difference, however, is the presence of granules located specifically in atrial fibers. The granules are round, dense, and membrane bound. They are 3.5 µm in diameter and are typically found in the sarcoplasm at the ends of the nuclei near a small Golgi complex. These atrial granules contain two polypeptide hor-

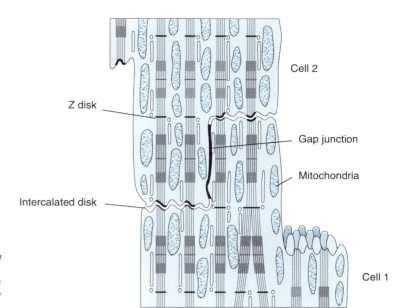

FIGURE 5-26. Intercalated disk. *The intercalated disk is formed when the sarcolemma traverses the cardiac muscle fiber. Note the changes in its structure that permits its identification as an intercalated disk. Note the gap junction between two cardiac fibers.*

mones: *cardionatrin,* a diuretic that stimulates the excretion of sodium ions by the kidneys (natriuretic effect), and *cardiodilatin,* which causes the smooth muscle of blood vessels to relax resulting in vasodilation.

The polypeptide-containing granules appear to be more abundant in the right atrium than in the left. Atrial fibers, unlike ventricular fibers, are considered to have a contractile function as well as a myoendocrine function.

Myocardial Pacemakers and Stimuli-Conducting Fibers

The heterogeneity of the myocardium also includes a system of fibers that carry stimuli from specific pacemaker areas of the heart to more distal areas to initiate meaningful function of the heart as a pump. The system consists of three parts: the sinoatrial node (Keith-Flack node), the atrioventricular node (node of Tawara), and the atrioventricular bundle (His's bundle).

The sinoatrial node is found in the epicardium at the junction of the superior vena cava and the right atrium. The nodal fibers are indistinguishable from ordinary atrial myocardium, with which they are continuous via intercalated disks. These fibers ultimately join with those forming the atrioventricular node.

The atrioventricular node is composed of highly branched myocardial muscle fibers located beneath the endocardium in the lower part of the right interatrioventricular septum, near the ostium of the coronary sinus and the septal leaf of the tricuspid valve (Fig. 5-27).

The nodal fibers are continuous with long, narrow (8 to 10 μm), unbranched bundle fibers that enter the fibrous part of the interventricular septum, where they divide into the right and left ventricular branches. These bundle fibers form an extensive plexus beneath the endocardium, where they join a group of very large fibers of distinctive structure known as Purkinje fibers (Figs. 5-28 and 5-29). Purkinje fibers have few myofibrils and one or two nuclei and are rich in mitochondria and glycogen. It is Purkinje fibers that join the ordinary ventricular muscle fibers, thereby completing the linkage of the heart as a functional whole.

Nodal muscle fibers are richly supplied by parasympathetic and sympathetic nerve fibers. The parasympathetic vagal preganglionic nerve fibers synapse with postganglionic cells within the heart, which ultimately innervate the nodal muscle fibers to regulate the rate at which excitatory impulses leave the node. The innervating nerve fibers of the sympathetic nervous system are postganglionic and do not synapse in the heart. The parasympathetic system slows the heart rate, and the sympathetic system accelerates it.

The nerve terminals on nodal fibers are different from those found on skeletal muscle fibers. The terminals are slender, nonmyelinated axons that pass over the surface of the nodal muscle fibers. These axons possess numerous vesicles similar to those found in the nerve terminals at the motor end-plates of skeletal muscle and at synapses in the central nervous system.

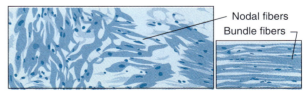

FIGURE 5-27. Atrioventricular node. *Exceptional branching of cardiac fibers in all directions in the wall of the atrium near the opening and valve of the coronary sinus locates the atrioventricular node. The nodal cardiac fibers join unbranched, small (7 to 9 μm) muscle fibers, which form the atrioventricular bundle fibers. The bundle fibers are next joined to Purkinje fibers in the interventricular septum, and finally, Purkinje fibers are joined to ordinary cardiac fibers by intercalated disks.*

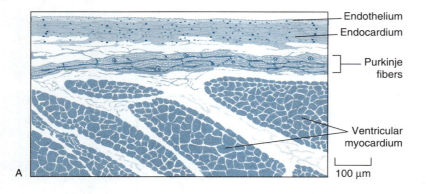

FIGURE 5–28. Cardiac muscle Purkinje fibers. *A, Purkinje fibers, located beneath the endocardium, are characterized by their large size and their seemingly empty sarcoplasms containing few myofibrils. The sarcoplasm usually contains large amounts of stored glycogen stainable by the PAS reaction. B, Purkinje fibers ultimately join ordinary cardiac muscle fibers near the apex of the heart to spread excitatory impulses.*

SMOOTH MUSCLE

Smooth muscle fibers are distributed widely throughout the body. They are found in the digestive system and associated glands and are essential for moving digesting food and secretory products of glands along the digestive tract (Fig. 5–30). In the reproductive tract, smooth muscle fibers move sperm, ova, and the mature fetus. They are found in the walls of the respiratory tract from the trachea to the alveoli. In the skin, smooth muscle fibers raise hair, wrinkle the scrotum, and cause erection of the nipple (Fig. 5–31). In the iris, they constrict and dilate the pupil; in the ciliary muscle, they adjust the tension on the lens.

Smooth muscle fibers are fusiform (Fig. 5–32). They are generally small but relatively long in respect to their cross-sectional diameter. They range widely in size from about 0.5 mm to 20 μm in length and are about 10 μm in diameter. Unlike other smooth muscle fibers, those of the uterus are under the influence of hormones that increase their size and functional activity. In the pregnant uterus, smooth muscle fibers hypertrophy to become the largest smooth muscle fibers in

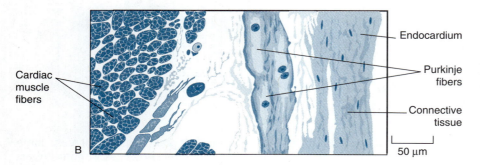

FIGURE 5–29. Purkinje fibers and ordinary cardiac fibers. *In both Purkinje fibers and ordinary cardiac fibers, the muscle nuclei are located centrally, within the sarcoplasm of the muscle fiber. A, Purkinje fibers. B, Purkinje fibers in cross-section. C, Ordinary cardiac fibers.*

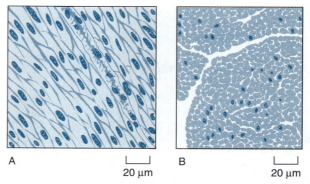

FIGURE 5–30. Smooth, nonstriated muscle. *Smooth muscle fibers are found in layers or bundles in blood vessels, the digestive tract, and skin. In these small, unbranched, elliptical muscle fibers, the nuclei are centrally located. A, Longitudinal section. B, Cross-section.*

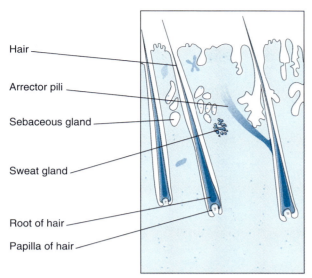

FIGURE 5–31. Skin muscle. The arrector pili muscle is a small bundle of smooth muscle fibers that cause piloerection. Hair is pulled into the erect position in situations of fear ("hair-raising" situations) and in cold weather. The arrector pili muscle is smooth muscle, except in the tenrec (a small mammal of Madagascar), in which certain specialized hairs (used for communication) have striated skeletal muscle arrector pili muscles; this is the only known exception.

the body; they are the smallest in small blood vessels. Each fiber is surrounded by a basal lamina and a fibrous network composed of reticular fibers (type III collagen) (Fig. 5–33). Each smooth muscle fiber has a single centrally located nucleus and, in the sarcoplasm at each nuclear pole, mitochondria, free ribosomes, elements of both ribosome-studded and smooth endoplasmic reticula, a pair of centrioles, and a small Golgi complex.

Smooth muscle fibers generally are arranged in concentric sheets and are tightly packed except in the skin, where small bundles are associated with hair follicles. Because the fibers are fusiform (thick in the middle and tapered at the ends), they are arranged so that the middle or thickest part of one fiber is adjacent to the thin distal end of adjacent fibers. Hence, when

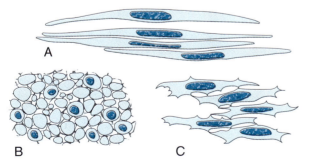

FIGURE 5–32. Smooth muscle; intercellular contacts. Smooth muscle fibers are generally described as elliptical or cigar-shaped. The electron microscope has revealed numerous areas of membrane contacts (gap junctions) between smooth muscle cells. It is through these gap junctions that excitation is spread from cell to cell. A, Idealized smooth muscle fiber. B, Smooth muscle in cross-section. C, Smooth muscle fibers normally exhibit processes that contact adjacent fibers.

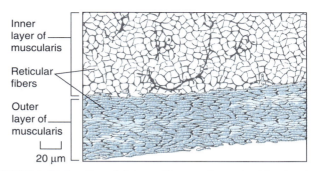

FIGURE 5–33. Smooth muscle in layers. The smooth muscle of the digestive tract is arranged in two layers. Centrally (inner layer), it is circularly arranged, as shown here in cross-section. The outer layer is longitudinally arranged, and here is seen cut in the long axis of the cell. The cells are held together by a connective tissue network of reticular fibers.

viewed in cross-section, the fibers are tightly packed, and profiles of variable diameter are seen (Fig. 5–34).

As with skeletal and cardiac muscle fibers, smooth muscle fibers contract and become shorter and thicker (Fig. 5–35). There are no highly ordered arrays of permanent filaments, such as are seen in the myofibrils of skeletal and cardiac muscle. The filaments are transient. When seen by electron microscopy, they criss-cross obliquely through the sarcoplasm and join the plasmalemma (sarcolemma). The thinner filaments are about 6 nm in diameter and are composed of actin and tropomyosin; the thicker filaments are about 15 nm and are composed of myosin. The thinner filaments are joined to so-called *dense bodies* found within the sarcoplasm. The dense bodies apparently serve the same function as Z lines in skeletal and cardiac muscle fibers. Desmin, an intermediate filament, is found in both the Z line and dense bodies. When contraction occurs, there is relative movement of actin and myosin in opposite directions owing to cross-bridge action. The force generated is transmitted from the dense bodies to the sarcolemma and to the connective tissue associated with the fiber and muscle mass.

It is thought that the level of calcium ion in the cytosol controls the contraction of smooth muscle, but unlike in skeletal and cardiac muscle, troponin is not the site of control. Troponin is not even a component of the contractile mechanism in smooth muscle. It is thought that contraction is initiated by myosin light-chain phosphorylation. One of the two myosin light chains is phosphorylated and controls the interaction of actin and myosin. The phosphorylation is catalyzed by the enzyme myosin light-chain kinase, whose action depends on the binding of calcium ions to calmodulin. As a result, contraction is controlled by the level of cytosolic calcium. It is thought that phosphorylation occurs slowly, causing contraction to occur slowly. The myosin of smooth muscle hydrolyzes ATP about one tenth as fast as that of skeletal muscle, yielding a slow cross-bridge cycle. Smooth muscle is therefore designed for slow contraction sustained over considerable time but hydrolyzing significantly less ATP than skeletal muscle would hydrolyze over the same time.

Intermediate filaments, 10 nm in diameter, course

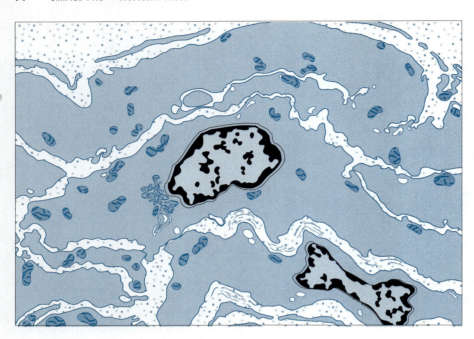

FIGURE 5–34. Smooth muscle. *At the level of the electron microscope, the highly irregular surface of the smooth muscle cell is seen. Although some intercellular contacts may be tenuous, others are actually gap junctions, a region of sarcolemma specialized for intercellular transmission of excitatory stimuli.*

throughout the cytoplasm of smooth muscle fibers. Desmin is the major protein in intermediate filaments that links together the dense bodies in the sarcoplasm. Vimentin also occurs in the intermediate filaments of vascular smooth muscle.

Molecular Basis of Smooth Muscle Function

Smooth muscle function is controlled by a variety of stimuli, including those arising from the autonomic nervous system and several hormones. Epinephrine increases cyclic AMP levels and induces phosphorylation by myosin light-chain kinase, which reduces the affinity of the kinase for the calcium ion–calmodulin complex; light-chain kinase phosphorylation is thus inhibited, and smooth muscle fibers relax. The action of hormones on uterine smooth muscle is also of interest. Estrogen not only initiates the hypertrophy of smooth muscle but also increases cyclic AMP activity and promotes the phosphorylation of myosin and the subsequent contractile activity of the muscle. On the other hand, progesterone decreases cyclic AMP activity and promotes the dephosphorylation of myosin, thereby inhibiting contractile activity.

Nerve Supply

Smooth muscle is innervated by both sympathetic and parasympathetic nerves of the autonomic nervous system (Fig. 5–36). There are no motor end-plates similar to those seen in skeletal muscle. Autonomic nerve fibers commonly terminate in a series of dilatations of axons in the endomysial connective tissue. These dilatations possess vesicles containing either acetylcholine or norepinephrine. Because the nerve endings (dilatations) are a variable distance from the muscle fibers, their excitation depends on diffusion through the endomysium to reach the muscle fibers.

There are two basic types of smooth muscle fibers, visceral (i.e., functionally syncytial) and vascular (i.e., functionally unitary). Visceral fibers are functionally linked together by gap junctions that permit ionic interchange between muscle fibers and the transmission of excitatory impulses from fiber to fiber. The activity is rhythmic, peristaltic, and tonic, all characteristic of the smooth muscle in the digestive system. Vascular fibers are activated by axons of the autonomic nervous system

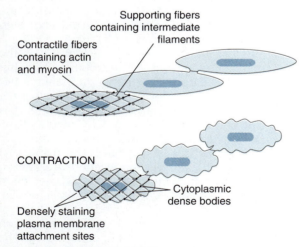

FIGURE 5–35. Smooth muscle contraction. *Smooth muscle is usually a very slowly contracting muscle. The arrangement of proteins of muscular contraction is not as orderly as that in skeletal and cardiac muscle. Nevertheless, the myosin and actin filaments interact in a similar fashion, and the force developed is directed to small patches of what is considered Z line protein. The Z line protein is both intracellular and located on the sarcolemma of the fibers. Contraction therefore makes the fiber shorter and thicker, resulting in muscle shortening.*

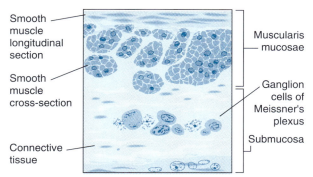

FIGURE 5-36. Smooth muscle of digestive tract. Smooth muscle of the muscularis mucosae and ganglion cells of Meissner's nerve plexus are seen. These nerve cells initiate muscular contraction, but the transmission of the excitatory impulses is from smooth muscle cell to smooth muscle cell, through gap junctions.

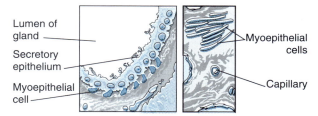

FIGURE 5-37. Myoepithelial cells. Myoepithelial cells are found in relation to certain secretory cells. Their function appears to be to express the viscous contents of glandular secretion to and through the ducts of the gland.

that regulate the size of blood vessel lumens, thereby controlling blood movement and pressure.

MYOEPITHELIAL CELLS

All cells show some capacity to change shape. This capacity depends on the cytoskeleton, which is a complex network of protein filaments that extends throughout the cytoplasm. The epithelium known as *myoepithelium* is intimately associated with glands. Myoepithelial cells encompass acini and ducts and appear to aid in the discharge of viscid secretory products through their contractile activity (Fig. 5-37).

Myosin is present in nearly all cells but is found as preformed thick filaments only in skeletal and cardiac muscle. Myosin molecules in smooth muscle and nonmuscle cells form smaller filaments of myosin for contractile activity. The molecular aggregation of myosin depends on its phosphorylation by myosin light-chain kinase, which affects the ATPase activity of the myosin and its ability to assemble into functional units. Dephosphorylated myosin becomes soluble, and filaments disappear.

Transient myosin assembly is important for cell division in nonmuscle cells, because it forms a contractile ring that constricts the middle of the cell, leading to cleavage into two cells.

Contraction in smooth muscle and nonmuscle cells is triggered by an increase of calcium ion in the cytosol. In these cells, troponin is absent, and calcium binds with calmodulin, a calcium-binding protein. The calcium-calmodulin complex activates myosin light-chain kinase, the enzyme that effects the phosphorylation of myosin, resulting in the assembly of myosin filaments and contractile activity.

CHAPTER SIX

BLOOD CELLS

AND

HEMATOPOIESIS

RED BLOOD CELLS 97

WHITE BLOOD CELLS 98
    Agranulocytes 99
    Granulocytes 100

PLATELETS 102

BLOOD PLASMA 103

ORIGIN OF BLOOD CELLS 103
    Erythropoiesis 103
    Granulocytic Development 105
    Megakaryocytopoiesis 108

GROWTH FACTORS 108

Peripheral blood is a dynamic organ in which cell production is under homeostatic control and the number of each cell type is maintained within a relatively narrow range.

Blood is a connective tissue whose matrix is fluid. It is composed of red corpuscles (erythrocytes), white cells (leukocytes), platelets, and plasma. It is estimated that a 150-lb (68.2-kg) adult has about 5 liters of blood. Blood is transported throughout the body within blood vessels. When blood is taken out of the body, as in venipuncture, it undergoes clotting (coagulation) unless the container in which it is kept contains an anticoagulant, such as heparin. The supernatant–clear, yellow fluid–of coagulated blood is called *serum*. *Plasma* is the term used to describe the supernatant fluid obtained upon centrifugation of whole blood. Below the plasma is a thin layer of cells (leukocytes and platelets) and a larger compartment of cellular elements (erythrocytes). The erythrocyte compartment represents approximately 43% to 45% of the blood volume. The thin layer of leukocytes and platelets interposed between the erythrocytes below and the plasma above constitutes about 1% of blood volume and is known as the *buffy coat*.

RED BLOOD CELLS

Red blood cells are also known as *erythrocytes* or *red blood corpuscles*. In humans, mature red blood corpuscles do not contain a nucleus and are therefore incomplete cells. They are incapable of cell division, or reproduction, and of self-maintenance and have very little metabolic activity. Red corpuscles are usually biconcave discs, but they are flexible and can bend and fold depending on specific circumstances as they circulate throughout the body. The biconcave shape favors the rapid absorption and release of oxygen and carbon dioxide by providing a large ratio of surface to volume. Absence of a nucleus allows additional room for the carrier protein hemoglobin, which also facilitates respiratory function.

Circulating red blood corpuscles average about 8.0 μm, whereas in dried blood smears, they are approximately 7.5 μm (Fig. 6–1). In fixed and sectioned tissues, red blood cells may shrink further, but they can still be regarded as roughly 6 μm for estimating internal size of cells and other structures, because of their widespread histologic availability. In human males, there are about 5.5 million red blood corpuscles per mm^3 of blood. In females, the number is about 5.0 million per mm^3.

Massed red blood corpuscles are red because of the presence of the respiratory pigment hemoglobin. Mature red blood corpuscles are membrane bound and normally devoid of a nucleus, nucleolus, cell organelles, and inclusions.

The membrane of an erythrocyte contains lipids, proteins, and carbohydrates. About half of the proteins are integral membrane proteins. One such integral membrane protein, glycophorin, is the determinant of the MN blood group. The ABO blood group is determined by oligosaccharide sugars on membrane glycoproteins and glycolipids. Peripheral proteins such as spectrin and actin serve to form the shape of the erythrocyte and, in association with other membrane proteins, contribute to the changes in the shape of erythrocytes when they pass through capillary walls. A small number (about 0.5% to 1.5%) of immature but circulating red blood corpuscles *(reticulocytes)* contain ribonucleoprotein (RNA) in the form of ribosomes. Because of their RNA content, they can be stained with nuclear dyes such as brilliant cresyl blue; the RNA appears as a reticular network, hence the name reticulocyte (Fig. 6–2). A circulating reticulocyte proportion in excess of 1% signals a demand for an increase in oxygen-carrying capacity, owing perhaps to hemorrhage, to a change in altitude above sea level, or to pathologic changes in the vital capacity of the lungs. It is well established that the life span of red blood corpuscles is approximately 120 days. This means that about 25×10^{10} corpuscles are replaced daily, a turnover rate of 2.5 million per second. Both damaged and normal but "worn out" erythrocytes are removed from the vascular system by macrophages, which are found primarily in the liver, spleen, and bone marrow. Breakdown products of hemoglobin are used in the formation of bile (bilirubin), and the iron is conserved and used to produce new red cells.

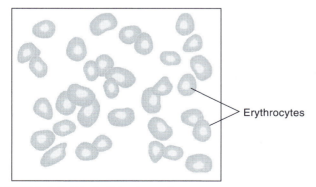

FIGURE 6–1. Red blood cells (erythrocytes). Usually biconcave and circular, erythrocytes are devoid of a nucleus when mature. Their number varies between 5 and 5.5 million per mm^3.

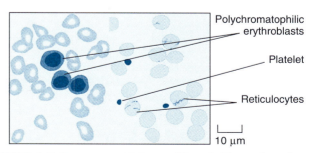

FIGURE 6–2. Bone marrow: polychromatophilic erythroblasts and reticulocytes, blood platelets. Polychromatophilic erythroblasts *(rubricytes)* are derived from basophilic erythroblasts *(prorubricytes)* (see Fig. 6–11). *Reticulocytes* are immature red blood cells found in circulating blood. Fixation resulting in clumping of ribosomes gives them a reticulated appearance. They can be seen and identified with cresyl violet stain (see also Fig. 6–9). Platelets *(thrombocytes)*, derived from megakaryocytes found in the bone marrow (see Fig. 6–10), are minute round or ovoid structures important in blood coagulation.

Red corpuscles are filled with a self-synthesized protein-iron complex, *hemoglobin*. Hemoglobin is a conjugated protein linked to an iron-containing heme group. Normal hemoglobin values for adult males are 13.2 to 17.7 g/dL, and for adult females are 11.9 to 15.5 g/dL. Hemoglobin value in the neonate is higher–15.0 to 24.0 g/dL. Hemoglobin combines with oxygen and carbon dioxide in a reversible reaction. This complex is thus capable of carrying carbon dioxide from cells and tissues to the lungs, where it is exchanged for oxygen. Both exchanges, in tissues and lung, take place at the capillary level. The cycle of gaseous exchange is repeated about 200,000 times during the life of each corpuscle. Red blood corpuscles, normally devoid of nucleic acids (DNA and RNA), stain with acid dyes because of their content of strongly basic hemoglobin. They stain red with the widely used hematoxylin and eosin stain (H&E) as well as other stains. The red corpuscle may therefore also be called *eosinophilic* or an erythrocyte ("red cell").

Because red blood cells are normally found only within blood vessels, any extravascular red cells may be an artifact of tissue preparation or the result of disease or a vascular accident (hemorrhagic stroke).

Clinically, erythrocyte volume is determined by centrifugation of heparinated blood. The proportion of packed erythrocytes per unit volume thus measured is the *hematocrit*. Normal hematocrit values are: for adult males 40% to 50%, and for adult females 35% to 45%. The hematocrit in the newborn is higher, at 45% to 60%.

Disease states can affect erythrocyte size or number. Erythrocytes whose diameter is greater than 9 μm are called *macrocytes*. Those with diameters of less than 6 μm are called *microcytes*. *Anisocytosis* refers to variation in size of erythrocytes when they are examined in a blood smear. A decrease in the number of erythrocytes is associated with *anemia*. Anemia may be either *macrocytic* (as in vitamin B_{12} deficiency states) or *microcytic* (as in iron deficiency states). An increase in number of erythrocytes is known as *polycythemia*. Polycythemia may be a normal physiologic response, as occurs in mountain climbers or in inhabitants of high altitudes where oxygen tension is low. It may be pathologic, as an early manifestation of leukemia. A reduction in the hemoglobin value is associated with anemia. Reduction in hemoglobin value with normal erythrocyte count is known as *hypochromic anemia*. Anemia may result from insufficient production of erythrocytes, insufficient content of hemoglobin within erythrocytes, or excessive loss of erythrocytes, as in hemorrhage or red blood cell lysis.

WHITE BLOOD CELLS

White blood cells or *leukocytes* ("white cells") are complete cells because they each contain a nucleus and other vital organelles. Two distinct types are recognized on the basis of the shape of the nucleus and the type of cytoplasmic granules: So-called *agranular leukocytes (agranulocytes)* include lymphocytes and monocytes. Agranulocytes do not have cell type–specific granules. They are, however, not devoid of granules (as their name implies), but may contain varying numbers of azurophilic granules. Their nuclei are either round or kidney-shaped. *Granular leukocytes* include neutrophils, eosinophils, and basophils, each of which has its own type-specific granules from which it derives its names. The nuclei of these cells are lobulated. Thus, the agranular leukocytes may or may not have nonspecific granules, whereas the granular leukocytes always contain type-specific granules except in the earliest stages of their development.

The relative percentages and numbers (per mm^3) of each of the leukocytes in normal adult human blood are shown in Table 6–1.

The average number of leukocytes in a normal adult varies between 5000 and 9000 per mm^3. The number is higher (15,000 to 25,000 per mm^3) at birth and gradually decreases to reach adult levels by age 10 to 12 years. Most leukocytes at birth are neutrophils. Lymphocytes constitute the majority (60%) of leukocytes during infancy and early childhood. The adult percentages of granulocytes and agranulocytes are reached by age 12 to 14 years.

The number of white blood cells rises or falls in disease states. An increase over the normal values is termed *leukocytosis;* a decrease is termed *leukopenia.* As examples, neutrophils are known to increase in number in bacterial (pus-forming) infections, eosinophils in allergic conditions and parasitic infections, and basophils in certain inflammatory conditions of skin. Other diseases may result in changes in the number of more than one type of leukocyte.

The life span of white blood cells is considered to be shorter than that of red blood cells. The exact life span is not known, however, because these cells normally leave the vascular system through spaces between capillary endothelial cells and enter tissue spaces to perform their special functions. Aging leukocytes are removed from the circulation by macrophages located in the liver and spleen. They may die and disintegrate in the connective tissue, with remnants being phagocytized by histiocytes, or they may migrate through the epithelium of the gastrointestinal and respiratory tracts and be eliminated.

Some leukocytes can be recognized in tissue sections, but others are not seen to advantage with this method. A *peripheral blood smear* is the preferred method for identification of blood cell types. In this method, a drop of blood is spread thinly and evenly over a microscope slide. The thin layer of blood air-

TABLE 6–1. Leukocytes in Normal Adults Human Blood

Type	Percentage of Total Blood Cells (%)	No. per mm^3 of Blood
Neutrophils		
Bands	1–5	50–500
Segmented	50–70	2500–7000
Eosinophils	1–3	50–300
Basophils	0.5–1	0–100
Lymphocytes	20–40	1000–4000
Monocytes	1–6	500–600

dries rapidly, is fixed with methanol, and is stained with a Romanovsky stain.

Romanovsky (1891) discovered that certain dye mixtures stained blood cell components in a way that permitted accurate determination or differential counts of the variety of cells in the circulating blood and bone marrow. Some white cell cytoplasmic components (primarily inactive DNA and RNA) stain blue with methylene blue (hence, they are called basophilic); some (primarily lysosomes and a variety of other hydrolytic enzymes) may bind the azures (dye products of methylene blue oxidation) and appear light purple; some (primarily hydrolases, which digest phagocytized materials such as antigen-antibody complexes) may bind eosin (hence, they are called eosinophilic or acidophilic); and some (primarily hydrolytic enzymes related to phagocytic function) may bind another dye complex, which produces a dusty pink or violet color (and are called neutrophilic, in spite of the fact that the particles are not chemically neutral). Giemsa's stain is also widely used and is similar in its staining characteristics.

Leukocytes are relatively inactive while being passively carried in the blood stream, but because they are capable of ameboid movement, they concentrate in sites of infection and are always found in sites of "potential infection" in tissues and organs. Neutrophils and monocytes are the most phagocytic of the white blood cells; they ingest foreign particles, bacteria, and degenerating cells and cell fragments whether or not they can digest them. Monocytes are considered the most active phagocyte. Neutrophils provide the first line of defense against invading foreign bodies and organisms, and lymphocytes are believed to form antibodies, a function shared with plasma cells.

Agranulocytes

Lymphocytes

Lymphocytes (Fig. 6–3) are the major cell components of lymph and the second most prevalent leukocytes in peripheral blood. In children, lymphocytes constitute 30% to 70% of leukocytes in peripheral blood. In older children and adults, the percentage of lymphocytes in peripheral blood drops to 20% to 40%. The higher number of lymphocytes in younger children is related to the development of immunity against infection.

Lymphocytes vary widely in size. Small lymphocytes are 7 to 10 μm in diameter, and large lymphocytes are approximately 14 to 20 μm in diameter, although intermediate sizes may be encountered. Larger lymphocytes are thought to be involved in humoral immunity, because they are activated by specific antigens; they differentiate into B (bursa of Fabricius–dependent) lymphocytes and are formed in specific areas of the spleen and lymph node. B lymphocytes are less numerous (15%) in blood than T lymphocytes. When activated by the appropriate antigen, B lymphocytes undergo multiple cell divisions and differentiate into antibody-producing plasma cells. B lymphocytes that do not undergo cell division are called *memory B cells*. Further exposure of memory cells to the appropriate antigen usually induces a quicker and greater response.

Most (80%) lymphocytes, however, are T (thymus-dependent) lymphocytes, which are long-lived and are formed in different areas of the spleen and lymph node from B lymphocytes. T lymphocytes are involved in cellular immune response, such as occurs in the host after organ transplantation. T lymphocytes also provide the necessary help for B lymphocytes to differentiate into plasma cells. T lymphocytes are generally classified, on the basis of function, into helper T cells, suppressor T cells, and killer cells. *Helper T lymphocytes* enhance the response of other T lymphocytes and of B lymphocytes. *Suppressor T lymphocytes* suppress the response of other T lymphocytes and B lymphocytes to foreign antigens and self-antigens. *Killer (cytotoxic) cells* are T lymphocytes that secrete substances that destroy other cells including tumor cells. Some T lymphocytes produce lymphokines, substances that influence the activity of macrophages.

A small number of blood lymphocytes (5%) are neither B nor T lymphocytes. They carry no surface antigens and are referred as *null cells*. They may represent undifferentiated stem cells.

The nuclei of lymphocytes are usually round but may be slightly indented. Nuclear chromatin is clumped, inactive heterochromatin, which stains intensely with Wright's stain. The scanty cytoplasm immediately adjacent to the nucleus is agranular and poorly stained and appears as a perinuclear halo. The thin rim of remaining cytoplasm is usually intensely basophilic

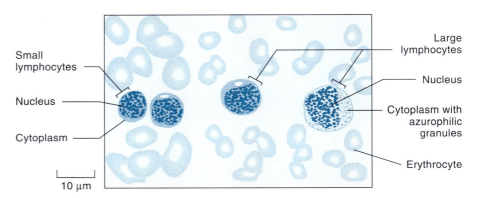

FIGURE 6–3. Peripheral blood: lymphocytes. By light microscopy, two populations of lymphocytes can be identified. Small lymphocytes are more common. They have large, dense, round nuclei and a thin rim of basophilic cytoplasm, and they are capable of ameboid movement and produce plasma cells. Uncommon in normal blood, large lymphocytes have indented nuclei and a more abundant cytoplasm. Azurophilic granules are readily found in large lymphocytes but are less commonly detected in small lymphocytes.

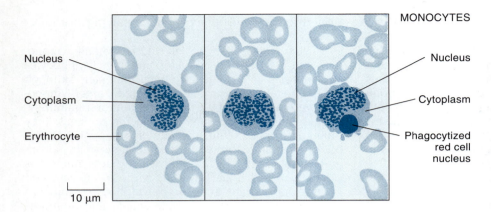

FIGURE 6–4. Peripheral blood: monocytes. *Monocytes are the largest cells found in circulating blood. The nucleus is centrally or peripherally located, is indented, and is ovoid or horseshoe shaped. The nuclear chromatin is not as dense as that of lymphocytes. Abundant cytoplasm contains azurophilic granules that tend to be smaller than those in lymphocytes. Monocytes are voracious phagocytes. Small pseudopodia extend from the monocyte on the right. Note the phagocytized red cell nucleus.*

but may stain variable shades of blue. Some lymphocytes possess a few azurophilic granules, but they are not evenly distributed. The cytoplasm contains few mitochondria and a small Golgi complex. Lymphocytes are produced in lymphoid tissues.

Monocytes

Monocytes (Fig. 6–4) are phagocytic leukocytes of the peripheral blood. Together with tissue macrophages and neutrophilic leukocyte, they play a major role in the first line of defense of the organism against infection. Monocytes constitute 1% to 6% of peripheral blood leukocytes, and less than 2% of bone marrow cells.

The largest cells in normal blood, monocytes are approximately 15 to 25 μm in diameter. They are round or oval but may have pseudopodia. The nuclei of monocytes are usually kidney-shaped, indented, or lobed. They are peripherally placed and their chromatin is not as dense as that in lymphocyte nuclei. The cytoplasm of monocytes is gray-blue and contains azurophilic granules, which generally are evenly distributed. Vacuoles are often demonstrable in the cytoplasm. Monocytes commonly show evidence of ameboid movement and are voracious phagocytes. Monocytes are also produced in lymphoid organs.

Granulocytes

Granulocytes are neutrophils, eosinophils, and basophils. These cells are also known as *polymorphonuclear cells* because of their characteristic segmented nucleus. The three polymorphonuclear cell types are produced in the bone marrow. Table 6–2 lists sizes, numbers, and functions of the granulocytes.

Neutrophils

Neutrophils (Fig. 6–5) constitute 60% to 70% of circulating white blood cells. They are 12 to 15 μm in diameter and possess a characteristic segmented nucleus consisting of two to five lobes joined by fine strands of chromatin; hence the name *polymorphonuclear neutrophils* (PMNs). The stainable heterochromatin is inactive DNA; there are no nucleoli. Immature "polymorphs" have a nonsegmented, oblong or rectangular nucleus; hence they are called *bands*. In females, the X chromosome may appear as a "drumstick-like" appendage on one of the lobes of the nucleus (Fig. 6–6). Neutrophils have abundant cytoplasm with two

TABLE 6–2. Granulocytes

Cell Type	Size (μm)	Number (per mm³ of blood)	Function
Neutrophil	12–15	300–700	Phagocytosis (cellular debris, bacteria, fungi, viruses, etc.)
Eosinophil	12–15	120–400	Phagocytosis (antigen-antibody complexes), antiparasitic agent
Basophil	12–15	30–100	Immediate hypersensitivity reaction

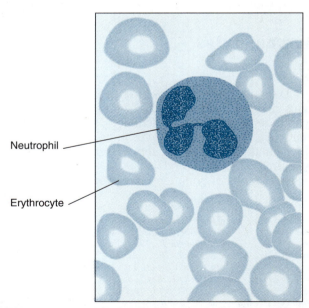

FIGURE 6–5. Peripheral blood: neutrophils. *The neutrophil has a lobulated nucleus (of two to five lobules) connected by thin bridges. The cell type–specific cytoplasmic granules are small. Neutrophils constitute 40% to 75% of the total white cell count. The number of neutrophils increases in inflammation, and these cells are the first line of defense against invading pyogenic organisms. Compare sizes of neutrophils and erythrocytes.*

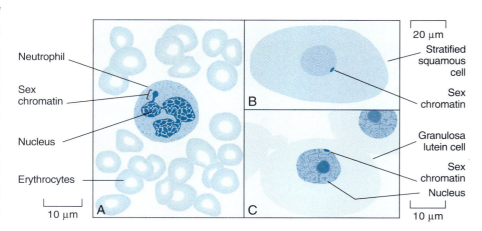

FIGURE 6–6. Sex chromatin in blood and somatic cells. The female sex chromatin is seen in a neutrophil (A), a buccal smear (B), and a corpus luteum cell (C). Sex chromatin (Barr body), composed of one of the X chromosomes that remain indented in interphase, is usually seen as a discrete structure in the nucleus. In peripheral blood, a drumstick-shaped projection may be found on one of the multilobed segments of the nucleus; this is found in about 3% of neutrophils in females. Buccalsmear of stratified squamous nonkeratinized epithelium frequently shows a dense body attached to the nuclear membrane. The same density can also be found in sections of other somatic cells (granulosa lutein cell, for example) adhering to the nuclear membrane.

types of granules of different size and staining characteristics. When stained with Romanovsky-type stains, the cytoplasm appears dusty rose because of cell type–specific (secondary) granules that are near and below the resolving power of the light microscope (about 0.2 μm). These *specific granules* contain vitamin B_{12}, binding proteins, lactoferrin, and several enzymes: alkaline phosphatase, collagenase, and lysozyme.

The second type of granules are not cell specific (primary or *nonspecific*). They are azurophilic, are about 0.5 μm in diameter, and stain metachromatically (light purple or violet). They contain acid hydrolases, neutral proteases, cationic proteins, lysozyme, acid mucopolysaccharide, and, most important, myeloperoxidase. Specific granules outnumber the nonspecific granules by a ratio of 2 or 3 to 1.

Although not seen with the light microscope, neutrophils have few mitochondria and utilize anaerobic pathways to degrade glycogen for their energy requirements. Neutrophils survive 1 to 4 days in tissues once they leave the blood stream. They traverse the connective tissues by ameboid movement and are the most active phagocytes of the three granulocytes. The azurophilic granules or lysosomes contain numerous enzymes that are capable of hydrolyzing bacteria, cellular debris, fungi, and viruses. Ameboid movement and, to a lesser degree, phagocytosis are seen in eosinophils and basophils.

Approximately 100 billion mature neutrophils are released daily from the bone marrow. The bone marrow reserve contains up to ten times the normal daily mature neutrophil requirement. This reserve is used to meet the increased demand for neutrophils in infection. If the bone marrow reserve is depleted, immature neutrophil precursors appear in the peripheral blood; this is referred to as "a shift to the left." About 10% of mature neutrophils are in the intravascular space. Half of this number is in the circulating pool, the other half in the marginating pool. The latter comprises neutrophils along the vascular endothelium, primarily in the venous circulation. The half-life of circulating mature neutrophils is 6 to 8 hours. In addition to infection, neutrophils increase in the peripheral blood after corticosteroid administration, stress, exercise, epinephrine administration, and hypoxia. The increase in neutrophil numbers under these circumstances is brought about by compartmental redistribution of available neutrophils. Prominent purplish granules designated *toxic granules* are demonstrable in the cytoplasm of neutrophils in severe infection. Toxic granules resemble the granules seen in the cytoplasm in the early stages of granulocyte development.

Eosinophils

Eosinophils (Fig. 6–7) constitute 2% to 4% of circulating white blood cells. They increase in number *(eosinophilia)* in allergic states and parasitic infestations. They decrease in number *(eosinopenia)* in shock, severe burns, and severe infection. The eosinophil is 12 to 15 μm in diameter and usually has a bilobed nucleus. The cell is easily identified by the presence of

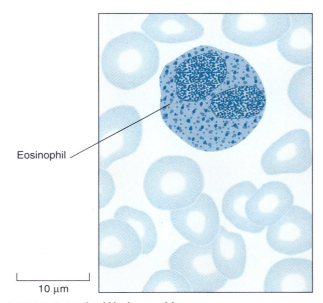

FIGURE 6–7. Peripheral blood: eosinophils. The nucleus is most commonly bilobed in peripheral blood. Cell type–specific granules are large and uniform in size. They stain intensely red with acid dyes. They constitute 1% to 3% of the total white blood cell count, and they increase in number in allergic states and parasitic conditions.

many (about 250) large, spherical, refractile cell-specific granules that fill the cytoplasm. These stain red with Romanovsky-type stains. The granules stain with the dye eosin; hence the name *eosinophil*, which means "eosin-loving." In the eosinophil, unlike in the neutrophil, specific granules are primary lysosomes. Specific granules have a unit membrane, a central dense core (internum) that contains the proteins responsible for the eosinophilia, and a less dense matrix (externum) containing several enzymes, including acid phosphatase, arylsulfatase, peroxidase, phospholipase and beta-glucoronidase. Eosinophils are produced in the bone marrow and are present only briefly (about 12 hours) in the blood before they enter tissues. The eosinophil is primarily a tissue cell.

Basophils

Basophils (Fig. 6–8) constitute less than 1% of the circulating white blood cells and usually require patient examination of a blood smear to locate, but they are worth the search when found. They are 12 to 15 μm in diameter but may be smaller. They possess an irregularly lobed nucleus most often obscured by the large, metachromatically basophilic granules; hence, the name basophil. The specific granules vary in size from 0.2 to 1.0 μm. Most granules are round and stain metachromatically owing to the presence of heparin. They also contain histamine. Basophils play a role in the immediate hypersensitivity reaction. Unlike neutrophils and monocytes, basophils are not phagocytic.

PLATELETS

Blood platelets are nonnucleated fragments of the cytoplasm of megakaryocytes (Figs. 6–9 and 6–10).

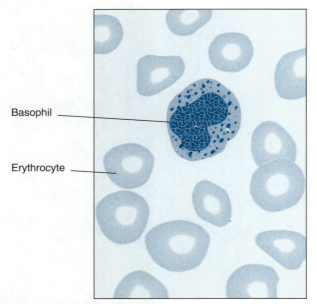

FIGURE 6–8. Peripheral blood: basophils. *In this cell type, the nucleus is large and strikingly less lobated than in the other two granulocytes. Cell type–specific cytoplasmic granules are large and variable in size and have a strong affinity for basic dyes. Basophils constitute 0.5% to 1% of the white blood cell count. They synthesize and release heparin and histamine into the circulating blood.*

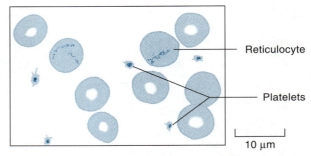

FIGURE 6–9. Peripheral blood: reticulocytes and platelets. *Reticulocytes are found in circulating blood in small numbers (0.5% to 1.5% of red blood cells). They must be specially prepared and stained to reveal the ribonucleoprotein (RNA) in the form of clumped ribosomes. The reticular nature of ribosome clumping gives the cells their name. When their circulating number exceeds 1%, a greater oxygen-carrying capacity may be indicated, owing to an increase in total red blood cell count. The higher red cell count may indicate a hemorrhage, a move to high altitude, or pathologic changes in the vital capacity of the lungs.*

Platelets are small discs, about 2 to 4 μm in diameter, and they number between 200,000 and 350,000 per mm^3 of blood. In general, two to six blood platelets or thrombocytes are seen in an oil immersion field, but their distribution is variable, and they may appear in large clumps. Under light microscopy, each platelet appears to have a peripheral, lightly staining region *(hyalomere)* and a central, densely staining granular region *(granulomere)*. The hyalomere region contains irregular, dense tubular structures and actin microfilaments. The microfilaments play a role in platelet movements. The granulomere region contains a variety of granules. Delta (δ) granules take up and store serotonin. Slightly larger alpha (α) granules contain fibrinogen and other proteins. Lambda (λ) granules, small compared with the other two types, contain lysosomal enzymes. The cytoplasm of platelets contains canaliculi that open into the plasma membrane and serve as channels for extrusion of substances stored within platelets. Outside the plasma membrane is a layer of glycosaminoglycans and glycoproteins that promote adhesion of platelets. Platelets' function relates to the clotting of blood both inside and outside blood vessels.

In response to endothelial damage, platelets aggregate to the damaged endothelium and release the contents of their granules. Factors secreted by the aggregated platelets, along with other factors from plasma and from the injured vessel wall, contribute to the formation of fibrin from plasma proteins. Fibrin thus formed traps blood cells and platelets, resulting in formation of a *thrombus* (blood clot). In addition to their role in thrombus formation, platelets function to assist clot retraction and removal. Clot retraction is induced by an interaction between actin, myosin, and ATP of platelets. Clot removal is effected by a series of steps consisting of activation of plasma plasminogen by factors produced by the endothelium. Activated plasminogen then forms plasmin, a proteolytic enzyme that removes the clot. Platelets' role in clot removal consists in the release of lysosomal enzymes from lambda granules.

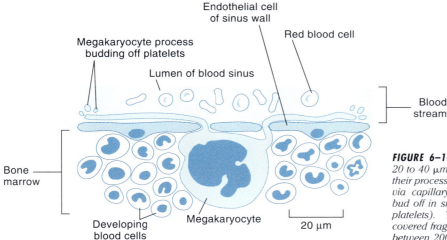

FIGURE 6–10. Bone marrow: megakaryocyte. *Megakaryocytes, 20 to 40 μm in diameter, are found in the bone marrow, but their processes leave the marrow and enter the blood sinuses via capillary pores. The ends of the processes break or bud off in small segments, forming thrombocytes (or blood platelets). The thrombocytes are therefore membrane-covered fragments of megakaryocyte cytoplasm and number between 200,000 and 350,000 per mm^3.*

BLOOD PLASMA

The fluid in which the blood cells reside within blood vessels is called *blood plasma*. Plasma constitutes 55% of whole blood, whereas the cellular components total 45%. Blood plasma contains gases, proteins, carbohydrates, amino acids, lipids, inorganic salts, enzymes, and hormones. The plasma proteins are albumin (main protein component), globulins (alpha, beta, and gamma) and fibrinogen. *Albumin* plays a major role in maintaining osmotic equilibrium across the blood vessel wall. *Gamma globulins* are antibodies important in the immune response. *Fibrinogen* plays a role in the clotting process. Blood plasma serves an important role in coagulation, temperature regulation, respiration, regulation of blood pH (as a buffer), and fluid balance. Hormones, absorbed nutrients, and metabolic wastes are carried in the plasma to sites of action, utilization, or elimination. When blood clots, the supernatant fluid is called *blood serum*.

ORIGIN OF BLOOD CELLS

Because blood cells have short life spans, they must be constantly replaced in vast numbers. The term applied to the replacement process is *hematopoiesis* (Fig. 6–11). In the adult, it occurs in the bone marrow and lymphoid tissues. In the embryo and fetus, various organs are active in hematopoiesis, including the yolk sac, liver, spleen, thymus, and lymph nodes, as well as bone marrow. Since the 1960s, a conceptual framework for the hematopoietic system and a better understanding of the factors that control hematopoiesis has emerged.

Erythropoiesis

Red blood corpuscles undergo their maturation *(erythropoiesis)* within bone marrow, and several "stages" can be recognized (Fig. 6–12). The stages are differentiated on the basis of changes in cell size, nuclear diameter, nucleolar size, chromatin density, and cytoplasmic basophilia. As they mature, the cells decrease in volume, nuclei decrease in diameter and are ultimately extruded, nucleoli diminish in size, chromatin becomes more dense, and cytoplasmic basophilia is replaced by acidophilia. The earliest (stem) cells of this series are large (14 to 19 μm in diameter); they have a large round nucleus, reticulated chromatin, and one or more small nucleoli. The cytoplasm is seen as a thin rim, which stains a royal blue color (basophilic) with Wright's stain. These cells are called by several names—*proerythroblast, rubriblast, pronormoblast,* and *megaloblast.*

Electronmicrographs of rubriblasts reveal a cytoplasm rich in ribosomes and ferritin. The abundance of ribosomes gives the cytoplasm its intense basophilia. Ferritin (iron) in the cytoplasm is found in its free form or within vacuoles *(siderosomes).* Iron enters the cytoplasm by a process of *pinocytosis* from specific receptor sites on the cell membrane. An iron-binding plasma protein, transferrin, provides iron particles to the specific receptor sites.

As the proerythroblast matures, the cell becomes smaller (12 to 17 μm in diameter), the nucleus becomes smaller, chromatin coarsens, and nucleoli become ill-defined or disappear. The cytoplasm remains basophilic (RNA-rich) and stains blue. The intense basophilia obscures hemoglobin content in the cytoplasm. These cells are termed *basophilic erythroblasts, prorubricytes, basophilic normoblasts, early erythroblasts,* or *early normoblasts.*

The next recognizable stage involves further decrease in cell size (12 to 15 μm in diameter), coarsening of nuclear chromatin, and reduction of nuclear size. Nucleoli are absent. Relatively, the cytoplasm appears to occupy more of the cell and is seen to contain a mixture of eosinophilic (red) and basophilic (blue) purplish cytoplasm, hence the name polychromatophilic erythroblasts. The eosinophilic areas in cytoplasm reflect hemoglobin formation; the decreasing basophilia is due to declining ribonucleoprotein content.

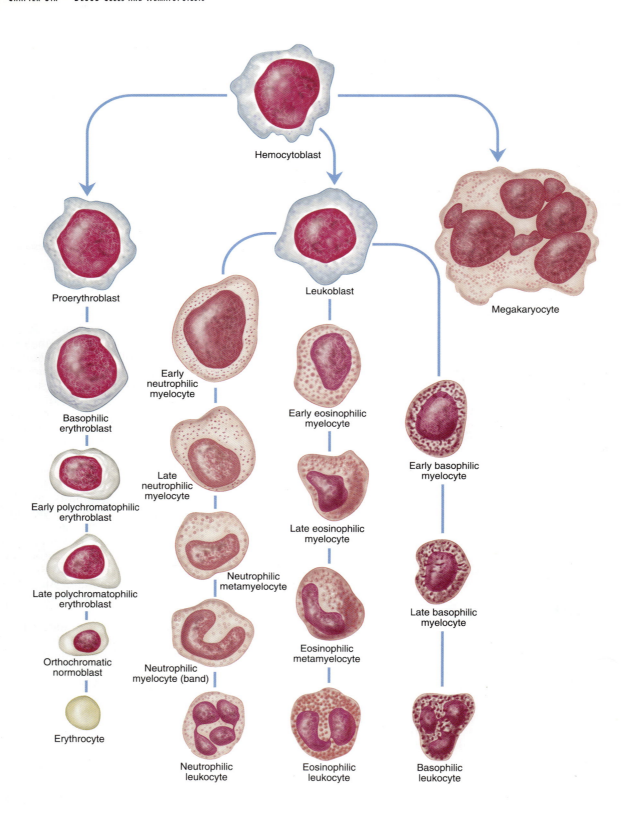

FIGURE 6–11. Bone marrow: blood cell development. *The cells of human bone marrow in air-dried smears. Note the progressive differentiation of mature cells from progenitor cells in the production of both erythrocytes and leukocytes. See subsequent figures for detailed descriptions.*

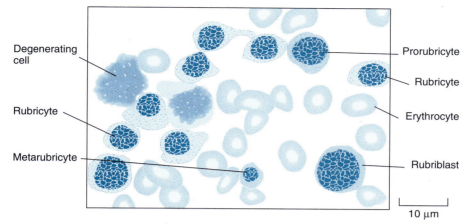

FIGURE 6-12. Bone marrow smear: red cell development.
The rubriblast (proerythroblast, hemocytoblast, myeloblast) is a stem cell of the erythroid series with a large rounded nucleus and basophilic cytoplasm.
The prorubricyte (basophilic erythroblast) develops from the rubriblast. It is smaller than the stem cell, and its nucleus has coarser chromatin. RNA-rich cytoplasm is densely basophilic. Basophilia obscures hemoglobin content. The prorubricyte undergoes mitotic division, giving rise to rubricytes.
The rubricyte (polychromatophilic erythroblast), a product of mitotic division of prorubricytes, is smaller than the mother cell. Nuclear chromatin is more compact, cytoplasmic basophilia is less marked, and hemoglobin content is greater than in the mother cell. Rubricytes have an affinity for both acid and basic dyes (because of their content of hemoglobin and RNA, respectively), which determines their polychromatophilic staining characteristics.
The metarubricyte (normoblast) arises by cytodifferentiation of rubricytes. The nucleus is small and pyknotic, and the cytoplasm is distinctly acidophilic owing to increased hemoglobin content.
The erythrocyte is nonnucleated (nuclei of metarubricyte has been extruded) with a circular outline. In side view, erythrocytes appear dumbbell-shaped because of the biconcave nature of their surfaces. Their number varies in humans from 5 to 5.5 million per mm^3. Erythrocytes carry oxygen from lungs to tissue and carbon dioxide from tissue to lungs, and are filled with hemoglobin. Immature stages in development (reticulocytes) have a diffusely basophilic cytoplasm because of the residual content of RNA.
Degenerating cells are often found in bone marrow. Remnants of damaged corpuscles, megakaryocytes, or myeloblasts, degenerating cells are primarily artifacts of a marrow smear preparation.

Cells at this stage are named *polychromatophilic erythroblasts, rubricytes, polychromatophilic normoblasts, polychromatic erythroblasts, polychromatic normoblasts, intermediate erythroblasts,* or *intermediate normoblasts.*

The nucleus of the next stage is still smaller than in the preceding stage and stains solid blue-black. The nucleus is now nonfunctional and ready to be discarded. The cytoplasm is predominantly acidophilic, with some residual basophilia. The hemoglobin, which is eosinophilic, dominates; only minimal amounts of residual ribonucleoprotein stain the cytoplasm purplish. These cells are termed *orthochromatic normoblasts, metarubricytes, acidophilic erythroblasts, acidophilic normoblasts, orthochromatic erythroblasts, normochromatic erythroblasts,* or *late erythroblasts.*

The nuclei are extruded in the next stage, and the anuclear cells are termed *reticulocytes, diffusely basophilic erythrocytes, polychromatic erythrocytes, polychromatophilic erythrocytes,* or *proerythrocytes.* Clumping of ribosomes when stained with supravital dyes gives them a reticulated appearance. Because they are nonnucleated, reticulocytes are incapable of protein synthesis. Reticulocytes normally constitute 1% of red blood cells. Their percentage increases in situations of increased demand for oxygen, as in bleeding. Reticulocytes leave the bone marrow for the blood, where they complete maturation.

The final stage of maturation consists of the disappearance of cytoplasmic ribonucleoproteins. The resulting cell is a biconcave, flexible eosinophilic disc 6 to 8 μm in diameter, the *erythrocyte.* It takes about 7 days for a stem cell of the erythropoietic series to become a mature erythrocyte. This period may be shortened to as little as 2 days in acute anemia. The process of erythropoiesis may be accelerated by the hormone *erythropoietin.* Erythropoietin is produced largely by the kidney. Its production is stimulated when there is an increased demand for reticulocytes and erythrocytes, as in hypoxia. The average life span of a human red blood cell is approximately 120 days. This means that approximately 5×10^4 red cells must be produced per day per μl of blood.

Granulocytic Development

Granulopoiesis

Granular leukocytes (granulocytes) develop in the bone marrow from undifferentiated (stem) cells and from precursor cells called *leukoblasts.* The process of maturation from stem cells to mature neutrophils (Fig. 6–13), eosinophils (Fig. 6–14), and basophils (Fig. 6–15) is characterized by a decrease in size of the cell, changes in configuration of nucleus from round to segmented and then lobulated, and development of specific granules with varying affinity to various dyes. Cells whose granules have affinity for basic dyes are called *basophils*; those whose granules have affinity to acidic dyes are *acidophils*; and those whose granules

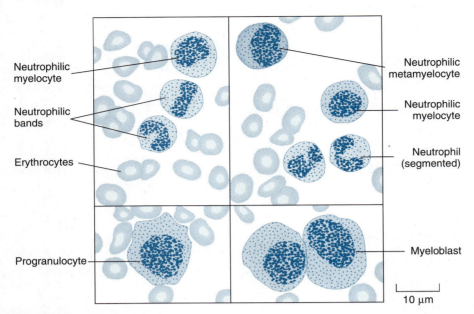

FIGURE 6–13. Bone marrow smear: neutrophilic cell development.

The myeloblast *is the stem cell of the leukocytic series. It has lightly basophilic cytoplasm, and its nuclei are large and rounded. The chromatin is in the form of moderately coarse interconnected strands. Myeloblasts constitute 0.3% to 0.5% of marrow cells, and their numbers increase in leukemia.*

The progranulocyte, *also called the promyelocyte, arises and differentiates from the myeloblast. The cells are large; their nuclei are rounded with coarse chromatin. The cytoplasm is basophilic, with some azurophilic granules. Progranulocytes constitute about 4% of marrow cells. These cells divide and give rise to myelocytes. The further differentiation of a neutrophilic myelocyte is outlined below.*

The neutrophilic myelocyte *arises from the progranulocyte. It is smaller, with less basophilic cytoplasm containing differentiated granules and a nucleus with more compact chromatin.*

The neutrophilic metamyelocyte *arises from division of the neutrophilic myelocyte. It has a kidney-shaped nucleus and is not capable of division. It differentiates into mature neutrophilic myelocytes.*

Neutrophilic bands *are immature neutrophils. Their nuclei are shaped like horseshoes or drumsticks.*

A segmented neutrophil *is a mature cell. Its nucleus is markedly lobulated, and the lobules may be connected with a thin chromatin thread. The chromatin is compact, and there is abundant cytoplasm. Granules in the cytoplasm are small and may be inconspicuous.*

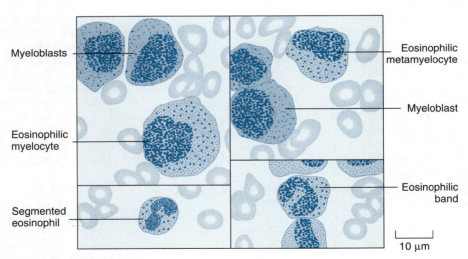

FIGURE 6–14. Bone marrow smear: eosinophilic cell development.

The myeloblast *is the stem cell of the leukocytic series. It has a rounded large nucleus and lightly basophilic agranular cytoplasm.*

Eosinophilic myelocytes *develop from myeloblasts. Specific acidophilic granules appear in the cytoplasm, and the nucleus is rounded or oval. The chromatin of the nucleus is coarser than in myeloblasts. Eosinophilic myelocytes are capable of division.*

The eosinophilic metamyelocyte *is no longer capable of cell division. Its nucleus is kidney-shaped or indented, and its cytoplasm contains acidophilic granules.*

Eosinophilic bands *are immature or juvenile eosinophils. The nucleus is shaped like a horseshoe or drumstick, and there are eosinophilic granules in the cytoplasm.*

Segmented eosinophils *are mature. The nucleus is lobulated (generally two lobules), and the lobes are connected with thin chromatin threads. There is abundant granular cytoplasm.*

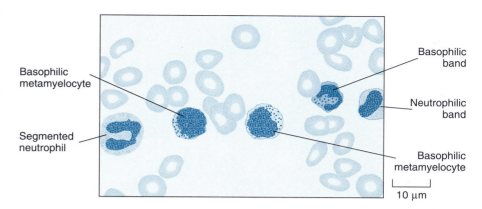

FIGURE 6–15. Bone marrow smear: basophilic cell development.
Basophilic metamyelocytes *are derived from basophilic myelocytes, which are not represented in this figure. Basophilic myelocytes are scarce and may not be seen in a single marrow smear preparation. It is believed that their granules are water soluble. They are no longer capable of cell division. The nucleus is oval to kidney shaped, and the cytoplasm has basophilic granules.*

A basophilic band is an immature basophil with a horseshoe-shaped nucleus. There are basophilic granules in the cytoplasm. See Figure 6–8 for the mature basophil.

do not stain intensely with either basic or acidic dyes are called *neutrophils.*

As cells mature, they are called progressively *myelocytes, metamyelocytes, banded cells,* and *segmented cells.* Leukoblasts are similar in appearance for the neutrophils, eosinophils, and basophils. Differentiation among these three cell types commences with the myelocyte stage. Leukoblasts are approximately 15–20 μm in diameter and constitute 0.3% to 0.5% of marrow cells. The nucleus is round, stains purple, and contains two or more nucleoli. The chromatin strands are well-defined and evenly stained. The scanty cytoplasm is basophilic, and when stained with Wright's stain, it appears agranular and pale blue.

In the next recognizable stage, the cell is the same size as or larger than the leukoblast, but the nucleus is round or oval and smaller. Chromatin becomes more coarse, bluer and not as red as in the leukoblast, and is unevenly stained. The cytoplasm is blue with a relatively light zone adjacent to the nucleus. Nucleoli may be visible but are usually indistinct. This cell now contains distinct granules that stain variably from red to purple-blue and is designated a *progranulocyte* or a *promyelocyte.* Most granules are round, but some are elongated, curved, or irregular. Progranulocytes constitute 4% of marrow cells.

A progranulocyte becomes a *myelocyte* when the granules become sufficiently differentiated in size, color, and shape to be positively identified as the specific granules of neutrophils, eosinophils, or basophils. The subsequent developmental stages are identical for the three types of granulocytes or polymorphonuclear cells. The primary changes are a reduction in cell size and alterations in nuclear shape. Myelocytes are smaller than promyelocytes and have a relatively large cytoplasm. The nucleus of the myelocyte tends to be slightly flattened. The chromatin becomes increasingly coarse and evenly stained. Nucleoli are usually indistinct or absent. The next stage, the *metamyelocyte,* is slightly smaller than the myelocyte and contains an indented, kidney-shaped, smaller nucleus with a well-defined chromatin structure. Additional folding results in a horseshoe-shaped nucleus, which stains deeply with basic dyes. In the *band* (nonsegmented) *cell stage,* nuclear indentation becomes more marked, and the cell is smaller than the metamyelocyte.

The final developmental "stage" results in a cell with a lobed nucleus, the lobes being united by narrow filaments or strands of chromatin. These cells are called *segmented granulocytes* or *polymorphonuclear granulocytes.* The mature polymorphonuclear granulocyte is approximately 15 μm in diameter.

It takes about 11 days for the maturation cycle to be completed. The transition through the various stages of granulocytes is gradual. Many cells are difficult to distinguish from one another. Neutrophilic band cells normally constitute 1% to 5% of granulocytes in peripheral blood. Their number rises in bacterial infections; as mentioned previously, increase in the number of bands and other immature neutrophils is known as a "shift to the left."

Lymphocytopoiesis

All lymphocyte progenitor cells are believed to originate in the bone marrow. They leave the marrow to develop in the thymus to form T lymphocytes, which will leave the thymus to populate other lymphoid organs. Other bone marrow lymphocyte progenitor cells become B lymphocytes, which leave the marrow to populate yet other specific areas of lymphoid tissue. T and B lymphocytes cannot be distinguished by means of ordinary histologic or cytologic methods; their identification requires use of immunocytochemical techniques.

The stem cells of circulating lymphocytes are large cells, the *lymphoblasts.* They have thin, evenly stained chromatin strands. One or several nucleoli are present. Lymphoblasts undergo division to form prolymphocytes. The process of maturation is characterized by a decrease in cell size, condensation of nuclear chromatin, and decreased prominence of nucleoli. Mature lymphocytes display characteristic antigenicity at their surface membranes.

Monocytopoiesis

The stem cells of circulating monocytes are monoblasts. They divide to form promonocytes. The process of maturation *(monocytopoiesis)* is similar to lymphocytopoiesis. Mature monocytes leave the blood stream for connective tissue, where they develop into

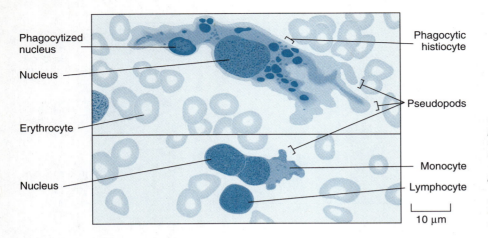

FIGURE 6–16. Bone marrow smear: wandering phagocytes. *The phagocytic histiocyte is a large cell with an irregular outline with many short cell processes (pseudopods). There is abundant cytoplasm containing phagocytized material. The nucleus is oval. The monocyte is also a large cell, but with a prominent eccentric nucleus. It has a highly ameboid cytoplasm containing various inclusions.*

fixed-tissue macrophages, a category comprising the alveolar macrophages, hepatic Kupffer's cells, dermal Langerhans' cells, osteoclasts, peritoneal and pleural macrophages, and possibly brain microglial cells (Fig. 6–16).

Megakaryocytopoiesis

The stem cell of megakaryocytopoiesis is the *megakaryoblast*. It is a large cell (15 to 50 μm in diameter) with strongly basophilic, nongranular cytoplasm, a large oval nucleus, and several nucleoli. Nuclear chromatin strands are distinct. The next stage in development is the *promegakaryocyte*. Larger than the megakaryoblast it has a horseshoe-shaped nucleus and slightly granular cytoplasm.

The megakaryocyte is the next stage in development (Fig. 6–17). It is a giant cell, with a diameter of 35 to 150 μm, a finely granular, large cytoplasm, a prominent multilobulated nucleus, and no nucleoli. With further maturation, pseudopodia extend from the plasma membrane of megakaryocytes and later detach

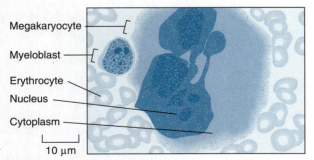

FIGURE 6–17. Bone marrow smear: megakaryocyte. *A megakaryocyte is a giant cell characteristic of bone marrow, with a conspicuous multilobed nucleus. Its cytoplasm contains fine granules. Pseudopodia extend from the cell surface and later detach to form the blood platelets. Blood platelets participate in the blood-clotting mechanism by contributing to the formation of thromboplastin, by "plugging" abnormal breaks in the endothelium of blood vessels, and by inducing the constriction of damaged blood vessels.*

Red blood cells *are nonnucleated corpuscles having a circular or dumbbell-shaped (biconcave) appearance. They contain hemoglobin. See also Figure 6–10.*

to form blood platelets. The average life span of platelets is 7 to 10 days. Their daily production rate is 2×10^4 platelets per μl of blood.

GROWTH FACTORS

The processes of hematopoiesis depend on stimulation by growth factors. Six such growth factors are identified: erythropoietin, interleukin-3 (IL-3), interleukin-5 (IL-5), granulocyte-macrophage colony–stimulating factor (GM-CSF), granulocyte colony–stimulating factor (G-CSF), and macrophage colony–stimulating factor (M-CSF). Erythropoietin has been shown to stimulate red cell production, G-CSF to stimulate neutrophilic leukocyte production, and GM-CSF to stimulates neutrophil, monocyte, and eosinophil production.

The different growth factors are grouped into three classes: The class of lineage-restricted colony-stimulating factors (class 1) includes G-CSF, M-CSF, erythropoietin, and interleukin-5. These cytokines stimulate the final mitotic divisions and the terminal cellular maturation of partially differentiated hematopoietic progenitors (those committed to blood cell production within a single lineage). Class 2 growth factors stimulate the proliferation of progenitor cells from more than one hematopoietic lineage. Also called pluripotent/oligopotent colony-stimulating factors, they are interleukin-3 and GM-CSF. They affect less mature progenitors than class 1 growth factors. There is evidence to suggest that interleukin-3 targets a more primitive stem cell than GM-CSF. Class 3 hematopoietic growth factors exhibit little or no intrinsic colony-stimulating activity but act synergistically with colony-stimulating factors to augment colony development. Interleukins 1 and 6 belong to this class.

On the basis of the interactions between growth factors and progenitor cells, a model of stem cell development has emerged. According to this model (Figs. 6–18 and 6–19), recruitment by interleukin-1 or interleukin-6 (class 3 growth factors) targets a primitive, multilineage progenitor that is predominantly unresponsive to colony-stimulating growth factors. After recruitment,

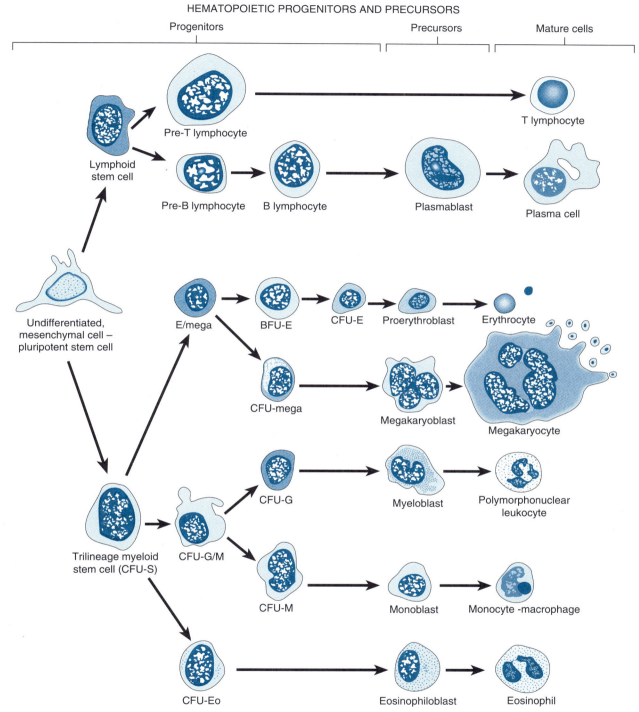

FIGURE 6–18. Hematopoiesis. *Schematic diagram of the process of hematopoiesis from an undifferentiated pluripotent stem cell to fully differentiated mature circulating blood cells. The progressive stages of maturation of the lymphoid, erythroid, and myeloid series are shown from left to right. E/mega, erythrocyte/megakaryocyte progenitor cell; BFU-E, burst-forming unit–erythroid; CFU-E, colony-forming unit–erythroid; CFU-mega, colony-forming unit–megakaryocyte; CFU-G, colony-forming unit–granulocyte; CFU-S, colony-forming unit–stem cell; CFU-G/M, colony-forming unit–granulocyte/macrophage; CFU-M, colony-forming unit–macrophage/monocyte; CFU-Eo, colony-forming unit–eosinophil.*

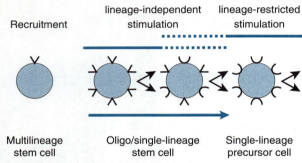

FIGURE 6–19. Hematopoiesis. *Schematic diagram of the hematopoietic process, showing main steps of transforming a multilineage, undifferentiated stem cell into a single-lineage precursor cell. Recruitment of the multilineage stem cell by interleukin-1 or interleukin-6 results in progenitor cells with receptors on their cell membranes for lineage-independent colony-stimulating factors (V). Cell divisions result in the acquisition of committed precursor cells with receptors on their cell membranes for lineage-dependent colony-stimulating factors (U); these latter cells develop into mature circulating blood cells (not shown).*

progenitors express receptors for class 1 factors, which primarily stimulate proliferation and expansion. Class 2 growth factors play a role in this stimulation. Cell division results in increasing commitment, with loss of multiple lineage and the acquisition of single-lineage growth factor receptors. The single-lineage committed stem cell is stimulated through its final mitotic and maturation stages by the appropriate lineage-specific colony-stimulating factor (class 3 growth factors).

In addition to regulating hematopoiesis, growth factors play a role in the stimulation of their own production. Central in this process is interleukin-1. Furthermore, the different hematopoietic growth factors are likely to have important therapeutic application in human disease. Colony-stimulating growth factors have exhibited efficacy in treatment of the leukopenia associated with aplastic anemia, leukemia, cancer chemotherapy, and other conditions.

CHAPTER SEVEN

Neural Tissue

CELLULAR COMPONENTS 112
   Neuron 112
   Neuroglia 117

GANGLIA 119
   Craniospinal Ganglia 119
   Autonomic Ganglia 119

NERVE FIBERS 119
   Myelinated Nerve Fibers 121
   Unmyelinated Nerve Fibers 122
   Conduction of Nerve Impulses 122
   Axonal Transport 122

SYNAPSE 122
   Neuromuscular Junction 124

RECEPTOR ORGANS OF SENSORY NEURONS 126
   Free Nerve Endings 126
   Encapsulated Endings 126

REACTIONS OF NEURONS TO INJURY 129
   Cell Body and Dendrites 129
   Axon 129
   Nerve Growth Factors 130
   Classification of Nerve Injury 131
   Neuronal Plasticity 132

The cells that constitute the nervous system are vast in number and complexity. As components of the peripheral and central nervous systems, they are distributed to every part of the body. Their function is to receive stimuli from the external and internal environments and to transmit (by electrochemical processes), modify, coordinate, integrate, and translate these stimuli into meaningful conscious experiences or coordinated motor activity through muscular and glandular tissues.

The cells of the nervous system can be divided into two general categories: nerve cells (*neurons*) and supporting cells (*glia*). Nerve cells are intricately linked to one another and to effector organs such as muscle and glands. Nerve cells influence one another through specialized areas of contact, the synapses. The complexity of the synaptic relationships among the billions of neurons provides the basis for the behavioral complexity of the human.

Students of the nervous system have revealed many aspects of the structure and function of cellular components, their organization into functional groups, and the pathways emanating from or projecting onto them. A wide variety of anatomic and physiologic methods have been developed to demonstrate the component parts of the nervous system and their interrelationships in normal and disease states. This chapter is concerned with the structural components of the nervous system.

CELLULAR COMPONENTS
Neuron

A neuron or nerve cell consists of a cell body (*perikaryon*) and all its processes (*axon* and *dendrites*).

Neurons vary remarkably in size and shape. The diameter of the cell body may be as small as 4 μm (granule cell of the cerebellum) or as large as 125 μm (motor neuron of the spinal cord). The overall configuration of a cell body may be pyramidal, flask-shaped, or stellate, depending on the number and organization of its processes (Fig. 7–1). In general, three types of neurons are recognized (Fig. 7–2): *Unipolar* or *pseudo-unipolar neurons* have spherical cell bodies with single processes that later bifurcate. Such cells are found in the dorsal root ganglia. *Bipolar neurons* are spindle-shaped, with one process at each end. They are found in certain peripheral ganglia, such as the spiral ganglion of the acoustic nerve and the ganglion of Scarpa of the vestibular nerve, as well as in olfactory and retinal receptor cells. *Multipolar neurons* have polygonal cell bodies and multiple processes. Such neurons are encountered in autonomic ganglia and the central nervous system.

The most remarkable features of the neuron are its processes. In humans, the axon may be a meter or more in length, extending from the spinal cord to the fingers or toes, or from the cerebral cortex to the distal extent of the spinal cord. The dendrites vary in number and in pattern of branching, which in some instances, enormously increases their surface area (see Fig. 7–1).

Perikaryon

The cell body contains the nucleus and a number of organelles (Figs. 7–3 and 7–4). The nucleus generally is round and usually is centrally located. The nucleoplasm is homogeneous and stains poorly with nuclear stains (basic dyes), indicating that the deoxyribonu-

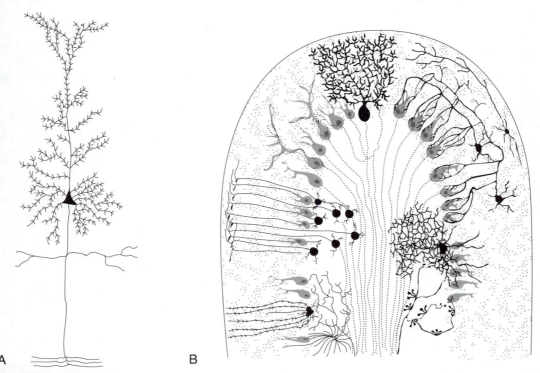

FIGURE 7–1. Schematic diagram of neuronal types. A, *The pyramidal neuron with its apical and basal dendrites, perikaryon, axon, and axon collaterals.* B, *Different cell types in the cerebellum.*

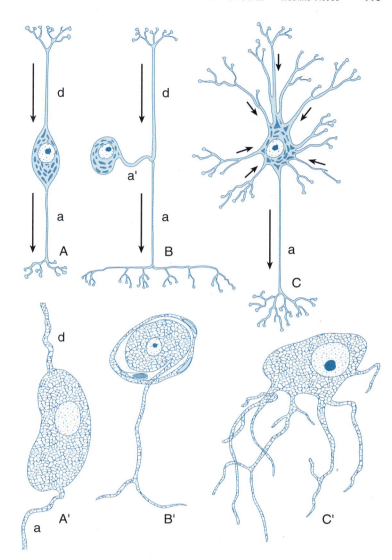

FIGURE 7–2. Schematic diagram of neuronal types. d, *Dendrite;* a, *axon;* a′, *process common to axon and dendrite. Arrows indicate direction of impulse conduction. A and A′, bipolar neuron. B and B′, pseudo-unipolar neuron. C and C′, multipolar neuron.*

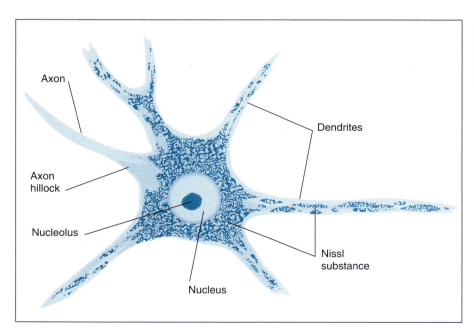

FIGURE 7–3. Schematic diagram of anterior horn cell. *Central round nucleus, Nissl substance in the cell body and dendrites, multiple dendrites, and one axon are shown. The axon hillock (site of origin of axon) is devoid of Nissl substance.*

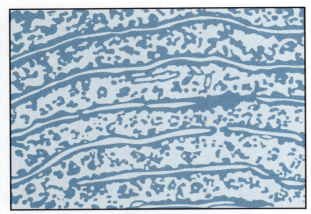

FIGURE 7-4. Schematic diagram of Nissl substance.

cleic acid (DNA) is in the dispersed or active euchromatin form. In stark contrast, one deeply stained nucleolus, composed in part of ribonucleic acid (RNA), is normally present within the nucleus. The nuclear contents are enclosed within a distinct nuclear membrane.

The cytoplasm is filled with various organelles and inclusions. Prominent among the organelles is the chromophil (Nissl) substance or *Nissl bodies*, which are particularly prominent in somatic motor neurons, such as those in the anterior horn of the spinal cord, and in some motor cranial nerve nuclei. Nissl bodies are composed of membrane-bound ribonucleoproteins (granular endoplasmic reticulum). The roles of the nucleus, nucleolus, and cytoplasmic RNA in protein synthesis are well established. The cell body generates the cytoplasmic proteins and other essential constituents, which are then distributed throughout the neuron. Nissl bodies are found not only in the cell body but also in the dendrites. They are absent from the *axon hillock* (the part of the perikaryon from which the axon arises) and axon. Nissl substance undergoes definite changes in response to axonal injury.

Mitochondria are dispersed throughout the cytoplasm of the nerve cell and play a vital role in the metabolic activity of the neuron. The *Golgi apparatus*, originally discovered in neurons, is highly developed (Fig. 7–5). It is composed of flattened, ovoid, and round agranular vesicles. The Golgi area of the neuron is the site where carbohydrates are linked to protein in the synthesis of glycoproteins. Small vesicles arising from this organelle may be the source of synaptic vesicles found in axon terminals.

Neurofibrils are found in all nerve cells and are continuous throughout all their processes (Fig. 7–6). They are composed of subunits (*neurofilaments*) that are 7.5 to 10 μm thick and thus beyond the limit of resolution of the light microscope. Neurofilaments are composed of type III intermediate filaments, related to others in other types of cells. In addition to neurofilaments, neuronal cytoplasm contains microtubules similar in external diameter (about 25 μm) to those observed in other types of cells. They are involved in the rapid transport of protein molecules through axons and dendrites. Most large nerve cells contain lipochrome pigment granules (Fig. 7–7), which appear to accumulate with the advancing age of the organism. In addition, certain nerve cells in specific locations contain melanin granules, which are black (Fig. 7–8). The perikaryon of a neuron is its trophic center. The separation of a process from the perikaryon results in the death of the process.

Axon

The axon usually arises from the cell body at the axon hillock; it is a slender cylindrical process of variable length. It may be extremely long, as indicated earlier. The axon hillock and axon proper are devoid of Nissl substance. Below the cell membrane of the axon hillock is a dense layer of granular substance about 200 Å thick. Within the hillock, there is a confluence of microtubules that exhibit clustering and cross-linkage. The junction between the perikaryon, axon hillock, and axon is termed the *initial segment*. Short, narrow, and devoid of myelin, the initial segment is the area in which the nerve impulse is initiated. Immediately beyond the axon hillock, the nerve becomes myelinated, increases greatly in diameter, and maintains this size until it terminates at the end organ. Mitochon-

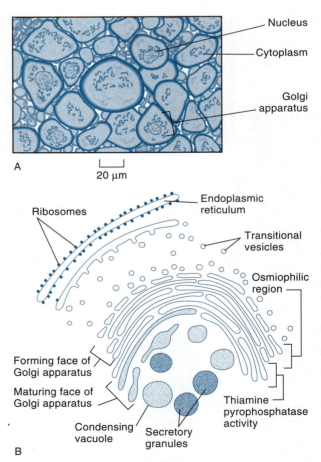

FIGURE 7-5. *Schematic diagram of Golgi apparatus.* A, *The location of Golgi apparatus in the cytoplasm.* B, *Golgi apparatus, associated endoplasmic reticulum, and vesicles transporting secretory material from the endoplasmic reticulum to the Golgi apparatus.*

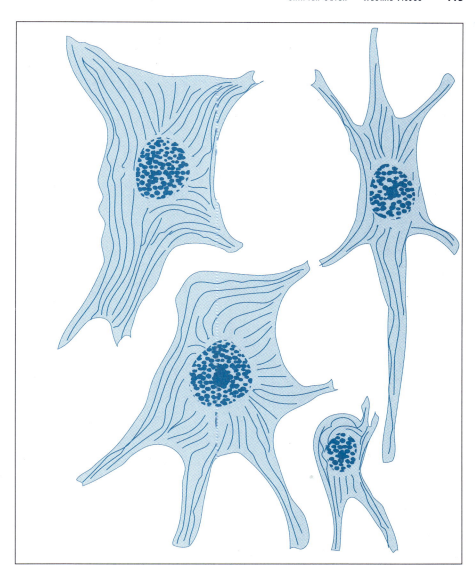

FIGURE 7–6. Schematic diagram of neurofibrils in different types of neurons. Note that neurofibrils are found in all nerve cells and are continuous through all of their processes.

dria, microtubules, microfilaments, neurofilaments, neurotubules, smooth endoplasmic reticulum, lysosomes, and vesicles are contained within the axoplasm (Fig. 7–9).

The axon, unlike the cell body (perikaryon), lacks any of the structures associated with protein synthesis or assembly (i.e., ribosomes, rough endoplasmic reticulum, and Golgi complex). The smallest axoplasmic components are the microfilaments, which are paired helical chains of actin. They are generally confined to the cortical zone near the axolemma; their contractile actin protein may play a role in intra-axonal transport. Neurofilaments are larger (7.5 to 10 μm in diameter) and more prevalent. They occupy the area within the axoplasm not occupied by other organelles. Neurofilaments are composed of three proteins with the molecular weight of 68,000 to 200,000 daltons. They are digested readily by intrinsic proteases, accounting for their rapid disappearance in damaged axons. Microtubules are longitudinally arranged, hollow cylinders measuring 23 to 25 μm in diameter and of indefinite length. They are composed of subunits of the protein tubulin. The number of microtubules along the axon varies in direct relation to axonal mass and type of nerve. Microtubules are more numerous in unmyelinated axons.

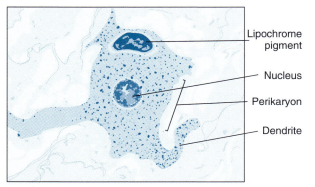

FIGURE 7–7. Schematic diagram of multipolar neuron with lipochrome pigment.

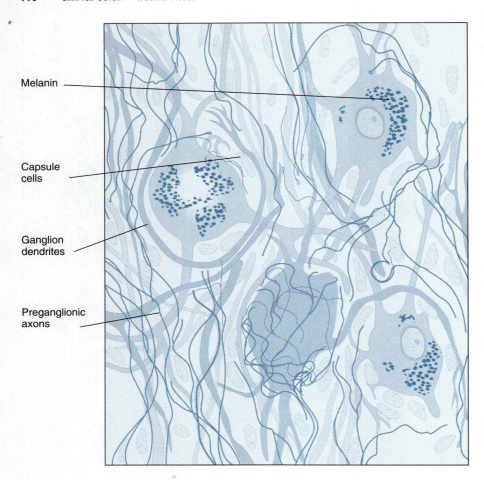

FIGURE 7-8. Schematic diagram of autonomic ganglion cells. Note the melanin aggregates within the cytoplasm and capsule cells surrounding the ganglion cells. Dendrites appear tangled.

Mitochondria vary in number in an inverse ratio to axonal cross-sectional area. They are often associated with one or more microtubules. The smooth endoplasmic reticulum gives rise to secretory vesicles along the axon. It is associated with transport of material along the axon. The secretory vesicles range in size from 40 to 100 μm. Concentrations of vesicles are seen along nodes of Ranvier and within nerve terminals. Lysosomes usually are observed near nodes of Ranvier and accumulate in abundance during the degeneration of nerves after an injury. Axons retain a uniform diameter throughout their length. They may have collateral branches proximally, and they usually branch extensively at their distal ends (*telodendria*) before terminating by synaptic contact with dendrites and cell bodies of other neurons or on effector organs (muscles and glands).

Axons may be myelinated or unmyelinated (Fig. 7-10). In either case, they are ensheathed by supporting cells; these are Schwann cells in the peripheral nervous system and oligodendroglia in the central nervous system. Myelinated axons are wrapped in multiple layers of the external membrane, or myelin, of these supporting cells (Fig. 7-11); the process of myelin formation is considered later in this chapter. The myelin sheath is discontinuous at the distal ends of each cell involved in the ensheathing process. This area of discontinuity, termed the *node of Ranvier*, is the site of voltage-gated sodium channels and ionic movements of impulse conduction. The flow of an electrical impulse along the nerve fiber thus skips from one node of Ranvier to the next (*saltatory conduction*). Between nodes of Ranvier, myelin sheaths serve to insulate axons.

Myelin is composed of a lipid-protein complex. Some of the lipid is usually lost during tissue preparation, leaving behind a resistant proteolipid, neurokeratin. In addition to myelin sheaths, peripheral nerve fibers are surrounded by connective tissue, the

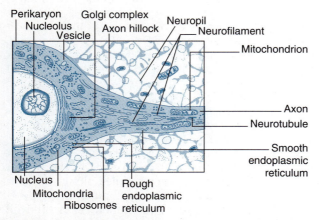

FIGURE 7-9. Schematic diagram of the perikaryon, axon hillock, and axon.

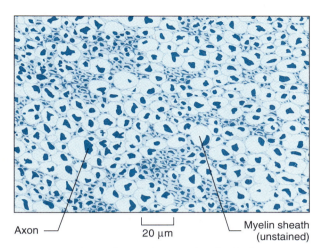

FIGURE 7-10. Schematic diagram of axons and myelin sheaths. *Note that the dark staining axons are of varying sizes. Unstained (clear) myelin sheaths surround the axons.*

endoneurium. The endoneurium is continuous with the *perineurium,* which contains more abundant connective tissue and envelops each bundle of nerve fibers. Nerve trunks are ensheathed in turn by the *epineurium.*

Myelinated axons range in diameter from 1 to 20 μm, whereas unmyelinated axons are less than 2 μm in diameter. The diameter of the nerve fiber (axon and myelin sheath) bears a direct relationship to the rate of impulse conduction. Large myelinated fibers conduct faster than small unmyelinated ones.

Dendrites

Although neurons possess only a single axon, they usually have more than one dendrite, which is tapered distally and may be highly branched. The dendrites may increase tremendously the surface area of the cell body from which they arise. Dendrites usually are covered by a large number of spines or *gemmules,* which are small projections representing sites of synaptic contact. They contain all the organelles found within the neuroplasm of the perikaryon except the Golgi apparatus. Neurons that receive axon terminals or synapses from a variety of sources in the nervous system may have an extremely complex dendritic organization (e.g., Purkinje's cell of the cerebellum). Most cells of the central nervous system and the autonomic ganglia have dendrites extending from their perikarya. This type of neuron is called *multipolar.* Those that possess only axon-like processes extending from each end of the cell are termed *bipolar;* bipolar neurons are found in the retina of the eye, olfactory receptors, and the peripheral ganglia of the vestibulocochlear nerve (eighth cranial nerve, or CN VIII). Sensory neurons located in the dorsal root of spinal nerves are termed *pseudo-unipolar,* because only a single process leaves the cell body before bifurcating to form proximal and distal segments (see Fig. 7-2). The processes of bipolar and pseudo-unipolar neurons are axon-like in structure and have a limited or specific receptive capacity; however, they usually retain the diversified terminal axonal branchings within the central nervous system. Certain cells of the retina, the amacrine cells, generally are regarded as axonless.

Neuroglia

The interstitial supporting cells of the central nervous system are termed *neuroglia* (Figs. 7-12 and 7-13). The several varieties of neuroglia are:

- Astrocytes—fibrous or protoplasmic
- Oligodendroglia
- Ependymal cells
- Microglia

Astrocytes and oligodendroglia are known as the *macroglia.*

Astrocytes

Astrocytes, largest of the neuroglia, are branched stellate cells. The nuclei of these cells are ovoid, centrally located, and poorly stained, with little heterochromatin and no nucleoli. Their cytoplasm may contain small rounded granules and glial filaments composed of glial fibrillary acidic protein (GFAP). Their processes are closely applied to capillaries (perivascular end feet, or footplates) or to the pia mater.

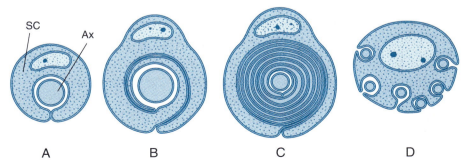

FIGURE 7-11. Schematic diagram of myelin sheath formation. *A and B, The myelin sheath is formed by concentric double layers of Schwann cell (SC) membranes wrapping themselves around the axon (Ax). C, The protoplasmic surfaces of the membrane become fused together, forming the major dense lines. In the peripheral nervous system, one Schwann cell produces myelin around a single axon. D, In contrast, unmyelinated axons are contained within the infoldings of a single Schwann cell.*

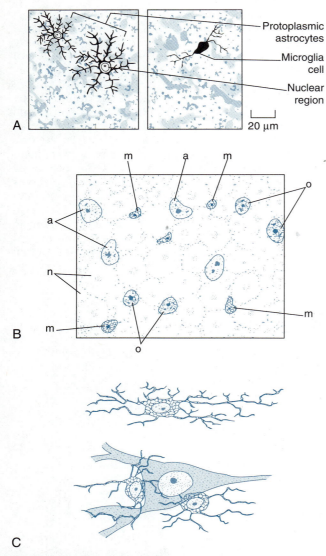

FIGURE 7–12. Schematic diagrams of neuroglia. A, Protoplasmic astrocytes with thick and numerous processes are contrasted with the microglia, which have slender and less numerous processes. B, Nuclei of astrocytes (a), oligodendroglia (o), microglia (m), and neuropil (n). C, The relationship of protoplasmic astrocytes to neurons.

FIBROUS ASTROCYTES. Fibrous astrocytes have thin, spindly processes that radiate from the cell body and terminate with distal expansions or footplates that are in contact with the walls of blood vessels lying within the central nervous system (see Fig. 7–13). The foot processes form a continuous glial sheath, the *perivascular limiting membrane*, around blood vessels. The cytoplasm of fibrous astrocytes contains filaments that extend throughout the cell as well as the usual cytoplasmic organelles. Fibrous astrocytes, found primarily within the white matter, are concerned with metabolite transfer and with repair of damaged tissue (scarring).

PROTOPLASMIC ASTROCYTES. Branches of protoplasmic astrocytes are thicker and more numerous than those of fibrous astrocytes (see Fig. 7–12). They are in close association with neurons and may partially envelop them; thus, they are considered satellite cells. Because they have a close relationship with neurons, they are found primarily in the gray matter of the brain and spinal cord. They may serve as metabolic intermediaries for nerve cells.

Oligodendroglia

Small cells, oligodendroglia have fewer and shorter branches than astrocytes (see Fig. 7–12). The nuclei are round and have condensed, stainable chromatin. The cytoplasm is less extensive and more dense than that of astrocytes and contains mitochondria, microtubules, and ribosomes; however, it is devoid of neurofilaments. Oligodendroglia are found in both gray matter and white matter. They usually are found lying in rows among the axons in the white matter. Electron-microscopic studies have implicated the oligodendroglia in central nervous system myelination. Within the gray matter, these cells are closely associated with neurons, as are the protoplasmic astrocytes (perineuronal satellite cells).

Ependymal Cells

Ependymal cells line the central canal of the spinal cord (see Fig. 7–13) and the ventricles of the brain. They are cuboidal to columnar and may possess cilia. Their cytoplasm contains mitochondria, a Golgi complex, and small granules. These cells are thought to be associated with the formation of cerebrospinal fluid. A specialized form of ependymal cell is seen in some areas of the nervous system, such as the subcommissural organ.

Microglia

The microglia, unlike other nerve and glial cells, are of mesodermal origin and enter the nervous system early in its development. Their cell bodies are small, dense, and elongated (see Fig. 7–12). They possess elongated nuclei and have few processes (occasionally two) at either end of the cell. The spindly processes may bear small, thorny spines. Under normal conditions, the function of the microglia is uncertain. When destructive lesions occur in the nervous system, the cells enlarge and become phagocytic and mobile. They are thus scavenger cells of the central nervous system.

Glial Cell Function

Glial cells have been classically described as the electrically passive elements of the nervous system. Recent studies have, however, demonstrated that glial cells in culture can express a variety of ligand-gated and voltage-gated ion channels that previously were believed to be properties of neurons. Sodium, calcium, chloride, and potassium channels have been described in glial cells; their functional significance remains unclear. Oligodendrocytes have been shown to change the potassium gradient across their membrane surprisingly quickly and then to have the potential to serve as

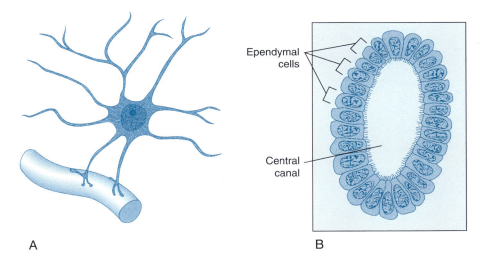

FIGURE 7–13. Schematic diagrams of neuroglia. A, *Fibrous astrocyte with its footplates in contact with blood vessel.* B, *Ependymal cells lining the central canal of the spinal cord.*

highly efficient potassium buffers. Receptors for many neurotransmitters and neuromodulators (GABA, glutamate, noradrenaline, substance P) have been demonstrated on glial cells, particularly astrocytes. Patch clamp studies have revealed that these glial receptors are similar in many respects to those on neurons.

GANGLIA

Ganglia are collections of nerve cell bodies located outside the central nervous system. There are two types of ganglia: craniospinal and autonomic.

Craniospinal Ganglia

The craniospinal ganglia are found in the dorsal roots of the 31 pairs of spinal nerves or in the sensory roots of the trigeminal (CN V), facial (CN VII), vestibulocochlear (CN VIII), glossopharyngeal (CN IX), and vagus (CN X) nerves. The dorsal root ganglia and the cranial nerve ganglia are sensory. They receive stimuli at their distal ends and transmit nerve impulses to the central nervous system. The ganglion cells of the spinal group are pseudo-unipolar neurons (see Fig. 7–2), whereas those of the vestibular and cochlear nerves are bipolar neurons. Dorsal root ganglion cells range in diameter from 15 to 100 μm.

In general, craniospinal ganglia can be divided into two groups. The smaller cells have unmyelinated axons, whereas the larger cells have myelinated axons. Each ganglion cell is surrounded by connective tissue and supporting cells, the perineuronal satellite cells or capsule cells, and from each, a single process emerges to bifurcate, forming an inverted T or Y, into proximal and distal axon-like processes. The intracapsular process may be coiled (so-called glomerulus) or relatively straight. The bipolar ganglion cells of the vestibular and cochlear cranial nerves are not encapsulated by satellite cells.

Autonomic Ganglia

Autonomic ganglia are aggregates of neurons extending from the base of the skull to the pelvis, usually in close association with and on either side of the vertebral bodies (sympathetic) or as part of the cranial-sacral nerves with ganglia located within the organ innervated (parasympathetic) (see Fig. 7–8). In contrast to cranial-spinal ganglia, the ganglion cells of the autonomic nervous system are multipolar and receive synaptic input from various levels of the nervous system. Autonomic ganglion cells are surrounded by connective tissue and small perineuronal satellite cells located between the dendrites in close association with the cell body.

Autonomic cells range in diameter from 20 to 60 μm and possess clear spherical or ovoid nuclei; some cells may be binucleate. The cytoplasm contains neurofibrils and small aggregates of RNA, Golgi apparatus, and mitochondria.

The dendritic processes of two or more cells often appear tangled and may form dendritic glomeruli; such cells are enclosed in a single capsule. The terminal arborizations of the ganglionic axons synapse on these dendritic glomeruli as well as on the dendrites of individual ganglion cells. In general, the preganglionic arborization of a single axon brings it into synaptic contact with numerous ganglion cells. The axons of these ganglion cells are small in diameter (0.3 to 1.3 μm).

Autonomic ganglion cells located within the viscera (intramural ganglia) may be few in number and distributed widely. They are not encapsulated but are contained within connective tissue septa in the organ innervated. The cells of the autonomic ganglia innervate visceral effectors such as smooth muscle, cardiac muscle, and glandular epithelium.

NERVE FIBERS

A *peripheral nerve* is composed of nerve fibers (axons) that vary in size, are myelinated or unmyeli-

TABLE 7-1. Some Properties of Mammalian Peripheral Nerve Fibers

Nerve Fiber Type					
Letter Designation	Number Designation	Function and/or Source	Fiber Size (μm)	Myelination	Conduction Velocity (m/sec)
A-alpha (α)	Ia	Proprioception, stretch (muscle spindle, annulospiral receptor), and motor to skeletal muscle fibers (extrafusal)	12–22	Yes	70–120
	Ib	Contractile force (Golgi tendon organ)	12–22	Yes	70–120
A-beta (β)	II	Pressure, stretch (muscle spindle, flower spray receptor), touch, and vibratory sense	5–12	Yes	30–70
A-gamma (γ)	II	Motor to muscle spindle (intrafusal muscle fibers)	2–8	Yes	15–30
A-delta (δ)	III	Some nerve endings serving pain, temperature, and touch	1–5	Yes	5–30
B		Sympathetic preganglionic axons	<3	Yes	3–15
C	IV	Other pain, temperature, and mechanical receptors; sympathetic, postganglionic axons (motor to smooth muscle and glands)	0.1–1.3	No	0.6–2.0

nated, and transmit nerve impulses either to or from the central nervous system. A peripheral nerve is often called a *mixed nerve,* because it is composed of both motor and sensory fibers. Nerves containing only sensory fibers are called *sensory nerves;* those that contain only motor fibers are called *motor nerves.* The structure of a nerve changes along its length because of the repeated division and union of different fascicles to form complex fascicular plexuses.

The nerve fibers that constitute a peripheral nerve have been classified according to size and other functional characteristics (Table 7–1). A-alpha axons range in diameter from 12 to 22 μm, A-beta axons from 5 to 12 μm; A-gamma axons from 2 to 8 μm; and A-delta axons from 1 to 5 μm. Preganglionic sympathetic fibers are less than 3 μm in diameter and are designated B-fibers. All of these are myelinated nerve fibers. The smallest axons (0.1 to 3 μm in diameter), designated C-fibers, are unmyelinated.

A peripheral nerve may contain thousands of axons invested in a connective tissue sheath. A study of nerve cross-sections shows that the proportion of connective tissue varies from 25% to 85%. The proportion of connective tissue stroma is greater at points where nerves cross joints or where there are relatively greater numbers of smaller nerve fascicles. The connective tissue elements are largely responsible for the tensile strength of nerve fascicles.

Three parts of the sheath are recognized (Fig. 7–14). The outer sheath, the *epineurium,* is generally thick, is composed of loose (areolar) connective tissue, and contains blood vessels and lymphatic vessels. It is continuous with the connective tissue of the dura mater. The epineurium gives the nerve its cordlike appearance and consistency and separates it from surrounding tissues. The epineurium acts as a shock absorber that dissipates stresses set up in the nerve when pressure is applied to the nerve. Nerves composed of closely packed fasciculi with little supporting epineurial tissue are more vulnerable to mechanical injury than nerves in which fasciculi are more widely separated by a greater amount of epineurial tissue. A larger amount of epineurial connective tissue exists where the number of nerve fascicles is higher and in areas where nerves cross joints.

From the epineurium, collagenous septa join with the dense *perineurium,* which separates and encompasses groups of axons in fascicles of different sizes. The perineurium partitions the fascicle and follows the nerve branches to the periphery, where it eventually may become a single cell layer of connective tissue (the sheath of Henle). Small blood vessels traverse these septa to reach the nerve fibers. The perineurium is continuous with the pia-arachnoid membrane and gives tensile strength and elasticity to the nerve. The perineurium is also considered a specialized structure that provides active transport of materials across the perineurial cells from and into the nerve fascicles. It also acts as a diffusion (blood-nerve) barrier similar to the pia-arachnoid with which it is continuous.

The inner sheath of connective tissue, the *endoneurium,* invests each axon and is continuous with the connective tissue forming the perineurium and epineu-

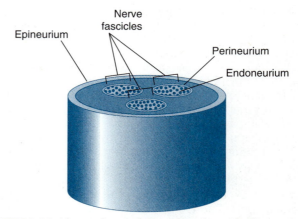

FIGURE 7–14. Schematic diagram of the structure of a peripheral nerve. *Nerve fascicles are separated by perineurium and surrounded by epineurium. Within each nerve fascicle, endoneurium separates individual axons.*

rium. This connective tissue provides a tough, protective, tubular sheath for the delicate axons. Within the endoneurium and surrounding each myelinated or unmyelinated axon are the Schwann cells. It is the Schwann cell that produces the myelin sheath (Fig. 7–15). This nucleated sheath of peripheral nerve fibers is also known as the *neurolemma* or *sheath of Schwann*.

In general, large axons are myelinated, and the smallest axons are unmyelinated. It is not known what factors determine the selection of fibers for myelination, but axon caliber and trophic influences on the Schwann cell from the axon have been implicated. The conduction velocity of axons is directly related to axon diameter and the thickness of the myelin sheath. Conduction is progressively faster in axons with larger diameters and thicker myelin sheaths.

Nerves are well supplied by a longitudinally arranged, anastomosing system of blood vessels that originate from neighboring large arteries and veins, muscular perforators, and periosteal vessels. These vessels ramify within the epineurium and reach the perineurium and endoneurium. Anastomoses are common between arterioles, between venules, and between arterioles and venules. There are also numerous anastomoses between epineurial and perineurial arterioles and endoneurial capillaries (Fig. 7–16). Electron-microscopic studies reveal structural differences between epineurial and endoneurial vessels. Endothelial cells that make up epineurial vessels have cell junctions of the open variety, allowing extravasation of protein macromolecules. Small amounts of serum protein can diffuse out into the epineurium but cannot pass through the perineurium. Endoneurial vessels, in contrast, have endothelial cells with tight junctions, which prevent extravasation of pro-

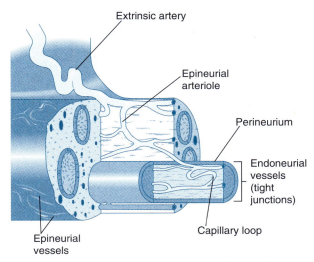

FIGURE 7–16. Schematic diagram of vascular supply of peripheral nerve. *Note the longitudinally arranged anastomosing system of epineurial, perineurial, and endoneurial vessels. The last have endothelial cells with tight junctions, which prevent extravasation of proteins within the endoneurial space.*

teins within the endoneurial space. These vessels, along with the perineurium, constitute the *blood-nerve barrier*.

Myelinated Nerve Fibers

Electron-microscopic studies have shown that most axons larger than 1 μm are myelinated. The myelin sheath, a proteophospholipid complex, is formed by many concentric double layers of Schwann cell membrane. The cell membrane is tightly wound, and the inner or protoplasmic surfaces of the membrane become fused, forming the dense, thicker lamellae of the myelin sheath (major dense lines) seen in electronmicrographs. The inner, less dense lamellae (intraperiod lines) are formed by the outer surfaces of the membrane. The sheath is not continuous but is interrupted at either end of the Schwann cell. A gap always exists between adjacent Schwann cells; this gap is termed the *node of Ranvier*. Sodium channels are known to be clustered at the nodes of Ranvier but are present in low density in the internodal axonal membrane. Interdigitating processes of Schwann cells partially cover the node. The internodal distance varies between 400 and 1500 μm, depending on fiber diameter and species. The axon at the node of Ranvier shows variations unique to this area. The number of mitochondria in the axon at the node is five-fold that in other areas. Lamellated autophagic vesicles, smooth endoplasmic reticulum profiles, glycogen granules, and lysosome-like granules are more numerous at this site. There is also an overall narrowing of the axon at the node.

Ultrastructural studies of the node of Ranvier reveal that the entire paranodal region, adjacent Schwann cell membranes, and the nodal axon constitute a single functional unit.

Occasionally, areas of incomplete fusion of the Schwann cell membrane occur, and small amounts

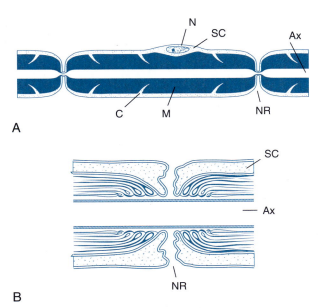

FIGURE 7–15. Schematic diagrams of myelinated peripheral nerve structure. A, *The central axon (Ax) is surrounded by myelin sheath (M) and Schwann cell cytoplasm (SC). Within the myelin sheath are the Schmidt-Lanterman clefts (C). Two nodes of Ranvier (NR) are shown. A nucleus (N) of Schwann cell is also shown.* B, *The ultrastructure of one node of Ranvier (NR) with interdigitating processes of Schwann cell (SC) cytoplasm. Ax, axon.*

of Schwann cell cytoplasm are trapped between the membranes. These areas of incomplete fusion are called *Schmidt-Lanterman clefts*. Their significance is not understood; they may be shearing defects in the formation of the myelin, or they may represent a kind of distention of the myelin sheath in which Schwann cell cytoplasm is left behind as the cell winds around the axon. Axonal myelin ends near the terminal arborization of the axon. It is now established that the axon provides the signal for myelination to take place. This signal seems to be carried by molecules located on the axonal membrane.

Myelination within the central nervous system is accomplished by oligodendroglia cells in a manner similar to that in the peripheral nervous system; however, the internodal distance and gap are smaller. In the peripheral nervous system, one Schwann cell produces myelin around a single axon. In the central nervous system, one oligodendroglial cell produces myelin around an entire group of axons in its vicinity, ranging from 3 to 200 axons.

Unmyelinated Nerve Fibers

Unlike their larger counterparts, several (8 to 15) small axons may be contained within the infoldings of a single Schwann cell, from which they are separated by a constant periaxonal space. The invested axon appears in cross-section to be suspended by a short segment of the invaginated outer membrane, which after encircling the axon is folded back and closely approximated. The similarity in appearance to the intestine within its mesentery has led to the term *mesaxon* for this membranous arrangement. Unmyelinated nerve fibers do not have nodes of Ranvier. Within the central nervous system, glial cells serve the same function as Schwann cells by ensheathing the nonmyelinated axons.

Conduction of Nerve Impulses

The cell membrane plays a key role in nerve impulse transmission. In unmyelinated fibers, the impulse is conducted as a spreading wave of change in membrane permeability that moves along the axon and induces the release of a transmitter substance at the axon terminal. The change in membrane permeability is associated with an influx of sodium ions and an efflux of potassium ions. In myelinated fibers, permeability changes occur only at the nodes of Ranvier; the insulating effect of myelin along the internodes prevents the propagation of the impulse. The impulse in such nerves jumps from one node to the next. This process, known as *saltatory conduction,* is faster than the process of continuous conduction of unmyelinated nerves. The loss of the myelin sheath, called *demyelination,* can disrupt conduction and thereby produce profound neurologic deficits.

Axonal Transport

Proteins synthesized in the perikarya of neurons are transported along the axon to its terminal. Axonal transport flows in two directions, anterograde from the perikarya to the synaptic terminal and retrograde from the terminal to the perikarya (Fig. 7–17). The retrograde transport system is very important for the recycling of intra-axonal proteins and neurotransmitters and for the transmission of extraneural materials from nerve endings to the neuron, the mechanism by which trophic influences from end organs reach neurons. Anterograde transport flows primarily at two rates, fast (100 to 400 mm/day) and slow (0.25 to 3 mm/day). Retrograde axoplasmic transport is fast and occurs at about half the velocity of the fast anterograde component. There is no slow retrograde transport component. There is no difference in rate of material transport between sensory axons and motor axons.

Microtubules are involved in fast anterograde and retrograde transport; thus, microtubule-disrupting drugs, such as colchicine and vinblastine, prevent fast axonal transport. In the case of fast anterograde transport, a distinctive protein, *kinesin,* is known to provide the motive force driving organelles along microtubules. A different protein, *dynein,* may be involved in fast retrograde transport. Substances moved by fast axonal transport are contained in the mitochondria or small vesicles of smooth endoplasmic reticulum. They include enzymes of neurotransmitter metabolism as well as peptide neurotransmitters and neuromodulators. Fast axoplasmic transport requires energy in the form of high-energy phosphate compounds; therefore, it is necessary for the neuron to be oxygenated adequately. Any interruption of mitochondrial oxidative phosphorylation causes axoplasmic flow to cease.

Substances transported by the slow component are structural proteins such as tubulin, actin, and neurofilamentous proteins. The underlying mechanism of motility for slow transport is not yet known. On the basis of the concept of anterograde and retrograde axonal transport, neuroanatomic tracing methods have been developed to study neural connectivity. A radioactively labeled amino acid injected into a region of neuronal perikarya is incorporated into proteins and is transported anterogradely to the axonal terminal. Alternatively, a histochemically demonstrable enzyme, horseradish peroxidase, travels retrogradely from the axonal terminals to the somata. Different fluorescent dyes injected at two different sites travel retrogradely to the neuron or neurons that project on those sites. Somata sending axons to the two injected sites fluoresce in different colors. A neuron whose axon branches end in both injected sites will be labeled in in two colors.

SYNAPSE

The simplest unit of segmental nerve function requires two neurons, a receptor or sensory neuron and a motor or effector neuron (e.g., the patellar tendon

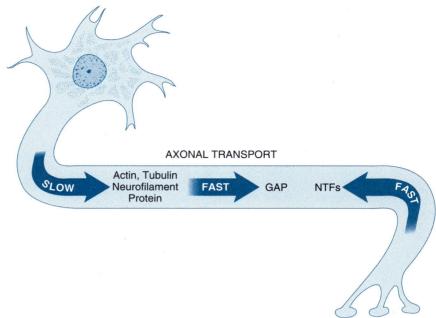

FIGURE 7-17. Schematic diagram of axonal transport. *The two types of anterograde transport are slow and fast. The only type of retrograde transport is fast. Substances transported in each direction are shown. GAP, growth-associated proteins; NTFs, neuronotropic factors.*

reflex or knee jerk). The structural-functional coupling of these two neurons is effected by a synapse. The terminal arborizations of the sensory neuron (axons) are dilated into small knobs or boutons (*boutons terminaux*), which lie on the dendrites, cell body, and axon of the effector neuron (Fig. 7–18). These small bulbs contain synaptic vesicles ranging in size from 300 to 600 μm. The vesicles may appear empty or clear but actually contain acetylcholine. In other kinds of synapses, the vesicles may contain a dense particle or core that is presumed to be catecholamine. Acetylcholine and catecholamine are among several chemical transmitter substances that facilitate the transfer of nerve impulses from one neuron to another or to a nonneuronal effector organ (muscle or gland). Electron microscopy has revealed the specialized structure of the synapse, which consists of thickened presynaptic and postsynaptic membranes separated by a synaptic gap (cleft) of about 200 μm. The thickness of presynaptic and postsynaptic membranes represents accumulations of cytoplasmic proteins beneath the membrane. Besides the synaptic vesicles, the synaptic terminal con-

FIGURE 7-18. Schematic diagram of nerve cell. *Nucleus, nucleolus, and cell organelles are shown. The axon hillock is devoid of Nissl substance. Axosomatic, axodendritic, and axoaxonic synapses are also shown.*

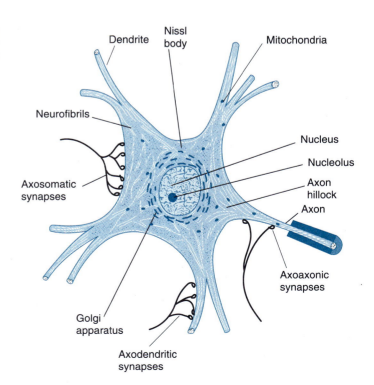

tains abundant mitochondria and infrequent neurofilaments (Fig. 7–19).

When an action potential arrives at an axon terminal, the membrane of the terminal is depolarized. Calcium ions enter the terminal and promote the fusion of synaptic vesicles with the presynaptic membrane. The neurotransmitter contained within synaptic vesicles is released by exocytosis into the synaptic gap (cleft), where it diffuses out and binds to receptors on the postsynaptic membrane. The ionic permeability of the postsynaptic membrane increases, leading to membrane depolarization and generation of an action potential in the target neuron.

Growing evidence indicates the importance of protein phosphorylation in the regulation of presynaptic nerve terminal function. Major synaptic vesicle–associated proteins include the *synapsins* (Ia and Ib, IIa and IIb), *synaptophysin*, and *synaptobrevin*. The precise physiologic functions of these phosphoproteins remains unknown, but that of synapsin I is becoming increasingly apparent. Phosphorylation of synapsin I occurs in response to nerve impulses and to a variety of neurotransmitters acting at presynaptic receptors. Dephosphosynapsin I binds to vesicles and inhibits their availability for release. Phosphorylation of synapsin I decreases its affinity for synaptic vesicles, which then become available for release. In addition to their role in neurotransmitter release, proteins of the synapsin family may also regulate the formation of presynaptic nerve terminals. Synapsin expression has been shown to correlate temporally with synapse formation during development and to play a causal role in synaptogenesis.

Functionally, synapses may be excitatory or inhibitory; transmission usually is unidirectional and not obligatory, except at the neuromuscular junction. Electron microscopy, however, has shown a wide variety of structural arrangements in synapses, suggesting that the transmission may be bidirectional in some.

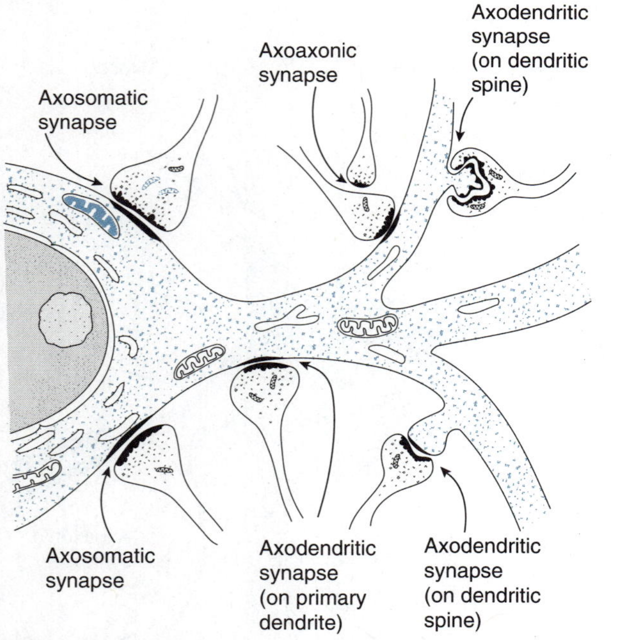

Some synapses, termed *electrical synapses*, have no synaptic vesicles, and the adjacent cell membranes are fused. The fused membranes of electrical synapses are called *tight junctions* or *gap junctions*. The transmission at these junctions is by electrotonic depolarization; it may be in either direction and is considered obligatory. These are not common in the mammalian nervous system.

Synapses have been classified according to their structural associations as follows:

- Axoaxonic: axon to axon.
- Axodendritic: axon to dendrite.
- Axosomatic: axon to cell body.
- Dendrodendritic: dendrite to dendrite.
- Neuromuscular: axon to muscle.

In chemical synapses, the following substances have been identified as transmitters: acetylcholine, monoamines (noradrenaline, adrenaline, dopamine, serotonin), glycine, γ-aminobutyric acid (GABA), and glutamic acid. Two natural brain peptide neurotransmitters, endorphins and enkephalins, have been shown to be potent inhibitors of pain receptors. They exhibit a morphine-like analgesic effect.

Other peptide hormones, such as substance P, cholecystokinin, vasopressin, oxytocin, vasoactive intestinal peptides, and bombesin, have been described in different regions of the brain, where they act as modulators of transmitter actions.

Although available data assign a role for peptides in chemical transmission that is auxiliary to that of classic neurotransmitters, peptides play the main role in certain neuronal systems. This is particularly apparent in hypothalamic neurosecretory cells, which produce and release the posterior pituitary hormones vasopressin and oxytocin.

In addition to their role in transmission, peptides seem to have a trophic function. Tachykinins have been shown to stimulate growth of fibroblasts and smooth muscle cells; vasoactive intestinal peptides affect bone mineralization and stimulate the growth of human keratinocytes.

During the last few years, increasing evidence seems to suggest a messenger role for peptides in the nervous system. It is now clear that peptides have their own receptors in the nervous system. Receptors for tachykinins, substance P, neurokinin A (substance K), and neurotensin have been cloned.

Neuromuscular Junction

The neuromuscular junction (myoneural junction, motor end-plate) is a synapse between a motor nerve terminal and the subjacent part of a muscle fiber. Motor neurons branch extensively near their terminations. One neuron may innervate as few as 10 or as many as

FIGURE 7–19. Synapses. *Schematic diagram of axosomatic, axoaxonic, and axodendritic synapses. Two varieties of axodendritic synapses are shown, those terminating on primary dendrites and those on dendritic spines.*

500 or more skeletal muscle fibers. A motor neuron and the muscle fibers it innervates constitute the *motor unit*. The motor unit, not the individual muscle fiber, is the basic unit of function. As the nerve fiber approaches the muscle fiber, it loses its myelin sheath and forms a bulbous expansion that occupies a trough on the muscle cell surface (Fig. 7–20). The terminal expansion of the nerve fiber is covered by a cytoplasmic layer of Schwann cells, the *neurolemmal sheath*. The endoneurial sheath of connective tissue that surrounds the nerve fiber outside the neurolemmal sheath is, however, continuous with the connective tissue sheath of the muscle fiber.

The end-plate is 40 to 60 μm in diameter and is usually located midway along the length of the muscle fiber. The axonal terminal contains synaptic vesicles (filled with acetylcholine) and mitochondria. The synaptic gap (cleft) between the nerve and the muscle is about 500 Å. The postsynaptic membrane of the muscle has numerous infoldings, termed *junctional folds* (see Fig. 7–20). When a motor neuron is fired, and the nerve impulse reaches the axon terminal, the contents of the synaptic vesicles (acetylcholine) in the terminal are discharged into the gap between the presynaptic and postsynaptic membranes. Once acetylcholine is released into the cleft, it diffuses very quickly to combine with acetylcholine receptors in the muscle membrane. The binding of acetylcholine to the receptor makes the muscle membrane (sarcolemma) more permeable to sodium. This results in the depolarization of the muscle membrane and the appearance of a propagated muscle action potential, leading to muscle contraction. This synaptic activity is always excitatory and is normally obligatory. The subneural sarcolemma or postsynaptic membrane contains the enzyme acetylcholinesterase, which breaks down the depolarizing transmitter, thus allowing the muscle membrane to re-establish resting conditions.

The most common disorder of the neuromuscular junction is a disease known as myasthenia gravis, which is characterized by the onset of muscle weakness after muscle use and improvement in weakness with rest. In this disease, antibodies bind to the acetylcholine receptors and render them less accessible to released acetylcholine. Many commercial pesticides and nerve gases interfere with neuromuscular transmission by inhibiting the hydrolysis (destruction) of acetylcholine, thus prolonging its effect on the muscle and thereby inactivating the muscle. Botulinum toxin interferes with neuromuscular transmission by blocking the release of acetylcholine from the presynaptic membrane.

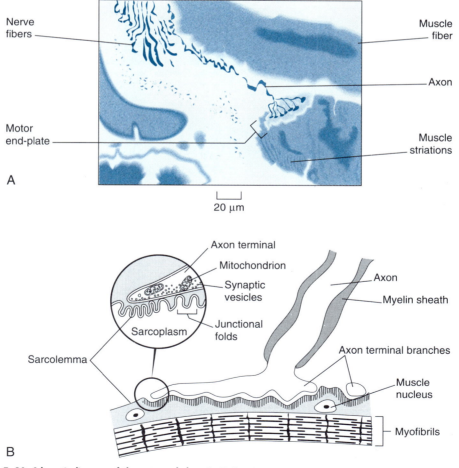

FIGURE 7–20. Schematic diagrams of the motor end-plate. A, *Light-microscopic appearance.* B, *Ultrastructural appearance.*

RECEPTOR ORGANS OF SENSORY NEURONS

The peripheral termination of a sensory neuron is differentiated into specialized dendrites. These dendrites are designed to change or transduce one kind of energy into another (i.e., the electrochemical or nerve impulses). Sensory receptors may be classified according to function (nociceptor, mechanoreceptor), structure (free or encapsulated), a combination of structure and function, or anatomic localization (skin, joints). Each receptor possesses different sensitivity and adaptive properties based on its response to continuous monotonic stimulation. Receptors may adapt quickly or slowly. Quickly adapting receptors produce impulses that gradually decrease to baseline values in response to a constant, unvarying stimulus. Slowly adapting receptors continue their response throughout the duration of the stimulus. Slowly adapting receptors are of two types. Type I receptors have no spontaneous discharge at rest and are more sensitive to vertical displacement; type II receptors maintain a slow regular discharge at rest and are more sensitive to stretch.

Free Nerve Endings

The free nerve ending is the type of receptor with the widest distribution throughout the body, being most numerous in the skin. Such receptors are also found in mucous membranes, deep fascia, muscle, and visceral organs. The distal arborizations are located in the epithelium between the cells, skin, and mucous membranes lining the digestive and urinary tracts, as well as in all the visceral organs and blood vessels. In addition, they are associated with hair follicles and respond to movement of hair. Certain specialized epithelial cells (neuroepithelium), such as are found in taste buds (Fig. 7–21), olfactory epithelium, and the cochlear and vestibular organs (hair cells), also receive free (receptor) nerve endings. Tendons, joint capsules, periosteum, and deep fascia may also be supplied with this type of nerve ending. Free nerve endings probably respond directly to a wide variety of stimuli, including pain, touch, pressure, and tension, and indirectly through so-called neuroepithelia to sound, smell, taste, and position. The sensory receptor axons may be either myelinated or unmyelinated.

MERKEL'S CORPUSCLES. Slowly adapting type I mechanoreceptors, Merkel's corpuscles are distributed in the germinal layer (stratum basale) of the epidermis. Groups of five or ten such corpuscles are interspersed among the basal layer cells. Unmyelinated free nerve endings form an axonal expansion *(Merkel's disk)* closely applied to a modified epidermal cell *(Merkel's cell)*. Merkel's cells are found in glabrous skin and in the outer sheaths of hairs in hairy skin. They are also found in areas of transition between hairy skin and mucous membrane. Synapse-like junctions have been observed between Merkel's disks and Merkel's cells; their functional significance, however, is uncertain. Merkel's cor-

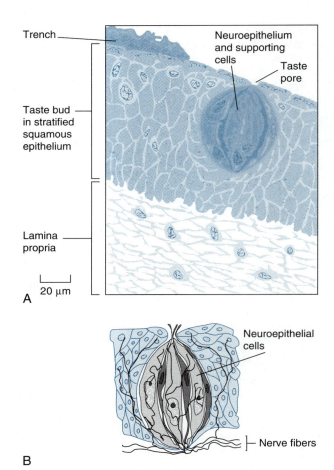

FIGURE 7–21. Schematic diagrams of taste bud. A, *The taste bud embedded in the stratified squamous epithelium of the tongue.* B, *Dark and light neuroepithelial cells of the taste bud and sensory nerve fibers.*

puscle subserves the sensory modality of constant touch or pressure and is responsible for tactile gnosis of static objects. The discharge frequency of Merkel's corpuscles is temperature dependent. Cooling the skin increases discharge, and warming it inhibits discharge.

Encapsulated Endings

Encapsulated nerve endings (Fig. 7–22) include the corpuscles of Meissner, Vater-Pacini, Golgi-Mazzoni, and Ruffini, the so-called end bulbs, neuromuscular spindles, and the tendon organ of Golgi.

MEISSNER'S TACTILE CORPUSCLES. Elongated, rounded bodies, Meissner's corpuscles are fitted into dermal papillae beneath the epidermis and are about 100 μm in diameter. Each corpuscle possesses a connective tissue sheath enclosing stacks of horizontally flattened epithelioid cells. The endoneurium is continuous with the capsule. The myelin sheath terminates, and the axon (A-beta fiber) arborizes among the epithelial cells. From one to four myelinated axons, as well as unmyelinated axons, enter the capsule.

These receptor organs are distributed widely in the skin, but they are found in greatest number in the hairless (glabrous) skin of the fingers, palm of the hand,

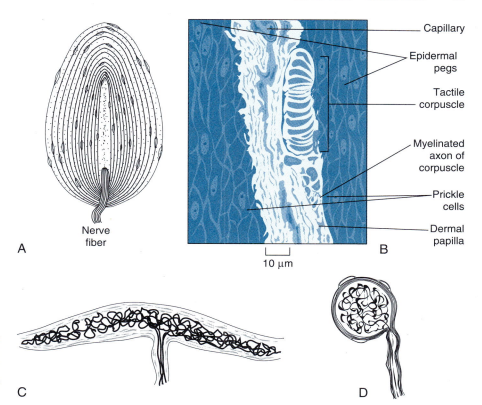

FIGURE 7–22. Schematic diagrams of four types of encapsulated nerve endings. A, Vater-Pacini (pacinian) corpuscle. B, Meissner's (tactile) corpuscle. C, Ruffini's corpuscle. D, Krause's corpuscle (end bulb of Krause).

plantar surface of the foot, toes, nipples, and lips. They are rapidly adapting mechanoreceptors. The sensory modality subserved by Meissner's corpuscles is low-frequency (30 to 40 Hz) flutter-vibration and moving touch. Under sustained pressure, an impulse is produced at the onset, removal, or change of magnitude of the stimulus.

VATER-PACINI (PACINIAN) CORPUSCLES. Pacinian corpuscles are the largest and most widely distributed of the encapsulated receptor organs. They may be as long as 4 mm and are the only macroscopic receptor organs in the body. The capsule is elliptical and is composed of concentric lamellae of flattened cells (fibroblasts) supported by collagenous tissue that invests the unmyelinated distal segment of a large myelinated (A-beta) nerve fiber. The interlamellar spaces are filled with fluid. These corpuscles receive their own blood supply.

Vater-Pacini corpuscles are mechanoreceptors sensitive to vibration. They are maximally responsive at 250 to 300 Hz. They are rapidly adapting receptors that respond only transiently at stimulus onset and offset or at the end of a step change in stimulus position. The recovery cycle of this receptor is extremely short (5 to 6 msec). The rapid adaptation of pacinian corpuscles is a function of the connective tissue capsule that surrounds central neural elements. The removal of the connective tissue capsule transforms the pacinian corpuscle from a rapidly adapting receptor to a slowly adapting one.

These ubiquitous receptors are distributed profusely in the subcutaneous connective tissue of the hands and feet. They are also located in the external genitalia, nipples, mammary glands, pancreas and other viscera, mesenteries, linings of the pleural and abdominal cavities, walls of blood vessels, periosteum, ligaments, joint capsules, and muscle. Of the estimated 2000 pacinian corpuscles in the human skin, more than one third are in the digits, and more than 100 may be found in a single finger.

GOLGI-MAZZONI CORPUSCLES. Quickly adapting receptor organs, Golgi-Mazzoni corpuscles are lamellated (like the pacinian corpuscles), but instead of a single receptor terminal, the unmyelinated receptor is arborized with varicosities and terminal expansions. These corpuscles are distributed in the subcutaneous tissue of the hands, on the surface of tendons, in the periosteum adjacent to joints, and elsewhere. Their function is uncertain, but it is probably related to the detection of vibration with maximal response under 200 Hz.

RUFFINI'S CORPUSCLES. Ruffini's corpuscles are elongated and complex receptors found most readily in the dermis of the skin, especially the fingertips, but they are widely distributed, especially in joint capsules. The receptor endings within the capsule ramify extensively among the supporting connective tissue bundles. These type II slowly adapting receptors have been associated with sensations of pressure and touch, as velocity and position detectors. The discharge of Ruffini's corpuscles is temperature dependent. It increases with skin cooling and decreases with skin warming. Three types of Ruffini's corpuscles have been identified in joint capsules on the basis of their position-related discharge. All maintain constant baseline output, but each type responds maximally at a different joint position: one at extreme flexion, another at extreme extension, and the third midway between flexion and extension of the joint.

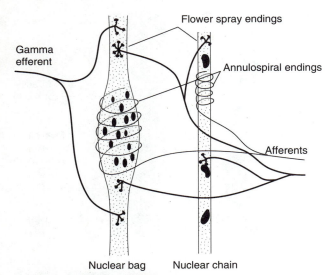

FIGURE 7-23. Schematic diagram of muscle spindle. *Two types of intrafusal muscle fibers (nuclear bag and nuclear chain), two types of afferent endings (flower spray and annulospiral), and the gamma efferent input are shown.*

END BULBS. The end bulbs resemble Golgi-Mazzoni corpuscles. They have a connective tissue capsule enclosing a gelatinous core in which the terminal, unmyelinated endings arborize extensively. The end bulbs of Krause (see Fig. 7-22) (Krause's corpuscles) are associated with sensations of temperature (cold) and are located strategically and distributed widely. The structural complexity of these end bulbs varies remarkably, as does their size. It is likely that they serve a wide variety of different functions; their size and distribution, however, preclude easy analysis. Much confusion has arisen regarding the end bulbs of Krause, because Krause identified and named two morphologically different structures "end bulbs."

NEUROMUSCULAR SPINDLES. Found in skeletal muscle, neuromuscular spindles are highly organized. Muscle spindles are distributed in both flexor and extensor muscles, but they are more abundant in muscles controlling fine movements. Each muscle spindle is less than 1 cm long and contains 2 to 12 specialized striated fibers (intrafusal fibers) in a connective tissue capsule parallel with the surrounding skeletal muscle fibers (extrafusal fibers).

Histologically, the muscle spindle is composed of two types of intrafusal muscle fibers (Fig. 7-23). The nuclear chain fiber, smaller in diameter and shorter in length, contains a single row of central nuclei. The nuclear bag fiber, larger and longer, contains a cluster of nuclei in a baglike dilatation in the central part of the fiber.

Each intrafusal muscle fiber is supplied with both efferent and afferent nerve fibers. The efferent fibers (gamma efferents), which are axons of gamma motor neurons in the anterior horn of the spinal cord, terminate on the polar ends of both the nuclear chain and nuclear bag fibers. The afferent nerve fibers originate from two types of receptor endings on the intrafusal fibers, the annulospiral (primary) endings and the flower spray (secondary) endings (see Fig. 7-23). The *annulospiral endings* are reticulated branching endings located around the central portion of both nuclear chain fibers and nuclear bag fibers; they are well developed, however, on the nuclear bag fibers. The *flower spray endings* are scattered diffusely along the length of the intrafusal fibers, but they are found especially on each side of the central portion adjacent to the annulospiral endings. Both nuclear chain fibers and nuclear bag fibers contain this type of ending.

The receptor endings of intrafusal muscle fibers respond to the stretching of extrafusal muscle fibers or their tendons. The activity of the spindle ceases with the relaxation of tension in the spindle, when the skeletal muscle contracts. The receptor endings may also be stimulated by the stretching of the intrafusal muscle fibers secondary to gamma motor nerve activity, which contracts the polar ends of intrafusal muscle fibers, thus stretching the receptor portions of the fibers.

A static stimulus, such as occurs in sustained muscle stretch, stimulates both the annulospiral and flower spray endings. Only the annulospiral (primary) endings, however, respond to a brief (dynamic) stretch of the muscle or to vibration.

The afferent nerves emanating from the receptor endings project on alpha motor neurons in the spinal cord, which in turn supply the extrafusal muscle fibers. Thus, when a muscle is stretched by tapping its tendon, the stimulated receptor endings initiate an impulse in the afferent nerves, which stimulates the alpha motor neurons and results in reflex muscle contraction. As soon as the muscle contracts, the tension in the intrafusal muscle fibers decreases, the receptor response diminishes or ceases, and the muscle relaxes. This is the basis of all monosynaptic stretch reflexes (e.g., knee jerk, biceps jerk). Gamma-efferent activity plays a role in sensitizing the receptor endings to a stretch stimulus and helping to maintain muscle tone.

TENDON ORGAN OF GOLGI. Golgi tendon organs are slowly adapting receptors located in tendons close to their junction with skeletal muscles (Fig. 7-24) and in series with extrafusal muscle fibers. Each tendon organ consists of fascicles of tendon ensheathed by a connective tissue capsule. The capsule encloses the distal end of a large (12-μm) myelinated fiber, which divides repeatedly before it splits into unmyelinated (receptor) seg-

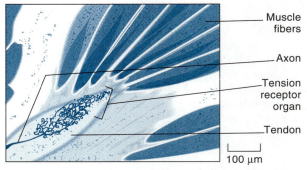

FIGURE 7-24. Schematic diagram of Golgi tendon organ embedded in muscle tendon.

ments. These branchlets terminate in ovoid expansions that intermingle with and encircle fascicles of collagenous tissue that compose the tendon. Tendon organs respond to tension in skeletal muscle fibers developed by stretching of the muscle or by active contraction of the muscle. The tension thus developed deforms the receptor endings. Afferent nerves emanating from Golgi tendon organs project on inhibitory interneurons in the spinal cord. Thus, when a muscle (and its tendon) is stretched excessively, the muscle relaxes.

REACTIONS OF NEURONS TO INJURY

The reaction of neurons to injury has been studied extensively in experimental animals and confirmed in humans; in fact, this reaction has become one of the methods employed in the study of cell groups and fiber tracts. Responses can be divided into those that occur proximal to the site of the injury and those that occur distal to it (Fig. 7–25). If death of the nerve cell does not occur, regenerative activity, in the form of nerve sprouts emanating from the proximal stump, may begin as early as 24 hours after the injury.

Cell Body and Dendrites

If an axon is severed or crushed, the following reactions can be found in the cell body and dendrites proximal to the site of the injury.

1. The entire cell, including the nucleus and nucleolus, swells; the nucleus shifts from its usual central position to the periphery of the cell.
2. The Nissl bodies undergo *chromatolysis* (i.e., they become diffuse), and the normally crisp staining pattern disappears. This process is most marked in the central portion of the cell (perinuclear), but it may extend peripherally to involve Nissl bodies located in dendrites. The process of chromatolysis reflects a change in metabolic priority from that geared to the production of neurotransmitters needed for synaptic activity to that geared to the production of materials for axonal repair and growth. The central cell must synthesize new messenger RNA, lipids, and cytoskeletal proteins. The components of the cytoskeleton most important for axonal regeneration are actin, tubulin, and neurofilament protein. These proteins are carried by slow anterograde axonal transport at a rate of 5 to 6 mm per day, which correlates with the maximum rate of axonal elongation during regeneration. Another group of proteins whose synthesis is increased during regeneration of nerve cells are growth-associated proteins (GAPs), which travel by fast axonal transport at a rate of up to 420 mm per day. Although GAPs do not initiate, terminate, or regulate growth, they are nevertheless essential for regeneration. Neuronotropic factors (NTFs) from the periphery signal to the cell body that an injury has occurred and travel by retrograde axonal transport (see Fig. 7–17).
3. The other organelles, including the Golgi apparatus and mitochondria, proliferate and swell.

The speed at which these changes occur, as well as their degree, depends on several factors, including the location of the injury, the type of injury, and the type of neuron involved. The closer the injury is to the cell body and the more complete the interruption of the axon, the more severe the reaction and the poorer the chances of full recovery. In general, this reaction is more often seen in motor neurons than in sensory neurons.

The reactions of the cell body and dendrites to axonal injury are termed retrograde cell changes. After about 3 weeks, if the cell survives the injury, the cell body and its processes begin to regenerate. Full recovery takes 3 to 6 months. The nucleus returns to its central location and is normal in size and configuration. The staining characteristics and structure of the organelles also return to normal. If regenerative efforts fail, the cell atrophies and is replaced by glia.

Axon

After an injury, the axon undergoes both retrograde (proximal) and anterograde (distal) degeneration. Retrograde degeneration usually involves only a short segment of the axon (a few internodes). Provided that the injury to the neuron is reversible, regenerative processes begin with the growth of an axon sprout as soon as new cytoplasm is synthesized and transported from the cell body. The regenerative sprouting of the proximal axon stump requires elongation of the axon. This process is mediated by a growth cone at the tip of the regenerating fiber (Fig. 7–26). Growth cones were first described by Ramon y Cajal, who compared their advance through solid tissue to a battering ram. Research has revealed that growth cones release a protease that dissolves the matrix, permitting their advance through

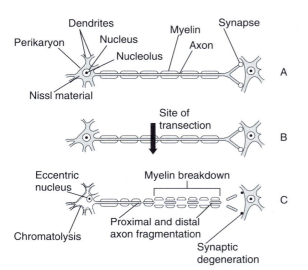

FIGURE 7–25. Reaction of neuron to injury. A, Normal neuron. B, Site of axon injury. C, Reaction to injury in the perikaryon, axon, and synapse.

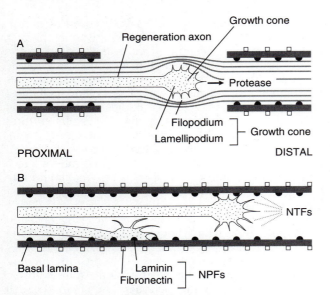

FIGURE 7–26. Schematic diagram of the process of axon sprouting and regeneration. A, Protease is released by the growth cone to facilitate its advance. B, The growth cone advances in response to clues from neurite-promoting factors (NPFs) (laminin, fibronectin) on the basal lamina of Schwann cells and from neuronotropic factors (NTFs) in the periphery.

tissue. Growth cones have mobile filopodia (extruding from a flattened sheet of lamellipodia), enabling them to move actively and explore the microenvironment of the regenerating axon. Growth cones play an essential role in axon guidance and are capable of responding to contact guidance clues provided by laminin and fibronectin, two major glycoprotein components of the basal laminae of Schwann cells.

Shortly after a nerve injury and before the onset of wallerian degeneration, severe degeneration of the tips of the proximal and distal stumps occurs. This injury is secondary to an influx of sodium and calcium and a massive loss of potassium and protein. This axonal debris may prevent the growth cone of the proximal stump from reaching a healthy distal stump.

Distal to the site of the injury, the severed axon and its myelin sheath undergo what is known as secondary or *wallerian degeneration,* so named in recognition of its description by Augustus Waller in 1852. The axon, deprived of its continuity with the supporting and nutritive substances from the cell body, begins to degenerate within 12 hours. The axon, which degenerates before its Schwann cell sheath, appears beaded and irregularly swollen within 1 week. The axonal reaction extends distally to involve the synapse. The fragmented portions of the axon are phagocytized by invading macrophages. This process may take considerably longer within the central nervous system.

Along with the degeneration of the axon, the myelin sheath begins to fragment and undergo dissolution within the Schwann cell. Macrophages also play an important role in the removal of myelin breakdown products. The degenerative process occurs within the endoneurium and is soon followed by mitotic activity in the Schwann cells, which form a tubelike sleeve within the endoneurium along the entire length of the degenerated axon. Endoneurial tubes persist after the myelin and axonal debris has been cleared. The proliferating Schwann cells align longitudinally within the endoneurial tube, creating a continuous column of cells called the bands of Büngner (Fig. 7–27). The growth of axons from the proximal stump begins within 10 hours and may traverse the gap between the proximal and distal ends of the axon and enter the Schwann cell tubes (neurolemma). Although many small axonal sprouts may enter a single tube, only one will develop its normal diameter and appropriate sheath; the others will degenerate. This process may occur within 2 or 3 weeks, because regenerative growth normally takes place at a rate of 1.5 to 4 mm per day. Failure to establish a pathway for regrowth may result in the formation of a *neuroma,* which is often a source of pain.

It must be pointed out that chance unfortunately plays an important part in this regenerative activity. If a sensory axon enters a sheath formerly occupied by a motor axon or vice versa, the growing axon will be nonfunctional, and the neuron will atrophy. Accurate growth and innervation of the appropriate distal target are thus of critical importance to the success of nerve regeneration. In this context, the target of innervation itself can exert a guiding "neurotropic" influence on a regenerating axon. Forrsman in 1898 and Ramon y Cajal subsequently have shown that the advancing tip of a regenerating axon is chemotropically attracted to its appropriate distal nerve target. Later experimental studies have confirmed this observation. In addition, although the process of degeneration is similar in both the central and peripheral nervous systems, there is a marked difference in the success of the regenerative process in the two systems. What has been previously described applies to regeneration in the peripheral nervous system. Degeneration of a neuron usually is limited to its perikaryon and processes. In certain areas of the nervous system, however, degeneration of a neuron is transmitted to the neuron with which it makes a connection. This type of degeneration is known as *transneuronal* degeneration.

Nerve Growth Factors

Successful nerve regeneration requires neuronal growth. Four classes of nerve growth factors are essential for optimal nerve growth:

- Neuronotropic factors (NTFs) or survival factors.

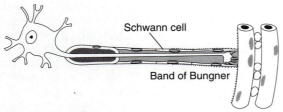

FIGURE 7–27. Schematic diagram of Schwann cell proliferation within the endoneurial tube to form a continuous column of cells, the band of Büngner.

TABLE 7-2. Sunderland Classification of Nerve Injury*

Degree of Severity	Wallerian Degeneration	Endoneurium Continuity	Perineurium Continuity	Epineurium Continuity	Nerve Fiber Continuity	Nerve Trunk Continuity
I	−	+	+	+	+	+
II	+	+	+	+	+	+
III	+	−	+	+	−	+
IV	+	−	−	+	−	+
V	+	−	−	−	−	−

*+ = present; − = absent.

- Neurite-promoting factors (NPFs), which control axonal advance and influence the rate, incidence, and direction of neurite growth.
- Matrix-forming precursors (MFPs), possibly fibrinogen and fibronectin, which contribute fibrin products to the nerve gap and provide scaffolding for the ingrowth of cells.
- Metabolic and other factors.

Neuronotropic factors (NTFs) are macromolecular proteins that promote the survival and growth of neuronal populations. They are present in the target of innervation, where they are taken up by the nerve terminals and transported by retrograde axonal transport back to the cell body. These factors exert a supportive or survival-promoting effect. The best-known NTF is nerve growth factor (NGF).

Neurite-promoting factors (NPFs) are substrate-bound glycoproteins that strongly promote neurite initiation and extension. Laminin and fibronectin, two components of the basal lamina, have been shown to promote neurite growth. Although NPFs were presumed to exert their neurite-promoting activity by increasing the adhesion of growth cones to the surface of the basal lamina, later studies have shown that NPFs promote neurite growth independent of growth cone adhesion.

After a nerve injury, a polymerized fibrin matrix is formed from the fibrinogen and fibronectin (thus the term *matrix-forming precursors*) found in exudates from the cut nerve ends. This matrix is important for the migration of Schwann cells and other cells into the gap between the cut ends.

Metabolic and other factors that promote nerve regeneration include sex hormones, thyroid hormone, adrenal hormones, insulin, and protease inhibitors.

Classification of Nerve Injury

Currently, there are two classifications of nerve injury based on the nature of the lesion in the nerve. The first classification, proposed by Seddon, recognizes three degrees of severity of nerve injury: conduction block (neurapraxia), loss of axonal continuity (axonotmesis), and loss of nerve trunk continuity (neurotmesis). The second classification, proposed by Sunderland, consists of five degrees of nerve injury (Table 7-2 and Fig. 7-28).

The *first* and least severe consists of a temporary physiologic conduction block in which axonal continuity is not interrupted. The conduction across the injured segment of the nerve is blocked. Conduction proximal and distal to the block is normal. The three connective tissue sheaths are intact. In the *second* degree of nerve injury, wallerian degeneration is present distal to the nerve lesion. Continuity of the endoneurial sheath is preserved, permitting regeneration of the distal segment of the nerve. The perineurial and epineurial sheaths also are preserved. The *third* degree of nerve injury is characterized by the loss of continuity of nerve fibers. Internal fascicular structure is disorganized, the endoneurial sheath becomes discontinuous, and wallerian degeneration is present. Perineurial and epineurial sheaths are, however, preserved. Axon regeneration in this type of injury is negligible because of the development of intrafascicular fibrosis and the loss of continuity of the endoneurial sheath. In the *fourth* degree of injury, fascicular nerve structure is destroyed. Endoneurial and perineurial sheaths are discontinuous. The epineurial sheath is intact. Regenerating axon growth is blocked by fibrous tissue scarring. This degree of injury requires excision of the injured nerve segment and nerve repair. The most severe, the *fifth* degree of injury, represents the complete loss of continuity of the nerve trunk. There is discontinuity of the axon and the endoneurial, perineurial, and epineurial sheaths.

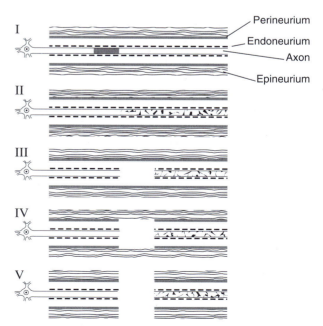

FIGURE 7-28. Schematic diagram of the five degrees of nerve injury. See Table 7-2 and text for explanation.

Neuronal Plasticity

Previously, it was thought that the mature central nervous system was incapable of recovering its function after an injury. Later studies have demonstrated that the central nervous system may not be so rigid or static. It has been shown that after an injury, the neuronal circuitry may reorganize itself by forming new synapses to compensate for those lost by injury. This property of forming new channels of communication after an injury is known as *neuronal plasticity*.

Neuronal plasticity is most dramatic after partial denervation. In such a situation, the remaining unaffected axons projecting on the partially denervated region develop axonal sprouts that grow and form new synaptic contacts to replace those lost by denervation. The ability of the mature central nervous system to form these sprouts and functional synapses varies from one region to another and from one species to another. The factor or factors that promote sprout formation and synaptogenesis in some, but not all, regions or species are not fully known and are the subject of intensive ongoing research. The identification of factors that promote neuronal plasticity in the injured mature central nervous system may have great impact on the recovery of function in such patients as paraplegics and stroke victims.

This discussion of plasticity has focused on the regenerative ability of the central nervous system after an injury. It should be emphasized, however, that plasticity in its broader sense is an ongoing phenomenon. Although all human brains are grossly similar anatomically, physiologically, and biochemically, human behavior differs from one person to another. This difference in behavior reflects the plasticity of the brain in adapting to its environment.

CHAPTER EIGHT

Cardiovascular System

Heart 134

Arteries 137
    Large Elastic Arteries 137
    Muscular Arteries 138
    Arterioles 138
    Capillaries 138

Veins 139

The cardiovascular system is composed of the heart and blood vessels.

HEART

The heart is a muscular organ that pumps blood into the arteries. Its wall is made up of three layers:

- The *endocardium* (the innermost layer, in contact with blood) is an endothelial cell–lined layer continuous with the tunica intima of blood vessels that enter and leave the heart. Beneath the endothelium is a layer of connective tissue and smooth muscles.
- The *myocardium* is composed of cardiac muscle and corresponds to the tunica media of the blood vessel wall. It is the thickest layer of the heart wall. Cardiac muscle fibers are of two types, contractile and conducting. Conducting muscle fibers generate and conduct electrical impulses that initiate cardiac rate and rhythm. Between the endocardial and myocardial layers of the heart wall is the *subendocardium*. This is a layer that contains impulse conducting muscle fibers and nerves. Muscle fibers in the myocardium are disposed in a variety of directions and orientation.
- The *epicardium* (the outermost layer) is covered by a reflection of the mesothelium-lined (serous or visceral) *pericardium*, contains coronary blood vessels and nerves, and corresponds to the tunica adventitia of blood vessels.

Between the epicardium and myocardium is the *subepicardial space*, which is filled with blood vessels, connective tissue, and fat (Fig. 8–1).

Projecting from the ventricular wall into the ventricular cavity are papillary muscles, which give origin to the chordae tendineae. The latter are attached to the cardiac valves (Fig. 8–2).

The mammalian heart has four chambers, two thin-walled *atria* and two thicker-walled *ventricles*. The central supporting structure is the *cardiac skeleton*, composed of dense white fibrous (collagenous) connective tissue into which the cardiac muscle fibers of the atria and ventricles insert and to which the heart valves are attached. The orifices of the four chambers are guarded by valves, which are endocardial folds supported by internal plates of dense collagenous and elastic connective tissue continuous with the cardiac skeleton. The right atrioventricular valve has three cusps; hence, it is called the *tricuspid valve*. The left atrioventricular valve has two cusps and is called the *bicuspid* or *mitral* (for the bishop's hat or miter) *valve*. *Semilunar valves*, located at the ventricular entrance to the aorta and pulmonary arteries, have three cusps each. The valves are arranged to prevent retrograde or reverse blood flow.

The heart pumps blood throughout the vascular system. Blood enters the right atrium from the inferior and superior venae cavae and coronary veins, which carry blood poor in oxygen and rich in carbon dioxide. Blood rich in oxygen and poor in carbon dioxide enters the left atrium from the lungs via pulmonary veins. This is the only instance in which oxygen-rich blood is carried in vessels called veins.

Contraction of the right and left atria forces blood past the right tricuspid and left bicuspid valves into the right and left ventricles, respectively. At the end of their contraction, the right and left atria begin to fill once again with blood. Contraction of the ventricles forces oxygen-poor blood from the right ventricle past the right semilunar valve into the pulmonary artery, and the oxygen-rich blood past the left semilunar valve into the aorta to supply the entire body and the heart itself. The pulmonary artery contains oxygen-poor blood, a situation opposite to that of the pulmonary vein and the only time oxygen-poor blood is carried in a vessel called an artery. A red corpuscle thus moves through the heart in the following way: right atrium, right ventri-

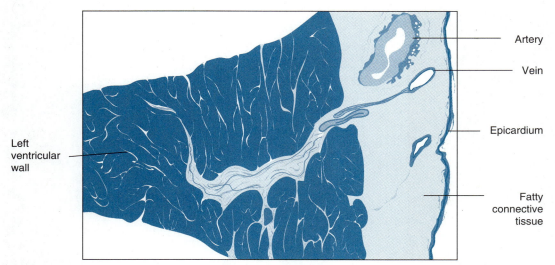

FIGURE 8–1. The heart muscle. *The left ventricular myocardium is shown separated from the pericardium by a subepicardial space filled with fatty connective tissue and blood vessels. The* epicardium *is the visceral layer of the pericardial sac in which the heart is located. It is covered by a single layer of mesothelial cells.*

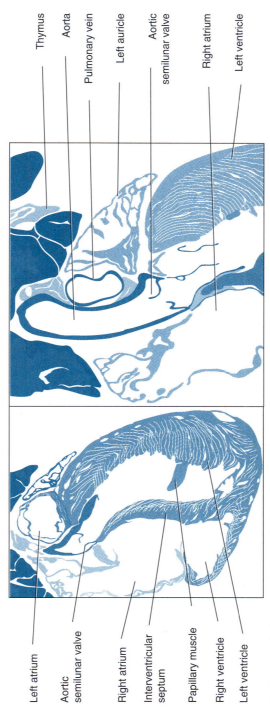

FIGURE 8–2. The four cardiac chambers and adjoining large vessels. Note the greater thickness of the wall of the ventricles compared with that of the atria, and of the wall of the aorta compared with that of the pulmonary vein. Note the papillary muscle protruding from the wall of the left ventricle.

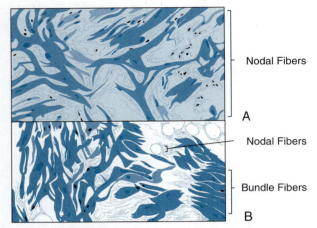

FIGURE 8–3. The specialized muscle fibers in the atrioventricular node and bundle. Note the irregular branched arrangement of nodal fibers (A) and their continuity with the small unbranched bundle fibers (B).

cle, pulmonary artery, lung capillaries, pulmonary vein, left atrium, and left ventricle; it leaves the heart to enter the aorta and systemic or coronary arteries. The contractile force required to move blood through the pulmonary system is less than that required to force blood throughout the entire body. This fact is reflected in the thickness of the myocardium of the right and left ventricles.

The mammalian heart possesses a special system of cardiac fibers that determine heart rate and coordinate contraction of the heart. These modified cardiac fibers lie beneath the endocardium. Two pacemakers are recognized: (1) the *sinoatrial node* (SA node), modified cardiac muscle fibers in continuity with and smaller than other atrial cardiac fibers, which lies at the junction of the superior vena cava and the right atrium, and (2) the *atrioventricular node* (AV node, node of Tawara), a mass of irregularly arranged, highly branched, specialized cardiac fibers (nodal fibers), located in the subendocardium of the right ventricle near the opening of the coronary sinus (Fig. 8–3). Extending from the AV node is a bundle of small unbranched cardiac muscle fibers called the *atrioventricular bundle (bundle of His)*, which passes to the midline of the heart to branch and form two larger bundles of *Purkinje's fibers* beneath the endocardium on either side of the interventricular septum. Purkinje's fibers (Fig. 8–4), functionally continuous with ordinary cardiac muscle fibers, are larger than ordinary cardiac muscle fibers and bundle fibers. They may be binucleate, having few myofibrils and a vacuolar cytoplasm rich in glycogen. Purkinje's fibers are linked to bundle fibers and to ordinary cardiac muscle fibers by gap junctions and desmosomes.

The sequence of impulse conduction in the heart is as follows: The SA node fibers are spontaneously active and transmit electrical signals to all other atrial muscle fibers, which are functionally linked to one another by intercalated disks (Fig. 8–5), resulting in atrial contraction. The electric signal then impinges on AV nodal fibers, which transmit the signal via small unbranched bundle fibers to Purkinje's fibers and finally to the ordinary ventricular cardiac fibers, which are also functionally linked by intercalated disks. Ventricular contraction begins at the apex of the heart and spreads upward to end at the midline skeleton between the atria and ventricles.

The myocytes of the right (and to a lesser extent the left) atrium contain specific, membrane-bound granules 0.3 to 0.4 μm in diameter. Two polypeptide hormones have been extracted from atrial muscle: *cardionatrium*, which has both diuretic and natriuretic effects, and cardiodilatin, which acts on vascular smooth muscle. Hence, it has been suggested that the atria be considered endocrine organs.

The heart is innervated by sympathetic and para-

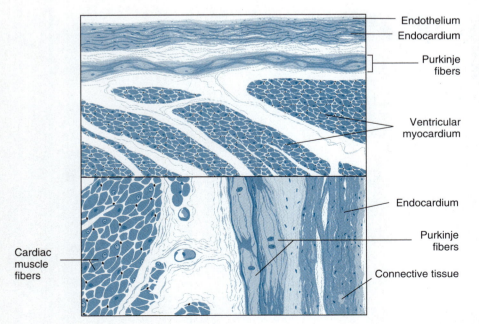

FIGURE 8–4. Purkinje's fibers adjacent to ordinary cardiac muscle fibers. Note that the Purkinje fibers are larger, may be binucleate, have vacuolar cytoplasm, and are located in subendocardial site.

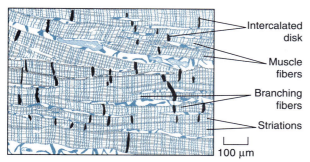

FIGURE 8–5. Cardiac muscle. *Note the branching pattern of the muscle fibers. The intercalated disks represent sites of termination and junction of adjacent cardiac muscle fibers.*

sympathetic fibers. The former accelerate heart rate, whereas the latter decelerate the rate.

ARTERIES

The wall of an artery usually has three tunics or coats:

- The innermost layer, or tunica intima, consists of an endothelial cell layer in contact with blood, a delicate subendothelial connective tissue layer, and an elastic tissue layer, the internal elastic membrane.
- The middle coat or tunica media, consists of smooth muscle fibers and variable amounts of elastic and collagenous tissues.
- The outer coat, or tunica adventitia, is composed primarily of loose collagenous connective tissue.

The exact structure and relative thickness of the three coats vary with the size of the artery.

In general, three different "types" of arterial vessels may be distinguished, but it must not be forgotten that these so-called types occur as part of a continuous, gradually changing vascular morphology based on functional requirements. The three types are: (1) large elastic (conducting) arteries, which leave the heart and are continuous with (2) medium and small muscular (distributing) arteries, which join (3) arterioles, which are continuous with capillary vessels. From the structural-functional point of view, elastic tissue is the most important component in the larger vessels, whereas smooth muscle is the most important in the smaller vessels.

Large Elastic Arteries

The aorta and pulmonary arteries constitute the large elastic type arteries (Fig. 8–6). They have a small endothelium-lined intima, which merges with a thick tunica media rich in concentrically arranged laminae of elastic fibers. Between elastic laminae are smooth muscles, reticular fibers, and chondroitin sulfate ground substance. The adventitia is small and devoid of an external elastic lamina; it contains elastic and collagenous fibers and nutrient vessels (vasa vasorum). The transition from one tunica to the other is indistinct.

Blood is ejected from the heart in a pulsating manner, and the aorta and the pulmonary arteries must expand to receive the bolus-type output *(systole)* of the right and left ventricles. The passive, elastic recoil between systoles *(diastole)* maintains the blood pressure, smooths the flow of blood, and forces blood through the coronary arteries while the ventricles are filling.

FIGURE 8–6. Elastic artery. *The tunica intima merges with a thick tunica media rich in concentrically arranged laminae of elastic fibers and smooth muscle fibers. The thin tunica adventitia contains nutrient vessels, the vasa vasorum.*

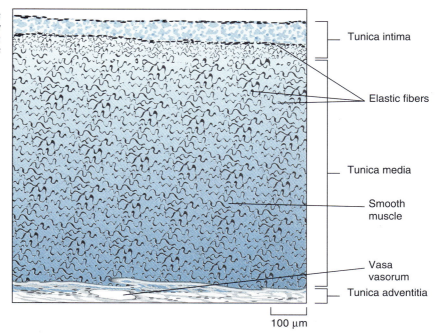

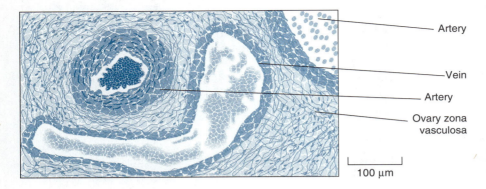

FIGURE 8–7. *A muscular artery and a vein from the human ovary.* Note the thick wall of the artery compared with that of the vein.

Muscular Arteries

Muscular (distributing) arteries regulate the blood flow to different parts of the body according to need—during exercise, to skeletal muscles; during and after eating, to the gastrointestinal tract (Fig. 8–7).

The intima of muscular arteries is small and endothelium-lined and contains few muscle cells. The internal elastic lamina is well developed. The tunica media consists of circularly arranged smooth muscle layers that decrease in number with reduction in size of the artery. Muscle fibers in the media are intermixed with elastic and reticular fibers. In the larger arteries, an external elastic lamina is present. The adventitia consists of collagen and elastic fibers, fat cells, and fibroblasts. It is equal to or smaller than the thick media. Nutrient vessels, nerves, and lymphatic vessels are located in the adventitia and may reach the outer limits of the tunica media.

Arterioles

Arterioles are small arteries, varying in diameter from 0.02 to 0.3 mm, with one to five layers of smooth muscle fibers (Fig. 8–8). Arterioles have a relatively thick muscular wall in comparison to their luminal diameter; the lumen of the smallest arterioles can accommodate about three to four red blood corpuscles. The lumen of arterioles is endothelium-lined. The intima is extremely small. Internal elastic lamina is absent except in large arterioles. The tunica media is made up of few layers of smooth muscle intermixed with collagenous and reticular fibers. The adventitia is thin. There is no external elastic lamina. Arterioles determine local blood flow with their precapillary sphincters (Fig. 8–9), located at the origin of capillary beds. Blood pressure falls sharply, and blood flow slows in arterioles.

Capillaries

Capillaries are endothelial cell tubes, 7 to 9 μm in diameter, whose walls appear as thin lines with bulging nuclei (Fig. 8–10). The cytoplasm contains a few mitochondria, ribosomes, endoplasmic reticulum profiles, Golgi complex, and intermediate filaments. The capillary is surrounded by a basal lamina.

Pericytes are located along the external surfaces of capillaries and small venules. Because they possess contractile proteins (myosin and actin), it has been suggested that these cells are contractile and may assist the movement of blood through sluggish, i.e., noncontractile, or poorly contractile, small blood vessels.

At the junction of an arteriole and a capillary, there is a ring of smooth muscle, the *precapillary sphincter,* which controls blood flow in the capillary. Because of their intimate relationship with the cells of the body and their special permeability characteristics, capillaries are functionally the most interesting of the blood vessels. Their thin walls and slow blood flow favor the exchange of nutrients and oxygen for metabolic wastes and carbon dioxide. In addition, hormones from endocrine glands enter and leave the vascular system through regionally specialized capillaries. Four types of capillaries have been recognized on the basis of endothelial structure and the presence or absence of a basal lamina (basement membrane) (Fig. 8–11):

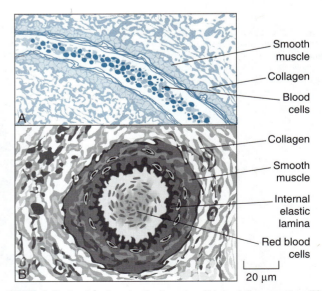

FIGURE 8–8. *Arteriole.* Longitudinal section (A) and Cross-section (B) of an arteriole showing the internal elastic lamina characteristically located between the tunica intima and media, the middle layer of circularly arranged smooth muscle fibers of the tunica media, and the outer tunica adventitia with collagen fibers.

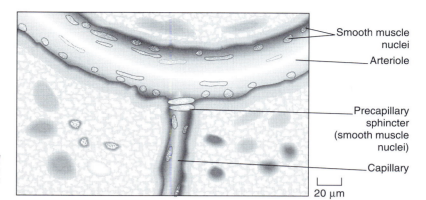

FIGURE 8–9. Precapillary sphincter between an arteriole and a capillary. Precapillaries contain smooth muscle fibers that encircle the vessels and act as sphincters to control blood flow in the capillary bed.

NONFENESTRATED (CONTINUOUS OR SOMATIC) CAPILLARIES. The endothelium does not have fenestrae, or open channels. This most common type is found in connective, muscle, nervous, and endocrine tissues. Transport of macromolecules back and forth across the cell occurs via pinocytotic vesicles approximately 70 nm in diameter. These capillaries have a basal lamina. It is of interest that the capillaries of the central nervous system do not transport by this mechanism, because pinocytotic activity is greatly reduced or absent in these vessels.

FENESTRATED (VISCERAL) CAPILLARIES. These capillaries possess large (60 to 80 nm in diameter) *fenestrae* or "openings." In one type of fenestrated capillary, the fenestrae are closed by a very thin diaphragm devoid of the typical trilaminar ultrastructure of other cellular membranes. These capillaries have a continuous basal lamina. The structural organization of these vessels is believed to favor rapid exchanges between blood and tissue spaces. This type of capillary is found in the kidney, intestine, and endocrine organs.

Fenestrated capillaries that do not possess diaphragms possess a thick basal lamina that separates the endothelium from the overlying epithelium (podocytes). These capillaries are type specific for the renal corpuscle (glomerulus).

SINUSOIDAL (DISCONTINUOUS) CAPILLARIES. Sinusoidal capillaries are large—about 30 to 40 μm in diameter. They also possess open fenestrations through their endothelium. This type of capillary normally has phagocytic cells attached to the endothelium within its lumen. The basal lamina characteristically is discontinuous. Sinusoids are found in the liver, spleen, and bone marrow.

Capillary Function

Capillaries have several important functions, including (1) selective control of what is exchanged, at what rate, and of what size between blood and tissue spaces, (2) production of "substances" that convert angiotensin I to angiotensin II and that can inactivate bradykinin, serotonin, prostaglandins, norepinephrine, and thrombin, (3) breakdown of lipoproteins to produce energy-yielding triglycerides and cholesterol used in membrane formation and hormone synthesis, and (4) production of arachidonic prostacyclin (prostaglandin 12), a significant inhibitor of platelet aggregation (blood clot).

VEINS

As with the arterial system, veins can be divided into three "types" according to size: venules, small

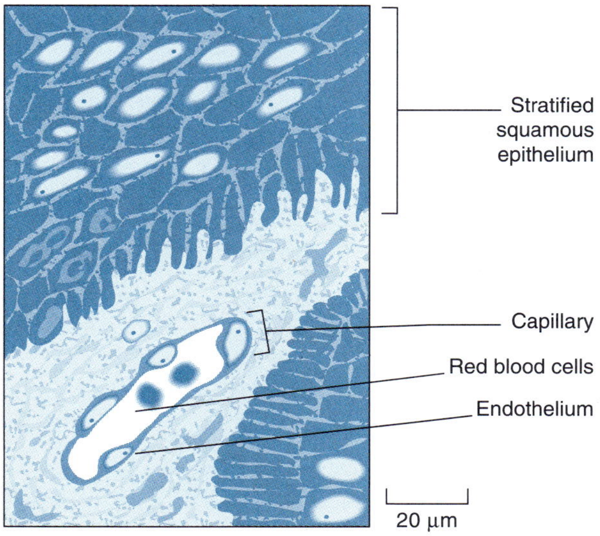

FIGURE 8–10. Capillary in a section of human skin. Note the extremely thin wall and bulging endothelial cell nuclei of the capillary.

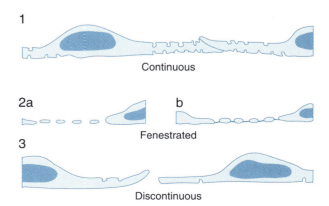

FIGURE 8–11. Capillary varieties. Schematic diagram showing the three types of capillaries: nonfenestrated or continuous; fenestrated or visceral; and discontinuous or sinusoidal.

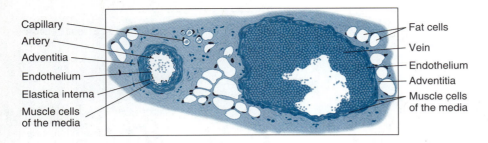

FIGURE 8-12. *Cross-section through a small artery and its accompanying medium-sized vein. Note the absence of elastic membrane and the thinner muscle layer in the vein.*

and medium-sized veins (Fig. 8–12), and large veins (Fig. 8–13).

Venules can be recognized when they are about 20 μm in diameter (about three red corpuscles across). They possess an endothelial lining, a thin layer of collagenous fibers with some fibroblasts. They have neither muscle fibers nor elastic fibers. With increasing size (about 45 μm), some elastic fibers appear in the tunica intima along with collagenous fibers, and smooth muscle begins to appear between the endothelium and the outer fibrous coats. With still greater increases in caliber, distinct intima, media, and adventitia become recognizable. The largest veins (venae cavae) possess some longitudinal smooth muscle and a delicate internal elastic membrane *(tunica intima)*; a thin smooth muscle coat that may be absent *(tunica media)*; and prominent bundles of smooth muscle separated by collagenous fibers that appear in the thickest of the three coats *(tunica adventitia)*, which also contains nutrient vessels *(vasa vasorum)*.

Many small and medium-sized veins contain valves that prevent retrograde blood flow and the pooling of blood in the limbs, where such valves are especially common. The erect posture of the human, in particular, necessitates this structural specialization in veins. *Valves* are paired folds of intima, which are commonly located just distal to the entry of a communicating vein. Some veins do not possess smooth muscle fibers and, as a result, do not have a tunica media. These veins are found in the maternal part of the placenta, the spinal cord pia mater, the retina, sinuses of the dura mater, most cerebral veins, trabecular veins of the spleen, and veins of the nail bed.

Other interesting veins are found in the penis; these veins possess specializations of their intima called *polsters* (Fig. 8–14). Polsters are local accumulations of fibroblasts and smooth muscle cells located beneath

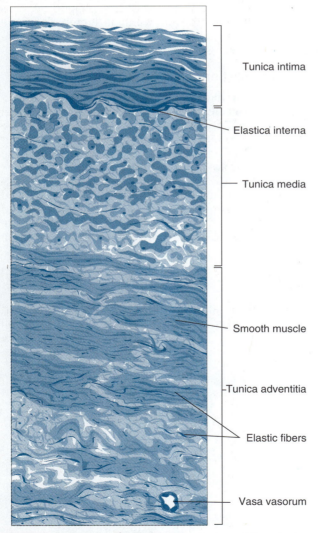

FIGURE 8-13. *Vena cava (large vein). Note presence of three tunics: a thick tunica intima containing elastic fibers, a relatively thin tunica media devoid of smooth muscle fibers, and a thick tunica adventitia containing smooth muscle and elastic fibers.*

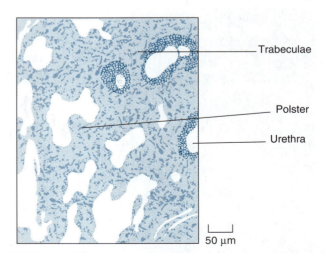

FIGURE 8-14. *Polsters. This schematic diagram of penile tissue shows the complex network of venous sinuses separated by trabeculae of smooth muscle and connective tissue. Note the specialization of the intimal lining of sinuses into polsters protruding into the lumen.*

the endothelium that form conspicuous longitudinal thickenings or ridges. They are believed to play a role in retarding venous outflow during erection.

Blood flow against gravity and toward the heart in the thin-walled veins is aided by the contraction of skeletal muscle and the system of valves. Blood pressure in the venous system is less than one tenth that in the aorta, and blood travels slowly and smoothly through relatively large, thin-walled vessels. In spite of the differences in blood pressure and velocity of flow, the venous return to the heart must equal the ventricular output. The vascular system contains approximately 5 liters of blood, which is pumped and circulated throughout the body about 3200 times daily.

CHAPTER NINE

Lymphatic System and Immunity

Lymphoid Tissue 143
    Diffuse Lymphoid Tissue 143
    Lymph Nodules 143
    Tonsils 143
    Lymph Nodes 143
    Thymus 145
    Spleen 147

Immune Response 149
    Cytokines 150
    Major Histocompatibility Complex 151
    Humoral and Cellular Responses 151
    Lymphocytes 151

The lymphatic system gives an organism immunity against injury by foreign substances and organisms. Specific cells of this system can distinguish between "self" and "nonself." They seek out and inactivate or destroy invasive foreign substances and organisms, "nonself." These cells are called *immunocompetent cells,* and the entire system is termed the *immune system.* Lymphoid tissue consists of reticular cells and their secretory product, collagen type 3 or reticular fibers, and supporting masses of lymphocytes, macrophages, antigen-presenting cells (APCs), and plasma cells.

Lymphoid tissue is remarkably variable in structure and distribution. It may appear as a diffuse infiltration into the lamina propria of mucous membranes or as well-defined organs, such as the thymus. A classification of lymphoid tissue, based on increasing structural-functional complexity, recognizes diffuse lymphoid tissue, lymph nodules, tonsils, lymph nodes, thymus, and spleen.

LYMPHOID TISSUE

Diffuse Lymphoid Tissue

The simplest form, diffuse lymphoid tissue, is found throughout the body but particularly in the alimentary and respiratory tracts. Located in the lamina propria, it underlies the surface epithelium, surrounds mucosal glands and their ducts, and is characterized by a loosely organized mass of lymphocytes.

Lymph Nodules

The diffuse form of lymphoid tissue grades into a more dense form, the lymph nodules, which are circumscribed masses of densely packed lymphocytes (mainly B lymphocytes). The lymph nodule constitutes the basic structural unit of lymphoid tissue. Each nodule may contain a light-staining central area, the *germinal center,* which is the site of active lymphocyte proliferation. The light staining of germinal centers is attributed to the presence of lymphocytes with abundant cytoplasm and large, pale-staining nuclei, the *lymphoblast* or *immunoblast.* Lymphatic nodules or lymph follicles are found in large numbers in the mucosa of the intestinal tract, notably in the ileum and vermiform appendix.

Tonsils

Groups of lymph nodules may be partially encapsulated as small organs with a definite lymphatic and blood vascular supply. Such is the case in the tonsils. The three distinct tonsillar masses, which form an incomplete ring, are the palatine, lingual, and pharyngeal (clinically, the adenoids). The palatine (Fig. 9–1) and lingual tonsils are covered with stratified squamous epithelium, whereas the pharyngeal tonsil is covered with pseudostratified columnar ciliated epithelium, with some goblet cells characteristic of the nasopharynx. In adults, some areas of the pharyngeal tonsil may also be covered by a stratified squamous epithelium. The palatine and lingual tonsils have numerous epithelium-lined pits, referred to as *crypts,* which may bifurcate. Surrounding the crypts is a single layer of lymph nodules with germinal centers. The pharyngeal tonsil has widened ducts of underlying glands rather than true crypts. The epithelium covering the tonsils is infiltrated extensively by lymphocytes, plasma cells, and polymorphonuclear leukocytes. The lingual, palatine, and pharyngeal tonsils form a ring of immunocompetent cells guarding the entrance to the digestive and respiratory tracts.

Lymph Nodes

Lymph nodes, completely encapsulated ovoid structures 1 to 25 mm in size (Figs. 9–2 and 9–3), are the immunologic filters of the lymph. They are composed of dense reticular meshwork ensheathed by stellate reticular cells and lymphoid tissue and cells. Each lymph node is surrounded by a connective tissue cap-

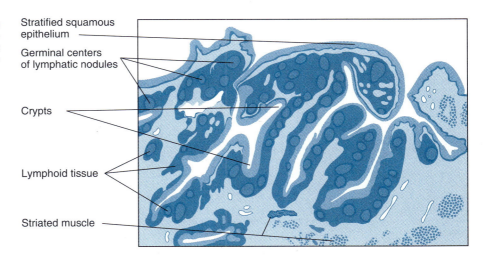

FIGURE 9–1. Schematic diagram of palatine tonsil. Note the epithelial invaginations (crypts) into the tonsillar substance. Crypts are surrounded by lymphatic tissue containing numerous germinal centers.

- Stratified squamous epithelium
- Germinal centers of lymphatic nodules
- Crypts
- Lymphoid tissue
- Striated muscle

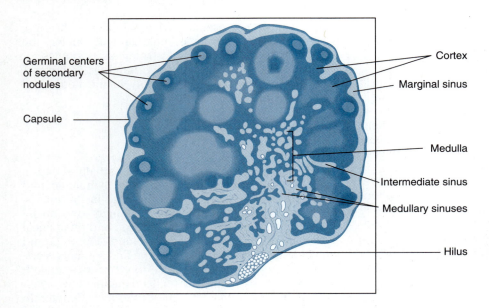

FIGURE 9–2. Schematic diagram of lymph node. Note the broad subcapsular marginal (cortical) sinus, superficial cortex, and deep medulla. Note germinal centers in secondary cortical nodules. In the medulla, note medullary sinuses separating medullary cords.

sule from which trabeculae penetrate and incompletely partition the substance of the node. Beneath its capsule, each node is composed of a cortex and a more deeply located medulla. The cortex is separated from the capsule by the subcapsular (cortical) sinus. The cortex contains primary and secondary lymphatic nodules or follicles.

Primary follicles consist of closely packed aggregates (0.2 to 1 mm in diameter) of lymphocytes and are devoid of germinal centers. Most cells in primary follicles are B lymphocytes. Other cells are T lymphocytes, reticular cells, macrophages, and follicular dendritic (antigen-presenting) cells (APCs). *APCs present antigen trapped on their surfaces to the B and T lymphocytes to induce an immunologic response.* Secondary cortical follicles are aggregates of lymphocytes with a lighter-staining center, the germinal center. Germinal centers contain activated lymphocytes (immunoblasts) and vary in size with age, being best developed in childhood. They develop when an antigen is present. Lymphocytes capable of responding to the antigen undergo mitosis (immunoblast) and subsequent differentiation into plasma cells or memory small B lymphocytes. *Memory B lymphocytes* ultimately reside in the mantle zone of secondary follicles, a zone of small lymphocytes surrounding the germinal center. Once formed, *plasma cells* leave the germinal center and go to the medulla (medullary cords), where they produce antibodies. Memory B lymphocytes leave the node with the lymph outflow to reach the peripheral vascular compartment. Memory cells readily leave the blood compartment for the connective tissue compartment if they encounter a stimulating antigen. In connective tissue, memory cells produce an antibody response to the antigen.

Between the cortical follicles and the medulla is the *paracortical region* of the lymph node. This region is composed of loosely aggregated lymphocytes (Fig. 9–4). Lymphocytes in the paracortical region are T lymphocytes, which are thymus dependent and disappear after a thymectomy.

The *medulla* consists of medullary cords composed of packed lymphocytes and numerous plasma cells. Around the medullary cords are the medullary sinuses, which join efferent lymphatic vessels.

The *capsule* admits valve-containing, afferent lymphatic vessels (Fig. 9–5) that provide one-way flow into the subcapsular sinus. The lymph circulates through sinuses located in the cortex and the medulla and leaves the lymph node via larger but fewer efferent lymphatic vessels. These efferent vessels also contain valves and emerge from a specific region of the node, the *hilus*. The passage of lymph through the cortical and medullary sinuses clears it of most of its antigens

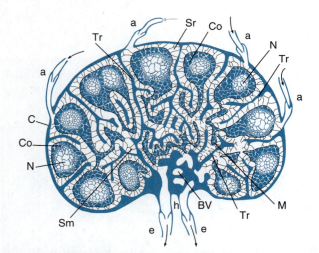

FIGURE 9–3. Schematic diagram of a lymph node. The connective tissue capsule (C), cortex (Co), and medulla (M) are identified. Afferent lymphatic vessels (a) enter the capsule to reach the subcapsular (cortical) sinus (Sr). From the cortical sinus, lymph circulates in the medullary sinuses (Sm) and into the efferent lymphatic vessels (e), which leave the node in the hilum (h). Blood vessels (BV) enter the lymph node in the hilum. Connective tissue trabeculae (Tr) incompletely partition the lymph node. Within the cortex are lymphatic nodules or follicles (N).

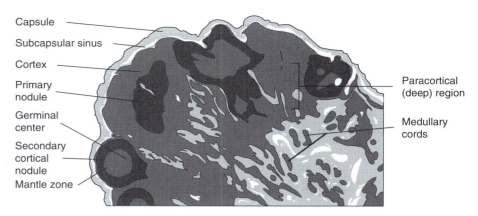

FIGURE 9–4. Schematic diagram of a part of a lymph node showing the capsule, cortex, and medulla. The subcapsular sinus separates capsule from cortex. Within the cortex are primary and secondary nodules (follicles). The latter contain germinal centers. Surrounding the germinal center is the mantle zone, a region known to contain small lymphocytes (memory cells). The medulla contains medullary cords. Between adjacent cortical nodes and between these nodes and the medulla is the paracortical region, containing loosely arranged lymphocytes of the T variety.

and cellular debris. These are phagocytosed by macrophages suspended in the sinuses.

A lymph node receives its blood supply only at the hilus. Arterial vessels enter both the trabeculae formed from the capsular connective tissue and the medullary cords. They regionally supply the node by giving off capillaries; they continue to the cortex, where an arterial branch penetrates each cortical lymph nodule and forms a capillary plexus around the germinal center. From the capillary beds, blood is carried by veins that follow a pathway similar to that of the arteries, leaving the node at the hilus along with efferent lymphatic vessels.

Thymus

The thymus develops from the third and fourth pharyngeal pouches. It changes in size and undergoes structural alterations with age. It grows rapidly until the end of the second year, after which time the rate of growth slows down until approximately the fourteenth year. The thymus then begins to involute, or decrease in size, and, gradually, the lymphatic tissue is largely replaced by fat and connective tissue. In old age, very little thymic tissue may be present.

The primary function of the thymus is to produce immunocompetent T lymphocytes. The organ is highly lobulated and is invested by a loose connective tissue capsule (Fig. 9–6). From the capsule, connective tissue septa containing blood vessels penetrate the substance of the organ, forming lobes. *Lobes* are composed of two distinct regions, cortex and medulla. The *cortex* contains densely and uniformly packed lymphocytes, but it lacks lymph nodules. It stains intensely with basic dyes, such as hematoxylin, and appears almost uniformly blue. In addition, the cortex is punctuated by stellate reticular cells, which do not take a stain and appear as empty spaces.

Lymphoblasts (stem cells) are immunologically incompetent, basophilic staining cells found at the periphery of the cortex. They divide by mitosis, producing small lymphocytes. The cortex contains small, medium, and large lymphocytes. The largest lymphocytes are about 9 μm and have nuclei with abundant euchromatin and a strongly basophilic cytoplasm that contributes to the intense staining of the cortex. *Stellate reticular cells* are part of the supporting framework of the organ and are not phagocytic cells (Fig. 9–7). They are, however, thought to secrete thymic hormones, which promote the differentiation of T cells. Also importantly, the reticular cell processes effectively isolate developing lymphocytes and completely ensheath blood capillaries (the only type of blood vessel in the cortex), thereby precluding the possibility of contaminating developing lymphocytes with antigens *(blood-thymus barrier).* Macrophages are found consistently in small numbers in the cortex. The cortex produces massive numbers of lymphocytes, but most do not survive to leave the organ. Those that leave the cortex do so via medullary postcapillary venules; they are immunocompetent T lymphocytes.

The *medulla* is less dense, as a result of the thinning of the concentration of lymphocytes, and contains eosinophilic structures (reticular fiber network and Hassall's corpuscles) (Fig. 9–8). It is in the medulla that reticular cells can be recognized. The medulla sends a projection to join the medulla of adjacent lobules. *Hassall's corpuscles*, named after a nineteenth century British physician, are diagnostic features of the thymus. They are formed of concentrically arranged polygonal or flattened cells with a hyalinized degenerative core. The diameter of Hassall's corpuscles ranges from 25 to 200 μm. The origin and nature of Hassall's corpuscles

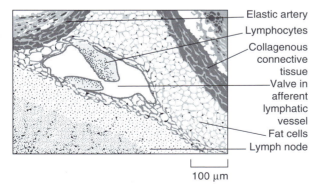

FIGURE 9–5. Afferent lymphatic vessels near a lymph node. The valve is formed of intimal folds of the vessel walls. Collagenous connective tissue forming the capsule of the lymph node, as well as fat cells and an elastic artery, are seen adjacent to the afferent lymph vessel.

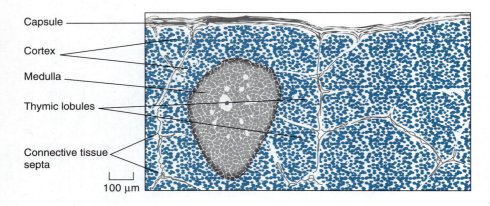

FIGURE 9-6. Thymus. Schematic diagram of the thymus showing the investing connective tissue capsule from which septa penetrate the substance of the thymus, dividing it into lobules. Each lobule is made up of a cortex and a medulla.

are unknown, but these cells may represent degeneration residue.

The thymic medulla contains primarily small, but fully mature T lymphocytes. The T lymphocytes leave the medulla via venules and efferent lymphatic vessels. These lymphocytes will populate specific regions of other lymphoid organs, such as lymph nodes (paracortical region) and spleen (periarterial sheaths of white pulp).

The thymus and its T lymphocytes play a major role in cell-mediated immune responses. Homologous and heterologous tissue and organ transplants are invaded by T lymphocytes (graft rejection cells), which will disrupt and destroy the transplanted tissue or organ. Nevertheless, T lymphocytes also promote the transformation of B lymphocytes into plasma cells. Defects in thymus maturation and development are associated with T-cell immunoincompetency.

Arteries supplying the thymus follow the connective tissue septa and give off branches that enter the lobular cortex and divide into capillaries, which supply the cortex. Epithelial reticular cells sequester developing lymphocytes and form a sheath covering capillaries and lymphatic vessels. The sheathing forms the

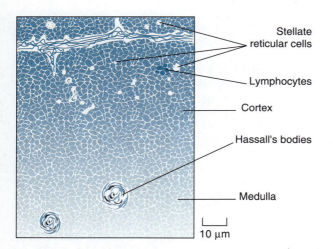

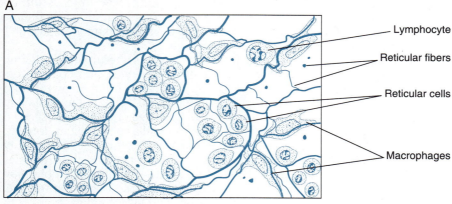

FIGURE 9-7. Thymic lobe. A, A schematic diagram of a thymic lobe showing the cortex and medulla. The cortex contains stellate (epithelial) reticular cells and small lymphocytes. The medulla characteristically contains Hassall's bodies (corpuscles). B, The supporting framework of reticular fibers within a lymph node is shown supporting clusters of cells of various types.

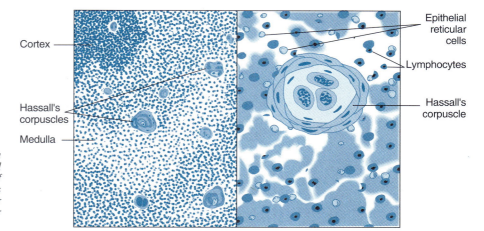

FIGURE 9–8. Schematic diagram of a thymic lobule composed of cortex and medulla. The cortex is composed of densely and uniformly packed lymphocytes punctuated by clear-appearing reticular cells. The medulla consists of looser lymphatic tissue and Hassall's corpuscles.

blood-thymus barrier, preventing antigen contamination of developing and programed T lymphocytes. The blood-thymus barrier is not found in the medulla, which appears to have a richer blood supply than the cortex. The capillaries terminate in thin-walled veins located in the connective tissue septa along with arteries. Lymphatic vessels arise within the thymic lobule and join to form larger vessels, which accompany the arteries and veins in the septa. In contrast to lymph nodes, the thymus contains no lymph sinuses or afferent lymphatic vessels.

Spleen

The spleen has attracted the attention of scientists and philosophers throughout the ages. Hippocrates and Aristotle commented on its anatomic relationships and shape. Galen described it as an organ full of mystery. The spleen was associated with merriment, and it was thought that great laughers have great spleens. During the seventeenth and eighteenth centuries, Harvey and others described in detail the structure of the spleen, Malpighi identified the bodies named after him, and Hewson suggested that the spleen was a lymphatic organ.

Developmentally, the primordium of the spleen is recognized in the dorsal mesogastrium at about 5 weeks of gestation. It assumes an active role as a hematopoietic organ by the fourth month of gestation. Germinal centers do not, however, develop fully in fetal life. At birth, the spleen weighs 11 g. The weight of the spleen, increasing in a linear fashion with body weight, reaches its maximum at puberty, after which it decreases.

The spleen is the largest lymphatic organ in the body and is the immunologic filter for the blood. Like the thymus, it has no afferent lymphatic vessels and no lymph sinuses. Splenic vessels enter and leave the spleen at the hilum of the organ and are located in thick trabeculae that extend inward from the capsule. The capsule and trabeculae are composed of collagen, elastic fibers, and some smooth muscle fibers (Fig. 9–9). A reticular fiber network and lymphocytes are found between the trabeculae.

Sections of fresh spleen reveal two different regions, the so-called red pulp and white pulp (Figs. 9–10 and 9–11). The red pulp, which constitutes the largest part of the organ, is loosely textured and is traversed

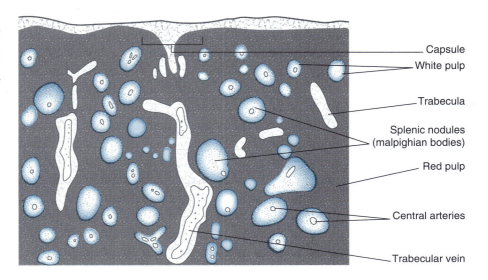

FIGURE 9–9. Spleen. Section showing the capsule of the spleen and the red and white pulps. Trabeculae with veins traverse the red pulp. Central arterioles are eccentrically located within the white pulp, also known as splenic nodules or malpighian bodies.

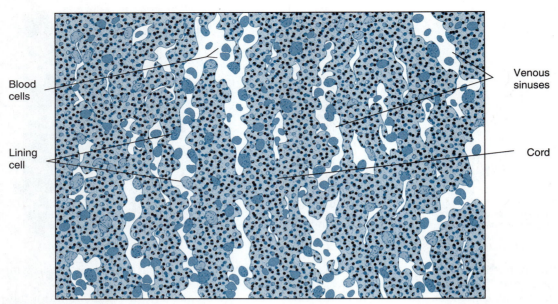

FIGURE 9-10. Schematic diagram of red pulp of the spleen. *Note the venous sinuses separating splenic cords. Sinusoids are lined by phagocytic reticular cells and contain red blood cells. The splenic cords are composed of lymphatic tissue.*

by a plexus of venous sinusoids separated by lymphatic splenic cords *(Billroth's cords)*. The venous sinusoids contain tightly packed red blood corpuscles when they perform a storage function. They are lined by phagocytic reticular cells. The red pulp also contains reticular cells, wandering macrophages, monocytes, plasma cells, and granulocytes.

The white pulp is composed of compact lymphoid tissue arranged in spherical or ovoid aggregations around arterioles *(central arterioles)*. The central artery (arteriole) of the nodule is invariably eccentrically placed. These aggregations, called *splenic corpuscles* or *malpighian corpuscles,* bear a resemblance to lymph nodules. Lymphatic nodules of the spleen may have germinal centers. They contain mainly B lymphocytes, plasma cells, macrophages, and other free cells. Lymphocytes around the central artery, the periarterial lymphatic sheath (PALS), are mainly T lymphocytes.

Between the white and red pulp is the *marginal zone* of venous sinuses and loose lymphoid tissue. This zone contains macrophages, B lymphocytes, and dendritic cells. Dendritic cells (APCs) present antigens on their surface to B and T lymphocytes removed from the blood in the marginal zone. These dendritic cells may, in the presence of the antigenically appropriate lymphocyte, initiate an immune response. The marginal zone, thus, is an important component of splenic structure for the immune process.

A knowledge of the vascular supply is critical to an understanding of the spleen. The splenic artery and its major branches enter at the hilum and are carried in, and branch with, the trabeculae *(trabecular arteries)*.

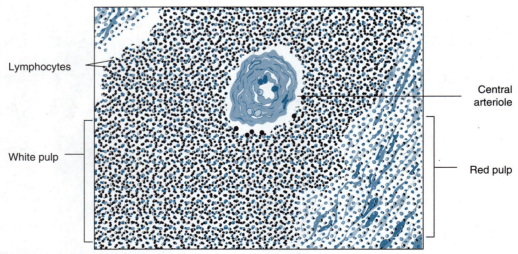

FIGURE 9-11. Schematic diagram of the splenic white pulp. *Note the spherical compact arrangement of lymphocytes around the central arteriole of the white pulp and the loose, cordlike pattern of the adjacent red pulp.*

Arterioles emerge from the trabeculae and pass into the splenic parenchyma (Fig. 9–12), where the adventitia of the arterioles *(central or white pulp arteries)* is infiltrated by lymphocytes to form splenic corpuscles. These arterioles supply capillaries to the white pulp, continue their course, lose their lymphatic investment, and enter the red pulp, where they subdivide into several branches called *penicilli*. These branches become smaller and are differentiated into three distinct regions: *pulp arterioles, sheathed arterioles,* and *terminal capillaries*. The nature of the termination of these capillaries and their ultimate union with venous sinuses is controversial. Some researchers think that the capillaries open directly into the sinusoids *(open circulation)*, whereas others believe that the blood remains within vessels *(closed circulation)* (see Fig. 9–12). Opinion favors the open type of circulation in the human. The venous sinuses are lined not by endothelium but by specialized reticular cells, which are fixed macrophages. The reticular cells are encircled by reticular fibers. The venous sinuses unite to form *pulp veins*, which are lined by endothelial cells. The pulp or collecting veins enter the trabeculae and leave the spleen at the hilum.

Ligation of the splenic artery usually does not result in infarction of the spleen because of the collateral arterial connections that exist between the splenic and gastric arteries throughout the splenic capsule. Splenic blood flow is estimated to be 150 mL per minute in humans.

Although the spleen is not essential for life, it carries out the following very important functions:

- Site of hematopoiesis: In fetal life, the spleen along with the liver functions as a hematopoietic organ. After midgestation, the bone marrow assumes a progressively more central role as the site for hematopoiesis. At term, only occasional small nests of hematopoietic cells are found in the spleen. The potential for splenic hematopoiesis persists postnatally, however, and under severe hematologic stress, the spleen may maintain or resume its hematopoietic function.
- Destruction of erythrocytes: Normally, worn-out and damaged red blood corpuscles are destroyed within the spleen and bone marrow. In pathologic states, intrasplenic red cell destruction increases markedly.
- Phagocytosis: The spleen removes particulate matter from the blood. The size of a particle determines whether or not it will be cleared by the spleen.
- Reservoir: The spleen acts as a reservoir for blood-borne elements, such as lipids and iron freed from the breakdown of hemoglobin, for reuse within the bone marrow to synthesize new hemoglobin. Other elements stored in the spleen are platelets and plasma proteins.
- Destruction of platelets and leukocytes: The spleen probably has a role in the normal destruction of lymphocytes, monocytes, and platelets. In hematologic disorders involving the destruction of platelets and leukocytes, removal of the spleen may improve the condition.
- Immunologic role: The spleen plays a role in the production of lymphocytes and monocytes in fetal life and after bone marrow failure postnatally (Table 9–1).

Accessory Spleens

Accessory spleens exist in about 16% of individual humans. Most are located in the hilum of the spleen or in the adjacent tail of the pancreas. They are usually small, measuring 1 to 2 cm in length.

IMMUNE RESPONSE

The immune system is composed of a large, complex set of elements that are distributed widely. It is designed to protect the organism against foreign elements (nonself) but to tolerate the organism (self). Although microorganisms are the principal nonself category encountered on a daily basis, tumors and transplants are viewed as nonself and are targeted by the immune system. The immune system consists of two interrelated systems. One is a *specific recognition system* inherent in the T and B lymphocytes. The cellular components of the specific immune system are lymphocytes (B and T), whereas its soluble components are the immunoglobulins. Its function is to learn, adapt, and remember. The second is a *nonspecific (innate) effector system* that amplifies the functions of the specific system. Its soluble components are complement proteins. Its cellular components are phagocytic cells in the blood (neutrophils and monocytes) and tissue macrophages (alveolar macrophages, Kupffer's cells of the liver, synovial cells in joint cavities, and perivascular microglial cells in the nervous system). The hallmark of the nonspecific immune system is that it reacts in the same manner to all encountered antigens. The specific and nonspecific immune systems constantly interact. Specific immune responses can facilitate nonspecific components, and nonspecific components may be

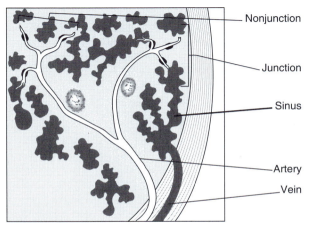

FIGURE 9–12. Splenic circulation. The sheathed arteries divide into arterioles, which are related to the venous sinuses either directly (closed system) or indirectly, across the red pulp (open system).

TABLE 9-1. Distinguishing Characteristics of Lymphatic Organs*

Structural Characteristics	Tonsils and Other Lymphatic Nodules	Lymph Node	Thymus	Spleen
Epithelial covering	+	−	−	−
Marginal sinus	−	+	−	−
Hassall's corpuscles	−	−	+	−
White pulp (splenic nodule, malpighian bodies)	−	−	−	+
Connective tissue capsule	−	+	+	+
Organized cortex and medulla	−	+	+	−

*+ = present; − = absent.

needed for the successful generation of specific immunity.

Cytokines

Work has focused on soluble factors that are made by or act on elements of the immune system but are not antigen specific. Collectively, these factors are called *cytokines*. Those produced by T lymphocytes are *lymphokines*, and those produced by monocytes are *monokines*. Cytokines are non–immunoglobulin, soluble proteins secreted by mononuclear cells in response to interaction with a specific antigen (in the case of lymphocytes), a nonspecific antigen (in the case of a macrophage), or a nonspecific soluble stimulus (as an endotoxin or another cytokine). Although the secretion of cytokines may be triggered by the interaction of a lymphocyte with its specific antigen, the cytokines themselves are not antigen specific. Thus, cytokines bridge the gap between the specific and nonspecific immune systems. Cytokines are divided into several subgroups: the interleukins (ILs), interferons (IFNs), tumor necrosis factors (TNFs), transforming growth factors (TGFs), and the hematopoietic colony-stimulating factors (CSFs). Cytokines, like the cells that produce them, act in concert, in tandem, or in conflict in a given immune response.

INTERLEUKINS. Mediators between leukocytes are called *interleukins*. Like lymphokines, interleukins are immunologically nonspecific. Eleven interleukins are recognized; the following interleukins are the best studied to date.

Interleukin-1 (IL-1), formerly called lymphocyte-activating factor (LAF), is produced primarily by antigen-presenting monocyte-macrophages. Antigen-presenting cells (APCs) produce interleukin-1 through antigen processing. Without IL-1, T-cell activation is suboptimal.

Interleukin-2 (IL-2), formerly called T-cell growth factor, is a true T-cell lymphokine secreted by some activated T cells. Under certain conditions, IL-2 secretion can be under the influence of IL-1.

Interleukin-3 (IL-3) is also made by activated T lymphocytes. It promotes the growth of many cells, particularly mast cells.

Interleukin-4 (IL-4) is also made by activated T lymphocytes. It is the same as the B lymphocyte–stimulating factor. It co-stimulates B-cell growth and, with IL-3, synergizes mast cell growth.

- Interleukin-5 (IL-5) is produced by activated T cells. It plays a role in eosinophil differentiation and immunoglobulin A (IgA) production and co-stimulates B-cell growth.
- Interleukin-6 (IL-6) is produced by monocytes. It enhances immunoglobulin production and synergizes with IL-3 in hematopoietic cell growth.
- Interleukin-7 (IL-7) is produced by bone marrow and thymus stromal cells. It plays a role in the proliferation of B-cell precursors and immature thymocytes.

Interleukin-8 (IL-8) is produced by monocytes, endothelial cells, and alveolar macrophages. It plays a role in neutrophil chemotaxis and activation and in T-cell activation.

INTERFERONS. Interferons were originally discovered in the supernatants of virally infected cultured cells. These supernatants interfered with the superinfection of cells by another virus; hence the name. Three major classes of interferons are delineated: alpha, beta, and gamma. Interferon alpha is produced by leukocytes, and interferon beta by fibroblasts. These two interferons have the same functions. They inhibit viral replication and tumor growth and modulate antibody response. Interferon gamma (immune interferon) is the most important in the immunologic response. It is produced by and modulates the function of B and T lymphocytes. Its effects may include both augmentation and diminution of the immune response.

TNFs. Tumor necrosis factors comprise two subclasses. TNF-α (cachectin) is produced by monocytes and macrophages. It induces the production of interleukin 1 and interferon gamma. TNF-β (lymphotoxin) is produced in T cells. It is a cytotoxic factor.

CSFs. Colony-stimulating factors are divided into three subclasses. Granulocyte-macrophage CSF (GM-CSF) is produced in T lymphocytes, macrophages, monocytes, and endothelial cells; it plays a role in the growth of granulocytes and erythroid progenitors and in macrophage activation and enhances monocyte tumoricidal activity. Granulocyte CSF (G-CSF), produced in monocytes and endothelial cells, promotes granulocyte growth. Monocyte CSF (M-CSF) is produced in monocytes and endothelial cells; it promotes monocyte growth.

TGFs. Transforming growth factors consist of two

subclasses. TGF-α, produced in monocytes and solid tumors, plays a role in tumor growth, bone resorption, and keratinocyte proliferation. TGF-β is produced in platelets, kidney, bone, and T and B lymphocytes. It inhibits T and B cell proliferation and enhances fibroblast proliferation.

Major Histocompatibility Complex

The ability of the immune system to differentiate self from nonself is determined, in large part, by products of the major histocompatibility complex (MHC), formerly called histocompatibility leukocyte antigen (HLA). Genes for the MHC are located on chromosome 6. This complex can be divided into two major classes. Class I MHC products (HLA-A, B, and C) have a wide distribution and are present on the surfaces of all nucleated cells and on platelets. Class II MHC products (HLA-D, DR, and DQ) have a more limited distribution and are present on B lymphocytes, macrophages, dendritic cells, Langerhans' cells, and activated T lymphocytes.

Although B lymphocytes can respond to soluble antigens, T cells rarely do so. T lymphocytes will recognize antigens only when presented in the context of MHC. Thus, the immune system needs a mechanism by which antigens can be processed, associated with MHC, and presented to the T lymphocytes. This task is accomplished by antigen-presenting cells (APCs), which include monocytes, macrophages, Langerhans' cells, follicular dendritic cells, and even B lymphocytes. The immune system is characterized by the following common attributes.

SPECIFICITY. Particular cells of the specific immune system respond to a specific type of antigen (A) or to a cross-reacting antigen with that specific antigen (A) but will not respond to another specific type of antigen (B) or to a non–cross-reacting antigen to A. Specificity is a function of antigen-specific receptors on the surfaces of T and B lymphocytes. The receptors are disulfide-linked heterodimers that can each react with only one antigenic determinant. The function of the antigen receptor on B lymphocytes is mediated by surface immunoglobulins (sIgs). B lymphocytes bind soluble antigens through their surface immunoglobulins. This interaction leads to a series of events (proliferation and differentiation) culminating in the secretion of the immunoglobulin (Ig) that is the antibody specific for that antigen. T lymphocytes do not have surface immunoglobulins (sIgs); they recognize antigens through their principal recognition tool, the T-cell receptor (TCR), as well as by other accessory adhesion molecules.

MEMORY. The exposure of the immune system to an antigenic stimulus leaves the memory of the immunologic response to that stimulus intact. A second exposure to the same antigenic stimulus would result in a boosted, more rapid, and more powerful immune response. This is the basis of booster immunization. There are two types of memory in the immune system. In *positive immunologic memory,* subsequent exposure to an antigen results in a boosted, more effective, and quicker response. Negative immunologic memory produces the reverse effect, whereby subsequent exposure to the antigen results in no response or a reduced response. Negative memory is often referred to as *acquired immunologic tolerance.*

MOBILITY. Elements of the immune systems, both specific and nonspecific, can circulate. They include T and B lymphocytes, immunoglobulins, complement cells, and hematopoietic cells. Because of this quality, local sensitization (via the respiratory tract) may result in systemic sensitivity.

REPLICABILITY. The cellular components of the specific and nonspecific immune systems can replicate when activated, allowing for an augmented immune response.

COOPERATIVITY. For the immune system to function optimally, specific cellular elements (lymphocytes) and cell products (immunoglobulins) should interact with each other and with nonspecific cells and molecules.

Humoral and Cellular Responses

There are two principal effector arms of immune responses: humoral and cellular. *Humoral responses* are mediated by antibodies and are concerned primarily with early protection from infection and soluble antigens (foreign proteins). *Cellular responses* are directed at infected cells and tumor cells. During the generation of an antigen-specific effector component of the immune response, an early step involves antigen presentation in an appropriate form to enable its recognition by receptors on B and T lymphocytes. The appropriate B and T lymphocytes then proliferate and differentiate into antigen-specific effector cells. Antigen-presenting cells (APCs) generally are derived from monocyte-macrophage lineage; these cells process antigens and express them on their surfaces.

Lymphocytes

There are two classes of lymphocytes, T lymphocytes and B lymphocytes. These cells are functionally different but structurally similar at the level of both light and electron microscopy. T lymphocytes are derived from the thymus and are involved with *cellular immunity,* in which they interact with and destroy foreign or nonself cells. The B lymphocytes are involved with *humoral immunity,* in which they interact with foreign substances, differentiate into plasma cells, and synthesize and secrete immunoglobulins. The two immune systems are assisted by macrophages and certain other cells known as antigen-presenting cells (e.g., Langerhans' cells of the skin and Kupffer's cells of the liver). Both T and B lymphocytes have subpopulations that play a role in the immune system.

T Cells

T cells are divided into two major subgroups: effector cells and regulator cells. *Effector T cells* include the cytotoxic T cells (Tc) and the delayed-type hypersensitivity T cells (Tdh). The *cytotoxic T cells* (Tc) are the best-understood subset of effector cells. They combine with the antigen to initiate the cytotoxic effect that kills the invading organism. The action requires direct contact with the target cells, which initiates a secretory process that results in a pore in the target cell membrane followed by osmotic lysis. Thus, cytotoxic T cells do not exist spontaneously but are generated on specific sensitization. There are three phases in the life of the cytotoxic T cell:

1. The precursor phase consists of a lymphocyte with the potential of becoming cytotoxic on appropriate stimulation.

2. The effector phase consists of a lymphocyte that has differentiated into a killer cell and that can lyse its appropriate target.

3. The memory phase consists of a cytotoxic T lymphocyte that is no longer being stimulated and has become quiescent; it circulates, however, as a long-lived memory cell ready to differentiate into an effector cell on appropriate stimulation.

Cytotoxic T cells are restricted by the major histocompatibility complex (MHC-restricted), in that they will kill only those cells that bear the same MHC haplotypes as the cells used for sensitization. A variety of nonspecific (non–MHC-restricted) cytotoxic (killer) cell has been reported that includes natural killer (NK) cells, lymphokine-activated killer (LAK) cells, and antibody-dependent cell-mediated cytotoxicity (ADCC) cells. The cytotoxic T cell is the most likely cause of chronic graft rejection. The *delayed hypersensitivity T cells* (Tdh) are responsible for initiating delayed-type hypersensitivity reactions. They carry out their effect through the production of T-cell cytokines, such as interleukin-2.

Regulator T cells include T helper cells (Th) and T suppressor cells (Ts). Regulator cells control the development of effector T and B cells; thus, they participate in T-T and T-B interactive mechanisms. *T helper cells* amplify the responses of other lymphocytes (B and T). Amplification is accomplished via secreted cytokines. T helper cells are necessary in the initial antigen responses, especially to generate IgG and IgA responses.

The immune response has good as well as harmful effects and should be modulated to prevent a hyperimmune response. The *T suppressor cell* serves this purpose. It modifies or suppresses T-cell activity and down-regulates the immune response. T suppressor cells are responsible for some forms of acquired immune tolerance. T suppressor cells do not have a direct effect on B cells. Instead, T suppressor cells function primarily to regulate the capacity of T helper cells to aid in the maturation of the B cell into an antibody secreting cell.

The T cell is the major immune factor involved in the rejection of organ transplants and is the culprit responsible for the graft-versus-host reaction. In addition, T cells are involved in the immune response to intracellular microorganisms (e.g., acid-fast bacteria, certain viruses and fungi). They are also the main mediators of the immunopathologic mechanism in contact dermatitis. The previous correlation of phenotypic subsets of T lymphocytes (T4, T8) to function (helper, suppressor) has been blurred as research into lymphocyte function has progressed.

The role of the T lymphocyte in the immune response can thus be divided into four phases: induction, regulatory, effector, and memory:

1. Induction phase: Antigen-specific T cells encounter antigens presented by antigen-presenting cells (macrophages). The recognition by the T cell of the specific antigen results in its activation. Depending on the conditions of antigen presentation, helper or suppressor T cells (regulators) are activated.

2. Regulatory phase: The effect of regulatory T cells on effector cells may be direct, as in the T cell–to–B cell interaction, or may be accomplished via an intermediate cell. In the latter instance, the T cell interacts with a monocyte, which then releases a product (interleukin-1 and other cytokines), which then affects the effector cell.

3. Effector phase: This phase arises from the interaction of helper and suppressor T cells with effector cells (cytotoxic T cell, delayed hypersensitivity T cell, and B cell).

4. Memory phase: The exposure of the immune system to an antigenic stimulus leaves the memory of the immunologic response to that stimulus intact. A second exposure to the same antigenic stimulus would result in a more rapid and more powerful immune response.

Studies on T-cell function have revealed that the interaction between T cells and B cells may be bidirectional. B cells have been shown to be capable of presenting antigens to T cells similar to those presented by monocyte-macrophages.

T cells and their products have also been shown to modulate monocyte-macrophage numbers and function. Interleukin-3 released by activated T cells enhances the maturation of monocytes and other myeloid and erythroid cells. Activated T cells also release the macrophage migration inhibitory factor, which keeps macrophages in the vicinity of activated T cells.

B Cells

Subpopulations of B lymphocytes have not been as well defined as those of T cells but are believed to exist on the basis of surface marker analysis. These surface markers have been designated "clusters of differentiation" (CDs). Seventy-eight CDs have been described to date. B-cell products, the immunoglobulins, are divided into five major classes (isotypes), each of which is produced by a different cell line. All immunoglobulin molecules are composed of chains of polypeptides connected to each other by various bonds and folded on themselves. They have attached carbohydrate moieties that do not contribute directly to antibody specificity. Heavy and light chains are basic building blocks for immunoglobulins.

Plasma cells produce five kinds of immunoglobulins, which have the following characteristics:

- Immunoglobulin G (IgG) is the most abundant immunoglobulin in the serum. It constitutes about 75% of serum immunoglobulin, which provides binding sites for antigens. It is the only immunoglobulin that crosses the placenta and thus provides passive immunity for newborns against infection for 3 to 6 months. IgG is an important antiviral and antibacterial isotype and a potent toxin neutralizer.

    There are four IgG subclasses: IgG1 to IgG4. Anti-Rh antibodies are usually IgG1 or IgG3. IgG2 antibodies develop in response to antitoxins. IgG4 antibodies may function as skin-sensitizing antibodies. In general, IgG1 and IgG3 may be involved in the response to protein (T-dependent) antigen, whereas IgG2 may be involved in the response to polysaccharide antigen. IgG1 to IgG3 can fix complement and thus are more efficient as opsonins. IgG is the main immunoglobulin in commercial gamma globulin. It is produced when IgM titers begin to fall after primary immunization, and is the major immunoglobulin produced after re-immunization.
- Immunoglobulin A. IgA is found in colostrum, saliva, and tears, as well as nasal, bronchial, intestinal, prostatic, and vaginal secretions. It is synthesized by mucosal epithelial cells. Another type of IgA and associated proteins are synthesized by plasma cells located in the mucosa of the digestive, respiratory, and urinary tracts. IgA is thus the main immunoglobulin in the secretory antibody systems of the respiratory, gastrointestinal, and genitourinary tracts. It is particularly effective in providing antimicrobial protection at various mucosal sites. There are two IgA subclasses, IgA1 and IgA2.
- Immunoglobulin M (IgM) is important for early immune responses. It may be bound to B lymphocytes or may circulate in the blood. The bound form (along with IgD) is a receptor for antigens, which leads to their differentiation into antibody-producing plasma cells. IgM can activate a group of plasma enzymes (complement) capable of lysing bacteria and other cells. Ten percent of serum immunoglobulins are of this type. Immunoglobulin M is a large molecule (macroglobulin). It is the isotype present in the cytoplasm and on the surface of B lymphocytes in the early stages of their maturation. Special antibodies such as cold agglutinins, heterophil antibodies, and isohemagglutinins belong to this class. IgM is the first antibody formed after primary immunization.
- Immunoglobulin E (IgE) is secreted by plasma cells and attaches itself to basophils and mast cells. When the antigen that induced IgE synthesis and secretion is once again encountered, the basophils and mast cells release their histamine, heparin, leukotrienes, and eosinophil chemotactic factor, engendering an allergic reaction. Leukotrienes are important compounds mediating allergic reactions (such as in asthma), which are produced by mast cells and, perhaps, other cells.
- Immunoglobulin D (IgD) is found on the surface membranes of B lymphocytes along with IgM, but its function is uncertain. IgD constitutes only 0.2% of serum immunoglobulins.

The mean serum concentrations and half-lives in days of the different human immunoglobulins are listed in Table 9–2.

Thus, of the immunoglobulins, IgM is considered the first line of defense. IgG has a long half-life and can cross the placenta; it is therefore ideally suited for passive immunization. IgA protects mainly the secretory surfaces (gastrointestinal, respiratory, and genitourinary tracts and eyes), where there are nonvascular exposures to antigens and conditions that may interfere with the usual antibody activity, such as acid secretion, intestinal motility, and proteolytic enzymes. IgE is important in the release of pharmacologically active agents from mast cells; it thus causes asthma and hay fever. It is also the major mechanism in the elimination of parasites. IgD is primarily a lymphocyte receptor; it is the strongest binding antibody and is important in directing antigens to B-cell surfaces to accomplish initial immunization.

B lymphocytes thus develop into *plasma cells,* which produce immunoglobulins. B lymphocytes in peripheral tissues respond to a limited number of antigens. The first interaction between the antigen and the B cell is known as the *primary immune response.* The B cells committed to respond to this antigen undergo differentiation and clonal proliferation. Some of these cells differentiate into antibody-synthesizing plasma cells, and others become memory cells. The primary immune response is characterized by a latent period before the appearance of the antibody, followed by the production of a small amount of antibody, which is initially IgM and then IgG, IgA, or IgE. The *secondary (anamnestic* or *booster) immune response* takes place on subsequent encounters with the same antigen. The secondary immune response is characterized by a rapid proliferation of B cells, their rapid differentiation into mature plasma cells, and prompt production of a large amount of antibodies, which are mainly IgG.

Interactions Between T and B Cells

B lymphocytes may respond to antigens in a T-dependent or a T-independent fashion. T-independent

TABLE 9–2. Human Serum Immunoglobulins

Immunoglobulin	Serum Concentration (mg/dL ± SD)	Half-Life (days)
G	1150 ± 300	
G1	615 ± 200	21
G2	295 ± 180	20
G3	90 ± 14	7
G4	20 ± 18	21
M	100 ± 25	5
A	200 ± 60	6
D	3	3
E	0.005	2

antigens primarily evoke an IgM response. Most natural antigens are T-dependent. They require antigen processing by antigen-presenting cells (APCs). APCs present the antigen to both T and B cells. T cells release cytokines, which cause B cells to respond to the processed antigen by making antibodies.

T lymphocytes that migrate into other lymphoid tissues are located in so-called thymus-dependent areas, such as the paracortical zone of lymph nodes and periarterial sheaths of the white pulp of the spleen. The paracortical area is an ill-defined band or zone that lies between the cortex and medulla. T lymphocytes are long-lived and constitute most of the lymphocytes in lymph and blood. B lymphocytes are located in the nodules of the spleen, lymph nodes, and lymphatic aggregations of the ileum (Peyer's patches).

When a microbe or a virus invades the body, white cells (including neutrophils) are among the first of the body's defenses to attack the invading organisms. White cells are short-lived scavengers, surviving only a few days. Macrophages, however, are long-lived scavengers that engulf cellular debris and foreign matter. Macrophages display specific markers from the invading organisms on their surfaces, known as antigens. Antigens signal T helper cells, which begin reproducing themselves. The T helper cells, in turn, produce chemicals (interleukins) to activate B cells. The B cells begin to reproduce and to mature into plasma cells. Plasma cells produce antibodies, which are intended specifically to destroy the invading organism either directly, by binding to it, or indirectly, by making it more vulnerable to macrophages and neutrophils. After the invader has been destroyed, T suppressor cells chemically notify B cells and helper T cells to return to a dormant state. B lymphocytes that do not produce plasma cells may produce small B lymphocyte memory cells. These cells circulate in the blood and enter lymphoid tissue, where they may encounter the antigen that initiated B lymphocyte proliferation; in such cases, they initiate a secondary and more effective immune response.

The capacity to mount a humoral immune response is determined in large part by heredity. Immune response genes regulate the ability of T cells to recognize antigen, the capacity of antigen-presenting cells (APCs) to present it, and the potential of the B cell to respond by producing antibodies. Thus, genetic factors are critical in determining the ability to respond to antigens. It is also critical, however, to control the magnitude of the mounted immune response in order to prevent unlimited production of antibodies, particularly to self-antigens, which could lead to destruction of self. This self-control is exerted by T suppressor cells.

CHAPTER TEN

INTEGUMENT

EPIDERMIS 156
    The Epidermal Epithelial Strata 156
    Nonepithelial Cells of the Epidermis 162
    Epidermal Basement Membrane 164

DERMIS 165
    Papillary Layer 165
    Reticular Layer 165

SKIN LINES 166
    Skin Creases 166
    Flexure Lines 166
    Papillary Ridges 166
    Externally Visible Striae 166

AGING SKIN 167

SKIN COLOR 167

NERVES OF THE SKIN 167

BLOOD SUPPLY TO THE SKIN 168

SKIN LYMPHATICS 168

HYPODERMIS (SUBCUTANEOUS TISSUE AND SUPERFICIAL FASCIA) 168

APPENDAGES OF SKIN 168
    Nails 168
    Hairs 170
    Skin Glands 173

The covering of the body, called the *integument, skin,* or *cutis,* is the largest organ of the body and is essential for life. The skin in adults forms about 8% of the body mass and has a surface area of 1.2 to 2.2 m². The skin varies regionally in thickness from 1.5 to about 4.0 mm (Fig. 10–1).

Because it serves as the interface between the internal and external environments, the skin is structurally complex and highly specialized. Though fundamentally the same over the entire body, it has many regional variations with respect to thickness, degree of keratinization, the absence or size and number of hairs, types of glands, pigmentation, vascularity, and innervation. Microscopically, skin is composed of two distinct parts (Fig. 10–2): the superficial *epidermis,* or keratinized stratified squamous epithelium of ectodermal origin, and a deeper layer of connective tissue, or *dermis* (corium), which may be more or less loosely organized and is of mesodermal origin (Table 10–1). Skin terminates at the superficial fascia or subcutaneous tissue, characterized by fat cells, which can form a thick layer (panniculus adiposus) beneath the skin in obese individuals.

EPIDERMIS

The epidermis is composed of keratinized stratified squamous epithelium. In this epithelium, there is a continual shedding of dead cells at its surface and continual replacement of those cells through mitosis at the base of the epithelium. As the newly formed cells progress toward the epidermal free surface, a number of changes in shape and cytoplasmic content occur. Newly formed cells are polygonal and exhibit a dynamic array of cytoplasmic organelles. They are destined to become flat, squama-shaped dead cells filled with the protein keratin by the time they reach the free surface of the epithelium. The cells undergoing this transformation, known as *keratinocytes,* constitute the greatest number of cells in the epidermis. Other cell types found in skin epithelium are (1) pigment-synthesizing melanocytes, which are of neural crest origin and invade the epithelium during the twelfth to fourteenth week of embryonic life, (2) phagocytic Langerhans's cells, (3) mechanoreceptor Merkel's cells or corpuscles, and (4) free nerve endings.

The epithelium is usually subdivided into specific zones or strata, which represent different stages in keratinocyte maturation. From the deepest to the most superficial layer these are (Fig. 10–3):

- Stratum basale
- Stratum spinosum
- Stratum granulosum
- Stratum lucidum (if present)
- Stratum corneum

The first two are metabolically active and may be referred to collectively as the *germinative zone* or malpighian strata. The stratum granulosum, stratum lucidum, and stratum corneum together constitute the *cornified zone* or strata.

In addition to the stratified epithelium, a variety of important structures are associated specifically with skin. These epithelial modifications, which are discussed subsequently, are glands, hair and hair follicles, and nails.

The Epidermal Epithelial Strata

Stratum Basale

The *stratum basale* is a single layer of cells in contact with the basal lamina. The keratinocytes are produced in this layer by division of the stem cells that constitute the stratum basale. These cells are in continual mitotic activity, because the epithelium is renewed every 2 to 4 weeks. The newly formed keratinocytes migrate toward the free surface and will themselves divide two or three times in the stratum spinosum.

The cells of the stratum basale are a heterogeneous layer of stem cells, keratinocytes in various stages of very early maturation, and other types of cells, some of which are migrating cells of the loose connective tissue. Cell types other than keratinocytes are also discussed in a subsequent section.

The majority of the stem cells are cuboidal or columnar (Fig. 10–3) and they are attached to the basal lamina by hemidesmosomes (Fig. 10–4). Their basal surfaces are usually highly infolded and interdigitate with projections of the basal lamina.

Ultrastructural examination of basal stratum keratinocytes reveals numerous free ribosomes and mitochondria. The nuclei of stem cells are primarily euchromatic, indicating intense metabolic activity. The cells also contain cytoskeletal filaments, including actin mi-

TABLE 10–1. Layers of the Skin

Layer	Composition
Epidermis	
Stratum corneum	Consists of many layers of keratinized, dead cells that are flattened and nonnucleated
	Cornified
Stratum lucidum	A thin, clear layer found only in the epidermis of the palms and soles
Stratum granulosum	Composed of one or more layers of granular cells that contain fibers of keratin and pyknotic nuclei
Stratum spinosum	Composed of several layers of cells with centrally located, large, oval nuclei, and spinelike processes
Stratum basale	Consists of a single layer of columnar cells that undergo mitosis
	Contains pigment-producing melanocytes
Dermis	
Papillary layer	Composed of type I and type II collagen, some elastic fibers
	Contains capillary loops in papillae and may contain mechanoreceptors in hairless skin
Reticular layer	Composed of type I collagen in thick bundles that intermesh with the collagen of the papillary layer, some elastic fibers
	This layer and the papillary layer accommodate ducts of sweat glands, hair follicles, nerves, and nerve endings, and blood and lymphatic vessels

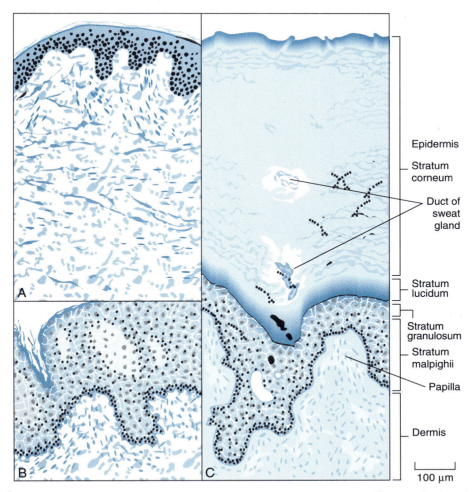

FIGURE 10-1. Skin thickness. Note the variation in different locations: shoulder (A), scalp (B), and foot (C). Note also how the keratinized stratified squamous epithelium varies in the three locations.

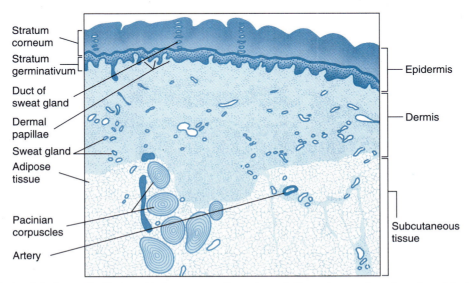

FIGURE 10-2. Stratification of the human skin. Various skin layers are well seen in particular regions, such as the palms of the hands and soles of the foot. These areas are heavily cornified. The skin consists of two parts, the epidermis and the dermis. The epidermis can be subdivided into a superficial cornified layer (stratum corneum) and a basal cellular layer (stratum germinativum), which gives rise to the other cellular layers of the epidermis. The dermis is composed of connective tissue. Its superficial or papillary layer joins the epidermis to the deeper layers of the dermis, which are composed of coarse collagen bundles but also ducts of glands, numerous blood vessels, and nerve fibers.

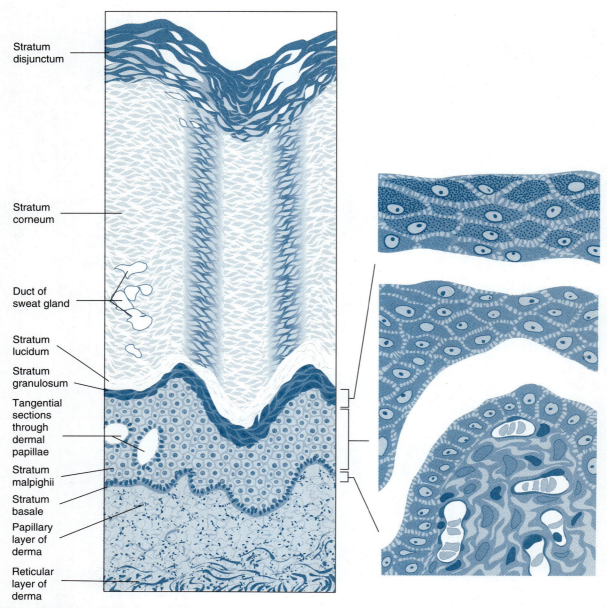

FIGURE 10-3. Thick skin of the sole of the foot. *The components of a highly keratinized skin are identified. The cellular layers are separated from the keratinized layers.*

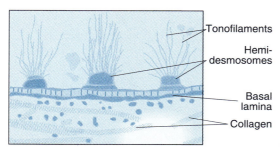

FIGURE 10–4. Hemidesmosomes. *These complex structures are believed to anchor the basal layer of the epidermis firmly to the extracellular matrix. The keratin filaments (tonofibrils) terminate in hemidesmosomes but only tangentially attach to desmosomes. The dense plaque labeled* hemidesmosome *is composed of various attachment proteins known as desmoplakins. The transmembrane proteins that link plaques with the basal lamina are glycoproteins called* desmogleins. *The mechanism whereby the hemidesmosomes hold the epithelium to the matrix is calcium ion–dependent.*

crofilaments and keratin filaments. The 10-nm keratin filaments may be anchored to desmosomes or to hemidesmosomes. The synthesis of keratin filaments is continuous during the migration of keratinocytes toward the stratum corneum. Melanin granules are also present in many of the cells of the stratum basale.

Excessive exposure to sunlight can cause basal cell carcinoma or even malignant melanoma. The skin permits passage of two wavelengths of ultraviolet (UV) rays, UV-A and UV-B. Nuclear DNA of basal cells can be damaged by the dangerous UV-B. Excessive exposure to UV-A may prevent repair of DNA damaged by UV-B.

Stratum Spinosum

The cells that compose the stratum spinosum are also known as *prickle cells*. They are maturing keratinocytes and are several layers deep. These polygonal cells are characterized by numerous projections from their surface that join those of adjacent cells. The projections are linked to each other by desmosomes (Figs. 10–5 and 10–6). Their spiny appearance on light microscopy led to the names prickle cell and aculeate cell (Fig. 10–7). Internally, the cells are filled with keratin filament bundles with many filaments being attached to the desmosomes at the ends of the cellular projections. It was once thought, before electron microscopy, that the projections were protoplasmic intercellular bridges and that the keratin filaments, formerly known as tonofibrils or tonofilaments, were actually continuous from cell to cell. It is now well established that prickle cells, although joined by desmosomes, do not communicate their cytoplasm.

The nuclei of the prickle cells are euchromatic, with prominent nucleoli. The cytoplasm contains numerous polyribosomes and vacuoles that in turn contain melanin pigment granules (melanosomes). In skin that is heavily pigmented, melanosomes are numerous, and each vacuole may have more than one melanosome. Melanin granules are produced and released from epidermal melanocytes, are ingested by prickle cells and other cell types, and are degraded as the

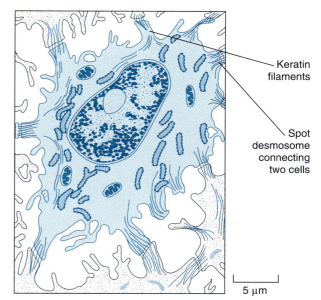

FIGURE 10–5. Cell of the stratum spinosum (prickle cell). *On electron microscopy, the exact nature of the intercellular projections can be ascertained. Each cell is connected to adjacent cells by spot desmosomes. Note that the bundles of keratin filaments inserted at the desmosomes help bind each prickle cell to its neighbor. The open spaces between cells permit the flow of nutrient-rich extracellular fluid. At the level of the stratum granulosum, the intercellular spaces contain a waterproofing seal. The secretion forming the seal is derived from the content of membrane-coating granules (lamellar granules) contained within the keratinocytes of this layer. The cells at the level of the stratum granulosum are beginning to die.*

maturation of keratinocytes continues. Melanin granules are absent from the outermost layers of the epidermis.

The stratum basale and stratum spinosum constitute the germinative or malpighian layers. Beyond the stratum spinosum, no keratinocyte cell divisions occur.

Stratum Granulosum

In the stratum granulosum, many structural changes culminate in keratinocytes that had their origin in the upper layers of stratum spinosum. The polygonal

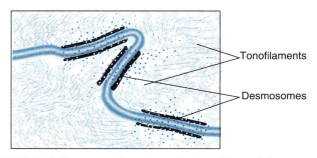

FIGURE 10–6. Desmosomes. *These button-like sites of intercellular contact essentially rivet cells together. Three are shown. Desmosomes also serve as anchoring sites for intermediate filaments (tonofilaments). Pemphigus vulgaris is a disease resulting from the action of autoimmune antibodies that localize and disrupt desmosomes of the skin; it is a potentially fatal disease, but it responds to corticosteroids. See also Figure 10–5.*

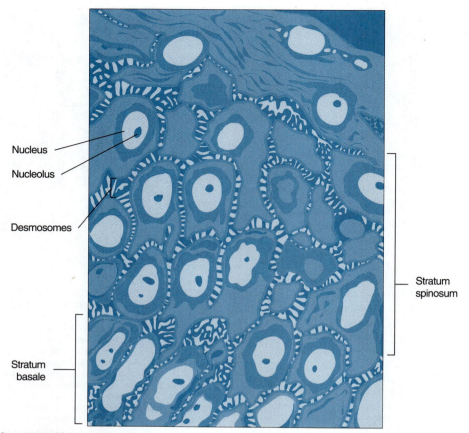

FIGURE 10–7. Stratified squamous epithelium (prickle cells). *The stratum spinosum is composed of so-called prickle cells that have numerous desmosomal, spikey attachment sites. Particularly in light-microscopic preparations, these spikey connections are readily seen. Beneath the stratum spinosum is stratum basale (stratum germinativum), where cell division is most active. The stratum germinativum and stratum spinosum together are termed the stratum malpighii. The cells of the stratum germinativum appear elongated and have prominent nuclei and nucleoli.*

cells of the lower strata become progressively flattened and accumulate many large, dense basophilic keratohyalin granules (many as large as 5 μm). At the level of the light microscope, the nuclei may appear shrunken, dense, and heterochromatic (pyknotic), signaling the cessation of cellular metabolic activity, which is further reflected in disintegration of organelles.

At the ultrastructural level, the granulosum cells accumulate networks of keratin filament bundles that enclose or entrap the large keratohyalin granules previously mentioned. The granules contain carbohydrate, lipid, and a highly phosphorylated protein rich in the amino acid histidine, so-called histidine-rich protein, also known as *stratum corneum basic protein* or *profilaggrin*. Electron microscopy also reveals small, finely granular, dense homogeneous granules, which may be elliptical, ovoid, or rod-like, in membrane-bound vesicles whose dimensions are about 0.1 by 0.3 μm. They have been named *membrane-coating granules, lamellar bodies,* and Odland bodies. These lamellar granules contain carbohydrate, lipid, and hydrolytic enzymes. The granules are discharged in the upper layers of the stratum granulosum and form a thick intercellular cement that serves both as a barrier to foreign substances and as a waterproofing material rich in lipids. The waterproofing material present here, as well as in the stratum corneum, permits life to exist in a dry terrestrial environment. It serves as an essential two-way barrier: (1) it prevents dessication by keeping extracellular fluid in the body and (2) it restricts many foreign substances from gaining access to the internal environment by crossing the epithelium of the skin.

Stratum Lucidum

The *stratum lucidum* is well defined in thick, hairless skin (e.g., palm of hand and sole of foot). Translucent (as indicated by its name), it is composed of flat, eosinophilic, dead cells. Nuclei and organelles are no longer present in the dead cells in this layer; desmosomes, however, can still be identified. The desiccated cytoplasm consists principally of densely packed filaments embedded in a matrix commonly referred to as *eleiden*. This layer constitutes a poorly understood stage of the keratinization process. The cells stain strongly with acidic dyes compared with the cellular remnants of the stratum corneum, which they resemble ultrastructurally. This layer is also more optically refractile than the stratum corneum.

Stratum Corneum

The stratum corneum varies in thickness and is very prominent in the thick, hairless skin of the sole of the foot and palm of the hand. It consists of closely packed layers of flat, dried, dead cells, termed *squames*. In thick skin, there may be 50 or more layers, and in thin skin only 5 to 10. The cells are compacted, and their cytoplasm is dominated by keratin filaments; these filaments lie parallel to each other and are 8 to 10 μm thick. Filaments of scleroprotein are embedded in a protein, *filaggrin*, originating from the histone-rich protein described for the stratum granulosum. The internal surface of the cell membrane of dead cells in the stratum corneum is coated with a dense 12-nm layer, the so-called *protein envelope*. The protein envelope is composed of cross-linked, chemically inert proteins, including keratolinin and involucrin. It is thought that these proteins arise from the dense homogeneous particles found in the stratum granulosum. The intercellular space is filled with the waterproofing material described in the discussion of the stratum granulosum. Only occasionally is a persistent desmosome found in the stratum corneum. The cells of this layer are continuously shed (desquamated) at the free surface of the epithelium. The cells of the stratum corneum are known as *horny cells* or *corneocytes*.

The superficial squames eventually loosen and become detached from the remainder of the epidermis. The loosening process may be due to friction and abrasion but may also be due to activation of lipases released by the membrane-coating granules found in the squames. The turnover rate of keratinocytes, depending on location, has been estimated to be 45 to 75 days, less (5 to 30 days) in thinner skin; in certain diseases of the skin, such as psoriasis, turnover occurs in only about 8 days.

The preceding discussion describes the histology of thick skin, such as that found on the sole of the foot and palm of the hand. Elsewhere, in thinner skin, the stratum corneum and stratum granulosum may be less well developed, with many fewer cells, and the stratum lucidum may be absent.

Keratinization

The tough, cornified squames of the keratinocyte contain only one of a large family of keratin filaments of similar size and type, which are characteristic of all types of epithelium. Immunocytochemical studies show that the maturation of keratinocytes involves a variable pattern of keratin filament chemistry. Keratins of the basal cells differ from those of young keratinocytes. The final form of keratin begins in the outer layers of the stratum spinosum. The free ribosomes of the keratinocytes produce the keratin filament protein. This protein is assembled into 8-mm to 10-mm filaments, which undergo progressive aggregation and contact with keratohyalin in the stratum granulosum. The process is completed when chemical changes occur, resulting in the formation of disulfide bonds. These stabilize the filament-filaggrin complex. The result is chemically inert keratin filament bundles embedded in a dense matrix. The cytoplasm of keratinocytes contains autophagosomes, the lysosomal enzymes of which apparently digest cellular organelles, thereby ending any nonessential metabolic activity (Fig. 10–8).

The keratin of hair and nails is chemically distinctive and harder than that of the cornified epithelium of skin. The differences are considered subsequently. The

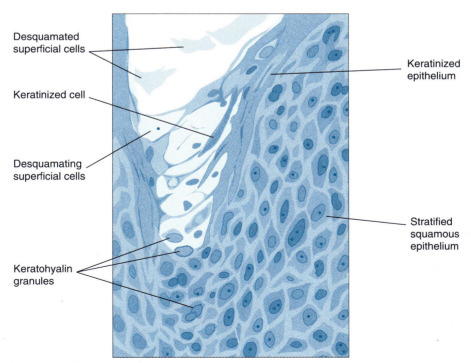

FIGURE 10–8. Stratified squamous epithelium: keratinization. *The structural changes in keratinization involve the aggregation and arrangement of microfilaments, the formation of keratohyalin granules, and a decrease in cell organelles. The cells continue to shut down metabolic activity, and they lose their nuclei, become clear of stainable organelles, elongate, and flatten. This process begins superficial to the stratum spinosum.*

thickness of the cornified epithelium is variable from person to person and depends on several factors, including abrasion or pressure in manual laborers (palmar callouses), walking bare-footed, and exposure to excessive sunlight.

Nonepithelial Cells of the Epidermis

Melanocytes and Melanosomes

The bases of the melanocytes (dendritic cells) lie near the stratum basale (germinativum) in contact with the basal lamina (Fig. 10–9). From the apices of the melanocytes, numerous cytoplasmic extensions arise, and they ramify extensively among surrounding cells. These dendritic projections extend into the stratum spinosum for a variable distance (Fig. 10–10).

As mentioned earlier, melanocytes migrate into the epidermis from the neural crest. Although melanocytes are attached to the basal lamina by hemidesmosomes, they do not form similar desmosomal attachments to adjacent cells. Their nuclei are round and their chromatin is euchromatic. The cytoplasm is typical of a secretory cell, containing granular endoplasmic reticulum, a Golgi complex, and numerous mitochondria. Cytoplasmic microtubules, intermediate filaments, and microfilaments extend into the dendrites.

The end product of the synthetic activity of the melanocyte is the melanosome. Melanosomes are contained within membranous sacs derived from the Golgi complex and are transported from the perikaryon to the ends of the dendrites. The terminal ends of the

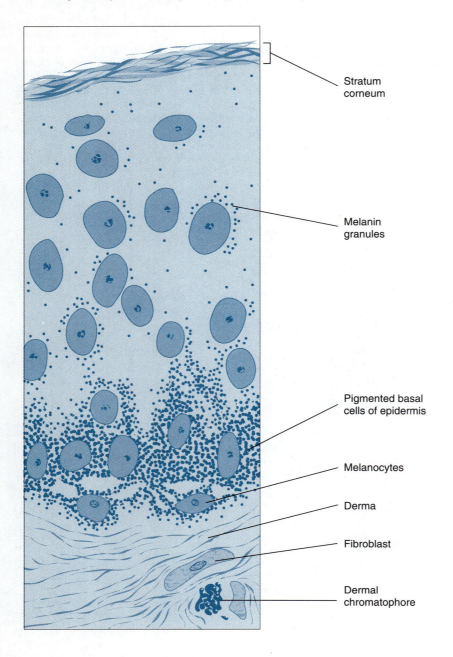

FIGURE 10–9. Stratified squamous epithelium: melanocytes. Section through skin of human mammary papilla. Note the high concentration of melanin granules in the pigmented basal cells. These are produced by the melanocytes and are transferred by cytoplasmic extensions to the basal cell layer by an injection process known as cytocrine secretion.

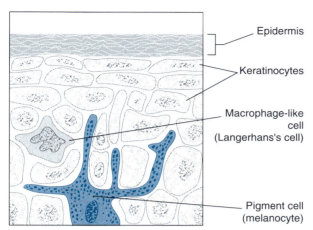

FIGURE 10-10. Melanocytes and Langerhans's cells. *Melanocytes, of epidermal neural crest origin, migrate to the skin in variable numbers and produce melanin granules. The granules are transferred to epidermal cells (keratinocytes) for storage. The process of transfer is known as cytocrine secretion. Langerhans's cells are found mainly in the stratum spinosum. They arise from bone marrow precursors and are believed to be a part of the mononuclear phagocytic system. Their role in the skin is believed to be concerned with processing and presenting skin antigens to lymphoid cells in the skin.*

dendritic, melanin-containing cytoplasm are shed and are engulfed and incorporated into the cytoplasm of neighboring keratinocytes and basal stem cells. This type of secretion, termed *cytocrine secretion*, is thought to be the mechanism whereby melanocytes protect germinal cell DNA from potentially harmful effects of ultraviolet light. It should be remembered that pigment is constantly being diluted and lost from the basal layer through cell division as well as through cell migration toward the epithelial surface. Hence, the synthesis of melanosomes is a continuous process. If melanosome synthesis is inadequate, basal cells and keratinocytes may die following prolonged exposure to intense ultraviolet light. In addition, epidermal neoplasms may occur if basal cell DNA is damaged. Squamous cell carcinoma may develop if the germinative cell layer is not protected by an adequate population of melanosomes.

Skin color or darkness depends upon several factors, including the number of melanocytes and the population and distribution of melanosomes. These factors vary according to genetic determination, hormonal activity, and exposure to ultraviolet light. The numbers of melanocytes are approximately equal in light and dark races, but the synthetic rate of melanin and the composition of the melanosome differ among races.

Melanocytes are most numerous on the face, external genital organs, nipples and areola of the breast, and mucosal orifices. Their number has been estimated to be between 800 and 2000 per mm^2.

Melanosomes are oblong to rounded, and are membrane-bound. They are composed of the brown pigment *eumelanin*. *Phaeomelanin*, another pigment, found in red hair, is reddish yellow and occurs in spheroidal granules called *phaeomelanosomes*. In blacks, melanosomes are rod-shaped, may be as large as 3 by 0.5 μm, and are dark brown. In Caucasians, the melanosome granules average about 0.5 μm in length with a range of 0.3 to 0.7 μm, and they vary widely in the density of their content of brown pigment.

Melanosome Synthesis

Melanosome synthesis takes place within the membranous sacs of granular (RNA) endoplasmic reticulum. Melanosomes "bud off" from melanocytes and remain within a granular membrane. The contents of the membranous bag are some "granular material" and a few cross-striated filaments; this is known as a *type I melanosome* or *promelanosome*. When the filaments increase in number, filling the bag, the structure assumes an elliptical shape and is termed a *type II melanosome*. Finely granular eumelanin is synthesized and is evenly distributed throughout the elliptical bag; this structure is then termed a *type III melanosome*. When the melanin becomes so dense that it obscures the striated filaments, the structure is designated a *type IV melanosome*. The type IV melanosome is relatively homogeneous, with some small spherical areas of lower density known as vesicular-globular bodies.

Phaeomelanosomes, containing reddish yellow pigment, differ from the elliptical variety in that they retain a spherical form. In addition, these bodies contain granular masses and appear less homogeneous than do the elliptical forms.

Of special interest are the striated rods contained within melanosomes and phaeomelanosomes. These have been identified as aggregations of the enzyme tyrosinase. They appear striated because the aggregation is in the form of a helix, 500 nm in length and 10 μm in diameter, with a 10-nm periodicity.

Eumelanin is an insoluble proteinoid polymer of dihydroxyphenylalanine (DOPA)-quinone. This pigment is synthesized by a series of reactions involving tyrosinase and other oxidative enzymes. Tyrosine, an amino acid, is converted in the melanocyte to DOPA. Several additional chemical reactions produce DOPA-quinone and, ultimately, eumelanin.

Melanocytes can be demonstrated in frozen sections of fresh epidermis by incubation of the sections with DOPA. The DOPA is converted to dark eumelanin by the enzyme systems within the melanocyte.

Phaeomelanin has a similar synthetic pathway but differs from that for eumelanin in using a cysteine-rich polymer of DOPA. This pigment is distinguished, accordingly, by its disulfide bonds.

Melanization

A variety of factors affect melanization. Genetics usually accounts for the variation in the number and kinds of melanosomes, rather than the number of melanocytes. Hormones also affect melanization, including the melanin-stimulating hormone (MSH) synthesized within the adenohypophysis (anterior pituitary). Estrogen and progesterone can also increase melanization during pregnancy. These effects occur primarily on the face but also in the genital area, nipples and areola, and abdominal skin. After pregnancy, the nipples and areola retain, permanently, the higher pigmentation.

Age and a variety of pathologic conditions also affect the degree of melanization.

Exposure to ultraviolet light increases melaninization primarily through two mechanisms. The first involves the increased synthetic and transfer activities of melanocytes; the second involves the multiplication of melanocytes by mitotic activity.

The degree to which these events occur depends upon the genetic characteristics of an individual as well as the amount and duration of exposure. In some individuals, only freckles occur, whereas in others, overall darkening results. In albinism, of which at least six biochemically distinct types are known, no melanosome production is possible because part of the enzymatic pathway is defective. Moles (melanocytic nevi), however, are rich in melanocytes and have a high density of dark brown melanosomes. Although most nevi are not dangerous, some may give rise to malignant melanomas, which become rapidly life threatening. Melanomas typically disrupt the skin around them and give rise to metastases that grow aggressively throughout the body. Hereditary leukomelanopathy is an autosomal recessive disorder characterized by decreased pigmentation in the skin, hair, and eyes and by abnormal white blood cells. Affected patients are generally susceptible to infections and early death.

The basis for general skin color is discussed later.

Langerhans's Cells (Epidermal Dendritic Cells)

Langerhans's cells are distributed throughout the epidermis and the epithelium of the buccal mucosa. They are derived from bone marrow precursor cells and are continually replaced (see Fig. 10–10). Langerhans's or epidermal dendritic cells are located in the deeper part of the stratum spinosum. The dendritic expansions of each cell extend between the surrounding cells. Unlike between the cells of the stratum spinosum, no desmosomal junctions occur between Langerhans's cells and adjacent cells.

The nucleus of each Langerhans's cell is euchromatic and indented or slightly folded, and the cytoplasm contains numerous mitochondria, a rough (or granular) endoplasmic reticulum, and a well-developed Golgi apparatus. The cytoplasm also contains lysosomes. The cells also possess membrane-covered Langerhans's bodies, which serve to specifically identify these cells. *Langerhans's bodies* are vacuoles varying in size from 0.5 μm in length and 30 nm in width with a central body marked with cross-striations at 9-nm intervals. They arise from the Golgi complex and are discharged from the cell. Their function is unknown.

Langerhans's cells appear structurally and functionally similar to other connective tissue macrophages, including in their immunochemical reactivity. Immunohistochemical research suggests that Langerhans's cells may belong to a group of dendritic immune cells that can also be found in lymph nodes and the medulla of the thymus.

Functionally, Langerhans's cells are important in cellular defense. They detect, find, bind, and present antigens to T lymphocytes and are an important part of the immune mechanism of the skin. It is believed that this system of cell-mediated immunity is effective in epidermal viral infections as well as in a diverse group of other "first line of defense" responses to a variety of organisms, such as ticks.

The cells arise from a progenitor located in the bone marrow but they may divide within the epidermis. In the mature adult, they number about 600 per mm^2 in the epidermis.

Merkel's Cells (Tactile Menisci)

Present only in thick, hairless skin at the base of the epithelium or at the dermal-epithelial junction, Merkel's cells usually protrude into the dermis and are the terminal attachments of mechanoreceptive (tactile) cutaneous nerve endings. They are variously described as interepithelial or dermal in location. In any event, they are located at or near the epithelial-dermal junction. The cells are roughly elliptical and possess several apical spikes of cytoplasm, which are inserted between epidermal keratinocytes to which they are attached by desmosomes. The cells contain numerous dense-cored vesicles and intermediate filaments. The nerve adjoining each Merkel's cell is an expanded disklike structure, suggesting a synaptic relationship. These cells are under active investigation and their function is still unclear. As an alternative to functioning as some form of tactile receptor, they have been shown to be a part of a diffuse neuroendocrine system.

Epidermal Basement Membrane

The basement membrane of the epidermis consists of a *basal lamina*, about 80 nm thick, together with an underlying layer of fine reticular fibers, the *lamina reticularis*. The epidermal cells of the stratum basale are attached to the basal lamina, as is the reticular lamina of the underlying dermis. The chemical composition of the basal lamina is thought to be unique to the skin. The reticular lamina is composed of a tough but delicate network of reticular fibers.

Similar to other basal laminae, the epidermal basal lamina is composed of two major parts. The lamina lucida lies immediately adjacent to the bases of epidermal cells; beneath it is an electron-opaque layer, the lamina densa. The *lamina lucida* is granular or filamentous and is composed of various macromolecules. The chemical composition includes laminin, heparan sulfate proteoglycan, and pemphigoid antigen (a unique skin protein). The *lamina densa* is composed of type IV collagen molecules, epidermolysis bullosa acquisita antigen (a glycoprotein), fibronectin, and a variety of proteoglycans. The lamina lucida is a significant adhesive to the epidermal cell membrane, and the lamina densa may have a regulatory function in limiting passage of macromolecules from the dermis to the epidermis.

The major function of the basement membrane is

to stabilize the epidermis through its hemidesmosomal attachments, by the fine filaments attached to the epidermal cell desmosomal plaques (which traverse the lamina lucida and insert into the lamina densa) and by delicate microfibrils of elastin-like proteins, such as oxytalan and elaunin, anchored into the dermis (see Fig. 10–4).

DERMIS

The dermis or corium is formed of irregular but rather dense connective tissue. It consists of collagenous networks, a variable number of elastin fibers, proteoglycans, fibronectin, blood vessels, lymphatics, nerve, and (in hairy skin) smooth muscle. The proteoglycans content of glycosaminoglycans consists of hyaluronic acid, dermatan sulfate, chondroitin 6-sulfate, and heparin sulfate. The dermis is not homogeneous, but varies from place to place in density and in elasticity. Because of its variable structure, the skin may be loose and elastic or taut and relatively immobile.

Tattooed designs on the skin owe their "permanence" to the fact that the dyes are injected into the dermis below the germinative layers of the epidermis. The dyes reside in the ground substance.

The dermis accommodates the blood vessels, lymphatics, wandering cells of the connective tissue, and nerves and their sensory receptors. The dermis can be divided into two distinct zones or layers: the superficial papillary layer adjacent to the basement membrane and a deeper, reticular layer (Fig. 10–11). The boundary between the two layers is not always distinct because of the gradation from the fine superficial to the coarser, more deeply placed collagenous bundles.

Papillary Layer

Located immediately beneath the epidermis, the papillary layer provides the epithelium with mechanical support. It is a richly vascular tissue containing numerous cells of the immune system and sensory nerves and their receptors as well. The surface adjacent to the epidermis is not smooth, but is markedly irregular, sending numerous projections (papillae) that fit into the base of the epidermis. The dermal papillae may have more than a single apex, or the apex may be rounded or flattened or composed of several cusps, or the tissue may form ridges rather than papillae. Dermal papillae, particularly those in the palm of the hand and sole of the foot, where the sensation of touch is highly developed, also contain sensory receptor nerve endings.

In thin skin, the dermal papillae are small and few. In thick skin, especially on the palmar aspect of the hand and plantar aspect of the foot, the papillae are much larger. The papillae in these locations run parallel to each other for variable distances; each, however, is a unique series of ridges and grooves typical of these skin surfaces. The dermal papillae alternate with an epidermal ridge through which the ducts of sweat glands reach the epithelial surface. Dermal papillae are composed of type I and type III collagen fibers, some delicate elastic fibers, and other microfibrillar structures. In addition, each papilla contains a capillary loop, and as discussed in a later section, they contain, in hairless skin, sensory receptors known as Meissner's "tactile" corpuscles (Fig. 10–12).

Reticular Layer

The collagenous tissue of the reticular layer merges with that of the papillary layer. In the adult, collagen is primarily type I, but initially during embryonic development, type III collagen predominates. The bundles are thicker than those found in the papillary layer, but they intermesh and form a very strong union between the two layers. The reticular layer, like the papillary layer, contains elastic fibers that vary in number from place to place. The coarser fasciculi of the reticular layer accommodate ducts of sweat glands, hair follicles, sebaceous glands, bundles of nerve fibers, and larger arteries, arterioles, veins, and venules (Fig. 10–11).

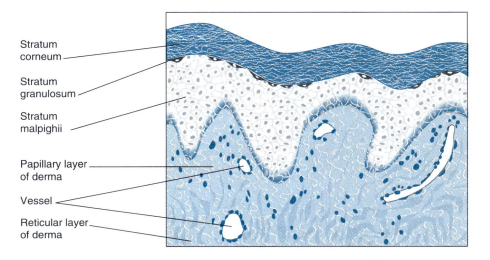

FIGURE 10–11. Thick skin. *The various parts of skin are identified (cf. Fig. 10–1).*

- Stratum corneum
- Stratum granulosum
- Stratum malpighii
- Papillary layer of derma
- Vessel
- Reticular layer of derma

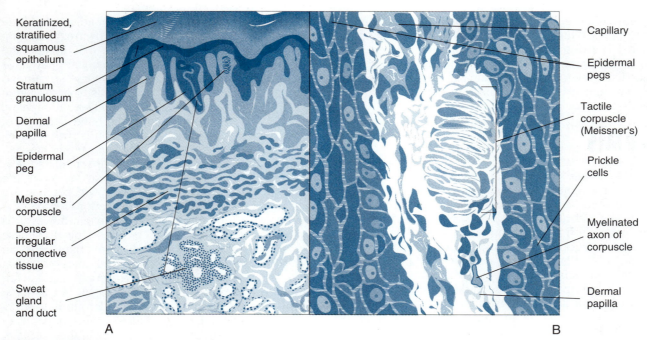

FIGURE 10-12. Skin: Meissner's corpuscle (touch receptor). A, Dermal papillae are formed from the superficial dermis and are composed of collagenous connective tissue. The papillae contain, in addition to Meissner's corpuscles and their myelinated axons, so-called free nerve endings and capillary blood vessels, which along with sweat glands, play an important role in temperature regulation in humans. Note the sweat gland duct within an epidermal peg (ridge) and its coiled glandular portion, seemingly unattached, deep in the dermis.

B, Meissner's corpuscles are located in the dermal papillae of skin and are usually in contact with the basal cells of the epithelium. They are surrounded by a thin connective tissue sheath. Nerve terminals within the corpuscle are not seen. Tactile corpuscles are common in hairless (glabrous) parts of the skin, but they are most numerous in the fingertips, palm of the hand, and sole of the foot. Meissner's corpuscles are rapidly adapting mechanoreceptors that subserve discriminative touch sensations.

SKIN LINES

There are numerous kinds of skin lines:

- Papillary ridges
- Externally visible striae
- Tension lines
- Skin creases
- Flexure lines

Some of these are discussed briefly.

Skin Creases

A simple pattern of skin creases is found on all areas of the body with the exception of the palm of the hand and sole of the foot. The pattern of creases is usually composed of polygons or parallelograms visible to the naked eye. These become divided into secondary triangular folds; tertiary creases are limited to the stratum corneum. Additional creases have been described. For the most part, creases and folds can increase the surface area when the skin is placed under tension. The expansion or stretch accommodates the stress and strain placed on skin under normal circumstances.

Flexure Lines

Flexure lines are found in the region of synovial joints, where the skin is strongly attached to the deep fascia associated with bony joints. The skin surfaces of the hands and feet provide examples of flexure lines, with the prominent creases superimposed on the tension line skin creases. Flexure lines are known to have a genetic component, owing perhaps to the connective tissue constituents, which are characteristic of some genetic defects (e.g., Down's syndrome individuals may have a prominent transverse palmar crease at the bases of the metacarpals).

Papillary Ridges

Located exclusively on the palms and digits of the hands and soles and digits of the feet, papillary ridges form whorls, loops, and arches separated by furrows. The ducts of sweat glands open onto the surface of each ridge at regular intervals. Each ridge corresponds to an underlying dermal papilla. These papillae and ridges have a constant pattern throughout life. Because the pattern is permanent and is unique to each person, finger-printing is a certain means of forensic identification. Clinically, some pattern formations may be affected by certain genetic disorders. It is not known why basic differences exist between females and males or why the fingerprints deviate consistently from the normal in the mentally handicapped.

Externally Visible Striae

If the skin is stretched more than can be normally accommodated, the reticular layer may tear, and the resulting repair by fibroblasts (scar formation) will ultimately leave lines that are paler than the surrounding skin. Such stretch marks may result from excessive stretching of skin by a rapidly developing fetus (striae gravidarum) or by rapid excessive weight gain or a tumor.

AGING SKIN

The fundamental structure and the unique organization of the papillary ridges are established in early fetal life. After birth, skin increases in size, becomes variably thicker, and, at puberty, undergoes changes in hair structure and distribution and glandular activity. These changes occur before the second decade of life. By the third decade, the skin begins the aging process. These alterations can be accelerated by excessive exposure to sun and other environmental factors.

As is true in other systems, the skin undergoes atrophy, which is seen microscopically and is reflected in the visible, macroscopic appearance. These changes are wrinkling, decreased elasticity, development of purpura (purpura senilis), pigmentation, and other epidermal and dermal aberrations. Epidermal projections and their counterpart dermal papillary ridges decrease in size. Alterations occur in both collagen and elastic fibers. These changes appear as a decreased extensibility, elasticity, and resistance to shear stress or tension. Collagen changes occur at about 65 years, with gradual shift to a relative increase in type III collagen over type I. The nature and significance of this change are not understood. It is clear that the changes occurring in aging skin result in a lowered tensile strength compared with that of young skin.

SKIN COLOR

Skin color is determined by several factors, including genetic skin color, vascular supply, and skin thickness. The pigments that color the skin are found in the epidermis and hair. The most common pigments are the brown-black melanin and the chemically related red-brown phaeomelanin found primarily in certain hair coloring. The density of these pigments varies according to body location, ultraviolet light, and genetic and other factors.

Early in fetal and postnatal life, melanoblasts of neural crest origin migrate and enter the epidermis from the dermis. If the melanoblasts remain in the dermis, bluish spots may be seen, and lines of demarcation (Voigt's lines) may mark boundaries between the darker dorsal aspect and lighter ventral aspect of the upper limb.

In the absence of large amounts of melanin, the primary contributor to skin color is the oxygenated hemoglobin of the superficial blood vessels and the dermis blood supply. When normally seen through the epidermis, the well-oxygenated hemoglobin gives the skin of Caucasians a pinkish hue. In congestive heart failure, for example, when the blood is poorly oxygenated, the skin has a bluish hue. In jaundice, the skin appears yellowish owing to an excess of bile pigment throughout the body and blood stream; jaundice is symptomatic of liver dysfunction, obstruction of bile excretion by pancreatic carcinoma, and other conditions.

Factors that affect blood flow, such as temperature, physical activity, emotional states, and general health, all play a role in skin coloration. In darker races, the coloration due to the vascular supply is diminished by the presence of varying concentrations of melanin.

NERVES OF THE SKIN

Besides being the physical interface between the internal and external environments, the skin is the most extensive sensory receptor organ and an important thermoregulator of the body. These functions are carried out by regional or spinal segmental nerves and by efferent sympathetic fibers of segmental craniospinal nerves.

The external environment impinges upon the epidermis, exciting receptors located in the epidermis, dermis, and deeper connective tissues. The receptors intercept rapid and continuous touch, pressure, vibration, stretch, and movement of hairs; they respond to hot and cold, extremes of temperature, and discomfort, including itch and pain. The receptors transmit their sensory information to nerve fibers, the cell bodies of which are located in spinal and cranial ganglia. Impulses are then transmitted to the central nervous system without conscious participation and may elicit reflex responses.

Autonomic nerve fibers are both noradrenergic and cholinergic. They innervate arterioles, arrector pili muscles (smooth muscles associated with hairs), the myoepithelial cells of sweat and apocrine glands, and smooth muscle associated with the scrotum and labia, nipples, and perineal skin. The functional nerve supply to these structures is primarily concerned with regulation of body heat in order to keep it constant and to control sweat glands and piloerection. The smooth muscle of the nipple is, of course, unrelated to thermoregulation.

Receptors that can be readily seen in sections of skin without resorting to special staining are the touch receptors of Meissner (Meissner's corpuscles) found in great numbers and located in the dermal papillae of the thick skin of the palms of the hand and soles of the feet (see Fig. 10–12). Deeper in the dermis and hypodermis, the larger, rounded pacinian corpuscles, which monitor pressure, vibratory activity and movement, can be found. In genital skin, small, encapsulated genital corpuscles monitor mechanical stimulation. Visualization of other receptor types, including those of pain and temperature and those involved with the movement of hairs, requires special staining techniques or electron microscopy. The density of sensory receptors varies greatly and is highest at the ends of the limbs (hands and feet), on the face, around the mouth, and in the anogenital regions. (See also Chapter 7.)

BLOOD SUPPLY TO THE SKIN

Although the skin itself does not have a high metabolic rate, various structures in it do require a rich blood supply. These are the epidermis, glands, hair follicles, and nerve fibers. The blood supply of the skin is shown in Figure 10–13.

Blood enters the skin as small arteries. These arteries penetrate the reticular layer, where they anastomose and ramify, forming the reticular plexus, or *rete cutaneum*, at the junction between the superficial fascia and the reticular layer of the dermis. From this plexus, some arterioles pass inward into the fatty superficial fascia below the dermis to supply sweat glands, sensory receptors (pacinian corpuscles), and hair follicles. Other arterioles pass into the reticular layer to form capillary beds around hair follicles, sweat gland ducts, sebaceous glands, and dermal smooth muscle. The majority of arterioles, however, form a secondary plexus at the reticular-papillary junction of the dermis; this plexus is known as the *papillary plexus, subpapillary rete*, or *superficial plexus*. Capillaries derived from the arterioles of this rete or plexus form dermal papillary loops that closely approximate the contour of the germinative zone of the epidermis. The capillaries are drained by veins into a venous plexus located beneath the arteriolar papillary plexus. This venous blood drains into a second, deeper, venous plexus.

Arteriovenous anastomoses occur in the deeper parts of the dermis. In the hands, feet, and other places, these arteriovenous anastomoses have an important role in thermal regulation. Through the autonomic nervous system, the vasomotor tone of the vascular bed is constantly regulated to adjust for gain or loss of temperature. In addition to nervous activity, humoral influences affect vascular smooth muscle. Prominent among the humoral agents are norepinephrine, angiotensin, and histamine.

The arteries and veins usually run closely parallel to each other, so that temperature control of arterial and venous blood can be maintained by a countercurrent or radiation mechanism.

SKIN LYMPHATICS

The origins, or blind ends, of lymphatic capillaries are numerous in the reticular layer of the dermis. These are drained by larger vessels in the reticular layer and progressively larger vessels in the superficial fascia. The lymphatics accept excess extracellular fluid produced by the capillary beds, and because of their structural organization, they usually appear dilated and filled with extracellular fluid. Larger lymphatic vessels have valves, as do vessels associated with lymph nodes, to direct the flow of lymph toward the venous drainage near the subclavian-internal jugular junction.

HYPODERMIS (SUBCUTANEOUS TISSUE, SUPERFICIAL FASCIA)

Underlying the dermis is a regionally thick layer of loose, fatty connective tissue, the *hypodermis*. This layer serves to give flexible attachment of the skin to underlying structures and conducts the vital nerve and blood vascular supply to the dermis. Over muscle, the hypodermis is coextensive with the superficial fascia *(tela subcutanea)*, and in regions such as the abdomen, breast, and buttock, the hypodermis serves as a rich depot of adipose tissue. It is into the loose fascial layer of the buttocks that hypodermic injections are made, for example (Figs. 10–14, 10–16, and 10–20).

APPENDAGES OF SKIN

The appendages of the skin are:

- Nails
- Hairs
- Skin glands: sebaceous, eccrine, apocrine

Nails

The nails of the fingers and toes are hard, semitransparent, horny plates somewhat rounded or rectangular and located on the distal end of each digit of the hand and foot. Nails appear as differentiations of the

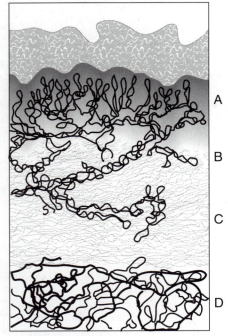

FIGURE 10–13. Skin blood supply. The blood supply is shown by injecting the blood vessels with a colored material. Four regions of blood supply are noted: A, papillary, B, subpapillary, C, reticular, and D, hypodermal. The papillary layer supplies the epidermis (epithelium) with nutrients and removes waste by diffusion; capillaries do not penetrate the epidermis.

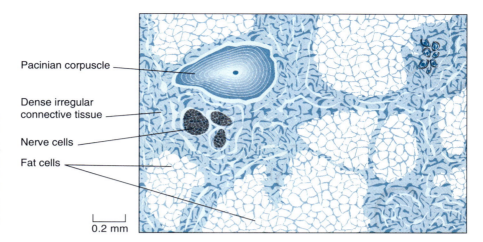

FIGURE 10–14. Superficial fascia. *Beneath the skin, epidermis and dermis, lies the superficial or fatty fascia (hypodermis). Within the superficial fascia, nerve fiber bundles, the large pacinian (Vater-Pacini) corpuscles (proprioceptive receptors of the peripheral nervous system), and sweat glands are found. The pacinian corpuscles, found in huge numbers in the palm of the hand and sole of the foot, appear elsewhere throughout the body.*

embryonic epidermis at the ninth week of gestation and are completely developed by about the twelfth week.

The nail has three distinct regions: the proximal root or radix, the exposed expanse of the nail, and the distal free border (Fig. 10–15). The nail is embedded in a deep fold of epidermis, the *proximal nail fold*. Where the stratum corneum of the epidermis folds over the nail is known as the *eponychium*, or more commonly, the *cuticle*. The sides of the nail are contained in the grooves of the lateral skin folds. The root of the nail lies on a thick plate of epidermal cells, the so-called *germinal matrix* (nail bed or sterile matrix), to which it is firmly attached. The germinal matrix is tightly bound to the deep fibrous tissue attached to the distal phalanx. The germinal matrix extends beyond the limits of the eponychium, where it appears as a pale, proximal crescentic area known as the *lunule*. The lunule is usually not seen on the fifth digit (or little finger). The nail bed's rich vascularity can be seen through the nail, although it is partially obscured by the lunule. The nail covering the lunule contains immature keratin and is not as transparent as other parts of the nail. The rapidity of capillary bed filling in a finger or toe is readily assessed by depressing and quickly releasing its nail.

Microscopically, the nails are homologous with the stratum corneum. They consist of dead, flattened, anuclear, keratin-filled squames. Nails are formed from what appear to be normal keratinocytes. The final keratinization takes place, however, without having passed through the granule cell (stratum granulosum) stage; the significance of this difference is not clear. The squames of the nail have tightly packed keratin filaments disposed transversely to the direction of nail growth. The squames are not shed but are embedded in a dense protein matrix. The dense protein matrix is cross-linked by disulfide bonds located between the packed layers of squames; desmosomes persist in joining adjacent squames.

Growth of the nail occurs only in the so-called root and lunule. The ventral surface of the nail is formed by the matrix, and the dorsal layers are formed from the epithelium of the proximal nail fold.

The nail bed has the same stratified columnar epithelium as skin, although the surface is only partially

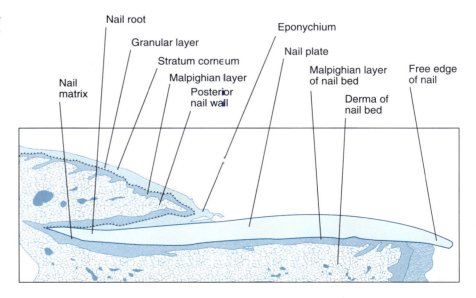

FIGURE 10–15. Fingernail. *Longitudinal section of a fingernail in situ, with its component parts identified.*

keratinized and the cells retain their nuclei. The surface cells of this epithelium are firmly coupled to the nail. They move forward with the growing nail and are shed at the distal edge of the nail bed. The surface cells do not contribute to the structure of the nail.

The rate of nail growth depends upon several factors, including the particular digit, age, and body temperature. The middle or longest digit has the fastest rate of nail growth, about 0.1 mm per day, and the last or smallest digit has the slowest. Fingernails grow faster than toenails by a factor of four.

Illness and damage to the germinative cells result in longitudinal or transverse ridges. Diet affects nail strength and growth. Any defect formed in the nail will appear and subsequently will move outward from the germinative and lunule area. Severe damage to the nail bed may result in loss of the nail. Subsequent return to normality will result in new nail formation. "Flattened" or thin nails are found only in primates and humans; other animals develop claws.

The nails can be a "window" into the general health of a person. The nails should appear pinkish. When depressed, each nail bed should blanch and upon release should quickly regain its normal pinkish hue. Poor filling of the nail bed by blood suggests cardiovascular problems. A prominent bluish tint indicates poor oxygenation of the circulating blood. Split nails indicate possible nutritional deficiencies. "Clubbing" or thickening at the base of a nail may indicate lung cancer.

Hairs

The *pili* or hairs are present over almost the entire body. They are absent, however, from the palms of the hands and soles of the feet and the flexor surfaces of the digits, and from nipples, glans penis, clitoris, labia minora, and the inner surfaces of the labia majora and prepuce. Hairs are filamentous and keratinized. Derived from the epidermis, they play a very marginal role in temperature regulation but a major role in touch sensation. They reduce friction or facilitate movements between covered surfaces, and they also play a role in the communication of a variety of cultural values.

With exposure to heavy metals such as lead, mercury, and arsenic, the concentration of the metals in hair is greater by a factor of 10 than that in urine or blood. Hair samples are useful in medicolegal investigations and in many clinical diagnostic tests. The hairs of malnourished individuals have a deficiency of zinc. The hair of children with cystic fibrosis may be deficient in calcium and contain excessive amounts of sodium.

Facial hairs are most numerous, numbering 600 per cm^2; the number of hairs on the body is typically found to be about one-tenth that on the face. Hair length is extremely variable, ranging from less than a millimeter for facial hair to potentially a meter or more for the hair on the head. Hair typically varies from 0.005 to about 0.5 mm in diameter. Hairs vary in shape, being curly, coiled, helical, straight, or wavy. They also differ in color, depending on the amount and presence of melanin or phaeomelanin granules. The type of hair varies from place to place on the body and also changes during the aging process. Racial differences are also present: in Caucasians, body hair is longer and coarser, and in Asians, it is shorter and finer.

Body hair is short and thin. In some places (the eyelid skin, for example), the hair does not extend beyond the end of the follicle. The terminal hairs of the scalp, eyelashes and eyebrows, moustache, beard, axilla, pubis, ear canals, and nose tend to be heavily

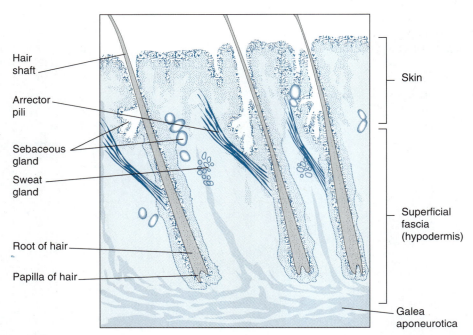

FIGURE 10–16. Scalp. *Section through three hair follicles. Note that the hair follicles extend into the superficial (fatty) fascia (hypodermis) below the dermis of the skin.*

pigmented except in old age. Straight hairs are round in cross-section, and curly hair tends to be flat. Curly hair is also weaker than straight hair.

Hair Structure

Each hair consists of a shaft and a root (Fig. 10–16). It is located in a *follicle*, a tubular invagination of the epidermis. The hair follicle may extend deeply into the dermis or even into the hypodermis. The proximal end of the follicle—the root of the hair—is enlarged and named the *hair bulb*. The hair is continuous with the epithelium at the hair bulb (Fig. 10–17). The hair bulb is indented by a cone-shaped dermal papilla that is richly vascular.

HAIR SHAFT. The hair shaft is composed of dead cells containing keratin strengthened by numerous disulfide bonds cross-linking the protein to produce a filament of high tensile strength. In cross-section, thicker hairs are found to possess three distinct zones: the outer cuticle, middle cortex, and inner medulla. Thinner hairs ordinarily do not possess a medullary layer.

The *cuticle* is formed of apically directed, keratin-filled squames. The *cortex* consists of elongated, tightly packed squames filled with keratin and a variable number of melanosomes or phaeomelanosomes, except in the white hair of older individuals. The dead cells forming mature hair shafts are devoid of nuclei; often, air spaces exist between the squames. The *medulla* is composed of loosely organized dead cells containing keratin, melanosomes, or phaeomelanosomes and often contains vacuoles. The cellular columns of rounded or discoidal cells may not be continuous. The apical ends of uncut hairs usually taper to a point (see Fig. 10–17).

HAIR FOLLICLE. Hair follicles extend for a variable distance through the dermis and, may, in long hair, extend

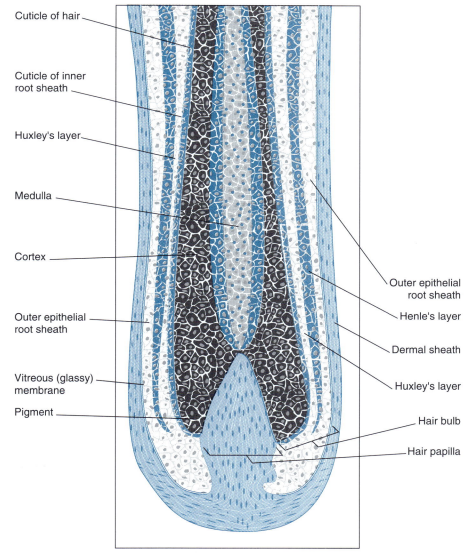

FIGURE 10–17. Hair follicle and connective tissue papilla. *The structural components of the hair and its various sheath coats are identified (see also Fig. 10–18). The connective tissue hair papilla contains essential blood supply, without which the follicle dies. Cells immediately adjacent to the papilla contain a variable number of melanocytes, which contribute pigment to the developing hair.*

into the hypodermis or superficial, fatty fascia. The follicles are arranged obliquely to the surface of the skin. At the proximal end of the hair, the follicle enlarges to encompass the hair bulb. Near the surface of the skin, the follicle opens to accommodate entry of the secretions of sebaceous glands. The area of a follicle between the sebaceous gland duct and the free surface is called the *infundibulum*. The region between the sebaceous gland duct and the attachment of the arrector pili muscle is known as the *isthmus*. That portion from the arrector pili attachment to the proximal end of the follicle (including the hair bulb) is the *inferior segment*. The follicle is embedded in a thick perifollicular dermal coat composed, in part, by type III collagen, elastic fibers, sensory nerve fibers, and blood vessels. The junction between the dermis and follicular epithelium is a periodic acid-Schiff-positive basal lamina known as the *glassy membrane*. Inside the glassy membrane, the outer and inner root sheaths are concentrically arranged around the hair shaft (Fig. 10–18).

The *outer root sheath* is an invagination of the epidermis, is also stratified, and is composed of basal and prickle cell layers that are usually rich in glycogen. Above the inferior segment, its surface cells undergo keratinization, although the granular layer (stratum granulosum) is not present. The follicle forming the inferior segment, which does not keratinize, forms a sheath a few cells thick (see Fig. 10–18).

The *inner root sheath*, found primarily in the region of the inferior segment, has three layers formed basally in the hair bulb. This three-layered sheath moves apically with the growing hair and disintegrates at the level of the isthmus of the follicle. The three zones, from outer to inner, are:

- The stratum pallidum epidermidis or Henle's layer, a single layer of keratinizing cells with pale, flattened nuclei
- The stratum granuliferum epidermidis or Huxley's layer, composed of two layers of partially keratinized cells containing the trichohyalin granules, which are very eosinophilic
- A single layer of flattened squames with pyknotic or atrophic nuclei known as the cuticle of the inner root sheath. This layer faces and loosely connects with the squames of the hair shaft cuticle.

The keratin in the squames and cells of the inner root sheath is relatively soft. The cells of the inner root sheath disintegrate at a level near but not beyond the entrance of the sebaceous ducts.

HAIR BULB. A hair is generated from the base of the hair bulb, which is composed of a germinative layer, with significant mitotic activity, and a keratogenous zone, where the hair cells undergo keratinization. The germinal layer is composed of pluripotent, tightly packed, polygonal cells. These cells move apically and, depending on their location, differentiate in several different ways. The medulla of the hair is formed of cells in the apex of the hair bulb. Away from the apex, successive rings of cells become the cortex and cuticle of the hair and the inner root sheath. The outer root sheath is not derived from the hair bulb. If the hair bulb is injured, the developing hair exhibits abnormalities or is lost.

Among the basal cells of the bulb are melanocytes, with their dendritic processes interspersed between the differentiating cells of the bulb. Hair color is produced by melanosomes (blond, brown, black) or phaeomelanosomes (red), which are synthesized and distributed as described earlier for epidermis. The absence of melanosome synthesis results in white hair.

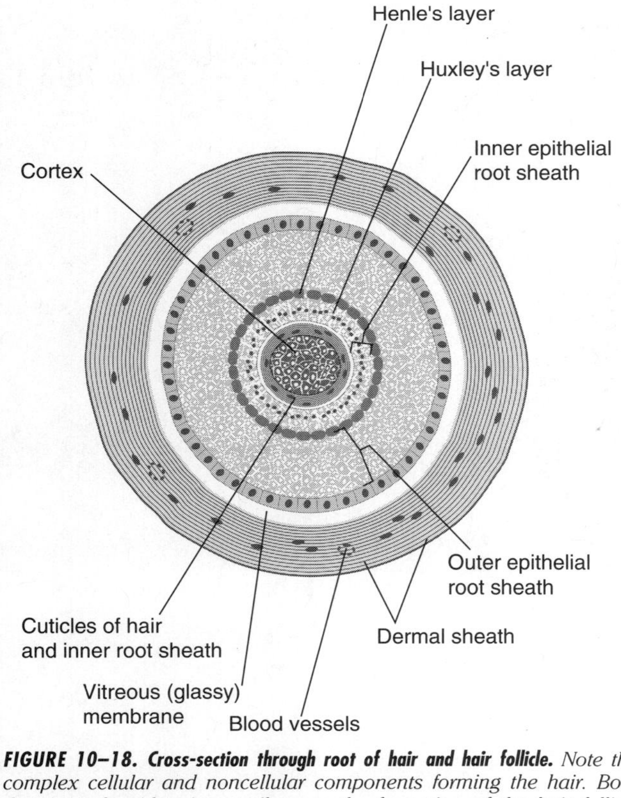

Hair Growth

Growth rates of hair are variable and depend upon hair size and location. They range from 1.5 mm per day for fine (thin) hair and about 2.3 mm per day for coarse (thick) hair, when hair is in its growth phase.

Hair growth and hair loss are cyclical. A phase of rapid hair growth is termed the *anagen*, a phase of growth cessation is called *catagen*, and a resting phase is known as *telogen*. A large scalp hair, for example, may survive for 10 years in the anagenic phase, 3 or 4 weeks in the catagenic phase, and 3 to 4 months in the telogenic phase. When this hair is finally shed, a new hair bulb is formed in the same follicle, and a new hair develops. For smaller hairs, the growth cycle may be as short at 6 to 10 months. Approximately 85% to 90% of scalp hairs in the human may be in the anagenic phase.

FIGURE 10–18. Cross-section through root of hair and hair follicle. *Note the complex cellular and noncellular components forming the hair. Both dermis and epidermis contribute to the formation of the hair follicle (see also Fig. 10–17).*

Development of Hairs

Hair follicles appear as solid, cordlike epidermal ingrowths of the epidermis into the mesenchyme at approximately the third month of gestation. Mesenchyme invades the cords at their base and forms papillae. Sebaceous glands and arrector pili smooth muscle differentiate at about the same time on one side of the developing follicle. At the fifth month, the fetus is covered with pigmented primary hairs known as *lanugo* hairs. These hairs are usually shed before birth and are replaced by secondary hairs, known as *vellus* hairs. Vellus hairs are not found on the scalp, eyebrows, or palpebral margins. Because no new hair follicles are formed after birth, their apparent number and concentration decrease as the body grows.

During puberty, hair growth and hair thickening occur, primarily on the axillae and pubes, in both sexes. In males, hair growth on the face and trunk is under androgen hormonal influence. Androgens also influence the transformation of terminal hairs of the scalp in males to the vellus type and subsequent baldness. The mechanism is still unsettled. In females, estrogen tends to maintain the fine vellus hairs. In the postmenopausal phase of life, with reduced estrogen production, a shift frequently occurs in hair type from vellus to the terminal thicker type. During mid to late pregnancy, hair growth is typically accelerated; this is followed by an extended telogenic phase and hair shedding before the usual growth cycle is restored.

Arrector Pili (Nonstriated Muscle)

Small bundles of smooth or nonstriated muscle originate on the dermal sheath of hair follicles, pass diagonally, and insert onto the connective tissue of the papillary layer of the dermis (see Fig. 10–16). Their orientation is specific; the muscle is directed obliquely and superficially from the same side that the hair follicle itself slopes. When this muscle contracts, the hair follicle is straightened or becomes more vertical, raising the hair itself (piloerection). This movement also elevates the skin around the follicle, which is said to appear like goose flesh or "goose bumps." The elevation of the hair occurs in cold and windy weather and in response to fright, emotional stimuli, and other sympathetic autonomic nervous system stimulation.

The arrector pili muscle is associated with body hair, hair of the upper and lower limbs, but not with facial hair, eyebrows and eyelashes, whiskers, moustache, nasal hair, or hair of the external auditory canal. The muscle also expresses sebaceous gland secretions into the follicle and onto the hair. Piloerection in some animals signals hostility, fear, and other social responses.

Skin Glands

Sebaceous Glands

Sebaceous glands are primarily associated with hair follicles. They are present wherever hair is found. The glands secrete an oily material called *sebum*, which coats hair and the surface of the skin surrounding a hair follicle (Figs. 10–16 and 10–19).

The sebaceous gland is composed of 5 to 20 secretory *acini* that open via a short duct into the apical part of the hair follicle. In certain regions, the duct opens onto the epidermal surface, e.g. the glans penis, glans clitoris, and the corners of the mouth. In addition, glands associated with the nipples, female mammary

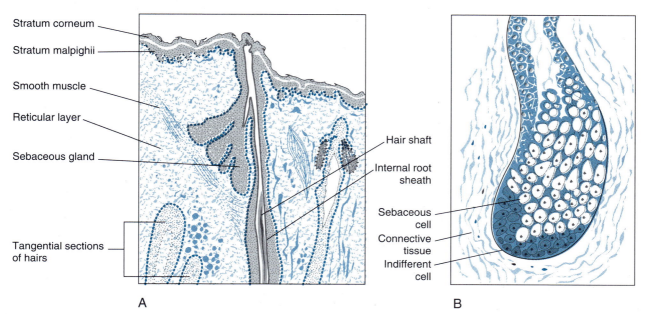

FIGURE 10–19. Hair follicle, sebaceous glands, and arrector pili (smooth) muscle. A, The structural arrangement of a hair follicle of the scalp. Contraction of arrector pili smooth muscles compresses the sebaceous glands, and their secretion is expressed into the follicle surrounding the hair, coating it with sebum. B, Sebaceous gland at high magnification. The arrector pili causes the hair to stand upright and the skin to rise, forming "goose bumps."

areolae (glands of Montgomery), labia minora, margins of the eyelids, inner surface of the prepuce (glands of Tyson), and the tarsal glands (meibomian glands) are all histologically related. These dermal glands have a frequency of about 100 per cm^2 except on the face, scalp, and the midline of the back, where there may be as many as 400 to 900 per cm^2. Sebaceous glands are not found in the hairless (glabrous) skin of the palms and soles.

Microscopically, the glandular acini are inverted in a basal lamina with support of dermal connective tissue and a rich capillary bed. Each acinus is lined with a single layer of polygonal cells. The nuclei are euchromatic and have large nuclei typical of secretory cells. In addition, they possess an agranular reticulum, free polyribosomes, rounded mitochondria, and keratin filaments. The polygonal cells are attached to each other by desmosomes. These basal cells divide and force the more superficial cells toward the center of the acini, where they complete their maturation into large, lipid-filled cells with pyknotic nuclei. These cells disintegrate, and the fatty cellular debris fills the duct of the gland. This form of secretion, which involves the destruction of the entire cell, is known as *holocrine secretion*.

The cellular debris passes into the hair follicle through a duct lined with stratified squamous epithelium or, less commonly, is secreted directly onto the surface of the stratified squamous epithelium. The cellular debris, known as *sebum*, is a complex mixture of every cellular component. The fatty component, however, is over 50% diglycerides and triglycerides, with some wax esters, squalene, cholesterol esters, and cholesterol. Bacterial action converts some glycerides to free fatty acids as the cellular debris is moved through the duct. The function of sebum is only incompletely understood, but it coats the hair and skin with oil and contributes to individualistic body odor.

DEVELOPMENT OF SEBACEOUS GLANDS. Sebaceous glands arise by invaginations of the epidermis between the thirteenth and fifteenth weeks of gestation. The glands are well developed at birth but regress until puberty. Under the influence of androgens, growth hormone from the anterior pituitary (adenohypophysis), and perhaps other influences, the glands enlarge at puberty and secretory activity increases. Excessive secretion, particularly around puberty, may plug hair follicles, cause damage and inflammation of the area, and result in acne, which is common at this age. Secretory activity does not appear to be under nervous control.

Sweat Glands

The sweat or sudorific glands can be divided into two types: eccrine glands, which are located almost universally over the skin, and apocrine glands, which are more highly restricted. Ceruminous glands of the external ear canal and the ciliary glands of the eyelids are modified sweat glands (see Figs. 10–10 and 10–21).

Eccrine Sweat Glands

A long unbranched tubular gland, an eccrine sweat gland has a coiled body usually larger in diameter than the long tubular duct. The coiled secretory portion lies deep in the dermis or upper hypodermis (see Figs. 10–16, 10–20, and 10–21). The walls of the duct join the epidermal pegs or papillae, and the lumen of the duct passes between the keratinocytes. The passage through the epidermis is usually accomplished in a tightly twisting spiral. In thick hairless (glabrous) skin, the rounded apertures of many eccrine sweat glands form a regular pattern along the center of the friction ridges, which account for the unique fingerprint patterns so useful for forensic purposes, as previously mentioned.

Eccrine sweat glands are absent from the very thin skin of the tympanic membrane, lips, nail beds, nipples, inner preputial surfaces, labia minoras, glans penis, and glans clitoris. The frequency elsewhere is about 80 to 600 per cm^2. The glands are most common on the plantar surfaces of the feet, palmar surfaces of the hands and digits, and the face. They are fewest on the limbs, with the exceptions already mentioned.

The eccrine duct cells form two layers. They are basophilic, and the inner cell has numerous microvilli projecting into the duct lumen. Duct cells become keratinized in the same manner as described for epidermal keratinocytes.

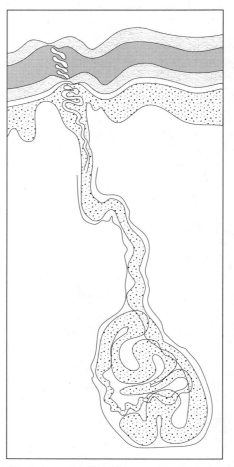

FIGURE 10–20. Eccrine sweat gland. *This drawing emphasizes the coiled nature of the secretory part of the typical sweat gland of skin, located in the superficial fatty fascia below the skin. The secretory product is carried to the skin surface by a single duct that traverses an epidermal peg and all of the layers of the epithelium.*

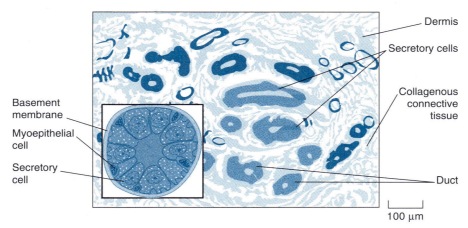

FIGURE 10–21. Eccrine sweat gland. *The secretory coils of an eccrine sweat gland are seen in this section. The secretory portion of the gland is surrounded by myoepithelial cells. The ducts lack this structural component. Sweat glands may be found in the deeper part of the dermis and in the underlying superficial (fatty) fascia.*

Microscopically, an eccrine sweat gland is surrounded by a fibrous dermal sheath and a basal lamina. The secretory part of the gland is composed of pseudostratified epithelium around a large lumen. Three cell types are recognized:

- So-called clear cells (the most common of the secretory cells)
- Dark mucoid-secreting cells
- Myoepithelial cells

CLEAR CELLS. Clear cells are roughly pyramidal, with their bases touching the basal lamina and the apices not reaching the lumen of the gland. The apices form small canaliculi that are continuous with the lumen of the gland. The apices of the cells bear microvilli, which are numerous and irregular in size. The bases of clear cells are highly infolded where they make contact with the basal lamina. The cytoplasm has a granular endoplasmic reticulum, a small Golgi apparatus, and many mitochondria; they also contain abundant glycogen. The nucleus is round and partially euchromatic.

DARK CELLS. Dark cells are also pyramidal, but their apices face the basal lamina and their broad surfaces face the lumen of the gland. The cytoplasm has the organelles of a typical secretory cell. Dense "carbohydrate-rich" secretory vacuoles are secreted into the lumen of the gland.

MYOEPITHELIAL CELLS (BASKET CELLS). Small muscle–like cells of ectodermal and endodermal origin, myoepithelial cells are numerous. They lie irregularly between the basal processes of the other two cell types and the basal lamina (Figs. 10–21 and 10–23). The cells receive a rich cholinergic sympathetic nerve supply. Stimulation of the myoepithelium by the sympathetic nerves causes an immediate secretory response.

ECCRINE GLAND SECRETION. The secretion of sweat glands is clear, odorless, and hypotonic to extracellular fluid. It contains sodium and chloride, bicarbonate, calcium, urea, lactate, amino acids, immunoglobulins, and other proteins in small amounts. The secretion is similar to extracellular fluid, but as it passes through the excretory duct, sodium, chloride, and water are reabsorbed by

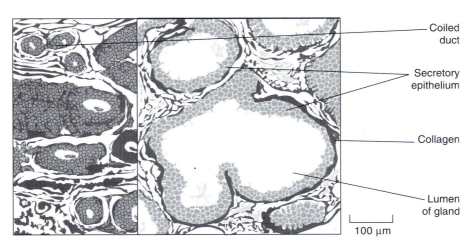

FIGURE 10–22. Axillary sweat gland. *(Redrawn from a section of an axillary apocrine sweat gland.) Characterized by wide lumens and thick-walled ducts, apocrine sweat glands differ significantly from the more numerous and smaller eccrine glands of the skin and hypodermis. These glands are similar in structure to the ceruminous (wax) glands of the external auditory canal of the ear.*

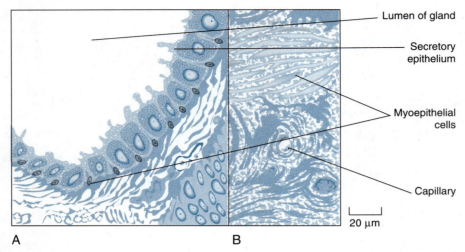

FIGURE 10–23. Apocrine sweat gland cells and myoepithelial cells. *The secretory epithelium is characterized by large buds extending from the secretory cells. The secretion is viscous and odorless but is readily degraded by bacteria to produce an unpleasant odor. The extrusion of the viscous product of these sweat glands is facilitated by myoepithelial cells that surround the glandular part of the gland. A, Myoepithelial cells in cross-section. B, Myoepithelial cells in longitudinal section.*

the duct cells. The adrenal hormone aldosterone increases the duct cell activity in reabsorption of ions.

Sweat gland secretion is stimulated by increased temperature; however, in some regions, cholinergic sympathetic innervation facilitates this facet of the emotional response. Affected areas are the hands, face, and axillae, in particular.

Apocrine Sweat Glands

Because of their especially large lumina, apocrine sweat glands look like enlarged eccrine sweat glands, but they secrete their product into the apical ends of hair follicles (Figs. 10–22 and 10–23). They extend into the dermis and hypodermis and are found in specific locations. Apocrine sweat glands are prominent in the axillae, perianal region, areolae, scrotum, labia minora, and mons pubis. The ceruminous glands of the external ear canal and the ciliary glands of the palpebral margins (so-called glands of Moll) are modified apocrine sweat glands. Although the secretion of each is very different, all are best considered specialized subtypes.

Apocrine glands superficially resemble eccrine glands, but the secretory region may be 2 mm wide and greatly distended with secretory product. The walls of the secretory part of the gland anastomose, unlike in eccrine glands. The walls are lined by a single layer of cuboidal or columnar epithelium. The nuclei are round and euchromatic. The free surface of the secretory cells have irregular and, frequently, globular projections containing secretory product. The base of secretory cells lies on a parallel array of contractile myoepithelial cells that are longitudinally arranged with respect to the tubular system (see Fig. 10–23). The myoepithelial cells, together with the whole secretory system, are surrounded by a basal lamina. Outside, the gland is supported by a dermal connective tissue capsule and a rich capillary bed.

The secretory cells of the apocrine gland have the typical array of organelles: granular and agranular endoplasmic reticula, Golgi complex, and secretory vacuoles varying in size and number. The types of secretion are not settled, but they include *merocine* secretion (of granules), *apocrine* secretion (by which large globules of cytoplasm are lost), and possibly *holocrine* secretion (disintegration of the entire secretory cell).

The secretions of these glands are rich in protein and cellular debris that is initially odorless. Rapid bacterial decomposition generates odorous, disagreeable compounds, including short-chain fatty acids.

Apocrine glands develop at about the same time as eccrine glands. Although abundant initially, by 5 months of gestation they progressively disappear, except in their future adult locations. Apocrine glands enlarge and become actively secretory at puberty.

CHAPTER ELEVEN

The Digestive System

Oral Cavity and Pharynx 178
   Mouth 178
   Pharynx 182
   Teeth 182

Digestive Tube (Organizational Plan) 188
   Esophagus 189
   Stomach 190
   Small Intestine 195
   Large Intestine 199
   Peritoneum 202
   Blood Supply to the Digestive Tract 202
   Lymphatics of the Digestive Tract 203

Salivary Glands 203
   Parotid Gland 203
   Submandibular (Submaxillary) Gland 204
   Sublingual Gland 205
   Ductal System 205

Pancreas 206

Liver 207
   Liver Parenchyma 207
   Liver Blood Supply 208
   Bile Ducts 210
   Liver Function 210

Gallbladder 211

The digestive tube is structurally and functionally differentiated in its several continuous parts. The oral cavity contains the cutting and grinding instruments (teeth) and adds glandular secretions that moisten the food and begin enzymatic digestion. The tongue mixes and moves the food and propels the "prepared" food into the pharynx, from which the bolus is automatically transported by the esophagus to the stomach. The stomach produces hydrochloric acid and acid-dependent enzymes, which further break down the foods to carbohydrates, small proteins, and fatty acids. When the food is sufficiently prepared, it is released into the small intestine (duodenum), and the acid is neutralized by alkaline secretions that activate pancreatic enzymes, which continue the digestive process. Bile secreted by the liver emulsifies fatty acids to small droplets for absorption. The duodenum moves the digested food to the jejunum, where the absorption of specific digested products occurs across the columnar epithelium into the extracellular space. Subsequently, these products are transported to the liver for processing, synthesis, and detoxification, after which the liver releases synthesized products into the blood for general distribution. The undigested materials are propelled into the ileum, where the process of water reabsorption into the blood begins. Resorption continues in the large intestine, where significant amounts of mucus are added. The fecal material is then expelled from the distal end of the digestive tube.

The entire gastrointestinal tract has a number of structural characteristics in common. Although the digestive tube varies regionally in length, size, and shape, it is composed of four primary layers: mucosa, submucosa, muscularis externa, and adventitia (or serosa, if the part of the digestive tube is enveloped in a mesentery) (Fig. 11–1).

The *mucosa* is composed of an epithelium consisting of columnar cells and unicellular glands of various kinds, which are discussed subsequently. The lamina propria, the next layer of the mucosa, is formed of loose connective tissue containing blood and lymphatic vessels, smooth muscle bundles, glands, numerous lymphoid and white blood cells, and, sometimes, lymphoid tissue. The muscularis mucosae usually consists of a thin inner layer of circularly arranged, and an outer layer of longitudinally arranged, smooth muscle fibers that separate the mucosa from the submucosa. The mucosa is frequently referred to as the *mucous membrane*.

The *submucosa* is also formed of loose connective tissue containing blood and lymphatic vessels, glands, and lymphoid cells and tissue. In addition, Meissner's submucosal nerve plexus—a part of the autonomic nervous system—which is composed of nerve cells and fibers, is also present.

The *muscularis externa* consists of smooth muscle organized in two layers. The inner layer is basically circularly arranged but with a slightly oblique twist; the outer layer is primarily longitudinally arranged but also with a slightly oblique twist. This organization facilitates the distal movement of ingested food. Located between the two muscle layers is Auerbach's myenteric plexus of nerve cells and fibers, which is also part of the autonomic nervous system.

The outermost layer is the *adventitia* or serosa. If the digestive tube is not contained in a mesentery, the outer layer is named *adventitia*; it is composed of loose connective tissue containing blood and lymph vessels, and lymphoid and adipose tissue. This part of the tube is considered retroperitoneal. If carried in a mesentery, the tube has, in addition to those components already mentioned, a mesothelial outer cell layer belonging to the visceral peritoneum. The part of the digestive tube possessing a mesothelial cell layer is said to possess a *serosa*, not an adventitia, and it is, by definition, intraperitoneal (see Fig. 11–1).

ORAL CAVITY AND PHARYNX

Unlike the rest of the digestive tube, the origins of the tube are firmly fastened to bone, so that in the mouth, the muscle layer has no uniform arrangement.

Mouth

The mouth is lined by stratified squamous nonkeratinized epithelium.

Lips and Cheeks

The lips are composed of three parts: a cutaneous area, a "red area," and oral mucosa. The *cutaneous area* is typical skin, containing hairs as well as sebaceous and sweat glands. The outer surface of the lips is stratified squamous keratinized epithelium (the epithelium of skin). In the *red area*, the superficial cells of the stratified squamous epithelium contain eleiden, render-

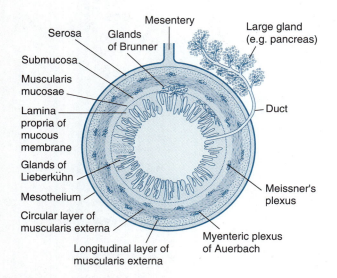

FIGURE 11–1. *Diagram of the generalized structural plan of the intestinal tract. Note the various features of the digestive tube.*

ing them translucent. The epithelium is deeply indented by vascular papillae, and the blood provides the red color. Glands are usually absent from the red area, accounting for the constant licking of the lips by the tongue to prevent excessive dryness. The red area is continuous with the outer, typical skin and the inner, mucous membrane of the lips (Figs. 11–2 and 11–3).

The inner epithelial surface of the lips and cheeks is composed of the stratified squamous nonkeratinizing type. The blood capillary–containing papillae in the connective tissue are not as deep as those in the red area.

The lamina propria beneath the epithelium is connected to underlying muscle by the submucosa. The muscles involved are the orbicularis oris in the lips and the buccinator in the cheeks. The thick submucosal connective tissue fibers are so organized as to prevent folds from forming, to reduce the chance of the cheek's being bitten during mastication.

Glands of the mucous type as well as mixed serous and mucous types are present in the submucosa of the lips and cheeks. The glands may even invade the buccinator muscles.

Gums

The gums have a stratified squamous epithelium that is variably keratinized (cornified) and usually possesses a stratum granulosum. Like the lips, the vascular papillae are long and deeply indented, giving the healthy gum a pinkish color. The lamina propria is composed of coarsely interwoven collagenous fibers bound to the periosteum of alveolar processes. The lamina propria is also firmly attached to gingival fibers of the periodontal membrane. The gums do not possess a submucosa or any glands.

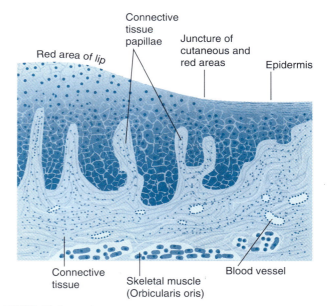

FIGURE 11–3. *Lip. Transverse section of the lip, showing the junction of the cutaneous region, and the red area (vermilion border).*

Hard Palate

The hard palate is lined by an epithelium, similar to that of the gums, that has a stratum corneum and a stratum granulosum. It, too, has long vascular papillae that indent the epithelium and give it a pink color.

The hard palate has a submucosa except in the area adjacent to the gums and in the midline. The submucosa is composed of coarse collagenous bundles that run vertically, binding the lamina propria to the periosteum of the hard palate. In the anterior part of the hard palate, fat is present in significant amounts in the submucosa, the so-called fatty zone; in the posterior two thirds, many mucous glands are present, the so-called glandular zone. In a narrow area on either side of the midline raphe, glands are absent.

Soft Palate

The soft palate and uvula are covered on their oral surface by a nonkeratinized stratified squamous epithelium. This epithelium extends for a variable distance onto the pharyngeal surface, where it meets the pseudostratified ciliated epithelium of that region. The submucosa is composed of loose connective tissue and contains numerous glands; these are mucous type on the oral side and mixed types (mucous and serous) on the upper or respiratory side. Several small muscles contribute to the formation of the soft palate and uvula.

The floor of the mouth is lined with a nonkeratinized stratified squamous epithelium except for the tongue. The submucosa is composed of loose connective tissue and contains the sublingual glands.

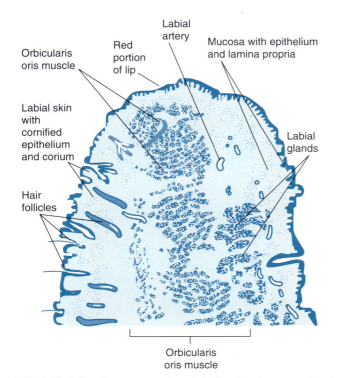

FIGURE 11–2. *Lip. Transverse section of the lip, showing external and mucosal surfaces.*

Tongue

Most of the tongue is striated muscle, particularly the anterior two thirds. The muscle fibers course variously in the longitudinal, transverse, and vertical planes, and they are interlaced. The arrangement of the muscle bundles gives the tongue great mobility and control of food during the chewing phase of eating. In the posterior third of the tongue, the lingual tonsils form somewhat large aggregations (Fig. 11–4).

The inferior surface of the tongue is covered by nonkeratinized squamous epithelium. Here, the lamina propria is thin and tightly bound to the underlying muscle.

The dorsal surface of the tongue is divided into two unequal parts; an anterior two thirds are separated from the posterior third by a chevron-shaped row of circumvallate papillae. The two regions are structurally different. The anterior part contains numerous lingual papillae, small organs with a central core of connective tissue and a covering layer of stratified squamous epithelium. The lingual papillae are described according to their shape as filiform, fungiform, or circumvallate (Fig. 11–5). The filiform papillae are the most numerous and are evenly spread over the dorsal surface of the tongue. Each papilla contains a connective tissue core and a keratinized stratified squamous epithelium, which forms one or more secondary projections.

The fungiform papillae resemble mushrooms in section, are relatively few in number, and are distributed among the filiform papillae. The apex of a fungiform papilla is rounded and broader than the base. It is covered by nonkeratinized epithelium and possesses a connective tissue core. The papillae of the core indent the epithelium and are highly vascular and contain sensory nerves. The fungiform papillae appear red because of their vascularity and the thinness of the epithe-

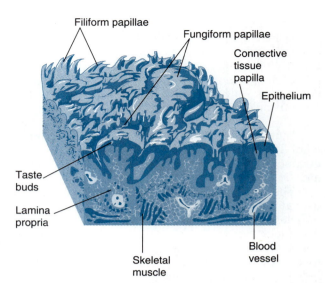

FIGURE 11–5. *Fungiform and filiform papillae. Note surface and sectional appearance of tongue.*

lium. The epithelium contains the organs of taste, so-called taste buds (Figs. 11–5 to 11–7).

Circumvallate papillae are large, are usually nine to ten in number, and are placed in a chevron or V-shaped row with the point of the chevron directed posteriorly. The papillae resemble fungiform papillae, but they are larger and are surrounded by a trench and a wall, hence their name (Figs. 11–8 and 11–9). These vallate or circumvallate papillae extend above their surrounding wall. A connective tissue core fills the papillae, except at their sides. The core contains blood vessels and many nerve fibers. Circumvallate papillae, the trench, and the wall are covered by nonkeratinized stratified squamous epithelium. In the epithelium of the walls of the papillae, and occasionally in the walls of the trench, the small oral taste buds are found. Along the posterolateral border of the tongue, folds of the mucous membrane, referred to as foliate papillae, may also contain taste buds. These papillae are not highly developed in humans (Fig. 11–10).

The dorsal part of the posterior surface of the tongue is without papillae, rather possessing mucosal ridges and lingual tonsils. The lingual tonsils appear as

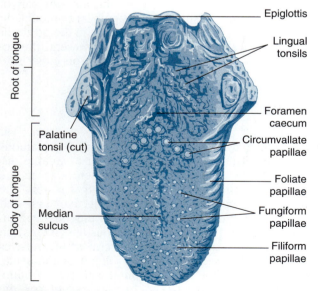

FIGURE 11–4. *Tongue. Diagram of the surface features of the dorsum of the human tongue, showing topographic distribution of the various lingual papillae.*

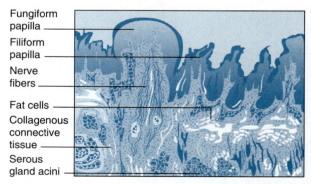

FIGURE 11–6. *Filiform and fungiform lingual papillae. Sagittal section of the tongue, showing relationship of papillae to deeper structures.*

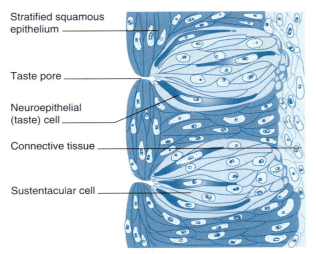

FIGURE 11–7. Taste buds. Longitudinal sections of taste buds, illustrating cellular detail.

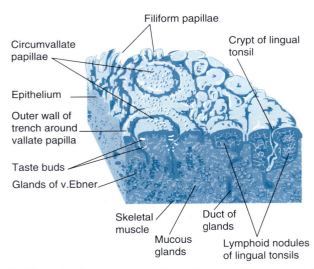

FIGURE 11–8. Circumvallate papillae. These papillae occur at the juncture of the dorsum and the root of the tongue. They contain numerous taste buds.

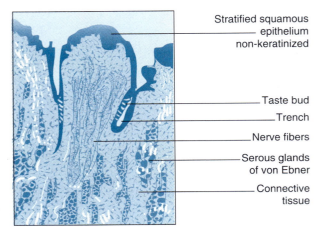

FIGURE 11–9. Detail of circumvallate papilla in longitudinal section. Note taste buds, trench (moat), and the serous glands of von Ebner.

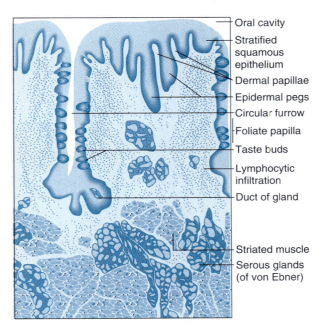

FIGURE 11–10. Detail of adjacent foliate papillae, in longitudinal section. These papillae are abundant in some animals but not in humans.

slight elevations or eminences owing to the underlying lymphoid nodules. Each eminence has a centrally placed pit or crypt. The covering and surrounding epithelium is normally highly infiltrated with lymphocytes and other immune cell types, plasma cells, and white blood cells.

Glands of the Tongue

The glands of the tongue can be separated into three types. A paired gland, composed of mixed mucous and serous secretory elements, is located in the anterior part of the tongue near its apex. These are the so-called glands of Nuhn. Embedded in muscle, they are closer to the ventral than the dorsal surface and their ducts open onto the ventral surface. Serous glands found in the region of the vallate papillae are known as the glands of von Ebner. These glands intrude into and between the muscle bundles, and their ducts open into the trenches of the vallate papillae.

Mucous glands are the most numerous type, and they are found in the posterior third of the tongue but extend far enough forward to intermingle with the serous glands. Their ducts open into the crypts of the lingual tonsils and between the tonsils.

No submucosa can be distinguished on the dorsum of the tongue.

Nerve Supply to Mouth and Tongue

The skeletal (striated) muscle of the lips and cheeks is supplied by the cranial nerve (CN) VII (facial nerve) and that of the tongue by CN XII (hypoglossal). The fibers carrying general sensation are in the lingual branch of CN V (trigeminal) and CN IX (glossopharyngeal). The nerve fibers carrying the special sense of taste are from the CN VII (facial) via the chorda tympani and from CN IX (glossopharyngeal).

Pharynx

The pharynx extends from the base of the skull to about the level of the cricoid cartilage, where it joins the esophagus. The pharyngeal cavity is also continuous with the cavities of the nose, mouth, and larynx and with the lumen of the esophagus. The eustachian or auditory tubes also open into the pharynx superiorly and laterally. The cavity of the pharynx is incompletely divided by the soft palate and uvula into two regions, an upper nasal part and a lower oral and laryngeal part.

The pharyngeal wall consists of three layers: mucosa, muscularis, and fibrosa. The only region of the pharynx having a submucosa is located near its junction with the esophagus.

The epithelium lining the pharynx varies. The epithelium lining the nasopharynx is ciliated pseudostratified columnar; near the oropharynx, where the soft palate and uvula come in contact with the posterior wall, the epithelium changes to the stratified squamous variety. The lamina propria of the pharynx is a strong fibroelastic layer, below which a well-developed elastic fiber layer is oriented longitudinally. Elastic fibers intrude between the skeletal muscle bundles and bind the lamina propria to muscularis. The muscle of the pharynx is skeletal and irregularly arranged in three so-called constrictor muscles. The outermost layer, a fibroelastic sheath of varying strength, binds the pharynx to adjacent structures.

The lymphoid tissue in the nasopharynx is normally abundant and is distributed both diffusely and in aggregations. The pharyngeal tonsils, when enlarged, become known as adenoids. Mixed glands (mucous and serous) are found, and they penetrate deeply into the muscular layer. In the oral and laryngeal pharynx, scattered nodules of lymphoid tissue are commonly seen. Glands in this region are uncommon but are of the mucous type.

Teeth

A tooth has three structural divisions: crown, root, and neck (cervix). The *anatomic crown* is that part of the tooth that is covered with enamel. The *root* has an outer layer of cementum. The *neck* or *cervix* is located at the junction of the crown and root (Fig. 11–11).

The *clinical crown* is the part of the tooth that is visible when the tooth is in situ. In early life, the gums cover part of the enamel, so the clinical crown is only a portion of the anatomic crown. As the aging process proceeds, the gums recede, and the clinical crown eventually includes all of the anatomic crown, the neck, and perhaps even a part of the anatomic root.

The root of the tooth is embedded in a bony cavity (alveolus or tooth socket) in the alveolar part of the maxilla and mandible. It is firmly attached to the bony wall of the alveolus by the connective tissue periodontal membrane.

The tooth is composed structurally of four parts: enamel, dentin, cementum, and pulp (see Fig. 11–11).

Enamel

Enamel is the hardest material in the body. It is composed (by weight) primarily of inorganic salts (90–97%), most significantly (about 90%) calcium phosphate, but by volume, the organic part is nearly as great as the inorganic part. Enamel is a brittle substance, but because of its internal structural organization and the underlying dentin, it survives normal occlusal stress. Enamel appears to be thickest on the cusps of permanent bicuspids and molars.

Enamel exists in the form of rods or prisms and interprismatic substance. Enamel prisms are very elongated, and they extend from the dentino-enamel juncture to the surface of the anatomic crown. They are oval, round, or hexagonal. The enamel prism (or rod) has a longitudinal groove on one side, into which an adjacent prism is fitted. From the shape of the crown, one can understand that the inner surface of the crown is less than the outer surface. As a result, the size of the prism increases as it extends from the dentinal to the outer free surface. Prisms average about 4 μm in diameter. Each prism or rod is composed of minute crystals of inorganic material, except for the rod sheath. The rod sheath contains more organic matter than most of the rod. Between prisms or rods, a small amount of calcified organic material known as *interrod substance* is found.

Enamel prisms or rods are striated transversely, and the striations occur regularly every 4 μm. It is believed that the striations occur because of a cyclic growth pattern during development. In addition, another striation pattern, variably spaced but continuous lines in the enamel, called *incremental lines of Retzius*, are found. Coronal sections of the crown of a tooth reveal these lines as concentric circles; in longitudinal sections, they appear as arches over the apex of the dentin. Incremental lines are formed because variations occur in the rate of enamel deposition during development.

Dentin

Dentin forms the bulk of the tooth, provides its main strength, and is elastic, hard, and yellowish. Chemically it contains more mineral salts (69%) than bone (46%) but less than that found in enamel (96%). Structurally, dentin resembles bone because it is composed of a mineralized, calcified ground substance deposited on collagenous fibers. It differs from bone, in that it contains no dentin cells (odontoblasts) but rather only the processes of odontoblasts whose cell bodies lie adjacent to the dentin in the pulp cavity (see Fig. 11–11).

In development, dentin deposition starts at the basement membrane separating the future enamel-forming cells (ameloblasts) and the mesodermal cells that will form dentin (odontoblasts). From this point, dentin is laid down centrally and apically in successive

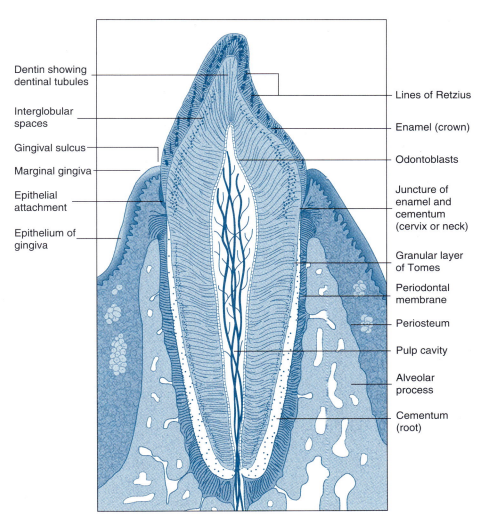

FIGURE 11-11. Tooth. Longitudinal section of a tooth (incisor) in situ. Note the various components of the tooth and supporting structures.

layers. A layer of odontoblasts is responsible for the deposition of dentin. The odontoblasts forming the layer of cells on the surface of the dentin are unlike osteoblasts, because the odontoblasts do not become embedded, but continue to line the surface as the layers of dentin are deposited. Each odontoblast, however, has branching processes that begin at the dentino-enamel or dentino-cementum junction. The cellular processes lengthen as the dentin is laid down, and they become embedded. Each process or dentinal fiber is contained within a minute canal, the so-called dentinal tubule. Because the inner part of the wall of a tubule stains more deeply than the remainder of the dentin, it is known as Neumann's sheath. In addition, parallel incremental growth lines (contour lines of Owen or incremental lines of von Ebner) result from the deposition of dentin in successive lamellar-like layers. In cross-sections of a tooth, they look like the annular rings of a tree.

The mineral salts are in the form of crystals. They have two types of organization: the long axes of the crystals are parallel to the collagenous fibers, and the crystals have a globular arrangement radiating from a center. The crystals in all cases lie in the matrix between collagenous fibers; this is also the case in bone.

Two regions of the dentin are consistently deficient in organic material. One of these regions is the root of the tooth near the dentino-cementum junction. The second is those interglobular areas found primarily in the crown but also in the root. Each of these areas has a granular appearance, the so-called granular layer of Tomes. Each of the areas is irregular in shape, and the interglobular areas are larger than the areas forming the granular layer of Tomes.

Odontoblastic processes describe a wavy course; they branch and may contact processes of other odontoblasts.

Dentin, unlike enamel, normally continues to be formed throughout life. The secondary dentin formed in later life, however, has dentinal tubules that are more irregularly wavy and are less numerous. The observed differences in form are thought to be due to functional stresses, which stimulate dentin formation in older people. More severe stimuli, caused by caries or functional erosion, contribute to a localized irregularly arranged dentin (known as *irregular dentin*). The continued deposition of dentin in response to destructive stimuli serves an important protective function.

Cementum

Cementum encases the dentin of the root and is another hard, bonelike substance. It is typically lighter than dentin but darker than enamel. Its chemical composition is actually quite similar to that of bone. Cementum may be free of cells (acellular cementum) or may contain cells similar to osteocytes (cellular cementum). Acellular cementum is usually adjacent to dentin except at the apex of the root. Cementum, like dentin, continues to be formed throughout life. The additional layers are irregular in thickness and may be either cellular or acellular. Exostoses of cementum are not uncommon. Connective tissue fibers extending from within the cementum into the adjacent tissue, known as Sharpey's fibers, make cementum similar to bone.

Cementum is a protective covering for dentin and is the bonding substance between dentin and the periodontal membrane. In the normal shifting teeth, cementum is less likely to be absorbed than the alveolar bone of the tooth socket (see Fig. 11-11).

Periodontal Membrane

The periodontal membrane is a layer of connective tissue found between the tooth root and the alveolus (see Fig. 11-11). It attaches the tooth to the wall of the alveolus, free margin of the gingiva, and the more superficial parts of the roots of neighboring teeth. In addition, some of its fibers continue into the cementum and into the alveolar bone, thereby anchoring the tooth to bone. The connective tissue fibers course in irregular directions, maintaining the tooth in its position; hence, the periodontal membrane serves as a suspensory ligament but allows physiologic movement of the tooth without structural alterations at the root or socket.

The periodontal (membrane) connective tissue contains fibroblasts, osteoblasts, and cementoblasts. There are also cells that are remnants of Hertwig's root sheath, a derivative of the enamel organ. In addition, blood vessels and nerve fibers are present.

The density and strength of a periodontal membrane vary with the stress placed upon it. In the absence of stress, the membrane weakens by thinning, a change associated with a decrease in alveolar bone.

Pulp and Pulp Cavity

The shape of the pulp cavity conforms to the shape of the tooth itself. It consists of a pulp chamber, which lies in the center of the crown and adjacent part of the root, and the pulp canal(s). The pulp cavity is relatively larger in the teeth of younger individuals, because dentin is deposited continuously throughout life. A pulp canal opens into the periodontal tissue by one or more foramina at or near the apex of the root (see Fig. 11-11).

The pulp filling the pulp cavity contains connective tissue, a variety of wandering cells, nerve fibers, and blood and lymph vessels. A layer of odontoblasts lines the pulp chamber. Each odontoblast has a peripherally directed process (Tomes's fiber) that extends into the periphery of the dentin. The bodies of the odontoblasts are variable in height, being columnar in the pulp cavity and becoming more cuboidal as they approach the apex. These cells have "intercellular bridges" or contacts and, at their dentinal ends, terminal bars or junctional complexes. The pulp tissues contain fibroblasts and macrophages, and the connective tissue consists of reticular and collagenous fibers. Reticular fibers are particularly abundant near the odontoblasts.

The pulp is highly vascular, usually having one arteriole, an extensive capillary bed, and two or three venules. The pulp has both myelinated and nonmyelinated nerve fibers serving general sensory and autonomic functions.

Attachment of Gingiva to Teeth

The gums are joined to the teeth by the attachment of the subepithelial connective tissue to the cementum and by the attachment of the gingival epithelium to the tooth (so-called epithelial attachment) (see Fig. 11-11).

With advancing age, an increasing proportion of the tooth becomes exposed owing to the normal recession of the gums. The relative size of the clinical crown increases. The epithelial attachment continually but slowly changes its site on the tooth. The epithelium grows apically as the gum line changes its position. In younger individuals, the attachment is on the enamel; with greater exposure of the crown, it moves onto the cementum; and in older individuals, the epithelium may be fully attached to cementum alone.

Tooth Development

Enamel is derived from the ectoderm. Dentin, cementum, and all the components of the pulp, except the nerve fibers, arise from mesoderm.

The first recognizable sign of tooth development in humans occurs during the sixth and seventh weeks of intrauterine life. At this time, the embryo is slightly over 1 cm in length. An epithelial ingrowth occurs into the underlying mesenchyme, along the future dental arch of each jaw. The epithelial ingrowth forms the dental lamina. In close association with the dental lamina, a continuous epithelial ingrowth is formed, the labiogingival lamina, into which a groove and a deep division will form. This lamina will divide the dental arch from the lip and cheeks. The dental lamina is initially of uniform thickness, but proliferations form at intervals on its outer side, close to the oral epithelium. These proliferations are the primordial enamel organs of deciduous teeth. They develop into cup-shaped and, later, bell-shaped structures (Fig. 11-12). Both within and beneath the concavity of the enamel organ, the dental papillae form from the proliferation and condensation of the mesenchyme; this is the primordium of the pulp. The peripheral cells of the dental papilla, adjacent to enamel organ, become the odontoblasts.

Later in development, the primordia of the enamel organs of the permanent teeth are formed. Each primor-

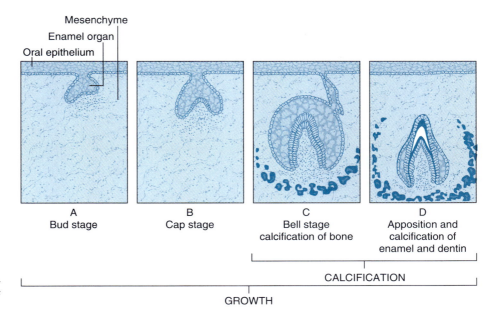

FIGURE 11-12. Human tooth development (1). Note the progressive stages in fetal tooth development.

dium arises as an inner or lingual growth from the dental lamina at a point coexistent with the enamel organ of a deciduous or milk tooth. As the dental arch lengthens, the dental lamina also grows dorsally, and from this dorsal extension arise the primordia of the enamel organs of the molars. It is not until the fourth or fifth year that the primordium of the last molar (wisdom tooth) is formed (Fig. 11-13).

The developmental processes of permanent and deciduous teeth are similar. During the development of an enamel organ, the dental lamina, which joined the enamel organ to the oral epithelium, disintegrates. Thus, the developing tooth becomes separated from the oral epithelium. The mesenchyme surrounding the enamel organ and the dental papillae play a role in tooth development. The mesenchyme thickens and forms a capsule-like structure named the *dental sac* or *dental follicle*. The segment of the dental sac adjacent to the papillae has the position of the future periodontal membrane. From the dental sac, cells associated with

FIGURE 11-13. Human tooth development (2). Section through the maxilla and mandible of a 50-mm CR (crown–rump) (10-week) human embryo. Note the positions of the enamel organs and dental papillae of the developing teeth.

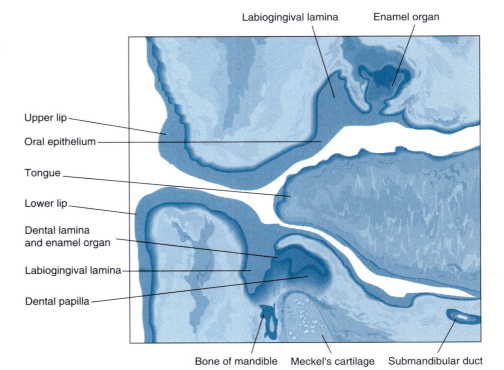

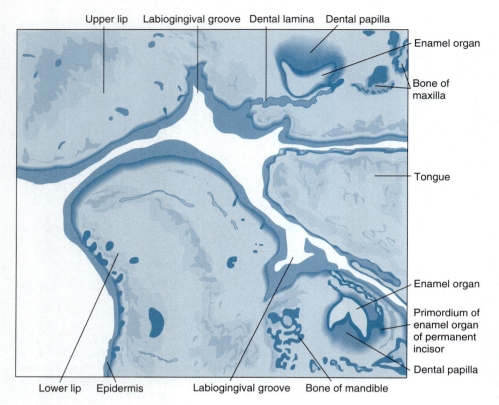

FIGURE 11–14. Human tooth development (3). Section through the maxilla and mandible of a 86-mm CR (3-month) human fetus. Note the primordia of both deciduous and permanent incisors.

the deposition of cementum arise. The peripheral part of the dental sac (follicle) serves as the periosteum of the bony wall of the future alveolus (Fig. 11–14).

All teeth are not at the same degree of development at any one time. The teeth located anteriorly are usually the most advanced in development. In any particular tooth, the future occlusal area develops more rapidly than more apically situated regions. The crown is fully formed at the time of eruption, but the root may still be in the process of development (Fig. 11–15).

Formation of Dentin

Dentin is the first hard material to be formed in a developing tooth. Several changes occur in the dental papilla before dentin is deposited. Reticular fibers appear in the papilla, especially in the peripheral zone adjacent to the enamel organ. The more peripheral of these reticular fibers (Korff's fibers) join the delicate basement membrane, which separates the papilla from the enamel organ. The thickened membrane thus formed (by the fusion of reticular fibers and basement membrane) is the *membrana preformativa*. The mesenchymal cells closest to this membrane enlarge and form a continuous layer of columnar cells, the odontoblasts. The Korff's fibers, which lie between the odontoblasts, become collagenous and change their direction so that they lie parallel to the membrana preformativa. A gel-like ground substance is deposited around these collagenous fibers. The final stage in the formation of dentin is the deposition of lime salts in the ground substance in lamella-like layers. The incremental growth lines of the lamella are known as contour lines of Owen or incremental lines of von Ebner (Fig. 11–16).

The apical ends of the odontoblasts are in contact with the membrana preformativa prior to the deposition of dentin. As dentin is deposited, the odontoblasts remain on its advancing surface. Each odontoblast forms processes, odontoblast processes (fibers of Tomes),

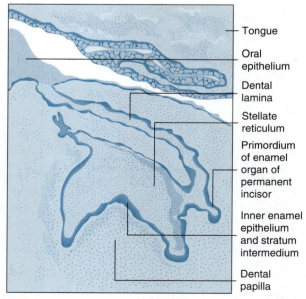

FIGURE 11–15. Human tooth development (4). Higher-power representation of developing lower incisor in 86-mm CR (3-month) human fetus.

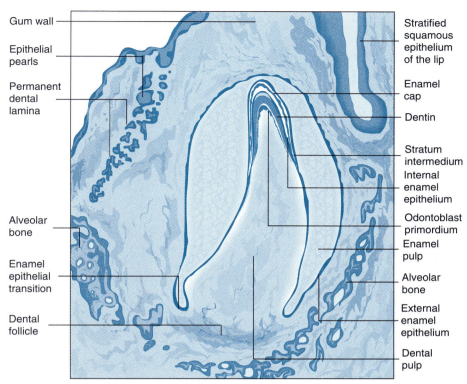

FIGURE 11–16. Human tooth development (5). Higher-power view of developing human incisor in 111-mm CR (approximately 14.5-weeks) human fetus.

which are embedded in dentin as it is deposited, and the processes extend through the entire thickness of the dentin. The odontoblasts remain functionally active throughout the life of the tooth. As a consequence of the functional longevity of the odontoblasts, secondary dentin can be deposited. The rate of deposition of dentin can be enhanced by mechanical stress and caries (Fig. 11–17).

Enamel Organ and Enamel Deposition

The enamel organ is usually described as having four layers. From its concavity outward they are:

1. Inner enamel epithelium. This single cell layer of columnar cells become the future ameloblasts. These cells are separated from the dental papilla by a basement membrane.
2. The stratum intermedium, which is composed of two or more layers of squamous or cuboidal cells.
3. The stellate reticulum, a loosely arranged group of branching cells.
4. The outer enamel organ, a single layer of cuboidal cells located adjacent to a rich vascular plexus in connective tissue.

The margin of the bell-shaped enamel organ, the cervical loop, does not have all four of these layers. After the crown of the tooth is formed, the enamel organ forms Hertwig's epithelial root sheath. This root sheath has an important role in determining the shape of the tooth root and in stimulating the differentiation of the odontoblasts of the root. The root sheath ultimately disintegrates, leaving nests of cells in the periodontal membrane (Fig. 11–18).

The deposition of enamel starts after a layer of dentin has formed and the ameloblasts have become tall columnar cells. The dentinal ends of the ameloblasts form processes (fibers of Tomes), which become incorporated into the developing enamel prisms. As the terminal ends of the processes of the ameloblasts are incorporated into enamel, the processes continue to grow so that they all remain approximately the same length.

There is a progressive deposition of mineral salts as prisms increase in length, but there is always an uncalcified portion adjacent to the ameloblasts. Between the prisms, interrod substance is deposited and calcified. Only about one fourth of the total amount of enamel mineral is deposited during this phase of development. Mineralization is completed after the rods or prisms reach their full length. Next, maturation of enamel matrix occurs, characterized by the dehydration and crystallization and final deposition of mineral. The maturation process starts at the occlusal part and progresses toward the cervix of the tooth.

Completion of enamel production does not end the functional role of enamel organ. The enamel organ involutes and becomes known as the *reduced enamel epithelium*. After eruption of the tooth, the enamel epithelium covering the exposed part of the crown becomes keratinized and, along with a thin calcified membrane (primary enamel cuticle) deposited on the enamel, becomes known as *Nasmyth's membrane*. That portion of the reduced enamel epithelium lying on the

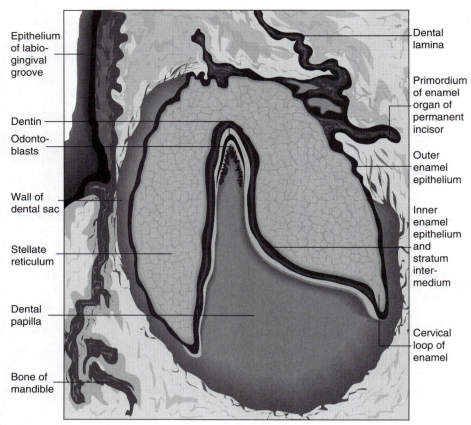

FIGURE 11–17. *Human tooth development at 5 months of gestation. Longitudinal section through the primordium of a developing incisor in a 5-month human fetus. Compare development and spatial arrangement of components at earlier stages of development.*

unexposed surface of the enamel forms the epithelial attachment. The epithelial attachment fuses with the epithelium of the gums at the gingival margin, and the two epithelia form a continuous layer. Continued eruption of the tooth results in an epithelial separation from the enamel at the gingival margin. Along with this separation, the epithelial attachment progresses apically on the tooth, so that the extent of the epithelial attachment does not decrease significantly as the tooth erupts.

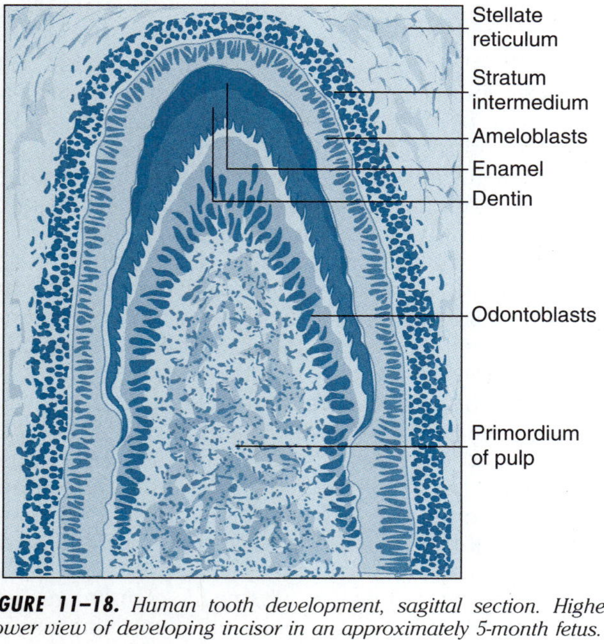

Cementum Deposition

Surrounding the developing tooth is a capsule-like grouping of the embryonal connective tissue, which forms the dental follicle or sac. That part of the follicular wall adjacent to the papilla becomes the position of the future periodontal membrane. It is separated from the papilla by the apically directed projection of the enamel organ, the so-called Hertwig's epithelial tooth sheath. After the first deposition of dentin of the root of the tooth, the epithelial root sheath disintegrates, and the cells of the dental sac wall differentiate into cementoblasts. Cementum then appears on the root. The cells of the outermost part of the dental sac differentiate into osteoblasts in the periosteum of the alveolus. In addition, fibroblasts produce fibers, forming the fibrous part of the periodontal membrane (Fig. 11–19).

DIGESTIVE TUBE (ORGANIZATIONAL PLAN)

Starting with the esophagus, four characteristic layers are a constant feature of the digestive tube: mucosa,

FIGURE 11–18. *Human tooth development, sagittal section. Higher-power view of developing incisor in an approximately 5-month fetus.*

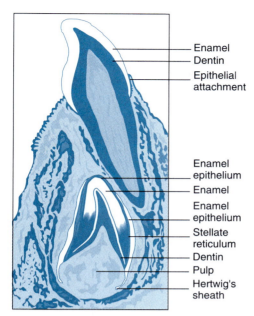

FIGURE 11–19. Deciduous tooth, in situ. Note the corresponding permanent tooth germ beneath the deciduous tooth.

submucosa, muscularis externa, and adventitia or serosa (peritoneum). In the different segments of the tube, modifications most commonly occur in the mucosa and are of great significance. Smooth muscle fibers, organized primarily in the longitudinal direction, form a constant component of the mucosa, the muscularis mucosae. Variations in the structure of the submucosa involve the presence or absence of glands. The muscularis externa is formed of two regularly arranged layers of smooth muscle, an inner circular and an outer longitudinal part, except in the stomach. The wall of the saccular stomach exhibits three muscle layers. At and near the junction of the esophagus and stomach and in the fundus, the muscle is more irregularly arranged.

The autonomic nervous system is represented by two nerve plexuses beginning with the esophagus. The myenteric plexus (of Auerbach) is located between the layers of the muscularis externa and it is readily located. The submucosal plexus (of Meissner) is located in the submucosa but is less prominent than the myenteric plexus (see Fig. 11–1).

Esophagus

The esophagus extends from the pharynx at the level of cricoid cartilage in the neck, passes through the thorax, and becomes continuous with the stomach immediately below the diaphragm. It is 25 to 30 cm in length. The esophagus has a well-developed muscularis mucosae, and except during the passage of food and/or water, its lumen is small. The circular muscular layer constricts the organ, resulting in characteristic longitudinal folds (Fig. 11–20).

Mucosa

The mucosa is lined with stratified squamous epithelium but it is not keratinized. The lamina propria is composed of loose connective tissue fibers, fibroblasts, and macrophages and may be infiltrated by variable numbers of lymphocytes and other immune cells (Fig. 11–21).

The muscularis mucosae is smooth muscle oriented primarily in the longitudinal plane but with some inner circular smooth muscle. The muscularis mucosae is thicker in the esophagus than elsewhere in the digestive tube.

Submucosa

The submucosa consists of loose connective tissue but with course bundles of collagenous connective tissue fibers that are interwoven and are so arranged to permit the formation of the characteristic longitudinal folds seen in sections of the esophagus.

Muscularis Mucosae

This layer of the esophagus is composed of striated muscle for about the first 6 or 7 cm, and the fibers are more orderly the further (distally) they are from the pharynx. The skeletal muscle forms inner circular and outer longitudinal layers. The striated muscle is then infiltrated by smooth muscle in each of the two layers. Past the middle of the length of the organ (actually quite variable), the striated muscle is completely replaced by smooth muscle.

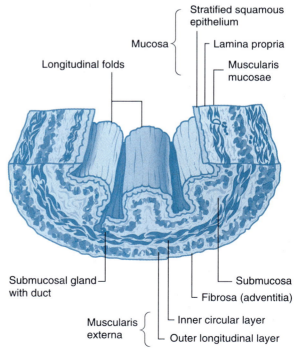

FIGURE 11–20. Esophagus. Camera lucida drawing showing the structural components of the human esophagus.

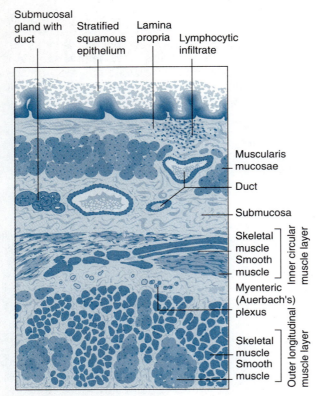

FIGURE 11–21. *Esophagus. Overview of the upper third of the human esophagus.*

Adventitia (Fibrosa)

This layer of connective tissue fibers is loosely arranged and binds the esophagus to surrounding structures. The small segment of the esophagus that extends below the diaphragm is covered with peritoneum, hence it is there covered by a serosa.

Glands of the Esophagus

Glandular tissue is found in the submucosa, the so-called submucosal glands, and in the mucosa, the mucosal or cardiac glands. In the human, the presence of submucosal glands is highly variable. Submucosal glands are composed of typical mucous cells arranged in alveoli. Small numbers of alveoli open by short ducts into a main duct, which is usually dilated. In the lamina propria, the duct walls change from a simple cuboidal to a stratified epithelium with surface cells being either squamous or columnar. Ultimately the duct opens between two adjacent mucosal connective tissue papillae. Very commonly, lymphatic cell infiltration occurs adjacent to ducts in the mucosa.

Cardiac glands of the esophagus are usually found in the most distal part, and lie in the lamina propria. The cardiac glands are similar to glands in the upper or cardiac region of the stomach, and are of the mucous type (Fig. 11–22).

Stomach

The stomach extends from the esophagus to the duodenum. When empty, the stomach is essentially tubular but has a bulge in its upper part that is usually directed to the left. At the esophagus-stomach junction, the epithelium changes from stratified squamous to a simple columnar type. Structures placed deeper do not have as sharp a line of demarcation, because certain glands of the stomach may extend under the stratified squamous epithelium of the esophagus; the muscularis mucosae is continuous from esophagus to stomach (Fig. 11–23).

Mucosa

The mucous membrane of the stomach is folded into ridges or rugae of variable number, depending upon the distention of the organ. They are most prominent in the empty stomach.

The epithelial surface is divided into small irregular areas, 1 to 5 mm in diameter, the so-called gastric areas. The surface of gastric areas is punctured with minute depressions, the gastric pits (*foveolae*). Their depth varies regionally. They are shallow in the fundus (one fifth the thickness of mucosa) and are deep in the pyloric region (one half the thickness of mucosa). Gastric glands secrete into the bottoms of the gastric pits (Figs. 11–24 and 11–25).

The epithelium lining the stomach is of several types. The epithelium that covers the entire surface of

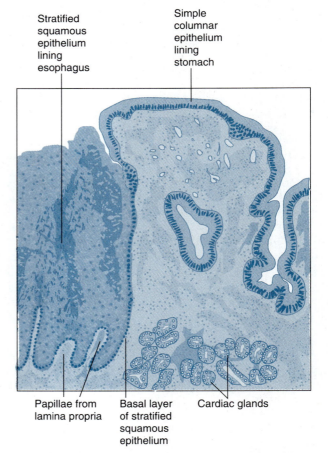

FIGURE 11–22. *Esophagus/stomach. Longitudinal section through the junction of the esophagus and stomach.*

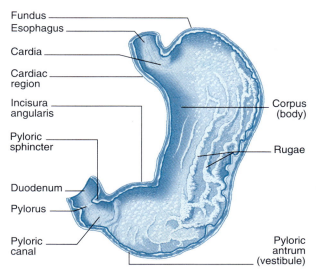

FIGURE 11-23. Stomach. Internal surface features of the human stomach. Note particularly the longitudinal folds, the rugae.

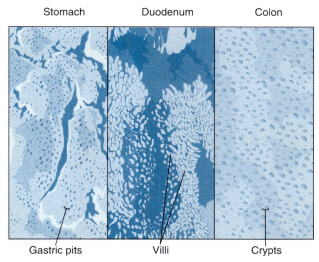

FIGURE 11-24. Distinguishing surface features of the three regions of the gastrointestinal tract. Note: in the stomach, the presence of gastric pits; in the duodenum, villi; and in the colon, the openings of the crypts of Lieberkühn.

the stomach mucosa and extends down into the pits consists of simple columnar, mucus-secreting gland cells. The apical end of such a cell (facing the lumen) contains mucus, and the basal end contains a spherical or, more frequently, a flattened nucleus if the cell is filled with mucus. The amount of mucus depends on the stage of the mucus synthetic activity.

As the epithelium extends deeper into the gastric pits, the cells become more cuboidal, and deeper-lying cells may show mitotic activity. These cells are destined to replace cells that are desquamated from the surface of the stomach.

Lamina Propria

Gastric glands are located in the lamina propria, which is composed of interlacing connective tissue fibers, fibrocytes, and macrophages. As elsewhere, the lamina propria is infiltrated with lymphocytes and other cells of the immune system. In addition to a diffuse distribution of immune cells, lymphoid nodules (so-called solitary nodules) may be located in the pyloric region.

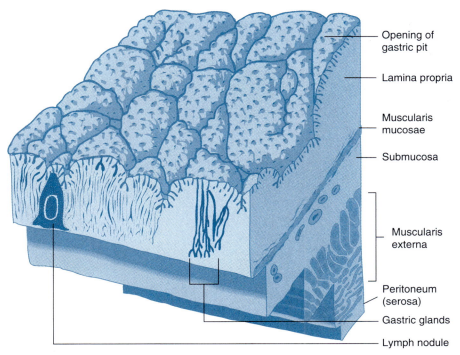

FIGURE 11-25. Overview of the gastric glands in this semidiagrammatic view of the gastric mucosa.

Muscularis Mucosae

The muscularis mucosae is a thin layer of smooth muscle cells distributed in both the circular and longitudinal directions. Thin strands of smooth muscle extend into the stroma between the glands.

Glands of the Stomach

The glands of the stomach begin at the bottoms of the gastric pits. Three types of glands, depending on their location, are recognized by histologists: gastric or fundic glands, having the widest distribution; pyloric

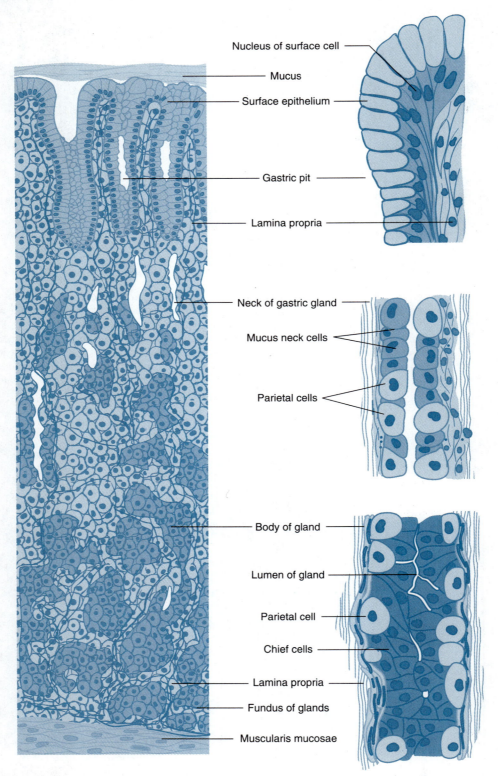

FIGURE 11-26. Cellular detail of the intestinal glands, the crypts of Lieberkühn. Note the distribution of the various cell types.

glands, confined to the pyloric region; and cardiac glands, found near the esophageal junction with the stomach, in the so-called cardiac region of the stomach. The gastric glands secrete hydrochloric acid and digestive enzymes, and the regionally specific pyloric and cardiac glands secrete primarily mucus.

Gastric Glands

Gastric glands are usually simple tubular glands that empty into a gastric pit. Each gastric pit may open into about five glands. The glands reach the muscularis mucosae by traversing the entire lamina propria. Each gland has a mouth or opening into a pit; a neck, or constricted part near the opening; a body, or main part of the tubular gland; and a fundus, a somewhat dilated and twisted end of the gland.

The gastric gland is composed of three types of cells: chief, parietal, and mucous neck cells (Fig. 11–26).

CHIEF CELLS. Chief cells, the most abundant secretory cells of the gastric gland, are located primarily deep in the body and fundic portions of the stomach. The cells are irregularly square or pyramidal. The bases of the cells lie on the basement membrane, and their apices face the lumen of the gland. The chief cell is a protein secretory cell, elaborating the enzyme pepsin, and is therefore rich in ribosome-studded endoplasmic reticulum, a Golgi apparatus, and numerous mitochondria. By virtue of its high concentration of RNA, these cells stain blue with the hematoxylin and eosin stains. The nuclei retain a rounded configuration even when packed with zymogen granules between meals or in the fasting state (see Figs. 11–26 and 11–27).

PARIETAL OR OXYNTIC CELLS. These cells are the largest and first described of the three cell types in gastric glands. They are usually described as hydrochloric acid secretory cells, but they actually secrete the acid precursor.

The cells are oval or polygonal, with a large spherical nucleus, which may be doubled and is usually centrally placed. The cytoplasm is strongly stained by acid aniline dyes; hence, they appear bright red when stained by hematoxylin and eosin and contrast significantly with chief cells.

Parietal cells are located primarily in the neck region and among the mucous neck cells. In the body and fundus of the gland, parietal cells are pushed away from the surface by crowding of the chief cells and lie peripherally placed against the basement membrane. Parietal cells in light-microscopic preparations commonly appear to have intracellular canaliculi, which have been shown by electron microscopy to be complex invaginations of the apical cell membrane. These cells are rich in mitochondria and smooth (ribosome-free) endoplasmic reticulum (Figs. 11–28 and 11–29).

The mechanism of secretion of hydrochloric acid depends on the presence of the enzyme carbonic anhydrase, which converts carbonic acid to carbon dioxide and water. A hydrogen ion from the carbonic acid is transported to the luminal (apical) end of the parietal cell, and bicarbonate is secreted into the extracellular

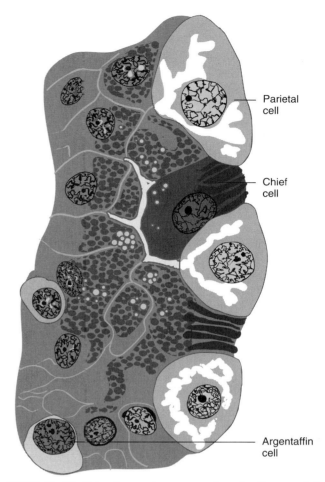

FIGURE 11–27. *Light-microscopic representation of cell types of the gastric gland. Note the secretory granules within the chief (zymogenic) cells and the intracellular canaliculi within the parietal cells.*

space and returned to the blood. Chloride ions are actively removed from the extracellular fluid, combined with hydrogen ions in the intracellular canaliculi, and discharged from the apical end of the cell into the lumen of the stomach.

In the gastric juice (succus gastricus), the so-called intrinsic factor is also found. The intrinsic factor facilitates the absorption of vitamin B_{12} (so-called extrinsic factor) by strongly binding to it for absorption in the ileum. Vitamin B_{12} is the important antipernicious anemia factor. It has been suggested that the parietal cell produces the intrinsic factor. Active parietal cell secretion of hydrochloric acid may result from the action of histamine and gastrin, a polypeptide, which are secreted by the gastric mucosa. In addition, the cholinergic nerve fibers of the parasympathetic nervous system stimulate secretion of hydrochloric acid.

Located near the bases of the tubular glands, individual cells, referred to as *argentaffin cells*, are found interspersed between other indigenous cells. These isolated cells have their apices facing the basement membrane rather than the lumen of the gland. Argentaffin cells are identified with the secretion of serotonin (5-hydroxytryptamine), which is secreted into the lamina

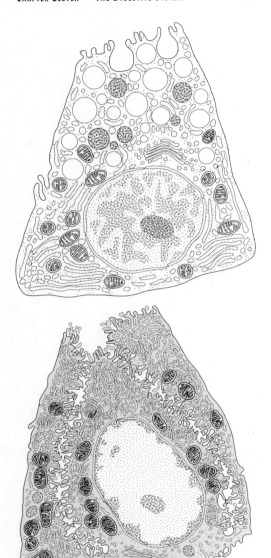

FIGURE 11-28. *Semidiagrammatic representation of electron micrographs of chief cell (top) and parietal cells (bottom) of the gastric gland. Note zymogenic granules within the apical cytoplasm of the chief cell and intracellular canaliculi; lysosomes; and nongranular reticulum within the parietal cells.*

propria. Serotonin is a powerful stimulant of smooth muscle, causing contraction of the muscle (Fig. 11-29).

A number of cells with specific functions are found throughout the digestive tract; see Table 11-1.

MUCOUS NECK CELLS. The mucous neck cell is cuboidal or low columnar. The cytoplasm contains finely granular mucigen. The nucleus is located basally and is commonly oval with its long axis perpendicular to the long axis of the cell and may be deeply indented on its apical side (Fig. 11-30).

Pyloric Glands

Pyloric glands are simple branched tubular glands that open deeply within the pyloric pits. These glands are short and markedly twisted, so that they are usually seen in oblique or transverse section. The mucous gland cells resemble mucous neck cells of gastric glands. The transition between gastric and pyloric glands is not sharply demarcated; glandular cells from both regions intermingle (Fig. 11-31).

Cardiac Glands

Cardiac glands, named for their regional location, are located in the transition area between esophagus and stomach and resemble glands in the lamina propria at the lower end of the esophagus. These cells produce mucus and resemble gastric glands and mucous neck cells. There is a transitional zone change in the appearance of the gland cells, which become more granular in the lamina propria of the stomach.

Submucosa

The submucosa of the stomach is composed of coarse but loosely arranged collagenous connective tissue. In addition, it contains larger blood vessels and nerve fibers, including Meissner's plexus of autonomic nerve cells and fibers.

Muscularis

The muscular layer is conventionally described as composed of three layers: inner oblique, middle circular, and outer longitudinal. In the fundus, however, the muscle bundles run in various directions that defy simple description. In the connective tissue that marks the boundary between the longitudinal and circular layers, a group of parasympathetic nerve cells and fibers homologous to Auerbach's plexus of the intestine is found (see Fig. 11-1).

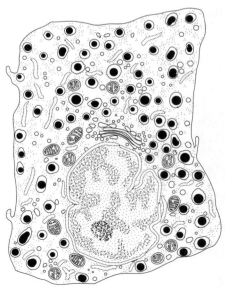

FIGURE 11-29. *Argentaffin cell of the gastric gland. Note the presence of dense-cored secretory granules within the apical cytoplasm.*

TABLE 11-1. Cells of the Digestive Tract

Cell	Location(s)	Product(s)	Function(s)
D	Stomach, jejunum, ileum, colon	Somatostatin	Inhibition of other endocrine glands
D1	Stomach, jejunum, ileum, colon	Vasoactive intestinal polypeptide	Increases intestinal motility, ion and water secretion
EC	Stomach, jejunum, appendix	Serotonin, substance P	Increased intestinal activity
ECL	Stomach	Histamine	Vasodilator, gastric secretion
C	Stomach, duodenum	Gastrin	Stimulates gastric secretion; neurotransmitter
GRP	GI system	Gastrin-releasing peptide	Releases gastrin
I	Jejunum, ileum	Cholecystokinin	Pancreatic exocrine secretion, gallbladder contraction
K	Jejunum, ileum	Gastrin, inhibitory peptide	Inhibits gastric acid secretion
L	Jejunum, ileum, colon	Glucagon-like	Hepatic glycogenolysis substance
Mo	Jejunum, ileum	Motilin	Increases gut motility
N	Ileum	Neurotensin	Myenteric plexus transmitter
P	Stomach, jejunum	Unknown	Unknown
PP	Stomach, colon	Pancreatic polypeptide	Pancreatic exocrine secretion
S	Jejunum, ileum	Secretin	Pancreatic and bile secretion
TG	Jejunum	C-terminal immunoreactivity	Neurotransmitter
X	Stomach	Unknown	Unknown

Serosa

The stomach has a mesentery, and hence is considered intraperitoneal. Because the stomach is contained in a peritoneal sling, it is covered by mesothelium. In the loose connective tissue of the serosa, blood vessels, lymphatics, and cells such as macrophages, mast cells, and wandering cells of the immune system can be found.

Small Intestine

The small intestine extends from the pylorus of the stomach to the cecum. It is divided into three regions: the proximal duodenum, the middle jejunum, and the distal ileum.

If the small intestine is opened in the longitudinal axis, a series of folds are found on the inner surface. Although generally parallel to one another, they have a circular or oblique course in the lumen of the tube. These mucosal and submucosal folds are known as plicae circulares, valves of Kerckring, or valvulae conniventes. These folds are absent in the proximal region of the duodenum. Tallest in the jejunum, they are almost absent in the ileum near the ileocecal valve. Unlike the rugae of the stomach, these plicae cannot be entirely eliminated by distention of the intestine. The mucosa also projects from the surface of the tube and from the plicae, in projections known as *villi*. Villi are made up of an epithelium-covered stroma into which smooth muscle cells from the muscularis mucosae project. The villi and plicae circulares are characteristic of the small intestine (Fig. 11–32). In distinction from the pits of the stomach, which are depressions in the mucous membrane, the villi are projections upward from the floor of the intestinal lumen. There are openings, however, between the villi that extend into the mucosa as far as the muscularis mucosae. These are simple glandular invaginations, the so-called crypts of Lieberkühn (or glandulae intestinales) (Fig. 11–33).

The wall of the small intestine has the same four coats or layers as are present in the stomach: mucosa, submucosa, muscularis externa, and serosa (except for that part of the duodenum, which is retroperitoneal and therefore does not have an outer mesothelial layer derived from the peritoneum).

Mucosa

The mucosa is composed of the lining epithelium, a lamina propria with its superficial glands, and its deeper muscularis muscosae. The most characteristic feature of the small intestine is the villus. In cross-section, the villus has a core of loose connective tissue normally infiltrated with plasma cells, lymphocytes, and white blood cells. In addition, cellular strands composed of smooth muscle cells from the muscularis mucosae are present. A single lymphatic capillary with a dilated blind end is also always present, as are blood capillaries (Figs. 11–34 to 11–36).

Epithelium

A single layer of columnar cells lines the villus and is attached to a delicate but tough basement membrane. Two types of cells constitute the epithelium: columnar absorbing cells and mucus-secreting goblet cells. A striking feature of the columnar absorbing cell is its striated or brush border composed of microvilli. The microvilli increase the food-absorbing surface enormously. In diseases of malabsorption, such as nontropical sprue, the microvilli may be lost from the columnar cell surface, essential food cannot be absorbed, and malnutrition and weight loss become significant problems. After treatment, the microvilli reappear, and proper absorption of food occurs once again. It has been shown that the striated brush border (microvilli) is the site of activity of disaccharidases, enzymes that convert disaccharides to monosaccharides, which are readily absorbed by the columnar cells (Fig. 11–37).

The columnar cells are acidophilic; hence, they stain with eosin. They are rich in mitochondria, Golgi apparatus, and smooth endoplasmic reticulum.

Scattered among the columnar absorbing cells are typical goblet cells. They vary in shape according to

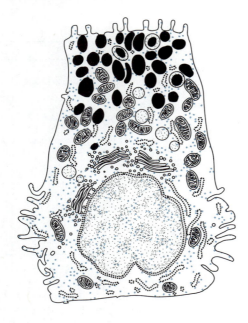

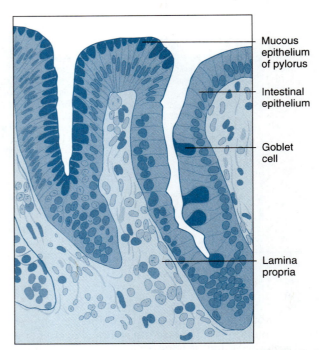

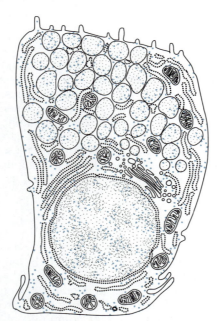

FIGURE 11–30. *Semidiagrammatic representation of electron micrographs of mucous gland cells. Note the two varieties,* mucous surface cells *(top) and* mucous neck cells *(bottom).*

FIGURE 11–31. *Epithelial junction between the pyloric stomach* (left) *and duodenum* (right). *Note the presence of surface mucous cells in the lining of the pylorus, and goblet cells in the duodenal lining, revealed by a special stain for mucus (mucicarmine).*

the content of mucin. These cells appear to be undergoing a continuous process of synthesis, accumulation, discharge, and resynthesis (Fig. 11–38).

The number of goblet cells increases progressively down the digestive tube from the duodenum, to the jejunum, ileum, and colon, where they are most abundant.

Villi move and change length and shape, depending on the contractile activity of the smooth muscle in the connective tissue core. These motions facilitate the movement of absorbed material into blood and lymphatic capillaries and transport out of the lacteal (lymphatic capillary) (see Figs. 11–35 and 11–36).

Crypts of Lieberkühn

These simple tubular glands are located in the mucous membrane. They open between the villi and extend as far as the muscularis mucosae. The epithelium of the gland is continuous with the surface epithelium of the villi but lacks a well-defined brush border of microvilli. It is believed that cells of the glands are undergoing differentiation and will migrate distally for renewal of the surface epithelium. This view is supported by the presence of dividing cells, especially in the midregion of the gland. Goblet cells also arise from undifferentiated columnar cells in the crypts.

In the depths of the crypts of Lieberkühn, coarsely granular cells, termed Paneth's cells, are found. These exocrine cells synthesize an enzyme (lysozyme) that is capable of antibacterial activity by destroying the cell wall of certain bacteria (Figs. 11–39 and 11–40).

Paneth's cells occur mainly in the crypts of Lieberkühn but may be encountered in the crypts of the large intestine.

Another cell located in the crypt but few in number is the argentaffin cell (see Figs. 11–27 and 11–39). Argentaffin cells are oriented toward the basement membrane rather than toward the lumen of the tubular gland. They are stained by silver and by chromium salts used either as a stain or in the fixative. They are believed to secrete serotonin (5-hydoxytryptamine), a powerful stimulant of smooth muscle that causes contraction. These cells may play a role in localized con-

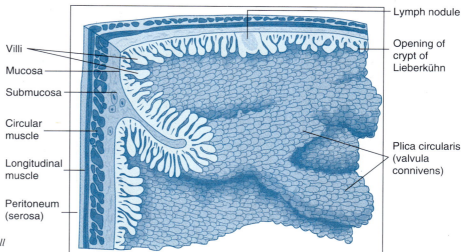

FIGURE 11-32. Organization of the small intestine. Note the component parts.

tractile activity, facilitating movement of fluid in lacteals (lymphatic capillaries) or blood capillaries.

Lamina Propria

Composed of a feltwork of reticular, elastic, and fine collagenous fiber bundles, the lamina propria fills the villi, the spaces between the crypts of Lieberkühn, and between the crypts located above the muscularis mucosae. Lymphocytes are very abundant in the lamina propria, and lymph nodules are commonly found. These are known as solitary follicles, to distinguish them from other groups of lymph nodules—Peyer's patches—found in the other parts of the small intestine. Solitary follicles are not as numerous in the stomach as in the intestine.

Peyer's Patches

Found mainly in the ileum, especially near its junction with the colon, Peyer's patches are aggregations of solitary follicles or groups of lymph nodules. They always lie on the side opposite the mesentery. Each patch contains from 10 to 70 nodules, which are found side by side in the long axis of the intestine. The patches are not covered by villi but rather by a single layer of columnar epithelium. The cells of the epithelium overlying the massive aggregations of B lymphocytes are called *M cells*. M cells are thought to endocy-

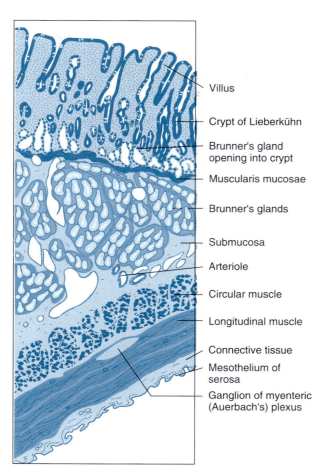

FIGURE 11-33. Human duodenum. Note the component parts of the proximal portion of the organ.

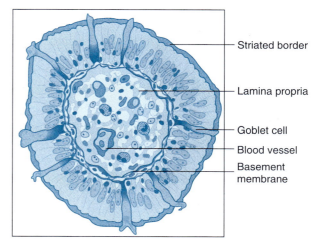

FIGURE 11-34. Cross-section of intestinal villus. This specimen is from human jejunum; note the blood vessels within the lamina propria, which forms the core of the epithelium-lined villus.

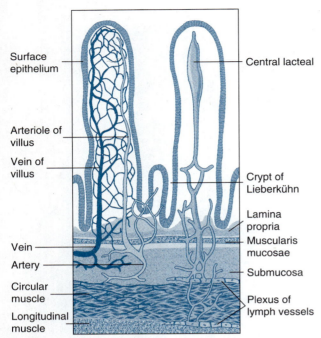

FIGURE 11–35. *Blood and lymphatics of the intestine. Note the plexiform arrangements of arterioles and venous channels within the intestinal villus. In addition, a lacteal of the lymphatic system is shown occupying the central core of the villus.*

tose antigens from the lumen of the intestine, transport them through their cytoplasm, and discharge them so that they make contact with active underlying lymphocytes. The bases of the lymphatic nodules are not confined to the lamina propria, but extend into the submucosa.

Muscularis Mucosae

The muscularis is thin, consisting of an inner circular layer and an outer longitudinal layer of smooth

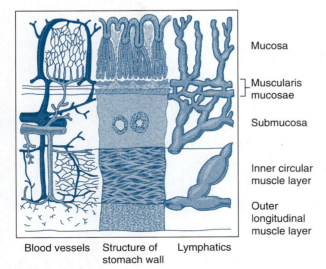

FIGURE 11–36. *Stomach wall. Note the relationship of blood vessels and lymphatics to the respective layers of the wall.*

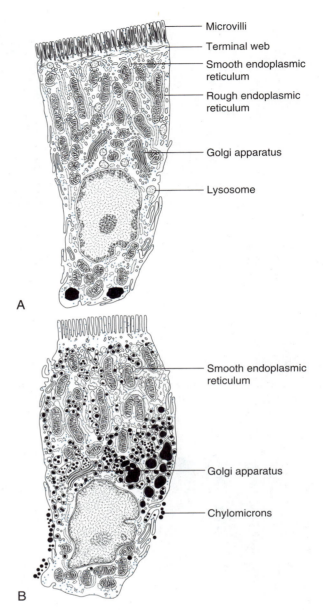

FIGURE 11–37. *Intestinal epithelial cells. A, Semidiagrammatic illustrations of electron micrographs of jejunal epithelium. B illustrates the route of vesicular lipid absorption across the epithelium, toward the base, and across the lateral cell membrane as chylomicrons.*

muscle. Small groups of smooth muscle extend from the muscularis mucosae into the core of villi.

Submucosa

The submucosa of loosely arranged connective tissue fibers also contains larger blood vessels, lymphatic vessels, and nerves.

The submucosa is free of glands except in the duodenum, where it contains the glands of Brunner. These duodenal glands are diagnostic for the duodenum but they are absent from the distal end of the duodenum. Brunner's glands are branched tubuloalveolar glands lined with columnar epithelium similar to

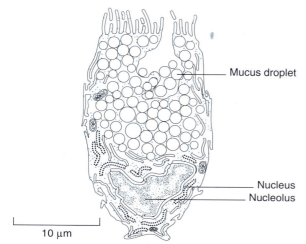

FIGURE 11-38. Goblet cell. Semidiagrammatic illustration of electron micrograph of a goblet cell. Note the accumulation of mucus within vesicles distorting the basally placed nucleus.

the pyloric glands of the stomach. The ducts are lined with simple columnar epithelium (Figs. 11–33 and 11–41). The glands empty typically into a crypt of Lieberkühn and less commonly on a surface between villi. Strands of smooth muscle (muscularis mucosae) are present among the acini.

Muscularis

The muscular component is composed of two layers: an inner circular coat and an outer longitudinal coat. Between the two muscular coats, a plexus of nerve cells and fibers (myenteric plexus of Auerbach) is located in the connective tissue septum, together with blood vessels and lymphatics.

Serosa

The outer serosal layer is composed of loose connective tissue covered by a layer of mesothelium (peritoneum). This applies for the entire small intestine, except for the distal two thirds of the duodenum, which is retroperitoneal and lacks the mesothelial outer layer of cells.

The outer connective tissue layer contains blood and lymphatic vessels, wandering cells of the immune system, and mast cells. Mast cells produce heparin, an anticoagulant that prevents blood clots. These cells also produce histamine, which increases permeability of capillaries. They are commonly found alongside or near blood vessels.

Large Intestine

The large intestine is usually divided into three primary segments: the colon, rectum, and anal canal. The wall of the large intestine is composed of the same four coats that have been described for the stomach

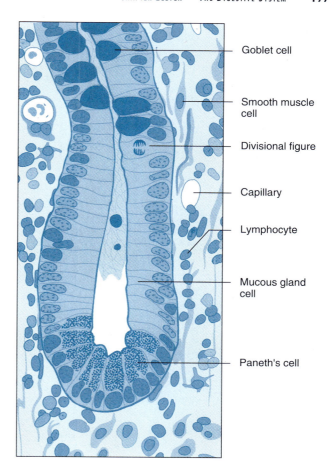

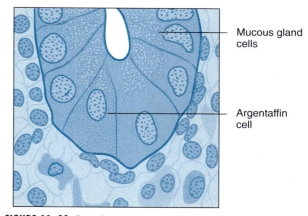

FIGURE 11-39. Paneth and argentaffin cells. Note the location of these cell types in the intestinal gland.

and small intestine: mucosa, submucosa, muscularis, and a serosa or an adventitia (fibrosa).

Colon

There is a striking change at the ileocecal junction, from the ileum to the colon. Grossly, a change in diameter is immediately obvious, but other differences are found in the various coats.

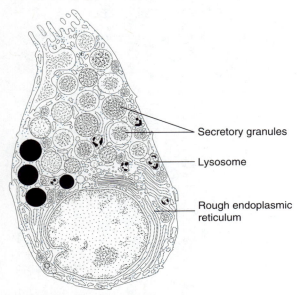

FIGURE 11–40. *Paneth's cell. Semidiagrammatic illustration of an electron micrograph of a Paneth's cell with its accumulated secreting granules. Frequently, these abundant granules obscure the nucleus in light-microscopic examination.*

Mucosa

The mucous membrane of the colon has a smooth surface as the plicae, and villi are found only in the small intestine (Figs. 11–24 and 11–42).

Long straight tubular glands descend from the surface and reach the muscularis mucosae on the floor of the mucosa. These glands form the crypts of Lieberkühn. The loose connective tissue of the lamina propria extends upward between the densely packed glands.

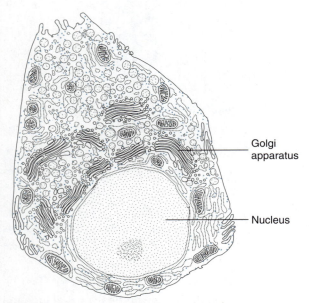

FIGURE 11–41. *Brunner's gland. Semidiagrammatic illustration of an electron micrograph of a mucous cell from the duodenal gland of Brunner. Compare this mucous secretory cell with the goblet cell and mucous cells from the stomach mucosa.*

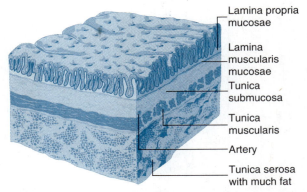

FIGURE 11–42. *Overview of the surface and internal structure of the colon. Note the opening of straight intestinal glands onto the surface of the folded mucosa; the presence in this section of only one layer of muscularis (the inner); and the thick, fatty serosa.*

Solitary lymph nodules, present in the mucosa, penetrate the muscularis mucosae to enter the submucosa (Fig. 11–43).

The surface epithelium is columnar, with a fine, short, brush (apical) border. Between the columnar cells are goblet cells. As the epithelium descends into the crypts, the columnar cells shorten and decrease in number and the goblet cells increase in number. The walls of the many glands appear to be composed entirely of goblet cells. At the base of the glands, undifferentiated cells divide and push the newly formed cells toward the surface to replace those that are constantly being lost. Paneth's cells and argentaffin cells are very rare in this glandular epithelium.

The mucous membrane has two chief functions; these are related to the absorption of water by the columnar cells and the production of large amounts of mucus to facilitate the movement of feces, which are usually being dehydrated.

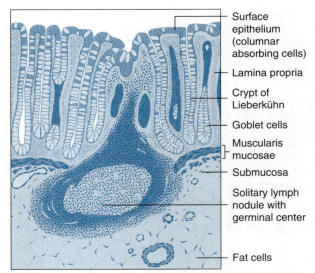

FIGURE 11–43. *Colonic lymph nodule. The lamina propria and submucosa are richly populated with solitary nodules and diffuse lymphoid tissue.*

Muscularis Mucosae

The muscularis mucosae is composed of an inner circular layer and an outer longitudinal layer of smooth muscle.

Submucosa

The submucosa is composed of loosely arranged connective tissue. As elsewhere, it contains blood and lymphatic vessels and Meissner's nerve plexus. Solitary lymph follicles lie primarily in the submucosa.

Muscularis

The muscularis externa shows a striking change. The circular layer is typical of the digestive system, but the longitudinal layer forms three strong, flat bands, the so-called taeniae coli. The three bands are equidistant and separated from each other by a much-thinned longitudinal coat. Nerve cells and fibers of Auerbach's plexus lie in the connective tissue separating the two muscle layers.

Adventitia and Serosa

The colon is both retroperitoneal and intraperitoneal. The ascending colon is retroperitoneal, the transverse colon intraperitoneal, and the descending colon retroperitoneal. The intraperitoneal part has a serosa, because it has a mesentery with a mesothelial surface. In either case, the connective tissue of the outer layer contains blood and lymphatic vessels and cells typical of the region and previously described for the small intestine.

Vermiform Appendix

The appendix is an appendage of the cecum. Its walls are continuous with the cecum and have the same four coats typical of the digestive system: mucosa, submucosa, muscularis, and serosa (Fig. 11–44).

The mucous membrane has the usual composition: epithelium, glands, lamina propria, and muscularis mucosae. The epithelium is columnar and the cells possess a brush border. The surface epithelium continues into the tubular glands, containing some goblet cells. The glands form typical crypts of Lieberkühn. The lumen of the appendix is very irregular owing to deep folds and may be entirely obliterated by them. The most conspicuous histologic feature of the appendix is the massive accumulation of lymphoid tissue. The lamina propria is completely infiltrated with lymphocytes and other cells of the immune system as well as rings of solitary lymphoid nodules. These nodules resemble the follicles seen in the palatine tonsils. The follicles are not confined to the lamina propria, but also divide the muscularis mucosae to lie in the submucosa as well.

The submucosa contains numerous fat cells, also characteristic of the appendix. In some instances in older people, the mucosa and some of the submucosa are replaced by fibrous connective tissue.

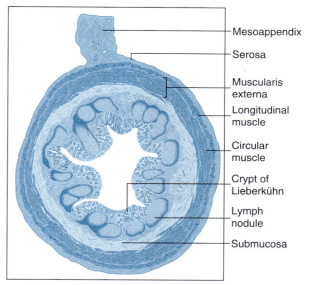

FIGURE 11–44. *Human vermiform appendix. Note the extensive lymph nodular tissue throughout the mucosa.*

The muscularis externa varies markedly in thickness and composition. The inner circular layer is usually well developed, and the outer longitudinal layer differs from the rest of the large intestine by having the longitudinal layer of uniform thickness; it does not possess the taeniae coli.

The muscular layers are covered by a thin feltwork of connective tissue covered in turn by mesothelium, a typical serosa.

Rectum and Anal Canal

The rectum is about 12 to 18 cm in length and is structurally identical to the colon. The rectum has no mesentery; it is, therefore, retroperitoneal and has an adventitia but not a mesothelial covering (Fig. 11–45).

The anal canal is 2.5 to 3.5 cm in length. It pierces the pelvic floor and is closed except during defecation. The mucous membrane has permanent longitudinal folds, the anal (rectal) columns that terminate distally about 1.3 cm from the anal opening. The columns contain smooth muscle and typically an artery and vein. The bases of the columns are joined by transverse folds of the mucosa, the so-called anal valves (Fig. 11–46).

Proximal to the anal valves, the mucosa is lined by simple columnar epithelium, composed of both columnar absorbing cells and goblet cells. At the level of the anal valves, the epithelium abruptly changes to stratified squamous nonkeratinized type. Crypts of Lieberkühn are not found below the anal valves. The nonkeratinized epithelium extends nearly to the anal orifice, but then it changes to the keratinized stratified squamous epithelium characteristic of the epidermis of skin. Typical appendages of skin appear at the anal orifice: hairs, sebaceous glands, and sweat glands. The sweat glands are of two types: typical body sweat glands and the very large circumanal glands that are similar in appearance to axillary and ceruminous glands. The secretory

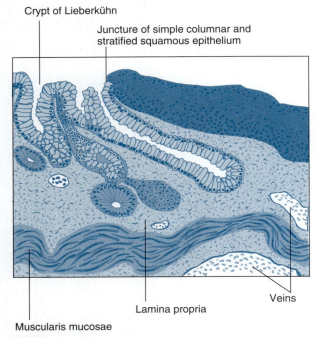

FIGURE 11-45. *Rectoanal junction. This specimen illustrates the distinctive and abrupt epithelial transition from simple columnar to stratified squamous epithelium.*

cells are usually filled with granules, and large myoepithelial cells are also found within the basement membrane.

At the level of the anal valves, the muscularis mucosae becomes discontinuous and then disappears.

The submucosa of the anal canal has an extensive plexus of blood vessels. The veins are often tortuous, and their size, arrangement, and absence of valves may result in the formation of hemorrhoids.

The circular smooth muscle of the anal canal is typically thick and forms the internal anal sphincter. The longitudinal muscle layer continues over the sphincter to end in connective tissue.

The external anal sphincter is composed of skeletal muscle, surrounded by an outer skeletal muscle layer derived from the (pubococcygeus) levator ani muscle.

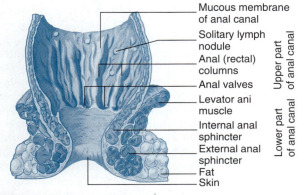

FIGURE 11-46. *Anal canal. Note the extensive internal and external sphincters at the distal end of the digestive tube, and the distinctive elevation of the rectal mucosa into the columns of Morgagni.*

Peritoneum

No description of the digestive system would be complete without mention of the peritoneum. The *peritoneum* is a serous membrane that lines the walls of the abdominal cavity (so-called parietal peritoneum) and becomes reflected over the viscera, which then are contained in peritoneal folds (so-called visceral peritoneum). The folds reflect upon each other and consist therefore of two layers (actually one continuous layer) of loose connective tissue and mesothelium. The peritoneum is supplied with blood vessels and lymphatics.

The reflected folds of peritoneum around the digestive tube form a sling called a mesentery, which carries blood vessels, lymphatics, and nerves to the digestive tube. The sling or mesentery is composed of loosely arranged connective tissue covered with peritoneum. If a part of the digestive tube has a mesentery, that part of the tube is said to be intraperitoneal.

The mesentery is richly supplied with lymph nodes and, usually, considerable amounts of stored fat.

Omenta and the visceral ligaments are similar in structure to mesentery.

Blood Supply to the Digestive Tract

Arteries reach the digestive tract through mesenteries, provide small branches to the serosa or adventitia, and pass through the muscular coats to the submucosa, where they form an extensive plexus of large vessels. Within the muscular layers, the main arteries provide small branches to the muscle.

In the submucosa, two sets of vessels arise, one passing outward to form the primary supply to the muscular coats, and the second passing inward to supply the mucous membrane.

The supply of the muscular coats results from larger vessels passing to the intermuscular septum, where a plexus is formed that provides smaller branches to the two outer muscular coats (tunics). Both short and long branches from the submucous plexus pass to the mucous membrane, where the shorter branch supplies the muscularis mucosae and the longer branches pierce the muscularis mucosae to form a capillary plexus around the glands in the lamina propria. The capillary plexus is most dense around the bodies and necks of the glands. A dense network of capillaries is also found beneath the surface epithelium. From the capillary plexuses, venules and small veins arise that pierce the muscularis mucosae to form a venous plexus in the submucosa. These then give rise to larger veins that accompany arteries to and in the mesentery.

In the small intestine, the blood supply is modified by the presence of villi. Each villus receives one to three small arteries, depending on its size. The artery passes throughout the length of the villus and provides a network of fine capillaries that lie just beneath the epithelial surface. From these capillary networks, one or two small veins arise to lie on the side opposite the artery (see Figs. 11–35 and 11–36).

Lymphatics of the Digestive Tract

Small lymph capillaries begin as blind channels in the stroma of the lamina propria in the mucous membrane. These lymph (chyle) capillaries occupy the center of the long axis of each villus, ending as blind ampullae beneath the surface epithelium. The walls of the lymph capillaries are composed of a single layer of large endothelial cells. Lymph capillaries are significantly larger than blood capillaries but are usually collapsed and almost invisible by light microscopy. The lymph vessels join to form a plexus of lymph vessels in the deeper part of the villus close to the muscularis mucosae. Vessels from the deep plexus pass through the muscularis mucosae and form a still larger plexus in the submucosa. In the submucosa, they often enlarge into sinuses surrounding lymphoid nodules. A third lymphatic plexus lies in the connective tissue that separates the two layers of muscle. From the submucosal plexus, branches pass through the inner muscular layer, receive vessels from the intermuscular plexus, and then pierce the outer muscular layer to reach the mesentery together with arteries and veins.

Larger lymph vessels have valves, and their walls may contain a variable thickness of smooth muscle. Lymph vessels are connected to lymph nodes ("in-line filters") as they traverse the mesenteries.

The primary function of the lymphatic system is the return of tissue fluids (lymph and extracellular fluid) to the blood stream. During digestion, lymph is a rich emulsion of fatty material (chylomicrons) distending the vessels and rendering them visible.

SALIVARY GLANDS

The parotid, submandibular (submaxillary), and sublingual glands compose the major salivary glands. They are compound tubuloalveolar glands whose ducts open into the oral cavity. They secrete proteins, glycoproteins, proteoglycans, electrolytes, and water and elaborate the major portion of the daily output of saliva, estimated in humans to be one liter. The bulk of this volume is elaborated by the submandibular (70%) and parotid (25%) glands. Saliva contains, in addition, gamma globulin (IgA) and peroxidase, both of which constitute defense mechanisms against pathogens in the oral cavity.

The secretion of salivary glands depends on innervation by the autonomic (sympathetic and parasympathetic) system. Stimulation of the sympathetic system produces secretions of a small volume of a viscous fluid rich in protein. Stimulation of the parasympathetic system, in contrast, results in the secretion of a large volume of watery saliva.

Secretions of salivary glands are delivered to the oral cavity via a branching system of ducts termed, progressively from the gland to the oral cavity, intercalated, secretory (striated), and interlobular (excretory). The intercalated ducts are longest in the parotid gland, and the secretory (striated) ducts are best developed in the submandibular gland. Both types of intralobular ducts are least conspicuous in the sublingual gland. The interlobular (excretory) ducts are, in contrast, similar in all three glands.

Each salivary gland is surrounded by a connective tissue capsule rich in collagen fibers from which septa extend into the gland, dividing it into lobes and lobules. Nerves, blood, and lymphatic vessels course through the connective tissue septa. Blood vessels form rich capillary networks within the lobules.

Two types of secretory cells are found in the three salivary glands, mucous and serous (Fig. 11–47). Mucous cells resemble intestinal goblet cells. On routine light microscopy, the nuclei are flattened and basal, and the cytoplasm appears empty or vacuolated, secretory droplets having been dissolved during the preparation process. On electron micrographs, the nucleus is basally located, and the supranuclear cytoplasm is filled with secretory droplets and Golgi complex. Mitochondria and rough endoplasmic reticulum profiles are located in lateral and basal cytoplasm. On light microscopy, serous cells are pyramidal, with a rounded basal nucleus, indistinct boundaries, and basophilic cytoplasm. On electron micrographs, the nucleus is basally located, the supranuclear cytoplasm contains numerous homogenous electron-opaque zymogen-secretory granules and Golgi complex, whereas the basolateral cytoplasm contains rough endoplasmic reticulum profiles and mitochondria. The secretory cells are organized into acini or alveoli. The parotid gland in humans is composed exclusively of serous cells. The submandibular and sublingual glands are composed of a mixture of serous and mucous cells. The former predominate in the submandibular gland, whereas the sublingual gland is composed primarily of mucous cells. Acini are separated by reticular connective tissue that contains plasma cells and lymphocytes.

Parotid Gland

The human parotid gland is formed almost exclusively of serous secretory cells arranged in acini around a central lumen that communicates with the ductal system (Fig. 11–48). Serous cells of the acinus are pyramidal, with a broad base resting on a basement membrane and a narrow apical surface facing the lumen and containing microvilli. Serous acinar cells have basal nuclei and indistinct cell boundaries. The apical cytoplasm contains secretory granules between the nucleus and the luminal surface. The secretory granules stain positive with periodic acid–Schiff stain (PAS), are rich in carbohydrates and proteins, and contain high amylase activity as well as peroxidase, DNase, and RNase. Myoepithelial cells are located between the serous cells and basal lamina. Their long cytoplasmic processes surround the serous acini in a basket-like

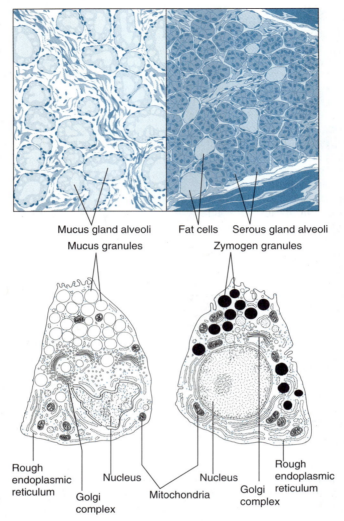

FIGURE 11–47. Secretory cells of the salivary gland. Two types of secretory cells (mucous and serous) are shown as they appear by light microscopy (top) and electron microscopy (bottom).

configuration; hence, the term basket cells. They are considered to have a contractile function, serving to expel the secretion of acinar cells into the lumen.

The parotid gland produces about one fourth of the daily output of saliva. The intercalated ducts of the parotid gland are long and well developed. The connective tissue around acini contains plasma cells and lymphocytes. The plasma cells produce the immunoglobulin IgA, which combines with a secretory component synthesized by acinar serous cells as well as the intercalated and striated duct cells to form the IgA–secretory piece complex. This complex is released into the saliva and serves as an immunologic defense function against oral pathogens. Septa that extend from the capsule separate lobes and lobules and carry secretory ducts, nerves, blood, and lymph vessels.

Submandibular (Submaxillary) Gland

The submandibular gland is a mixed serous and mucous tubuloacinar gland in which mixed seromucous acini predominate over the purely mucous acini (Fig. 11–49). The latter are uncommon in human submandibular glands. In the mixed acini, serous cells cap the mucous cells, forming crescent-shaped demilunes, whereas mucous cells are located closer to the intercalated duct. Serous cells in such acini are pyramidal and darkly staining with indistinct boundaries. Nuclei are rounded and basally located. Accumulations of rough endoplasmic reticulum are located in the basal third of the cell. The secretory granules, located apically in the cell, are PAS positive as well as rich in sialoglycoproteins and sulfated polysaccharides. They contain a lysozyme that serves to hydrolyze bacterial walls. Myoepithelial cells are located between the serous cells and the basal lamina. Serous cells of the submandibular gland are further characterized by elaborate infoldings of the lateral and basal membranes toward the vascular bed, which significantly increase the surface area and enhance electrolyte and water transport.

Mucous cells, in contrast, are cuboidal or columnar with flattened, oval nuclei pushed to the basal part of the cell by secretory droplets. They have little rough endoplasmic reticulum. Their secretory granules contain sialomucin, sulfomucin, or both. In routine histologic preparations, the cytoplasm of mucous cells appears empty or vacuolated because the secretory droplets have usually dissolved. The submandibular gland elaborates the majority (70%) of daily saliva output. Whereas the intercalated ducts are best developed in the parotid gland, the secretory (striated) ducts are best developed in the submandibular gland. A connective tissue capsule surrounds the gland. Septa containing nerves, blood, and lymphatic vessels divide the gland into lobes and lobules.

Sublingual Gland

The sublingual gland, like the submandibular gland, is a mixed serous and mucous tubuloacinar gland in which mucous acini predominate (Fig. 11–50). The sublingual gland, however, has a variable number of acini containing serous cells and serous demilunes in different parts. The mucous gland cells secrete viscid mucigen rich in sulfated polysaccharides. The serous gland cells secrete a watery product rich in sulfated glycoproteins. The histologic characteristics of mucous, serous, and myoepithelial cells are similar to those in other salivary glands.

The intralobular duct system (intercalated and secretory) are poorly developed. The intercalated ducts are composed primarily of mucous cells in the form of tubules and are linked to very short secretory (striated) ducts. Connective tissue septa extending from the connective tissue capsule carry nerves and vessels.

Ductal System

As previously mentioned, the secretory elements of the salivary glands are linked to the oral cavity via a system of ducts that are divided into three segments, intercalated, secretory (striated), and excretory (Fig. 11–51). The intercalated and secretory ducts are located in connective tissue septa within glandular lobules (intralobular), whereas the excretory ducts are

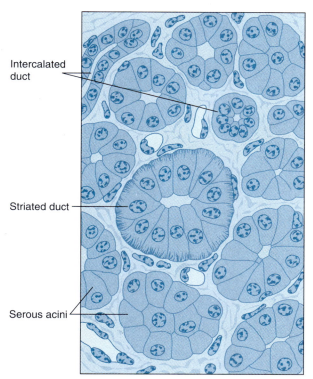

FIGURE 11–48. *Parotid gland. Note the almost exclusive presence of serous acini and the characteristically well-developed intercalated ducts. Note also the basal striations in the striated ducts.*

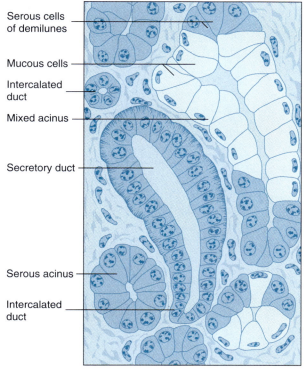

FIGURE 11–49. *Submandibular gland. Note the mixed seromucous acini that characterize this gland. Serous cells cap mucous cells in the form of demilunes. Well-developed secretory ducts characterize this gland.*

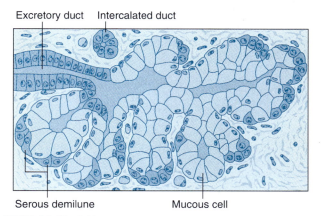

FIGURE 11–50. *Sublingual gland. Note the mixed seromucous acini that characterize this gland, and the poorly developed ductal system.*

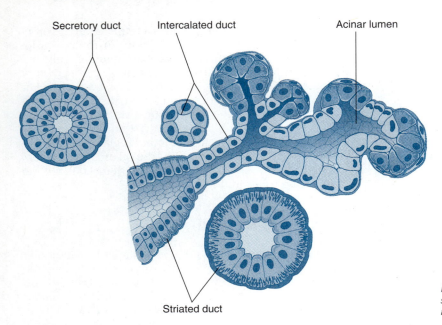

FIGURE 11-51. Ductal system of salivary glands, showing the progression from the lumen of the acinus into the intercalated and striated ducts.

located in connective tissue between lobules (interlobular). Of the intralobular ducts, the intercalated ducts are best developed in the parotid gland, but the secretory (striated) ducts are best developed in the submandibular glands. The interlobular ducts are well developed in the three salivary glands. The intercalated ducts are lined proximally by squamous cells and distally by cuboidal cells associated with myoepithelial cells within their basal laminae.

Several intercalated ducts join to form the secretory duct. The secretory ducts are lined by cuboidal to columnar cells with basal striations; hence the term striated ducts. The striations represent interdigitations or infoldings of basal plasma membrane and rows of mitochondria aligned parallel to the membrane infoldings (Fig. 11-52). These ducts are believed to be secretory and absorptive in nature and to contribute water and calcium salts to gland secretions. Secretory (striated) ducts drain into the excretory ducts. The excretory ducts are lined initially by simple columnar cells and then by pseudostratified columnar cells and stratified columnar cells; they terminate as tubes lined by stratified squamous epithelium continuous with the epithelium of the oral cavity. In addition to the lining epithelium, the ductal walls contain myoepithelial cells within their basal laminae.

PANCREAS

The pancreas is a mixed exocrine and endocrine organ. The exocrine, or digestive enzyme–producing, part of the gland is discussed in this chapter; the endocrine part is considered in Chapter 15.

The exocrine pancreas is a compound tubuloalveolar gland with purely serous acini (alveoli). The serous cells of the acini consist of pyramidal cells arranged around a central lumen. The cytoplasm is densely basophilic, reflecting specialization of these cells for protein synthesis. On electron micrographs, the basal part of serous cells contains abundant rough endoplasmic reticulum cisternae, free ribosomes, and mitochondria (Fig. 11-53). The apical cytoplasm is packed with zymogen granules. The number of zymogen granules reflects digestive activity and is highest in resting cells (fasting). The nucleus is spherical and basally located. A unique feature of pancreatic acini is the presence of centroacinar cells (Fig. 11-54); these are smaller than the serous cells, stain lighter, and are squamous to cuboidal. They are interposed between the serous cells and the lumen and are in continuity

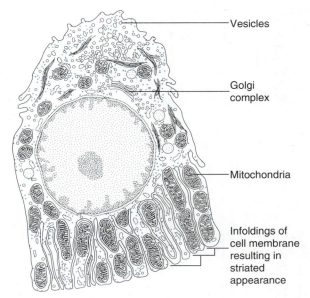

FIGURE 11-52. Striated duct cell as seen by electron microscopy. Note the formation of basal striations by interdigitations of basal plasma membrane infoldings and rows of mitochondria.

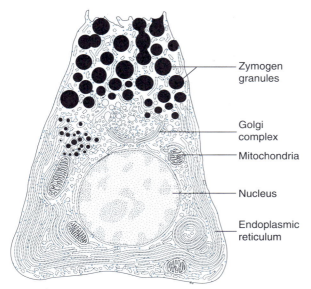

FIGURE 11–53. *Pancreatic acinar cell as seen on electron micrographs. Note zymogen granules in apical part of the cell, and condensation of endoplasmic reticulum in the basal cytoplasm.*

with intercalated ducts. They thus constitute the intra-acinar portion of the intercalated duct. The acini of the pancreas are surrounded by a basal lamina and are packed close together with an intervening delicate reticular connective tissue sheath and a rich capillary network. The pancreas is covered by a capsule of connective tissue from which thin fibrous septa extend into the gland and subdivide it into lobules and lobes. Nerve fibers, blood, and lymphatic vessels are present in the connective tissue stroma.

The ductal system of the pancreas consists of intercalated and excretory (interlobular) ducts. Secretory (striated) ducts are not present in the pancreas. The intercalated ducts are lined by cuboidal epithelium, and the excretory ducts by columnar epithelium. The main excretory duct empties into the lumen of the duodenum. The acinar cells produce the following enzymes and proenzymes: amylase, lipase, RNase, DNase, trypsinogen, chymotrypsinogen, (pro)carboxypeptidase, (pro)elastase, and (pro)phospholipase A_2. The centroacinar cells are responsible for elaborating bicarbonate-rich, slightly alkaline pancreatic fluid. The secretion of enzymes as proenzymes protects the gland from autodigestion.

Pancreatic secretion is regulated mainly by two hormones produced in endocrine cells in the base of the crypts of Lieberkühn, secretin and cholecystokinin. Both hormones are released to the circulation in response to entry of acidic gastric contents to the duodenum. Secretin stimulates the centroacinar cells and duct cells to produce copious alkaline fluid poor in enzyme activity. Cholecystokinin stimulates the acinar cells to extrude their enzymes and proenzymes into the lumen of the acinus. The alkaline pancreatic juice rich in enzymes thus serves to neutralize the acidity of gastric contents in the duodenum, allowing pancreatic enzymes to function at an optimal, neutral pH.

LIVER

The liver is the largest gland in the body. It is composed of four, incompletely separated lobes covered by a thin connective tissue capsule (Glisson's capsule) and incompletely invested by reflections of the peritoneum. The capsule is thicker at the hilum of the liver (the porta hepatis), where blood and lymphatic vessels and bile ducts enter or leave the liver. Connective tissue extensions from the capsule divide the liver into lobules and follow vessels and ducts throughout their courses in the liver up to the liver lobule, where a delicate reticular fiber network forms the supporting framework for the liver lobule.

Liver Parenchyma

The classic structural unit of liver parenchyma is the hepatic lobule, composed of anastomosing series of hepatic cords. Hepatic cords of cells radiate outward from the central vein (terminal hepatic venule) much like the spokes of a wheel (Fig. 11–55). The cells of the cords (hepatocytes) are arranged in sheets one and

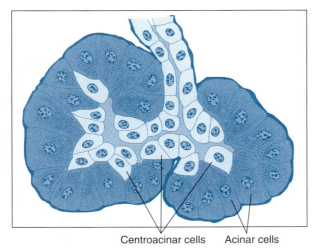

FIGURE 11–54. *Pancreatic acinus, showing the centroacinar cells that are unique to the pancreas. Note their smaller size, lighter shade, and interposition between serous acinar cells and lumen.*

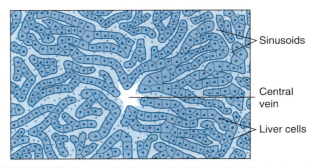

FIGURE 11–55. *Liver lobule. Note cords of liver cells radiating from the central vein and separated by sinusoids.*

two cells thick. Hepatocytes are large polyhedral cells of different sizes (Fig. 11–56). Nuclei are large, rounded, and centrally located and contain one or more prominent nucleoli and scattered clumps of chromatin. Polypoid nuclei and binucleated and multinucleated hepatocytes are found. The cytoplasm of hepatocytes varies in appearance, depending on the nutritional and functional state. It contains large amounts of ribonucleoprotein, abundant mitochondria, lipid droplets, lysosomes, and peroxisomes. Located between cellular sheets are vascular spaces (liver sinusoids) 9 to 12 μm in width. The spaces of Disse separate the surfaces of hepatic cells and endothelial cells in the walls of sinusoids. These spaces contain reticular fibers and microvilli of hepatocytes. At the interface between adjacent hepatic cells, minute bile canaliculi are formed (Fig. 11–57). The cell membranes near the canaliculi are joined by tight junctions. Thus, the surfaces of hepatocytes are in contact with other hepatocytes, bile canaliculi, or the spaces of Disse. Each hepatic lobule is a hexagonal unit with a central vein (the terminal hepatic venule) and three to six portal spaces containing a hepatic arteriole, portal venule, bile ductule, nerves, and lymphatic vessels embedded in connective tissue at the corners of the hexagon (portal triad) (Fig. 11–58).

The validity of the hepatic lobule as the basic structural-functional unit of hepatic function has been challenged. Two other structural-functional units have been proposed (see Fig. 11–58):

- The triangular or biliary unit *(portal lobule)*, the corners of which are formed of three central veins and the anatomic axis is the portal triad. It thus includes parts of three adjoining hepatic lobules.
- The *hepatic acinus*, an irregularly shaped mass of parenchymal tissue between two (or more) central veins. Its axis is a small radicle of the main portal canal between two adjacent hepatic lobules containing terminal branches of the portal triad. The acinus includes small segments of two adjacent hepatic lobules and may contain as much as one sixth of the hepatic lobule. The acinus has been subdivided into three functional zones (Fig. 11–58): Zone 1 is nearest to the blood supply (periportal). Zone 3 is nearest to and includes the central vein. Zone 2 is in between them. An oxygen gradient (from high to low) has been shown to exist between zones 1 and 3. Cells in zone 1 are thus the first to receive blood and nutrients, the first to regenerate, and the last to die. After a meal, glycogen is stored first in zone 1, later in zone 2, and last in zone 3. Conversely, glycogen is depleted first from zone 3, followed by zones 2 and 1. The administration of phenobarbital results in proliferation of smooth endoplasmic reticulum in zone 3. Continued administration spreads the effect to zone 2 and ultimately to zone 1. There is also a differential effect between zones with regard to liver damage. Zone 3 is affected by acetaminophen, halothane, carbon tetrachloride, and other agents. Fewer compounds selectively damage zone 1. Bile salts in high concentration damage zone 1 initially.

The concept of the hepatic lobule emphasizes endocrine function of the liver, whereas that of the portal lobule reflects exocrine function (bile) and that of the acinus the gradient of metabolic activity within the liver.

Liver Blood Supply

The liver receives dual blood supply from the hepatic artery and portal vein. Three fourths of the blood to the liver is supplied by the portal vein. The hepatic artery, a branch of the celiac trunk, carries oxygen-rich blood. The portal vein carries oxygen-poor, nutrient-rich blood that has already passed through the capillary beds of the gastrointestinal tract, spleen, and pancreas. These vessels enter the liver at the hilum (porta hepatis) and branch into interlobar, interlobular, and terminal vessels that travel within corresponding connective tissue septa. The terminal hepatic (perilobular) arteriole and terminal portal (perilobular) venules, located within the portal space (portal triad), contribute blood to the sinusoids either directly (hepatic arteriole) or via inlet venules (portal venule). Thus, oxygen-rich blood from the hepatic artery and oxygen-poor blood from

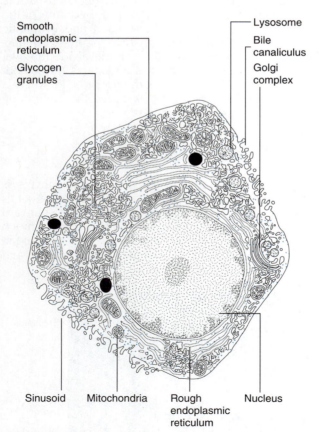

FIGURE 11–56. Hepatocyte showing a nucleus with a nucleolus and cytoplasm rich in endoplasmic reticulum, mitochondria and glycogen. Note bile canaliculi at the interface between hepatocytes.

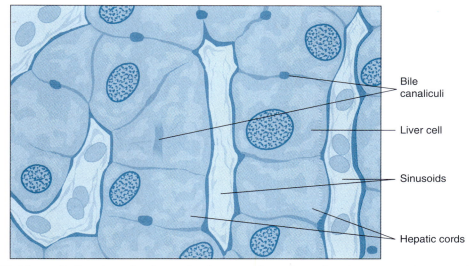

FIGURE 11-57. Bile canaliculi are located at the interface between adjacent liver cells, whereas sinusoids separate hepatic cords.

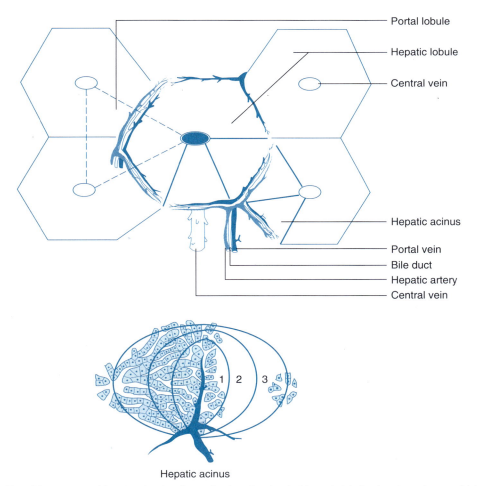

FIGURE 11-58. Liver. Top, Three structural-functional units of organization: the classical hepatic lobule, the triangular portal lobule, and the hepatic acinus. Bottom, The hepatic acinus is divided into three functional zones with diminishing oxygen gradients from zone 1 to zone 3.

the portal vein mix in the sinusoids. Sinusoids drain blood from the periphery of the hepatic lobule toward its center, the central vein (terminal hepatic venule). Outside hepatic lobules, central veins drain into the sublobular (intercalated) veins, which ultimately join the hepatic vein, which in turn drains into the inferior vena cava.

Sinusoids course between hepatic cell cords (sheets) and are lined by endothelial cells and Kupffer's cells (Fig. 11–59). The latter are large phagocytic cells belonging to the widely distributed system of fixed macrophages. They are located on the luminal surfaces of endothelial cells. The endothelial cells are separated from the adjacent hepatocytes by the space of Disse, which consists of reticular fibers, microvilli of hepatocytes, and occasional fat-storing cells (Ito cells). The function of Ito cells is not fully understood, although they have been implicated in vitamin A metabolism.

Bile Ducts

Bile is secreted by hepatocytes into bile canaliculi, minute anastomosing channels between hepatic cells (see Fig. 11–57). The bile canaliculi are lined by plasma membranes of hepatocytes. The flow of bile within canaliculi is toward the periphery of the hepatic lobule into bile ductules (Fig. 11–60) (canals of Hering), and from there into bile ducts in the portal canal. The bile ducts form the right and left hepatic ducts, which at the porta hepatis form the common hepatic duct. The latter is joined by the cystic duct to form the common bile duct (ductus choledochus), which empties into the duodenum.

Bile is secreted continuously by the liver, with a total daily output of about 500 ml, some of which is recycled once or twice during a meal rich in fat.

Liver Function

The liver is both an exocrine gland, secreting bile via a system of bile ducts into the duodenum, where it

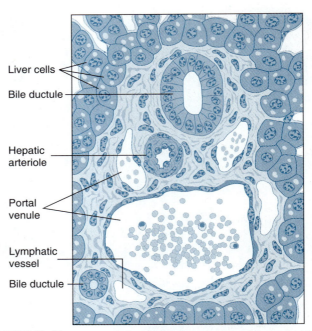

FIGURE 11–60. Portal triad showing the hepatic artery, portal vein, bile duct, and lymphatic vessel surrounded by small amount of connective tissue. Liver cells of adjacent liver lobules surround the portal area.

plays an important role in the digestive process, and an endocrine gland, synthesizing and releasing a variety of organic compounds into the blood stream. Bile is composed of water, bile salts, bile pigment, cholesterol, lecithin, fat, and inorganic salts. About a tenth of bile is synthesized by hepatic cells; the rest is simply trans-

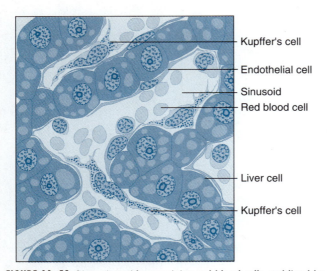

FIGURE 11–59. Liver sinusoids containing red blood cells and lined by endothelial and Kupffer's cells are seen between sheets of liver cells.

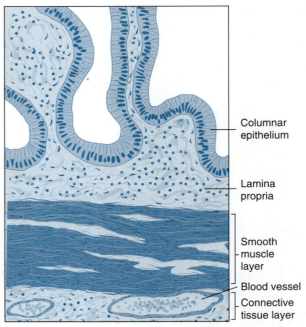

FIGURE 11–61. Gallbladder wall showing the columnar epithelium and abundant infolding of the mucosae, the loose connective tissue of the lamina propria, the smooth muscle layer, and the outer connective tissue layer with blood vessels.

ported from the blood compartment to bile canaliculi by hepatocytes. The secretion of bile into the duodenum accelerates the action of pancreatic and intestinal lipases and facilitates the absorption of fat from the intestine.

The functional importance of the liver can be appreciated by considering its blood supply. The blood supply of the liver brings to it, from the digestive tract, absorbed carbohydrates, amino acids, bile salts, and vitamins; from the pancreas, the hormones insulin and glucagon; and from the spleen, breakdown products of red blood cell destruction. The liver metabolizes digestion products, stores glycogen, fat, and vitamins (especially vitamin A), maintains blood glucose levels, synthesizes plasma protein, glucose, and bile, and degrades or detoxifies a variety of exogenous substances (drugs, toxins) and endogenous substances (steroids, other hormones). Lipids and amino acids are converted in the liver to glucose (gluconeogenesis), and amino acids are deaminated to urea.

GALLBLADDER

The gallbladder is a pear-shaped organ located on the undersurface of the right lobe of the liver. In humans, it has a capacity of 30 to 50 ml of bile. The gallbladder wall consists of the following layers: mucosa, lamina propria, muscularis, outer connective tissue layer, and serosa (Fig. 11–61).

The mucosa, composed of simple columnar epithelium, shows abundant folds when the gallbladder is empty. The apex of epithelial cells contains numerous microvilli typical of absorbing epithelium but with an added ability to produce small amounts of mucus.

The lamina propria contains loose connective tissue and small blood vessels. Near the cystic duct, the lamina propria contains mucus-secreting tubuloacinar glands, which are invaginations of the mucosa. The glands are sparse in normal tissue and increase in chronic inflammation of the gallbladder.

The muscularis is relatively thin and made up of circumferentially oriented smooth muscle.

A thick connective tissue layer binds the superior surface of the gallbladder to the liver. A typical serosa covers the surface of the gallbladder in contact with the peritoneum.

The main functions of the gallbladder are to store and concentrate bile. The process of concentration of bile is effected by osmotic absorption of water secondary to active transport of sodium (sodium pump).

Contraction of the gallbladder is induced by the hormone cholecystokinin, produced by enteroendocrine cells (I cells) located in the mucosal epithelium of the jejunum and ileum. The secretion of cholecystokinin is initiated by dietary fats.

CHAPTER TWELVE

URINARY SYSTEM

KIDNEYS 214
   Urine Production 215
   Renal Vascular System 216
   Renal Tubular System 217
   Juxtaglomerular Apparatus 222
   Renal Interstitial Tissue 222
   **The Histophysiology of Regulating
   Urine Concentration** 223

LOWER URINARY TRACT 223
   General Considerations and Epithelium 223
   **Characteristics of the Wall of the Lower
   Urinary Tract** 224
   Urethra 225
   Clinical Considerations for the Lower Urinary Tract 226

The regulation of body fluid and electrolyte balance is in large measure a function of the urinary system, which consists of paired kidneys and ureters, together with the urinary bladder and urethra. Metabolic wastes are removed from the blood by means of the glomerular filtration apparatus in the kidneys; water is conserved or excreted in this process, as dictated by tissue hydration and endocrine status. The fluid excretory product of the kidneys, urine, is transported via paired ducts, the ureters, to the urinary bladder, where it is stored. Urine is excreted to the body exterior via a single duct, the urethra, at the time of bladder constriction and emptying, a process termed *voiding*, or *micturition*. The system of urinary ducts is referred to as the *urinary tract*. In addition to the functions cited, the kidneys serve an endocrine function in the production of the hormones renin and erythropoietin. These hormones function in the regulation of blood pressure and the production of red blood cells (erythropoiesis), respectively.

In the adult, the organs of the urinary system lie within the abdomen and pelvis. During embryonic development, the kidneys and urinary tract arise in close anatomic proximity to the developing genital system; the term *genitourinary system* reflects this fact. This developmental synergy is particularly evident in the adult male, in which the urethral duct serves both the urinary and genital systems. Accordingly, *urology* is that medical specialty that treats disorders of the female urinary system and of the entire male genitourinary system.

KIDNEYS

The kidneys lie high within the abdominal cavity, beneath its peritoneal lining, spanning the level from the 12th thoracic vertebra to the 3rd lumbar vertebra. The superior pole of each kidney lies in relation to the suprarenal gland. The lateral surface is convex and smooth in the adult; the medial surface is concave and indented at the hilus, from which a connective tissue space, the renal sinus, extends deeply into the interior of the organ. As noted previously with other organs, the hilus of the kidney serves as the point at which the renal vasculature, its nerve supply, and the ureter enter and leave the organ (Fig. 12–1). The ureter has a greatly expanded upper end, the renal pelvis, which occupies most of the sinus and is supported by its connective tissue. The pelvis is subdivided into two or more intercommunicating compartments, the major calyces, which give rise to smaller subdivisions, the minor caly-

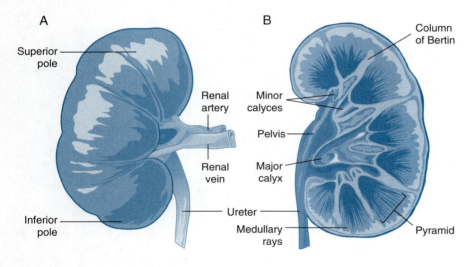
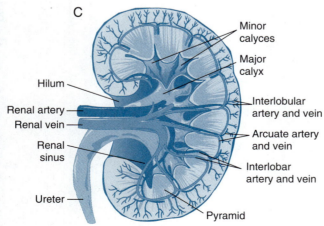

FIGURE 12–1. A, *Drawing of the right kidney, view of anterior surface. Note the relationship of the renal artery, vein, and ureter with one another at the region of the hilus.* B, *Drawing of the longitudinally hemisected human kidney. Note the anatomic relationships of the ureter with the renal pelvis, and the calyces with the medullary pyramids.* C, *Diagram of a longitudinally hemisected human kidney through the region of the hilus, showing the pattern of blood vessels within the renal sinus, medulla, and cortex.*

ces, each of which drains a single cone-shaped renal pyramid (see Fig. 12–1).

With the unaided eye, a dark brown (highly vascular) outer cortex is readily distinguished from the lighter medulla in the hemisected kidney. The cortex enfolds each conical pyramid; the cortical tissue that extends alongside the pyramids is termed a *renal column* (of Bertin). A renal pyramid, together with its overlying cortical tissue, constitutes a renal lobe. The renal lobule, however, is less readily visualized. Many tubular profiles within the cortex are collected within what appear to be radial extensions of renal medullary tissue into the cortex; these are traditionally, but inappropriately, termed *medullary rays* (Figs. 12–1 and 12–2). One of the components of the medullary ray is the collecting tubule, which drains the renal tubular system of the adjacent cortex. Consistent, therefore, with convention in defining a lobule in other organs as that portion of the parenchyma drained by a common duct, the renal lobule is centered upon a medullary ray and its collecting system, and consists of the renal tubular parenchyma that drains into it.

The tip of each pyramid is termed its *papilla*. The papilla is perforated (at the area cribrosa) by the openings of large collecting ducts (of Bellini), which drain collectively into a single minor calyx. The calyx encloses the papilla and is sealed at its margins by connective tissue and transitional epithelium. Thus, urine produced by each of the 10 to 18 lobes in the human kidney is delivered to the calyceal system of the ureter.

Urine Production

One of the principal functions of the kidney is the production of urine. Urine production depends on the

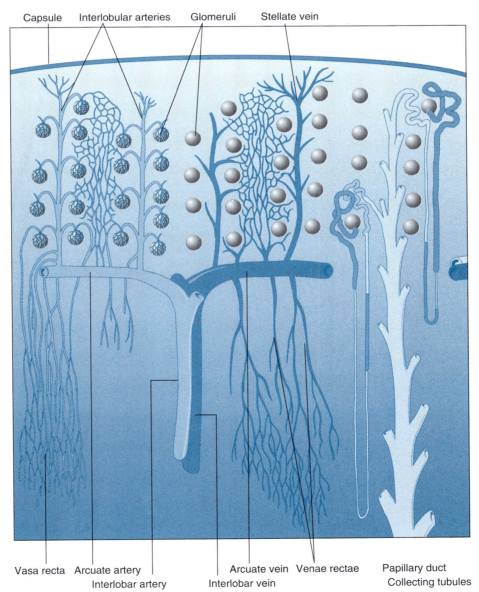

FIGURE 12-2. *Schematic diagram of a portion of kidney medulla and cortex. Note the topographical relationship of the tubular and vascular elements.*

process of filtration of the blood, with the production of a fluid ultrafiltrate. This fluid is further modified within the tubular system of the kidney by both the selective resorption and addition of ions, water, and organic molecules. Therefore, an understanding of the organization of both the renal vascular system and the renal tubular system is essential to appreciating the complex structure-function relations of these two systems in the production of urine.

Renal Vascular System

Some 1.2 L of blood flows through each kidney per minute, representing nearly one fourth of the cardiac output. Such a copious blood flow is consistent with the blood-filtering function of the kidney. The kidneys are supplied by renal arteries, direct branches of the abdominal aorta, which enter the organ at the hilus. Within the fatty connective tissue of the renal sinus, these arteries branch into smaller tributaries, which eventually course between the medullary pyramids as interlobar arteries, which in turn give rise to arteries that describe an arching course at the base of the renal pyramid (corticomedullary junction), parallel to the cortical surface. These are the arcuate arteries, and they serve as a useful topographic marker in the histology laboratory, therefore, to the division of renal cortex and medulla. Radial branches arise at regular intervals, which enter the cortical parenchyma between lobules, and are known as *interlobular arteries*. Short branches from these vessels enter the lobule as *intralobular arteries*, which, in turn, are continuous with the afferent arteriole leading to a renal glomerulus. A *glomerulus* (Fig. 12–3) is a knot or tuft of capillaries arising from the terminus of the afferent arteriole. Three-dimensionally, the glomerulus is more than loops of terminal capillaries; it is a complex branching and anastomotic network of vessels.

Blood is drained from the glomerulus by the efferent arteriole, which (in the outer cortex) gives origin to a second capillary network, the peritubular capillary network. This capillary bed supplies the cortical parenchyma and then drains via venous channels accompanying the arteries to the arcuate vein. Efferent arterioles arising from glomeruli situated in the region of the corticomedullary junction (juxtamedullary glomeruli) describe a unique course into the medulla, as straight vessels called *vasa recta* (see Fig. 12–2). The vasa recta are thin-walled, somewhat larger than usual capillaries, and they give rise to a capillary network within the medulla that supplies the medullary tubular parenchyma. The vasa recta recur, however, as hairpin loops at various levels within the medulla and return to the corticomedullary junction, where they drain to arcuate veins. A relatively few vasa recta arise directly from the

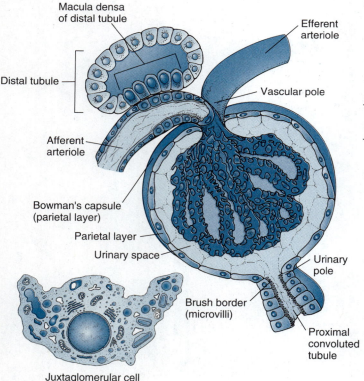

FIGURE 12–3. Top, Diagrammatic representation of the renal corpuscle. Note the vascular and urinary poles, and the relationship of the macula densa (of the distal convoluted tubule) and the juxtaglomerular cells (of the afferent arteriole) in the formation of the juxtaglomerular apparatus. Shown also are the visceral layer of podocytes covering the glomerulus and the continuity of the urinary space with the proximal convoluted tubule at the urinary pole. Bottom, Fine structural features of a juxtaglomerular cell. The cytoplasm contains secretory granules of varying size and shape, including some that contain crystalloids. Renin has been localized to the granules of the juxtaglomerular cell.

arcuate arteries, follow a similar course into and out of the medulla, and drain to the arcuate venous system (see Fig. 12–2).

Renal Tubular System

The Nephron

The *nephron*, together with the collecting tubule to which it drains, forms a structural and functional unit of the kidney, the *uriniferous tubule*. The nephron consists of several morphologically distinct portions. A dilated proximal portion, in the shape of a capsule, is Bowman's capsule. The space within the closed capsule is termed the *urinary space* (Bowman's space), which is continuous with the lumen of the subsequent portions of the nephron, respectively, the proximal convoluted tubule, the loop of Henle, and the distal convoluted tubule (see Fig. 12–6). Detailed consideration of the structure and function of the tubular portions of the nephron is deferred to a later section of this chapter.

The capsular portion of the nephron develops in close approximation with the renal glomerulus, and these two structures together form a renal (malpighian) corpuscle. It is this intimate association of the nephron with the renal blood supply that forms the basis for the renal filtration mechanism.

During fetal development, the glomerulus invaginates into the nephric capsule and becomes enveloped by a layer of specialized epithelial cells derived from the inner wall of the capsule, termed *podocytes* (Figs. 12–3 and 12–4). The outer wall of the capsule retains its unspecialized squamous epithelium and forms the parietal epithelial layer of the capsular (urinary) space. The podocyte layer is termed the *visceral layer* of the capsule (see Fig. 12–3). The site at which the afferent arteriole enters and the efferent arteriole exits the renal corpuscle is termed the *vascular pole* of the renal corpuscle, and that point of origin of the proximal convoluted tubule, 180 degrees from the vascular pole, is designated the *urinary pole* (see Fig. 12–3). Blood plasma is filtered across the glomerular capillary wall and its adherent podocyte layer, to form an ultrafiltrate that resides within the urinary space of the corpuscle and exits the corpuscle via the proximal convoluted tubule.

Electron-microscopic studies of the fine structure

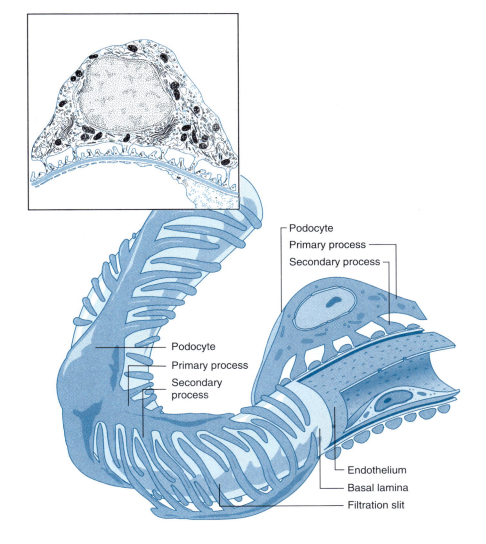

FIGURE 12–4. Schematic depiction of a scanning electron micrograph of the podocytes covering a fenestrated glomerular capillary. The branching of primary podocyte processes into secondary processes (pedicels) is shown, together with the manner in which pedicels from adjacent podocytes participate in the formation of the filtration slits that contribute to the glomerular filtration barrier. Inset, Diagram from a transmission electron micrograph of the interface between the glomerular endothelium and the overlying podocytic epithelium. The fenestrations of the capillary endothelium are shown adjacent to the thick, fused basal lamina between the endothelium and the pedicels of the podocyte.

of the renal glomerulus and the podocyte layer have defined the components of the renal filtration barrier. The cytoarchitecture of the podocytes is crucial to the formation of the barrier. Scanning electron-microscopic studies have shown elegantly that podocyte cell bodies give rise to primary and secondary cell processes, the latter being termed *pedicels* (see Fig. 12–4). Pedicels from adjacent podocytes interdigitate in their placement upon the glomerular endothelium, leaving 25-nm spaces or filtration slits between them, which are in turn closed by a thin diaphragm. The stability of the filtration slits is enhanced by the presence of numerous cytoskeletal elements (microfilaments and microtubules) within the pedicels. Cytoplasmic organelles of the podocytes also include a prominent Golgi apparatus and vesicles, elements of rough endoplasmic reticulum, and numerous free ribosomes. The basal lamina of the pedicel processes and that of the fenestrated glomerular capillary endothelium are fused, forming a thick (0.1 to 0.3 μm) layer, which exhibits a central dense zone (lamina densa) bounded on each side by a lamina rara. Electron-cytochemical studies have localized heparan sulfate, a polyanionic glycosaminoglycan, to the lamina rara.

The structural barrier to passage from blood into urinary space therefore, consists first of the fenestrated capillary endothelium (Fig. 12–5). The endothelium bears large fenestrae (70 to 90 nm) that lack the closing diaphragms typical of other fenestrated endothelia and offers little resistance to the passage of water, ions, and most small proteins. The second filtration level consists of the fused basal laminae of collagen type IV filaments of the endothelium and podocyte layer; and a third lies in the filtration slits between adjacent pedicel processes. In addition to these physical barriers, a charge barrier deriving from the anionic molecules in the basal lamina and from a polyanionic sialoprotein (podocalyxin) of the podocyte surface coat are hypothesized to impede the passage of charged molecules. Thus, the barrier becomes progressively more fine and discriminating as it is crossed: the formed elements of blood are excluded at the level of the endothelium, whereas water and ions pass the fenestrae unimpeded.

At the level of the basal lamina, the passage of particles greater in size than approximately 10 nm is impeded, as are negatively charged molecules, particularly those larger than 70 kD. Of clinical significance is the observation, in diabetes mellitus and membranous nephropathy, of a greatly thickened glomerular basement membrane that is disrupted in its structure and possibly altered in its charge characteristics. The filtration barrier is rendered leaky even to high-molecular-weight proteins. The condition of excessive loss of protein in the urine is known clinically as *proteinuria*. Also worthy of clinical note is the involvement of podocyte abnormalities in recognized kidney disease (nephropathy, or nephrosis). In a renal disease of childhood, minimal change nephropathy, the light-microscopic appearance of the glomerulus is little changed, but electron-microscopic examination reveals that the regular arrangement of pedicels is disrupted and a nearly continuous sheet of podocyte cytoplasm sheathes the glomerular capillaries. Polyanionic charge is also lost, perhaps explaining the leakiness of the barrier to protein.

A third population of cells that reside within the renal corpuscle are *mesangial cells* (also termed *lacis cells*). These cells are insinuated between adjacent loops of the glomerular capillaries and are enclosed within the basal lamina of the endothelium; they send cytoplasmic extensions between the endothelial cells that reach the capillary lumen. Their many processes are surrounded by a copious extracellular matrix, which bears a resemblance to the glomerular basal lamina, with which it becomes continuous at certain points of attachment to the glomerulus. Hypothesized functions include (1) support of the glomerular system of capillaries, (2) a possible role in the regulation of blood flow through the glomerulus (mesangial cells contain myosin-like filaments in their cytoplasm and have angiotensin II receptors), (3) a hypothesized phagocytic function of scavenging the basal lamina for particulates trapped during the filtration process, and (4) a possible role in maintaining the integrity of the basal lamina. These cells are also recognized as contributors to certain nephropathies, such as mesangial glomerulonephritis, in which the mesangial cells proliferate avidly, compressing the glomerular capillaries.

Proximal Convoluted Tubule

Glomerular ultrafiltrate leaves the urinary space of Bowman's capsule at the urinary pole, via the proximal convoluted tubule. The epithelium and basal lamina of the tubule are continuous with the simple squamous, parietal epithelium of Bowman's capsule and its basal lamina (see Fig. 12–3). The proximal tubule is the longest of the nephric tubules (some 14 mm) and therefore histologically is the most commonly observed tubular profile within the renal cortex. The tubule consists of a tortuous, convoluted portion, which is confined to the cortex, and a straight portion, which traverses the cortex within its adjacent medullary ray and becomes

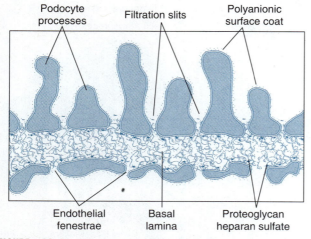

FIGURE 12–5. *Diagrammatic representation of the structural components of the renal glomerular filtration barrier. Note the interposition of the thickened basal lamina between the glomerular endothelium and the pedicels of the podocyte.*

the thick descending portion of the loop of Henle (Fig. 12–6).

The proximal tubule is lined with a simple cuboidal to columnal epithelium, which bears conspicuous, tall (1-μm) microvilli on its apical surface. Often following routine histologic fixation, the cross-sectional profiles of proximal tubules appear irregular and puckered, with the microvilli from opposite cells within the tubule obscuring the lumen. Electron-microscopic studies of optimally fixed tissue, however, demonstrate the open nature of the lumen of these tubules. The microvilli form such a distinct apical feature on these cells that early microscopists coined the term *brush border* to describe it. Lateral cell boundaries are indistinct, reflecting the presence of interdigitating lateral cell membranes between adjacent cells. Tight junctions occur between the apical lateral margins of adjacent cells, preventing the free intercellular passage of large molecules. Numerous apical canaliculi are evident between the bases of the microvilli; vesicles forming from the canaliculi transport macromolecules into the cytoplasm, where they fuse with lysosomal vesicles. Here, macromolecules (particularly low-molecular-weight proteins) undergo degradation. Amino acids are returned to the interstitium and the systemic circulation. Also, the basal plasmalemma of the epithelial cells exhibits infoldings from adjacent cells, often in association with elongated mitochondria. Such a configuration greatly increases the surface area of the basal membrane and is commonly associated with active transport of ions across epithelia. The cytoplasm is decidedly acidophilic, reflecting the presence within it of numerous mitochondria. Owing to the large size of the cells composing the epithelial lining of the proximal tubule, the spherical nuclei are frequently missing from one or more of the cells in a cross-sectional profile.

FUNCTIONAL CONSIDERATIONS. Normally, only 1 ml of the 125 ml of glomerular filtrate formed per minute is ultimately excreted as urine. This reduction in volume is accomplished by tubular resorption of vast quantities of fluid and macromolecules daily. It is within the proximal tubule that some 85% of the water and NaCl of the glomerular filtrate is resorbed, transported across the basal lamina to the interstitium, and returned to the systemic circulation. Likewise, all glucose is normally resorbed by the proximal tubule. In diabetes mellitus, however, the amount of glucose in the filtrate exceeds the ability of the proximal tubule to resorb it, and glucose is carried through the length of the uriniferous tubule to the collecting ducts, where it is released with urine, a condition termed *glycosuria*. The magnitude of this physiologic feat of tubular resorption is appreciated from the calculations of the amount of glucose, salt, and water resorbed from glomerular filtrate in one day

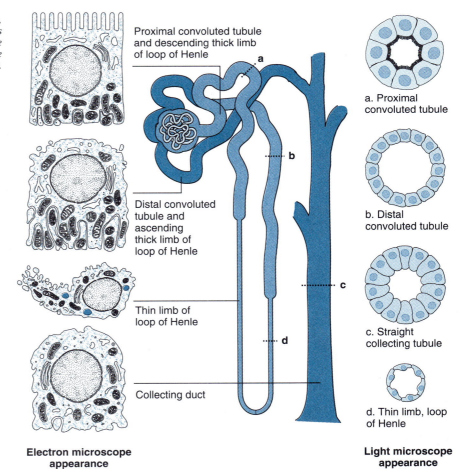

FIGURE 12–6. *Diagram of a uriniferous tubule, illustrating histologic and fine structural details of major portions of the tubule.* Right, *The light-microscopic appearance of transverse sections through various levels of the tubule.* Left, *details of tubular fine structure.*

in the human—an astounding half pound of glucose, over three pounds of sodium chloride, and nearly 160 L of water.

Fluid resorption across the proximal tubule is facilitated by the greatly increased surface area accorded the cell by its many apical microvilli, lateral interdigitations, and basal infoldings. Water moves into the proximal tubule from the tubular lumen as a consequence of the high osmotic pressure generated by the action of the laterally and basally located sodium-potassium (Na^+/K^+) ATPase pump. Water and solutes may utilize a paracellular route through the epithelium and across the apical junctional complexes, or a transcellular route of diffusion through the apex of the cell and then across the lateral cell membrane to gain access to the lateral intercellular space. This movement is osmotically driven by the active transport of sodium into the lateral intercellular space by the Na^+/K^+ ATPase pump. The pump itself is driven by means of energy supplied by the numerous mitochondria intimately associated with the membranous infoldings in the region of the pump. Among other moieties resorbed by the proximal tubule by the transcellular route are proteins, polypeptides, and amino acids, and larger carbohydrates. Glucose, however, is thought to be resorbed via the sodium pump route cited above.

It must be recalled that the nephron alters glomerular filtrate not only by resorption but also by secretion and excretion. For example, the proximal tubule actively secretes a number of molecules and detectable dyes (e.g., creatinine, para-aminohippuric acid [PAH], phenol red, and Diodrast) across its epithelium and into the tubular lumen. This feature facilitates clinical assessment of both kidney function and renal blood flow. The kidney removes other substances, the waste products of metabolism, from the body by excretion. For example, urea, uric acid, and creatinine are only partially resorbed, are allowed to pass through the uriniferous tubular system, and are excreted in the urine.

Loop of Henle

The loop of Henle is traditionally described as a U-shaped tubular structure consisting of thick descending and ascending limbs and an intervening thin limb. Typically, the loop descends out of the cortex within a medullary ray as the straight portion of the proximal tubule. The thin portion descends to a point within the medulla that is determined by the position of its renal corpuscle of origin within the cortex, and then the loop turns back upon itself in a hairpin loop and ascends toward the cortex within the same medullary ray as the straight portion of the distal tubule. There is great variation in the relative length of the thin limb in the human kidney, however, depending upon the location within the cortex of the nephron's renal corpuscle. Those nephrons originating closest to the medullary junction are termed *juxtaglomerular nephrons*. Approximately one seventh of the nephrons are so placed, and they are characterized as having exceedingly long, thin limbs that reach deep into the renal medulla before recurring (Fig. 12–7). The nephrons originating from

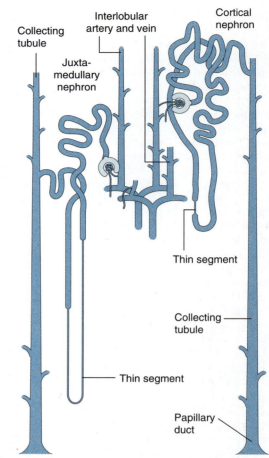

FIGURE 12–7. Schematic drawing of cortical and juxtaglomerular nephrons. Note the morphology and relative length of the loop of Henle in the two classes of nephron.

renal corpuscles more peripherally located in the cortex exhibit much shorter loops of Henle, so much so that a few may be contained entirely within the cortex. Their descending thin limbs are short, and they may exhibit no ascending thin portion (see Fig. 12–7).

The transitions between thick and thin limbs occur abruptly; the tubule is greatly reduced in overall diameter (to about 12 μm, one fifth the diameter of the proximal tubule), and its epithelium changes abruptly to simple squamous cells, lacking a brush border (see Fig. 12–6). The lumina of thin limbs are open and resemble in size the capillaries of the medulla, the vasa recta (see Fig. 12–6). The lining epithelial cells exhibit few surface and cytoplasmic specializations. The lining epithelia of the thick limbs within the medulla, however, retain those specialized features typical of the proximal and distal tubules with which they are continuous.

FUNCTIONAL CONSIDERATIONS. Formerly, the thin ascending limb was ascribed a function inconsistent with its fine structure, namely active transport of sodium. It is, rather, the epithelium lining the thick ascending portion of the loop of Henle that consistently exhibits the numerous deep basal and lateral infoldings of its plasma membrane, in association with mitochondria, that lodges an active transport system for chloride ion.

When Cl^- is pumped from the tubular lumen to the medullary interstitium, Na^+ follows passively. As discussed in a later section, this mechanism is crucial to the maintenance of the hyperosmolarity of the medullar interstitium and to the consequent ability of the kidney to produce a urine that is hypertonic to blood plasma.

Distal Tubule

The distal nephric tubule consists of three distinct portions:

- The straight portion, noted already as the ascending thick limb of the loop of Henle. It resides within the medulla and traverses a medullary ray as it hones on the cortex, specifically to its "parent" renal corpuscle—that from which its nephron arose.
- The macular portion, at the vascular pole of its originating renal corpuscle.
- The convoluted portion, which traces a circuitous route of short loops back to the periphery of the lobule. There it joins with the collecting tubule that descends from the cortex to the medulla in a medullary ray.

The straight and convoluted portions are similar in morphology, i.e., a cuboidal epithelium that lacks both the intense acidophilia and brush border of the epithelium in the companion proximal tubule. The distal tubules may be distinguished from the proximal in three ways: (1) their lumina are relatively more patent, (2) their epithelial cells are smaller, and (3) they show more nuclei per cross-sectional profile than proximal tubules. The basal specializations of the epithelium and their significance to the cytophysiology of the distal tubule have been noted previously in relation to the loop of Henle.

The cells of the macular region are distinct both topographically and fine-structurally from the remainder of the epithelium. The tubular profile is flattened on the side adjacent to the afferent arteriole, and the nuclei of the lining cells appear more numerous and crowded, thus giving the appearance of a dense spot (macula) within the distal tubule (see Fig. 12–3). The macula must be conceptualized in three dimensions as an elliptical disk of cells somewhat taller than those lining the adjacent portions of the distal tubule. The fine structure and hypothesized functional significance of these cells are considered in the section on the juxtaglomerular apparatus.

FUNCTIONAL CONSIDERATIONS. In the convoluted portion, as in the straight portion already considered, the epithelium functions in active ionic transport. It is within the convoluted portion of the distal tubule (as well as the proximal convoluted tubule) that aldosterone, a steroid mineralocorticoid from the zona glomerulosa of the adrenal cortex, exerts its principal effect on electrolyte and acid-base balance. In the presence of aldosterone, the cells of the distal convoluted tubule actively resorb Na^+ from the tubular fluid, and secrete K^+ into it. Likewise, bicarbonate ion is resorbed from the hypotonic urine of the distal tubule, and hydrogen ion is secreted, thus acidifying the urine. We have noted previously the remarkable 1.2 kg of sodium reclaimed daily by the kidney as a result of this mechanism, and the normal daily loss of only milligram amounts of sodium in the urine.

The uniqueness of the anatomy of the blood vascular network of the kidney (see Fig. 12–2), has already been described. The uriniferous tubules are almost exclusively dependent for their vascular supply upon the tubular network of capillaries arising from the efferent arteriole of the renal corpuscle. Thus, tubular hypoxia and damage can readily occur in the presence of arterial or glomerular disease that impairs glomerular blood flow. Severe chronic hypoxia may lead to the clinical condition of *chronic renal failure*, resulting in debilitating systemic electrolyte and fluid imbalance. Quite aside from glomerular disease, reduced blood flow to the tubular vascular bed is frequently seen clinically in the case of massive hemorrhage, low blood pressure resulting from cardiac failure, and reduced blood pressure following a myocardial infarction. Lowered blood volume or pressure significantly compromises glomerular filtration as well, resulting in reduced urine production (oliguria). Tubular hypoxia may impair active transport, secretory, and excretory functions of the nephric tubules noted earlier, precipitating the clinical condition of *acute renal failure*. Although no new renal corpuscles are thought to be produced postnatally, the nephron itself has remarkable potential for repair following ischemic episodes that may induce acute tubular necrosis or, for example, the hours of interrupted blood supply and tubular necrosis that occur during renal transplantation.

Collecting Tubules and Ducts

Acidified, dilute urine is transported from the distal convoluted tubule to a straight collecting tubule, via a short arched collecting tubule located at the periphery of the renal lobule, adjacent to the medullary ray in which the collecting tubule courses to the medulla. Deep in the medulla, the collecting tubules are confluent with others, resulting in the formation of progressively larger collecting ducts. These drain to straight, terminal papillary ducts of Bellini, which in turn perforate the surface of the medullary papilla at the area cribrosa and deliver urine into the minor calyx embracing the papilla (see Fig. 12–6).

The collecting tubules within medullary rays have an overall diameter somewhat less than that of the straight portions of the proximal tubule but also have a much lower, simple cuboidal epithelium devoid of apical microvilli and, consequently, a more patent lumen. The principal (clear) cells lining the tubules stain faintly with routine stains and exhibit a paucity of cytoplasmic organelles. A clear halo encircling the nucleus, together with a bulging (cobblestone) appearance of the apical cell surface, may represent helpful artifacts by which to distinguish collecting tubules from other segments of the uriniferous tubule within the medullary ray. The lateral cell boundaries of these cells are distinct, reflecting few lateral interdigitations of the adjacent cell membranes of the lining cells. Although basal infoldings of the plasma membrane are present in the smaller tubules, they are lost in the more distal portions of the collecting system. In addition to the majority of clear cells, dark or intercalated cells are found within the lining epithelium. Although they possess numerous mitochondria, exhibit numerous apical microvilli, and become more numerous in the distal portions of the collecting duct system, the significance of these dark cells has yet to be determined. The epithelium gradually increases in height as the terminal portions of the collecting system are reached; the ducts of Bellini exhibit a tall columnar epithelium at their terminations. Their lining epithelium is reflected onto the surface of the papilla at the area cribrosa.

FUNCTIONAL CONSIDERATIONS. The collecting tubules and ducts, once considered passive conduits of urine to the calyces, are vital to the final concentration of urine, and therefore, the regulation of body fluid balance. In the presence of sufficient levels of pituitary antidiuretic hormone (ADH, vasopressin), the collecting ducts are rendered permeable to water; water is thus moved osmotically to the exceedingly hypertonic medullary interstitium, where it is returned to the vascular system through the vasa recta. In the absence of sufficient ADH (as in diabetes insipidus), the epithelium is impermeable to water; water is retained in the collecting duct system, and vast quantities of dilute urine are produced and voided. Additional clinical conditions involving the collecting ducts are papillary necrosis (death and sloughing of the distal ends of the medullary papillae), infection (often retrograde from the bladder via the calyces and papilla), and the deposition of crystals within the ducts. This last condition is observed in gout and hypercalcemia, with the respective obstructive deposition of urate and calcium crystals. Because the nephron and collecting duct system develop from separate embryonic anlagen, the possibility exists that the proper joining of the two duct systems may fail. If such failure occurs, fluid-filled cysts form within the cortical tissue, giving rise to the condition known as *polycystic kidney*.

Juxtaglomerular Apparatus

The juxtaglomerular (JG) apparatus (or complex) is frequently described as comprising two populations of cells residing within the region of the vascular pole of renal corpuscles, namely, the macula densa and juxtaglomerular cells. Given their close topographic relationship with this same region, however, it is not unlikely that mesangial cells should be included, as well, in this functional complex.

Juxtaglomerular cells are myoepithelial cells derived from the smooth muscle of the tunica media of the afferent arteriole. The apices of JG cells lie in contact with the endothelium of the afferent arteriole; basally, they abut the attenuated basal lamina that lies between them and the cells of the macula densa. They contain fine structural features, including rough endoplasmic reticulum, a prominent Golgi complex, and conspicuous secretory granules, subpopulations of which may be distinguished at the electron-microscopic level. Degranulation of the cells may be induced experimentally by renal ischemia and altered salt intake, procedures that also promote increased systemic blood pressure. Conclusive evidence for the content of the secretory granules of JG cells has come from immunocytochemical studies, which have localized renin exclusively within them.

Renin is a hormone that acts upon angiotensinogen, a plasma protein (alpha$_2$ globulin of hepatic origin), to form an inactive decapeptide, angiotensin I. By means of a converting enzyme secreted within the lung, angiotensin I is converted to the octapeptide angiotensin II. This molecule is a potent vasoconstrictor of arterioles; resultant peripheral vascular resistance raises systemic blood pressure. Renin also stimulates aldosterone secretion from the adrenal zona glomerulosa, which augments sodium retention, promotes expanded fluid volume, and increases blood pressure. Decreased blood pressure deriving from such causes as dehydration activates this process, which has been termed the *renin–angiotensin II–aldosterone mechanism* of blood pressure regulation. Imbalances in this intricate system caused by renal disease may underlie the chronic clinical syndrome, renal hypertension.

The *macula densa* was defined previously as consisting of specialized epithelial cells of the distal tubule, where it lies in apposition with JG cells of the afferent arteriole. Interestingly, the Golgi of the macula densa cells is basally located, toward the JG cells, rather than apically toward the tubular lumen as it is in the lining cells of the remainder of the distal tubule. Changes in the enzymatic activities of the macula densa cells during experimental alterations of renin release from the JG cells strongly suggest the functional interrelatedness of these two cell populations. It has been hypothesized that the two cell populations act as a dynamic feedback circuit in which the arteriolar JG cells may serve as stretch or baroreceptors in monitoring reductions in blood volume or pressure and that the macula densa cells may integrate information about the osmotic pressure or ionic content of the fluid of the distal tubule.

Renal Interstitial Tissue

The interstitial (intertubular) connective tissue of the kidney cortex and medulla contains at least five specialized cell types not encountered in typical areolar connective tissue beds. Their function is not known, but several of these types exhibit a fine-structural morphology consistent with their serving a secretory function. They have been suggested in the past, without confirmation, as possible sources of medullary prostaglandins and antihypertensive factor. Additionally, interstitial cells (as well as cortical tubules and mesangial cells) have been cited as possible candidates for production of the hormone erythropoietin, which stimulates erythrocyte production in the bone marrow. The interstitium of cortical lobules has been shown in optimally preserved tissue to contain an extensive system of renal lymphatics, previously neglected morphologically and in hypotheses of renal histophysiology.

The Histophysiology of Regulating Urine Concentration

In the foregoing discussions of glomerular filtration and tubular function, it was observed that a crucial role of the ascending thick limb of the loop of Henle was to pump chloride into the medullary interstitium, thereby establishing and maintaining a gradient of hypertonicity within the surrounding interstitium. This mechanism of moving (1) water passively into the descending thin limb and (2) salt passively out of the ascending thin limb and actively out of the ascending thick limb is collectively termed the *countercurrent multiplier system.*

It is currently believed that the gradient established by the action of the pump in the ascending thick loop of Henle applies principally to the outer medullary and inner cortical regions, because of the anatomic placement there of the thick ascending limbs (see Fig. 12–7). The intense hypertonicity of the papillary region of the medulla, however, is better attributed to the *passive* movement to the interstitium of sodium and chloride ions from the *ascending thin limbs* placed there, augmented by the *passive movement of urea* from the *collecting ducts* into the interstitium (the collecting duct being permeable both to water and to urea). By such means, the papillary interstitium achieves a hypertonicity some four times that of blood plasma and serves as a powerful osmotic force to draw water from the collecting ducts into the interstitium. The crowning beauty of the system is contained in the anatomic superimposition of the loops of vasa recta over the loops of the limbs of Henle (Fig. 12–8), providing the basis for a *countercurrent exchange mechanism* between the collecting ducts and the blood vascular system. By means of this arrangement of "give on the downstroke and take on the upstroke," the gradient of hypertonicity established within the medulla is not disrupted as it would be if straight vessels served the medulla. Rather, on their downward course, the vasa lose water and gain sodium, and on the upward swing, they gain water and lose salt, achieving the required removal of water from the interstitium at no expense to the interstitial salt gradient. This interrelationship is summarized in diagrammatic form in Figure 12–9.

LOWER URINARY TRACT

The *lower urinary tract* refers to the closed system of spaces and ducts that collect, store, and excrete urine distal to the renal papilla. The term is a misnomer, because intrarenal structures (the renal calyces and pelvis of the ureter) are included in the designation in addition to the more distal ureters, bladder, and urethra. As mundane as these conducting and storage structures may seem in comparison with the complexities of the mechanisms of urine formation, they are

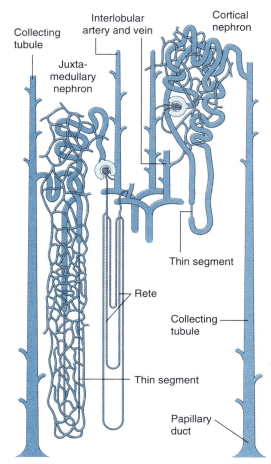

FIGURE 12–8. *Schematic representation of the relationship of the renal vasculature with those portions of uriniferous tubules depicted in Figure 12–7. Note particularly the relationship of the vasa recta and the thin limbs of the loops of Henle in the medulla.*

crucial to the excretory process as well as to social acceptability and are of clinical significance because of their susceptibility to obstruction and infection.

General Considerations and Epithelium

All of these organs have certain similarities in their structural organization. They are lined by an impermeable epithelium, *transitional epithelium* or *urothelium,* which successfully withstands the acidity and hypertonicity of urine and is capable of even heroic distention without compromised integrity. Details of the structure of transitional epithelium are given in Chapter 2; and it suffices here to note that the epithelium varies in thickness from two or three cell layers in the minor calyces to five or six layers in the undistended urinary bladder. In the undistended state, the surface facet (outer lining) cells have rounded apical contours, which tend to bulge into the bladder cavity. Depending upon the degree of distention, the number of cell layers within the bladder epithelium may be reduced to two or three

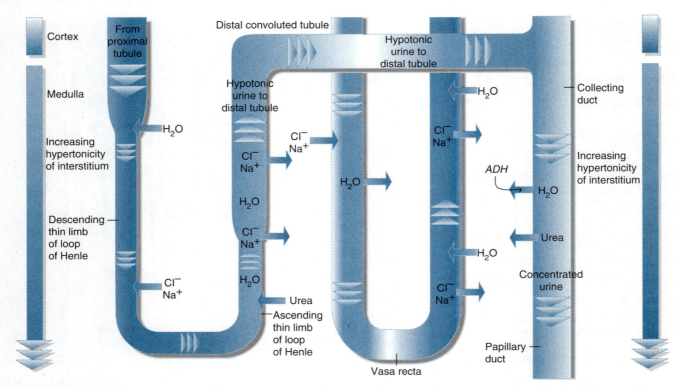

FIGURE 12–9. Schematic representation of the means by which the loop of Henle, collecting ducts, and vasa recta participate in the renal countercurrent multiplier and exchange mechanisms (see text). Note particularly (1) that Na^+ and Cl^- are transported to the interstitium passively from the ascending thin limb, and actively from the ascending thick limb of the loop of Henle, thus establishing a gradient of hyperosmolarity within the medulla which is greatest at the papilla; and (2) that urea also enters the medullary interstitium from the distal collecting ducts and augments the hyperosmolarity of the deep medulla, and recirculates to the nephron through the thin limb of the loop of Henle.

As a result of this countercurrent multiplication of medullary osmolarity, (1) water is drawn osmotically from the collecting duct into the hypertonic medullary interstitium (responsive to ADH control of the permeability of the collecting duct to water); and (2) interstitial fluid is drawn osmotically into the ascending (venous) loop of the vasa recta and thus is removed from the medulla. These countercurrent exchanges of ions and water between the interstitium and the loops of vasa recta concentrate the urine within the collecting ducts. The concentrated urine is excreted into the pelvicalyceal system through the papillary ducts.

layers of squamous cells. Such transitions in thickness and shape are the hallmarks for which this epithelium is named. Electron-microscopically, the free surface of the surface facet cells exhibits a scalloped appearance, owing to the presence of vesicles of various sizes and contour within the superficial cytoplasm (see Fig. 12–11). These vesicles and associated glycoprotein plates are hypothesized to serve as reservoirs of membrane for fusion with, or retraction from, the surface membrane of the surface facet cells as required.

Characteristics of the Wall of the Lower Urinary Tract

The epithelium is underlaid by a tunica propria; together they constitute the lining mucosa. In the ureter, the mucosa assumes a puckered appearance, which assists in its identification at low magnification (Fig. 12–10). No muscularis mucosae or distinct submucosa is present in the urinary tract, and intrinsic glands are lacking except in the urethra. Smooth muscle is present to a varying degree in all portions of the lower tract. The ureters propel urine distally by means of vigorous peristalsis, and the bladder contracts forcefully at the time of micturition. The ureters exhibit, in their upper and middle portions, a double layer of smooth muscle, arranged in what appears in histologic transverse section to be inner longitudinal and outer circular layers. Critical studies, however, have shown these to consist

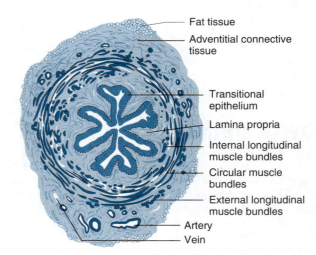

FIGURE 12–10. Depiction of the histologic features of the human ureter in cross-section, from its lower third. The stellate configuration of the mucosa is typical of the contracted ureter. Three layers of smooth muscle permit the generation of a powerful peristaltic wave.

of loose and tight helically arranged layers, respectively. A third, longitudinal layer is added to this pattern in the distal ureter where it meets the bladder (see Fig. 12–10). The outermost layer covering the lower tract is an adventitia, except for the superior portion of the urinary bladder, which is covered by a reflection of the peritoneum. Because of their shapes, both the pelvicalyceal region and the urinary bladder are difficult to characterize in terms of the arrangement in their walls of smooth muscle layers. The bladder is usually described as having three muscle layers: (1) an innermost layer, which is coextensive with the ureter's inner longitudinal layer, (2) a middle layer, which blends with the ureter's middle circular layer, and (3) an outer longitudinal layer. This arrangement is difficult to appreciate in histologic section, however, owing to the obliquity with which these layers are cut in a single section through the wall of a spherical organ (Fig. 12–11). The innermost (longitudinal) layer of smooth muscle forms a sphincter at the neck of the bladder that is under involuntary reflex control. Voluntary sphincters of striated muscle encircle the urethra, and coordinated relaxation of the voluntary and involuntary sphincters allows micturition to occur.

Urethra

Significant differences in the morphology of the male and female urethra exist. The female urethra is short (only 25 to 30 mm) and conducts urine from the bladder to the perineum. Its epithelial lining is principally the stratified squamous, mucosal variety. It is underlaid by a thick tunica propria rich in venous channels. Mucous glands occur as outpocketings within the mucosa and empty directly onto the mucosal surface. The prominent mass of smooth muscle in the urethral wall is organized into inner longitudinal and outer circular layers. Where it passes through the pelvic diaphragm, the wall acquires a sphincteric layer of skeletal muscle, representing the voluntary sphincter.

The male urethra serves as the common conduit for both the urinary and reproductive tracts. Some 20 to 25 cm long, it has three anatomically distinct portions

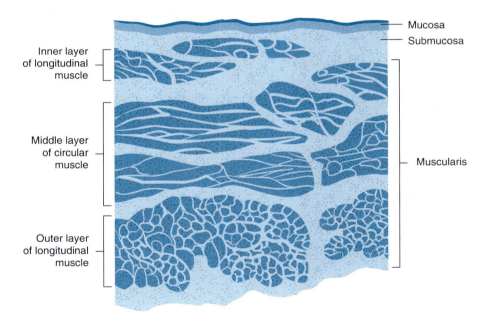
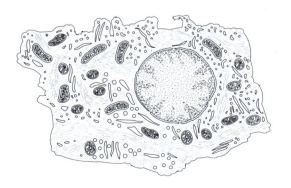

FIGURE 12–11. Top, Depiction of the histologic features of the bladder wall. A thin mucosa is present in this specimen fixed in the distended state; the three smooth muscle layers of the wall are shown clearly in this fortuitous section normal to their plane of orientation. Bottom, Drawing of the fine structural features of a surface facet cell as seen with transmission electron microscopy. Vesicles of various size and shape, together with microfilaments, are found in the peripheral cytoplasm; the vesicles may serve as a depot of membrane that facilitates epithelial distention and contraction.

and a more complex morphology than the female urethra. These named portions are the prostatic, membranous, and penile (pendulous; pars spongiosum).

In the male, the prostate gland abuts the bladder inferiorly at its neck, and the first portion of the urethra, the prostatic urethra, is completely enclosed by the gland (see Chapter 17). The posterior wall bears a central elevation, the colliculus seminalis (verumontanum), into which a small diverticulum, the utriculus prostaticus (male homolog of the female uterus) is inserted. The ejaculatory ducts course through the substance of the prostate gland and empty on either side of the utriculus. The prostatic ducts also empty into the prostatic urethra. The entire prostatic urethra is lined with urothelium. At the inferior margin of the prostate gland, the urethra emerges and courses as the membranous urethra through the pelvic diaphragm of skeletal muscle to the bulb of the corpus spongiosum of the penis. Skeletal muscle fibers form a sphincteric ring around the membranous urethra, the voluntary urethral sphincter. This portion is short—less than 20 mm in length—and receives the ducts of Cowper's glands (see also Chapter 17). The epithelium of the membranous urethra is variable, with the stratified or pseudostratified columnar type predominating. The penile urethra, some 15 cm in length, exhibits a similar epithelial morphology, interspersed with patches of stratified squamous mucosal variety. The penile urethra is surrounded by erectile tissue; the epithelium typically is thrown into many recesses, which assist in its histologic identification. Like that of the female urethra, the epithelium contains pockets of mucous secretory cells, named in the male the glands of Littre. A terminal dilatation of the penile urethra is the fossa navicularis, which is lined with stratified squamous epithelium coextensive with the surface lining of the glans penis (see Chapter 17).

Clinical Considerations for the Lower Urinary Tract

There is no anatomic valve or sphincter present at the site of entry of the ureter into the bladder (the vesicoureteric junction). Rather, the ureters pass through the posterolateral bladder wall obliquely, which normally assures closure of the ureteric lumen in the distended bladder as a result of both muscular compression and the acute angulation of the ureter as it enters the bladder wall. Urine is thus prevented from traveling retrograde up the ureter to the upper portions of the urinary tract. If the union of ureter and bladder is developmentally compromised or damaged owing to infection, however, such urinary reflux may occur up the ureter to the calyces. In this way, urine from an infected bladder may transmit infection to the kidney, resulting in pyelonephritis. If reflux is chronic, even in the absence of infection, stagnant urine may pool in the renal pelvis (hydronephrosis), and hydrostatic pressure is transmitted to the renal parenchyma, resulting in renal atrophy or necrosis and consequent severe impairment of renal function. Chronic obstruction of the ureter, such as in the case of renal calculi (kidney stones) lodged in the ureter, promotes the same end result, i.e., hydrostatic pressure atrophy of renal tissue. Tumors of the urinary bladder are not uncommon and are diagnosed in the vast majority of cases as carcinomas of the urothelium.

CHAPTER THIRTEEN

Respiratory System

Airway	228
Epithelium	228
Respiratory Tract	229
Nasal Cavity	229
Associated Nasal Sinuses	230
Nasopharynx and Oropharynx	230
Larynx	230
Vocal Apparatus	230
Trachea	231
Bronchi and Bronchial Tree	231
Bronchi	232
Bronchioles	232
Alveolar Ducts	233
Alveoli	234
Cells of the Interalveolar Septum	236
Pulmonary Protective Mechanisms	238
Pulmonary Blood Vessels	238
Pulmonary Lymphatic Vessels	238
Pulmonary Innervation	239

The primary and essential function of the respiratory system is to transport air, allowing the exchange of the oxygen in inspired air for carbon dioxide carried by the red blood cells in the vascular system. In order to accomplish this, the mammalian respiratory system is composed of two main parts: first, a system of progressively smaller structurally and functionally complex tubes, and second, a respiratory unit at the distal end of the airway where gases are exchanged between the airway and the circulating blood cells (Fig. 13–1).

The *airway*, or conducting part of the system, consists of the nasal cavity, nasopharynx, larynx, trachea, bronchi, and terminal bronchioles. The part of the system where gaseous exchange takes place comprises respiratory bronchioles, alveolar ducts, and alveoli.

TABLE 13–1. Types of Epithelial Cells Lining the Respiratory Tract

Respiratory Structure	Type of Epithelium
Nasal vestibule	Stratified squamous
Concha	Pseudostratified ciliated columnar; goblet cells
Sinuses	Pseudostratified ciliated columnar; goblet cells
Naso- and Oropharynx	
Above soft palate	Pseudostratified ciliated columnar; goblet cells
Distal to soft palate	Stratified squamous, nonkeratinizing
Epiglottis	
Proximal	Stratified squamous, nonkeratinizing
Distal, base	Pseudostratified ciliated columnar; goblet cells
Vocal apparatus (larynx)	Stratified squamous, nonkeratinizing
Trachea	Pseudostratified ciliated columnar; goblet cells
Bronchi and bronchial tree	Pseudostratified ciliated columnar
Bronchioles	Simple ciliated columnar or simple ciliated cuboidal
Respiratory bronchioles	Ciliated cuboidal and alveolar (squamous) type I cells
Alveolar ducts	Type I alveolar (squamous) cells
Alveoli	Type 1 (squamous) and type 2 ("cuboidal") alveolar cells

AIRWAY

The airway has two main functions: (1) to clean, moisten, and warm the inhaled air, and (2) to contain the air and conduct it to the site where respiratory exchange takes place. The movement of air within the respiratory system depends upon the lungs' being contained in a closed container (thorax) not open to the surrounding air and on a way to change the volume of the container. The volume changes are accomplished by means of movement of the ribs of the thoracic cage, intercostal muscles, and diaphragm. The elastic tissue of the lungs facilitates passive expansion and spontaneous contraction when the muscles of the thorax and diaphragm relax, thereby ending the negative or reduced pressure within the closed container (thorax).

Epithelium

As many as six different cell types have been reported in the epithelium that lines the tubes of the airway (Table 13–1). Most of the airway is covered by ciliated pseudostratified columnar epithelium (Fig. 13–2). This epithelial type is so widespread within the respiratory system that it is designated *respiratory epithelium*. The columnar cells all reach the basement membrane, and their free or apical surfaces are each covered by as many as 300 motile cilia. Beneath the cell surface, the ciliary basal bodies and numerous mitochondria fill the most apical region of the cytoplasm of the cell. The ATP synthesized by the mitochondria is essential to maintain functional cilia, and the topographic relationship between the energy source and the active cilia is a consistent structural-functional relationship. The base of the cell is in contact with a distinctive, very thickened basal lamina.

Insinuated into the pseudostratified columnar epithelium are *goblet cells*, unicellular glands that synthesize mucus. The apical ends of these goblet-shaped columnar cells contain polysaccharide-rich mucus droplets that stain with periodic acid–Schiff (PAS) stain. These cells are essential for respiratory airway protection, because they produce a continuous carpet of mucus that collects debris, which is then carried away from the functional surfaces of the airway by the ciliated epithelium. In addition, the mucus protects and prevents dehydration of the ciliated epithelial surface.

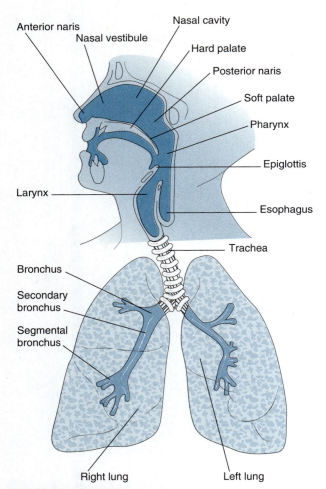

FIGURE 13–1. Human airway. *The airway system in humans comprises the nasal cavity, oral cavity, pharynx, larynx, trachea, bronchi, and lungs.*

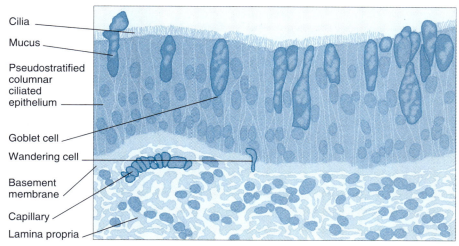

FIGURE 13-2. Ciliated pseudostratified epithelium. Pseudostratified *refers to the appearance of the epithelium in section. Although the cells appear to be stratified because the nuclei are found in several layers, the basal portions of all cells are actually in contact with the basement membrane.*

The cilia are motile structures that carry a carpet of mucus; the mucus collects inhaled debris and moves it to the pharynx, where it is either coughed out or swallowed.

Goblet cells are nonciliated, mucus-secreting cells; they are seen here in various stages of mucus synthesis and discharge.

The basement membrane is thickest in the trachea, but wandering cells of the immune system can be found traversing the membrane. Other cells of the immune system are also seen at various levels of the epithelium.

The lamina propria of the trachea is thin but contains small blood vessels and collagenous and elastic fibers.

Less numerous within the epithelium are *basal cells*, which are short and lie on the basal lamina but do not reach the free surface of the pseudostratified columnar ciliated epithelium. Basal cells are believed to be undifferentiated, multipotential cells that undergo mitosis and differentiate into other cell types.

Another intrinsic cell type found in respiratory epithelium is the *small granule cell*. This cell resembles the basal cell but is clearly distinguishable because it contains many dense core granules varying in size from 100 to 300 nm in diameter. These cells belong to the so-called diffuse neuroendocrine system. The role of these cells is not certain, but they may secrete factors that activate mucous and serous secretion. They are located among the epithelial cells lining the respiratory tract.

RESPIRATORY TRACT

The component parts of the respiratory tract are as follows:

- Nasal fossae
- Nasopharynx
- Larynx
- Trachea
- Bronchi of variable size (large and small)
- Bronchioles of variable size, including terminal and respiratory types
- Alveolar ducts
- Alveoli

A discussion of the distinctive structural features of each part follows.

Nasal Cavity

The nasal cavity is composed of the vestibule and the paired nasal fossa. Associated with the nasal cavities are the paranasal sinuses.

The *vestibule* is that part of the nose that receives air via the paired nares, or nostrils. The thin skin of the nose continues into the vestibule, loses its keratinization, and changes into nonkeratinized stratified squamous epithelium before entering the nasal fossae. The skin of the inner surface of the nares contains terminal-type hairs that are short and thick. The apparent purpose of these hairs is to block large particles and "flies" from entering the nasal fossae. The hairs are richly supplied with motion-sensitive sensory receptors that signal such an event and bring about a sneeze or other vigorous response.

Each *nasal fossa* is divided into two parts by the cartilaginous and osseous bony septum. Extending from the lateral wall of the nasal fossae are bony, shell-like projections termed *conchae*. Typically three, they may number as many as five. The lower two conchae have specialized lamina propria that contains large venous plexuses similar to the erectile tissue found in the reproductive system. The covering epithelium is the pseudostratified ciliated columnar type. The covering epithelium of the upper concha is also specialized epithelium serving the sense of smell. It consists of both supporting cells and neurosensory cells, which are sensitive to odoriferous substances adsorbed on the moist mucous surface. Associated serous glands of Bowman faciliate the sensory function of smell by continuously renewing the fluid-covered epithelial absorptive surface.

The erectile tissue covering the conchae periodically may "swell" on an alternative basis, effectively closing the airflow on one side of the nasal fossae and thereby directing inhaled air into the opposite nasal fossa (Fig. 13–3).

Associated Nasal Sinuses

The sinuses joined to the airway are the frontal, ethmoid, sphenoid, and maxillary. They are all lined with pseudostratified ciliated columnar epithelium and goblet cells. The lamina propria is thin and contains some seromucinous glands. The drainage of the mucus produced in the paranasal sinuses depends upon the activity of pseudostratified ciliated epithelium and also the position of the head during sleep.

Nasopharynx and Oropharynx

The nasopharynx is the superior part of the pharynx. The nasopharynx joins the oropharynx posteriorly. The nasopharynx and oropharynx are both lined, above the soft palate, by pseudostratified ciliated epithelium. Distal to the soft palate, the epithelium is nonkeratinizing stratified squamous epithelium.

The cuplike pharynx is joined to the larynx. The larynx contains the vocal apparatus and is joined to the trachea and, by its division, also to the esophagus.

Larynx

The larynx contains within its lamina propria several cartilages that serve three important and essential functions: (1) to keep the airway open, (2) to direct air into the trachea (the next distal part of the respiratory tree) and food and fluid into the esophagus, and (3) to serve as the origin and as a conduit for sounds produced by the vocal folds. The cartilages in this region are the thyroid, cricoid, arytenoids, cuneiforms, and corniculate, and the epiglottis. These cartilages articulate with one another (for details consult a book of gross anatomy) and all play a role in sound production or closure of the rima glottis (opening of the airway) when food or liquid is swallowed. The thyroid and cricoid cartilage also serve to keep the airway open (Fig. 13–4).

The larynx joins the pharynx with the trachea and esophagus and contains the vocal apparatus.

The lamina propria of the larynx contains several cartilages. These cartilages are primarily concerned with the vocal apparatus but also support the thin-walled larynx by keeping the airway open. The thyroid, cricoid, and arytenoid cartilages are hyaline cartilage and the epiglottis, cuneiform, corniculate, and the tips of the arytenoid cartilage are elastic cartilage.

Although the intricate structure of the larynx is usually studied in gross anatomy, it should be noted that the cartilages are articulated and bound together by ligaments. Movements of the cartilages are effected by striated muscle. With the exception of the epiglottis, the cartilaginous structures are involved with speech as well as with the opening and closing of the airway through muscle action. They all serve to prevent food and fluid from entering the airway.

The *epiglottis* projects from the anterior rim of the larynx, over the airway, and into the pharynx. Because of its location, the epithelium of the epiglottis is also continuous with that of the tongue. This is called the lingual surface of the epiglottis. The continuation of the epithelium over the apex of the epiglottis is also continuous with the larynx; hence, it has a laryngeal surface. On the lingual and apical surfaces, the epiglottis is covered by nonkeratinized stratified squamous epithelium. Near the base of the laryngeal surface of this elastic cartilage, the epithelium gradually changes to pseudostratified ciliated columnar epithelium. The lamina propria contains mixed mucous and serous glands.

Vocal Apparatus

Distal to the epiglottis, the laryngeal mucosa forms two pairs of folds. The superior pair form the so-called *false vocal cords* or vestibular folds (Fig. 13–5). These folds are covered by pseudostratified columnar ciliated epithelium, and the lamina propria contains seromucinous glands.

The inferior pair of folds constitutes the *true vocal folds* (cords). The vocal folds are covered by stratified squamous epithelium and contain large parallel bundles of elastic fibers. These elastic fibers constitute the vocal ligament. Parallel to the vocal ligament is the small vocalis muscle, composed of striated skeletal fibers. The vocalis muscle, along with others, regulates the tension on the vocal ligament (fold). Air passing

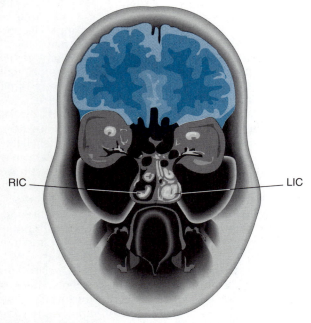

FIGURE 13–3. Nasal fossae. Diagram of a magnetic resonance image of the nasal fossae, showing the airway closed on the left side and open on the right.

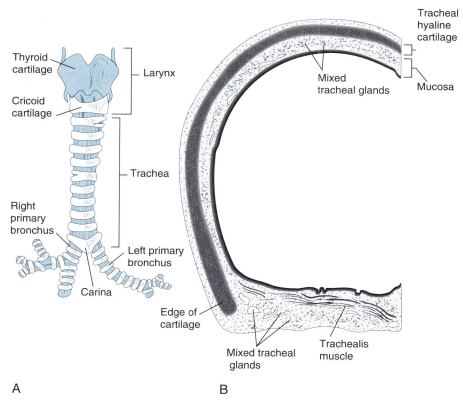

FIGURE 13-4. The cartilages of the airway. A, The important cartilaginous components of the airway are shown. B, The supporting cartilage of the long trachea is seen to be incomplete posteriorly. The two ends are joined by the trachealis muscle. The mucosa has numerous serous and mucous glands and a pseudostratified columnar ciliated epithelium.

over the vocal folds produces sound, which is varied by the amount of tension placed on the vocal fold (ligament).

Trachea

The trachea is a tube with incomplete, C-shaped rings of hyaline cartilage in its lamina propria. These cartilages vary in number, depending on the length of the trachea, from as few as 15 to as many as 20. Because the trachea is relatively thin walled, forceful air movement would collapse it if not for the cartilaginous rings. The "open end" of each C-shaped cartilage faces posteriorly, where the trachea and esophagus interface. The ends of the cartilages are spanned by a fibroelastic ligament and a bundle of smooth muscle named the trachealis muscle, inserting on the perichondrium of the ends of the cartilage. The fibroelastic ligament trachealis and muscle provide resistance to dangerous or exaggerated enlargement of the trachea in strenuous or forceful air movement. The fibroelastic ligament and trachealis muscle also provide a resilient and distendable cushion for boluses of food or fluid being carried in the immediately adjacent thin-walled esophagus. Contraction of the trachealis muscle reduces the resting size of the trachea, for example, during the cough reflex. The trachea is covered primarily by pseudostratified columnar ciliated epithelium and goblet cells (see Fig. 13-4).

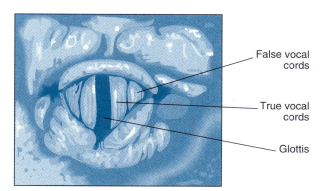

FIGURE 13-5. Vocal cords. Two sets of vocal folds, or cords, are found in the laryngeal part of the airway. The movement of air across the true vocal cords produces sounds interpreted as speech. This illustration is their appearance with the use of a laryngoscope.

Bronchi and Bronchial Tree

The trachea divides in the thorax into two primary or *mainstem bronchi*. The primary bronchi enter the substance or parenchyma of the lungs at a point designated the *hilum* (also called the root of the lungs). They accompany pulmonary arterial vessels that carry deoxygenated blood; at this same site, veins and lymphatics leave the lungs. The bronchi again subdivide within the lung, into three secondary or lobar bronchi on the right side and two on the left. Therefore, the right lung usually has three lobes and the left, two. The lobar bronchi divide into smaller segmental bronchi. There are commonly ten bronchopulmonary segmental bronchi in the right lung and nine in the left lung. These divide repeatedly.

The terminal branches of lobar bronchi, called *bronchioles*, branch into five to seven terminal bronchioles. The transitions between these named parts of the bronchial tree occur gradually and can be identified because each has a distinctive structural feature. Transitional parts, however, may not always be easy to categorize, and there is no particular reason to do so.

Bronchi

The mainstem bronchi have essentially the same structure as the trachea, except for modification in the arrangement of cartilaginous tissue (Fig. 13–6). Primary or mainstem bronchi divide 9 to 12 times, each branching resulting in smaller bronchi. At a diameter of about 5 mm, bronchi change their structure, function, and name, becoming bronchioles.

Bronchial cartilage is more variable in shape than that of the trachea and tends to completely encircle the larger bronchi. The smaller bronchi possess smaller plates, or so-called islands, of hyaline cartilage. The epithelium is typical pseudostratified ciliated columnar epithelium with mucus-secreting goblet cells (Fig. 13–7).

Beneath the epithelium, the bronchial lamina propria contains a layer of smooth muscle that is circularly arranged. Careful examination may show the smooth muscle layer to be discontinuous and irregularly arranged.

Contraction of the smooth muscle diminishes the size of the lumen of the bronchus. The lamina propria typically contains elastic fibers that are consistent with its function in that they resist expansion and contraction and return the bronchial lumen to its typical or usual diameter. The lamina propria also contains an abundance of mucous and serous secretory glands whose ducts empty onto the bronchial surface.

Because the "internal" environment, i.e., the cells and tissues below the surface epithelium, is separated from the septic external environment by the height of only a single cell (pseudostratified ciliated columnar epithelium), lymphocytes and other cells of the immune system are commonly found among the epithelial cells. In addition, lymphatics, capillaries, larger vessels, and small nodes accompany the branching bronchi and leave the lung at the hilum, where they join numerous large and small nodes, that aggregate at the root of the lung.

"Smoker's cough" is caused by paralysis of ciliary action by nicotine and other products of tobacco smoking. The resultant stasis and accumulation of mucus in the lower respiratory system in turn triggers the cough reflex in an effort to clear the distal airway. Bronchitis is a common sequel to such ciliary paralysis.

Bronchioles

The distinguishing feature of bronchioles is that they possess neither cartilage nor glands in their mucosa but they may have some goblet cells in their initial parts (Fig. 13–8). In addition, the pseudostratified ciliated columnar epithelium is progressively shorter in height, finally becoming simple columnar ciliated or simple cuboidal ciliated in structure, at which point the bronchioles are renamed terminal bronchioles.

Terminal bronchioles contain distinctive cells, so-called *Clara's cells* or nonciliated bronchiolar epithelial cells. The precise function of these interesting cells is unknown, but sparse facts and speculation lead to a conclusion that they are secretory in nature. Clara's cells have a rounded, dome-shaped apical surface without cilia. Their cytoplasm has a basally located nucleus that is typically deeply indented and contains membrane-bound granules, although these are not numerous. Radioactively labeled dipalmitoyl lecithin, a constitutent of surfactant, can also be localized to Clara's cell granules. These cells are probably a secondary source of surfactant material (the primary source being type 2 alveolar cells).

The bronchiolar lamina propria, devoid of cartilage, is composed of smooth muscle and elastic and reticular fibers.

The activity of the smooth muscle of the respiratory tree is under the control of both the parasympathetic (vagus nerve) and sympathetic parts of the autonomic nervous system. Stimulation of the vagus nerve produces contraction of smooth muscle and a reduction in the size of the bronchiole. Local release of naturally occurring serotonin, histamine, and leukotrienes may produce bronchiospasms, thereby impairing respira-

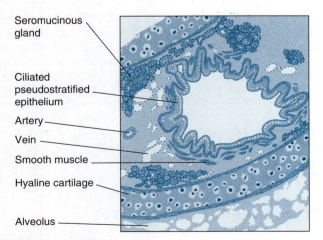

FIGURE 13–6. Bronchus. Note the hyaline cartilage, which appears platelike in this section. The lumen of the bronchus can be decreased by the contraction of the smooth muscle that surrounds the pseudostratified epithelium–lined airway. Seromucinous (seromucous) glands and blood vessels are found in the lamina propria.

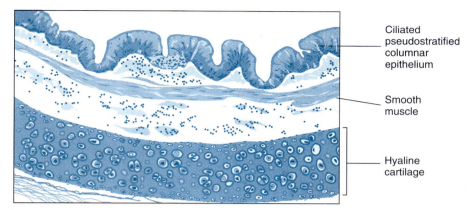

FIGURE 13-7. Bronchus in cross-section. *Part of the bronchus can be seen. Bronchi are lined by pseudostratified columnar epithelium with goblet cells. The thickness and layering of the epithelium decrease gradually with the decrease in size of bronchi. A smooth muscle layer encircles a thin connective tissue, lamina propria. In contrast to the trachea, the smooth muscle of the bronchus is arranged in interlacing spirals around the bronchus. Between the smooth muscle layer and the cartilage is the submucosa, which may contain seromucous glands, not seen in this preparation (see Fig. 13–6). The hyaline cartilage is arranged in discontinuous plates around the bronchus.*

tion. Sympathectomies inhibit the contraction of the smooth muscle and foster enlargement of the airway. Inhalers containing epinephrine also inhibit contraction and decrease the tone (tension) commonly found in smooth muscle.

Terminal bronchioles subdivide into *respiratory bronchioles*. Respiratory bronchioles can be considered relatively short transitional segments between the conducting and the respiratory parts of the airway (Figs. 13–9 and 13–10).

The mucosa of respiratory bronchioles is similar to that of terminal bronchioles, except for the presence of numerous "saccular" alveoli, which interrupt the wall of the bronchiole. It is within the alveoli that gaseous exchange takes place.

The epithelium, therefore, is also in transition at the level of the respiratory bronchiole. Ciliated cuboidal epithelium and Clara's cells disappear at the junction with alveoli. At this point, the epithelium becomes squamous and consists of cells designated as *type 1 alveolar epithelial cells*. As the respiratory bronchiole extends distally, the number of alveoli increases greatly. Between alveoli, ciliated cuboidal epithelium is still present. Near the distal end of this type of bronchiole, the cilia may disappear from the apical ends of the cuboidal lining cells. Smooth muscle and elastic fibers and some reticular connective tissue fill the lamina propria of respiratory bronchioles.

Alveolar Ducts

Distal to the respiratory bronchiole is the alveolar duct, characterized by numerous alveoli with little or no evidence of a bronchiolar wall, with the exception of small, characteristic segments of smooth muscle that bulge into the lumen of the duct, appearing similar to pegs with large heads or to doorknobs (see Fig. 13–10).

At the distal end of the alveolar duct, the smooth muscle pegs or knobs disappear. The lining epithelium is primarily type 1 squamous epithelium. Alveolar ducts

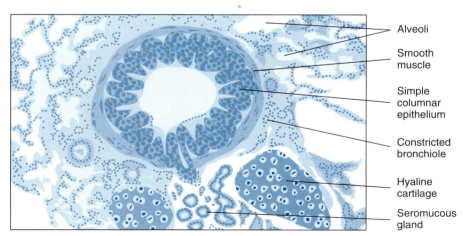

FIGURE 13-8. Bronchiole. *A bronchiole is seen in the midst of respiratory tissue. The epithelium is simple columnar, ciliated. The lamina propria is replaced by the muscle layer that encircles the bronchiole. In humans, cartilage and glands are characteristically present until bronchioles decrease in size to approximately 0.5 mm in diameter.*

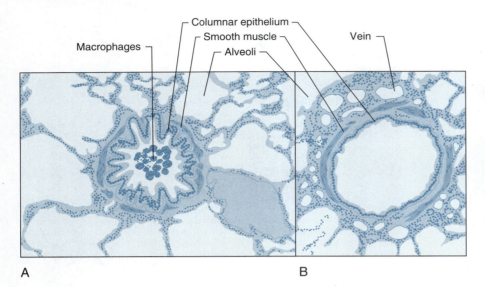

FIGURE 13-9. Bronchiole: contracted and relaxed. Cross-sections of contracted (A) and relaxed (B) bronchioles surrounded by respiratory tissue. Note the low columnar epithelial lining, the prominence of smooth muscle fibers in the lamina propria, and the absence of cartilaginous plates and glands. Macrophages filled with black carbon particles are seen in the lumen of the contracted bronchiole. The elastic spongework of respiratory tissue surrounding the bronchioles prevents their collapse during contracted inspiration. Every inspiratory movement exerts a pull on the wall of the bronchiole, protecting it from collapse; hence, there is no need for cartilage rings or plates.

terminate in atria, which divide to form two or more alveolar sacs.

Alveoli

Alveolar ducts become subdivided into atria, which, as their name implies, are the entryways into the terminal part of the airway, the alveoli (Figs. 13–11 and 13–12). Alveoli are the smallest and most numerous units of the airway. It is at the level of the alveoli that gaseous interchange takes place across the blood-air barrier. The saclike alveoli are about 200 to 300 μm in diameter and are so numerous that they give the lung a spongelike consistency. The repeated subdivision of the airway to form alveoli increases the surface area and thus facilitates gaseous interchange. Volumetric changes during respiration in the lung occur primarily in the alveoli.

Alveoli are thought to number about 300 million. The area of the interface between the epithelium of the alveolus and capillary blood is 1000 m² or more. One study found the alveolar surface area in a pair of lungs to be 143 ± m², the blood capillary surface area to be 126 ± 12 m², and the capillary volume to be 231 ± 31 m². An alveolus that varies between 200 and 300 μm in diameter may have as many as 1800 blood capillary contacts.

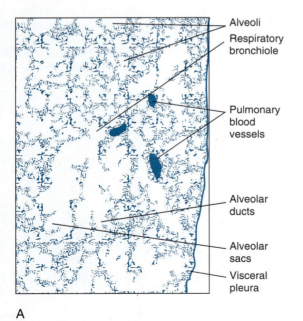
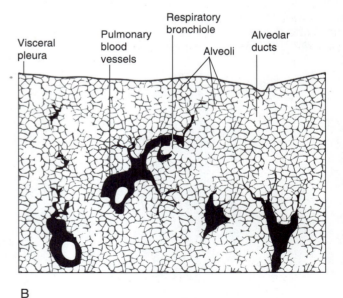

FIGURE 13-10. Section of human lung. A and B, These sections are at two magnifications. They show respiratory bronchioles and alveolar ducts. Note that these important components of the airway have a distinctive structural pattern, permitting their distinction from the alveoli.

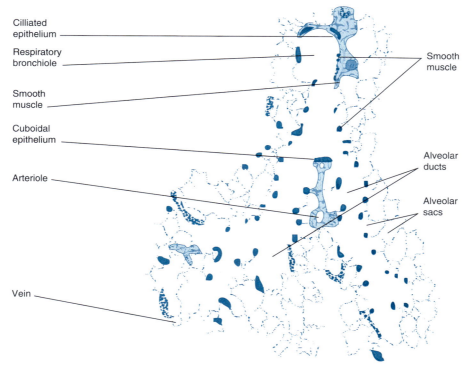

FIGURE 13–11. Respiratory bronchiole. *This section of a respiratory bronchiole has two alveolar ducts and is taken from human lung. The alveolar ducts lead into alveoli, where gaseous exchange takes place.*

Alveoli of the lungs are not developed sufficiently to sustain life until after the twentieth week of gestation. Thus, extrauterine life prior to that time is extremely difficult even with life-supporting devices. The first breath of life is arduous because the newborn must overcome large surface tension forces in order to inflate partially collapsed alveoli. The transpulmonary pressure required for the first breath is about 20 times that required for subsequent breaths, and an infant with respiratory distress syndrome must repeat the first effort with every breath. Many babies with this condition can be kept alive with mechanical ventilators long enough for their lungs to mature and manufacture sufficient surfactant for alveolar expansion (see later).

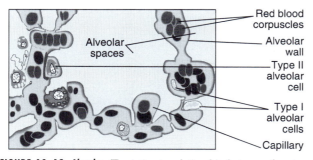

FIGURE 13–12. Alveolus. *The intimate relationship between the airway alveolus and the capillary bed is shown. On light microscopy, the nature of the cellular relationships cannot be appreciated fully. Note that type II alveolar cells project into the alveolus and that type I alveolar cells form most of the alveolar wall.*

Alveolar Wall

The alveolar wall is designed to enhance the gaseous diffusion between the external and internal environments. In general, the wall is composed of alveolar squamous cells, so-called *type 1 alveolar epithelial cells* or *type 1 pneumocytes*, which form a continuous layer about 0.05 μm in thickness. The basal lamina of this wall is doubled, at about 0.1 μm thick, and the capillary endothelial layer is another 0.05 μm. Hence, the total barrier to gaseous diffusion (blood-air barrier) could be as little as 0.2 μm in thickness. Actual measurements by electron microscopy, however, yield mean values of 2.2 μm in normal human lungs. The discrepancy between the theoretical and the actual thickness is due to the presence in large areas of wider spaces containing free fluid, fixed and free cells of the immune system, and connective tissue, both collagen and elastin.

The alveolar surface is usually covered by a film of pulmonary surfactant, composed primarily of a phospholipid secreted mainly by type 2 (great) alveolar cells and perhaps Clara's cells as well. Surfactant reduces surface tension and is essential in normal alveolar expansion and in the prevention of alveolar collapse during expiration. *Pulmonary surfactant* is a layering composed of different stages in the transformation of multilamellar bodies formed in the type 2 alveolar cells. The layers of human surfactant on the epithelial surface, from deep to superficial, are as follows:

- The most recent secretion of multilamellar bodies

- Paired lamellae rearranged to form tubules
- Mature tubular "myelin" surfactant
- The surfactant-air interface in the form of a single lipid bilayer
- Degraded surfactant, which is subsequently removed by macrophages

Cells of the Interalveolar Septum

These cells have already been noted above as those of the alveolar epithelium, capillary endothelium and, in addition, the interstitial space. Additional considerations include the following.

The alveolar epithelium is formed of at least two cell types.

Simple squamous type 1 alveolar epithelial cells (pneumocytes) cover over 95% of the alveolar surface. This cell's highly attenuated cytoplasm may be 0.05 to 0.2 μm in thickness, extending distally from a thicker region containing the cell nucleus. Cell division is not common, and damaged cells are replaced by the multiplication of "primitive" type 2 cells, which may later differentiate into type 1 cells. The cytoplasm of type 1 pneumocytes contains pinocytotic vesicles and a perinuclear cytoplasm with a few mitochondria, a scanty agranular endoplasmic reticulum, and, infrequently, some lysosomes. The edges of these squamous cells overlap with those of adjacent cells, and they are joined by tight or occluding junctions.

Type 2 alveolar epithelial cells cover about 3% of the alveolar surface and are, in fact, more numerous than type 1 cells. The type 2 cells are mainly concerned with the elaboration of surfactant. These cells project into the alveolar lumen, and their free surfaces are covered by numerous short microvilli. The cytoplasm of these cells contains abundant mitochondria, granular endoplasmic reticulum, lysosomes, and multilamellar bodies (secretory granules). The multilamellar secretory granules contain dipalmitoylphosphatidylcholine, cholesterol, and a protein. These are "stacked" in regular lamellae, each as phospholipid bilayer (Figs. 13–13 and 13–14).

In fetal development, surfactant, in the form of lamellar bodies in type 2 cells, is normally produced in the last few weeks of gestation. Premature delivery therefore may have serious consequences for the premature baby, who may have labored breathing and, because its lungs cannot expand, may be in respiratory distress. The condition is known as hyaline membrane disease or respiratory distress syndrome. Hyaline membrane disease is a respiratory disorder that accounts for about one third of neonatal deaths. Glucocorticoid administration stimulates the synthesis of surfactant and is useful clinically.

Pulmonary Capillary Endothelial Cells

The pulmonary endothelial cells of the vascular system of the lung may be extremely thin (0.1 μm) and very versatile functionally. In addition to their role in gaseous exchange, these cells:

- Play a role in removal of emboli and thrombi
- Assist in the metabolism of chylomicrons
- Convert angiotension I to angiotension II
- Produce thromboplastin
- Process hormones and prohormones that come in contact with the endothelium

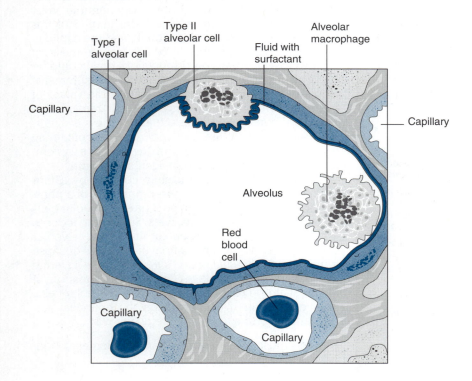

FIGURE 13–13. Alveoli, alveolar cells, and capillaries. *This illustration shows alveolar components; type I alveolar wall cells, type II cells producing surfactant, which keep the alveolus open, and alveolar macrophages, which keep the alveolus tidy.*

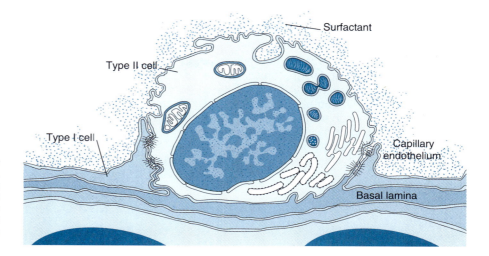

FIGURE 13-14. Alveolar type II cell. Alveolar type II cells are the source of surfactant, seen in this illustration as blue granules both within and outside the cell. Note the relationship to the flattened type I cell. The alveolar wall consists of the alveolar type I cell, basal lamina, and the capillary endothelial cell (unlabeled in illustration).

- Synthesize prostaglandins and related compounds
- Inactivate serotonin
- Perform other metabolic activities

The primary structural feature of pulmonary endothelial cells are the abundant transcytotic vesicles. The capillary endothelium is a simple continuous layer of very thin squamous cells.

If the human lung has 3×10^8 alveoli, each with as many as 1000 capillary segments in its walls, the pulmonary capillary bed may measure 1500 miles or more. The size of the capillaries indicates that 1.0 ml of blood would be contained in 10 miles of capillaries (Fig. 13-15).

Interstitial Space

Interstitial space is a misnomer, because it is not a space but rather is filled with fluid, collagen and elastic fibers, and a variety of cells that may be of a fixed or wandering type.

The most numerous fixed interstitial cells are fibroblasts and pericytes. These cells are structurally similar, but fibroblasts are the source of connective tissue fibers, and pericytes lie close to the capillary basal lamina. The pericytes are contractile, contain actin and myosin, and may be able to modify the extensibility of alveoli and thereby regulate lung compliance.

The free or migratory cells in the septa include macrophages, mast cells, lymphocytes and, less frequently, plasma cells.

Loss of elasticity and breakdown of interalveolar septa gives rise to emphysema, also often a sequel to long-term smoking. Smoking may cause a wide variety of pulmonary disorders quite apart from the well-documented correlation with the incidence of lung cancer.

Alveolar (Free) Cells

Cells are also found within the alveoli, the most common being alveolar macrophages. These macrophages are related to the tissue macrophages and monocytes, which are part of the mononuclear macrophage system. These scavenger cells migrate from capillaries through the epithelium to "prowl" on alveolar epithelial surfaces. They clear alveoli of inhaled and other debris and then migrate into lymphatic channels or move to the alveolar tree, where they are swept along the continuous carpet of mucus, at about 1 cm per minute, by the ciliated epithelium and are eliminated via the larynx by either swallowing or expectoration (see Fig. 13-13).

In a variety of unfortunate circumstances, red

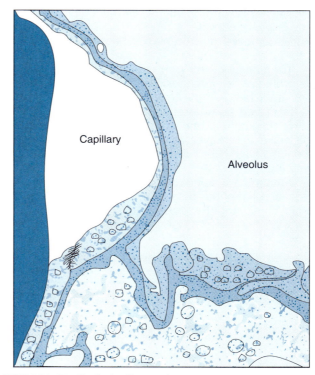

FIGURE 13-15. Alveolar/capillary interface. The capillary endothelial cells that form the capillary wall are separated from the alveolar epithelial cell (type I) wall by the basal lamina. Three structures are traversed during gaseous exchange. The capillary bed virtually surrounds each alveolus, which facilitates the exchange.

blood cells may escape from their capillaries. When this occurs, the macrophages, after engulfing the red blood cells, become a deep rusty red (brick-red). Such cells are frequently detectable in so-called rusty sputum, a condition that occurs in congestive heart failure; macrophages loaded with red blood cells are termed "heart failure cells." Sputum can be tested histochemically for iron, a constituent of red blood cells. Human alveolar macrophages have been shown to produce, paradoxically, both collagenase and a collagenase inhibitor. Hence, these cells also play a role in either altering or stabilizing the connective matrix, which is sensitive to collagenase.

Interalveolar Pores

Interalveolar pores, 10 to 15 μm in diameter, are found in the interalveolar septa. They allow air to pass from one alveolus to another, thereby equalizing air pressure between alveoli. The pores also provide an alternative entryway into an alveolus for air and cells if its normal entryway, the atrium, is blocked.

PULMONARY PROTECTIVE MECHANISMS

As a vital organ, the lung must be protected against the harsh variability of the inspired air and its contaminants. The surface area of the lungs is enormous, and they are vulnerable to desiccation and microbial infection. The air is warmed and humidified, and the epithelium is provided with a mucous coating that is constantly removed and replaced, thereby eliminating many inhaled particles regardless of their nature.

The glands of the respiratory tract secrete numerous protective compounds. The glands and their secretions are listed in Table 13–2.

Damaged alveolar epithelium has a limited regenerative capability, but normally, alveolar squamous cells have a turnover or life span of about 21 days. Alveolar phagocytes, on the other hand, are replaced every 4 days.

Numerous lymphoid nodules, so-called bronchus-associated lymphoid tissue, are found in the bronchial lining. These nodules provide local immunologic protection against infection by both cell-mediated (T cell) activities and by production of immunoglobulins, primarily IgA, by B cells. These immunoglobulins are distributed to gland cells for delivery to the epithelial free surface.

The cough mechanism is another important protective device. The irritation of afferent receptors, which are located at the laryngeal opening, are associated with taste bud–like epithelial receptors that probably trigger the cough reflex.

PULMONARY BLOOD VESSELS

The lungs have two kinds of blood supply: the blood supply for the lung tissue itself, and the blood that takes part in essential gaseous exchange.

Bronchial arteries carry oxygenated blood to supply the cells that constitute the lungs. These vessels accompany the bronchial tree and communicate with branches of the pulmonary artery. Some branches of the bronchial arteries form subpleural capillary plexuses. These arteries supply the bronchial wall as far as respiratory bronchioles. They anastomose with branches of the pulmonary artery in the walls of smaller bronchi and in the visceral pleura.

Bronchial veins are of two kinds, deep and superficial, but they do not receive all of the bronchial artery blood. Some drains into the pulmonary vein, and the remainder into the azygos, hemiazygos, or superior intercostal veins.

The greater volume of blood for gaseous exchange is carried in the pulmonary artery. The artery divides into branches that accompany segmental and subsegmental bronchi. These arteries subdivide many times, ending in very dense capillary networks in the walls of alveolar sacs, as mentioned previously.

Pulmonary veins, two from each lung, drain the pulmonary capillaries. The veins collect into larger and larger vessels that traverse the lungs independently of the pulmonary arteries and bronchi. The larger veins ultimately accompany arteries and bronchi to the pulmonary hilum. The pulmonary veins empty into the left atrium of the heart, for distribution by the left ventricle to the entire body.

PULMONARY LYMPHATIC VESSELS

Pulmonary lymphatic vessels arise from a plexus beneath the pleura and also from a deep plexus that runs with branches of pulmonary vessels and bronchi. In large and smaller bronchioles but not alveoli, the deep plexus has submucous and peribronchial parts. There are no lymphatic vessels in alveolar walls. Superficial efferents converge in the bronchopulmonary nodes, and deep efferents arrive at the hilum along pulmonary vessels and bronchi and end, primarily in the same bronchopulmonary nodes. Deep in fissures,

TABLE 13–2. Respiratory Tract Glands and Their Secretions

Gland/Cell	Secretion(s)
Goblet cell	Sulfated acid mucopolysaccharides
Mucous glands (lamina propria)	Carboxylated mucopolysaccharides—some sialic acid, others sulfated Lysozyme IgA antibodies (Possibly) interferon
Serous glands (lamina propria)	Neutral mucopolysaccharides Lysozyme IgA antibodies (Possibly) interferon

lymphatic vessels of adjoining lobes join; hence, vessels from upper lobes join the superior tracheobronchial nodes, and those from lower lobes join the inferior tracheobronchial nodes. At the lobar level, the lymphatic vessels follow both the central lobar artery and its lobar peripheral veins.

PULMONARY INNERVATION

The anterior and posterior pulmonary nerve plexuses are formed by sympathetic and parasympathetic (vagus nerve) branches. Rami from both systems follow the bronchial tubes and provide efferent branches to bronchial smooth muscle and glands. Afferent pain fibers arise from the bronchial mucous membrane and alveoli. It is generally thought that bronchoconstriction occurs with vagal stimulation and that the sympathetic supply is inhibitory to contraction and diminishes the tone of smooth muscle fibers. Relaxation also occurs in the absence of vagal stimulation.

Drugs that mimic the sympathetic nervous system, such as epinephrine and isoproterenol, act as vasodilators; they are used by sufferers of asthma attacks.

CHAPTER FOURTEEN

SPECIAL SENSES

OLFACTION 241
    Olfactory Epithelium 241
    Olfactory Mechanisms 242

TASTE 242
    Taste Buds 242
    Physiology of Taste 243
    Central Transmission of Taste Sensations 243

VISION 243
    The Sclera 244
    The Conjunctiva 244
    The Cornea 244
    The Uvea 245
    The Lens 246
    The Vitreous Body 246
    The Retina 246
    Visual Pathways 250
    Accessory Structures of the Eye 251

HEARING 251
    The Ear 251
    Mechanics of Audition 252
    Cochlea 252
    Auditory End Organ (Organ of Corti) 253
    Auditory Physiology 254
    Audiometry 255
    Deafness 255

VESTIBULAR SENSATION 255

The different sensations perceived by the human body are grouped into two major categories: those concerned with general sensations (touch, pressure, pain, and temperature) and those concerned with special sensations (olfaction, taste, vision, audition, and sense of position and movement). This chapter is devoted to a consideration of the organs of special senses. Whereas nerve endings concerned with general sensibility are widely distributed, those concerned with special sensations are limited to specific areas of the body.

OLFACTION

The olfactory organ is located in the mucous membrane lining the uppermost part of the roof of the nasal cavity. From the roof, the olfactory epithelium extends down both sides of the nasal cavity to cover most of the superior concha laterally and 1 cm of nasal septum medially. Humans are microsmatic animals in whom the surface area of olfactory mucous membrane in both nostrils is small (approximately 5 cm^2).

Olfactory Epithelium

The olfactory epithelium is a thick pseudostratified columnar epithelium that contains three types of epithelial cells: receptor cells, supporting cells, and basal cells (Fig. 14–1). Interspersed among epithelial cells are ducts of Bowman's glands. Epithelial cells are densely packed and their nuclei are layered, with those of supporting cells being the most superficial, followed by those of receptor cells and basal cells.

Receptor Cells

Olfactory receptor cells are bipolar sensory neurons. Their perikarya are located in the lower part of the olfactory epithelium. Each cell has a single dendrite that reaches the surface of the epithelium and forms a knoblike expansion that extends beyond the epithelial surface. From this expansion, 10 to 20 cilia project into a layer of fluid covering the epithelium. From the basal part of the perikaryon, a nonmyelinated axon emerges and joins with axons of adjacent receptor cells to form the *olfactory nerve* (first cranial nerve). Olfactory nerve bundles penetrate the cribriform plate of the ethmoid bone to reach the *olfactory bulb*.

It is estimated that there are more than 100 million receptor cells in the olfactory mucosa. The specialized nerve cells of the olfactory epithelium are highly sensitive to different odors. Olfactory neurons are continuously produced from basal cells of the olfactory epithelium and are continuously lost by normal wear and tear. The presence of these nerve cells at the surface exposes them unduly to damage; it is estimated that 1% of the fibers of the olfactory nerves (axons of olfactory neurons) is lost each year of life because of injury to the perikarya. The sense of smell thus diminishes in the elderly as a result of the exposure of the olfactory epithelium to repeated infections and trauma in life. The presence of olfactory neurons at the surface represents the only exception to the evolutionary rule by which nerve cell bodies of afferent neurons migrate along their axons to take up more central and well-protected positions. The surface of the olfactory epithelium is constantly being moistened by secretions of Bowman's glands. This moistening helps dissolve the gaseous substances, facilitating stimulation of the olfactory epithelium. The continuous secretion also prevents retention of dissolved odorous substances.

It is believed that different basic odors stimulate different olfactory neurons that are not evenly distributed throughout the olfactory mucosa. Stimulation of different combinations of receptors for basic odors is believed to be the basis for humans' ability to recognize all the varieties of odors to which they are exposed.

Supporting Cells

Columnar epithelial cells, supporting cells separate the olfactory receptor cells. Their nuclei are lined up toward the surface of the epithelium, above the perikarya of receptor cells. The surface of supporting cells is specialized into microvilli that project into the fluid layer covering the epithelium.

Basal Cells

Basal cells are polygonal cells limited to the basal part of the epithelium. They are the source of new epithelial cells. Mitotic activity persists in these cells through maturity.

Bowman's Glands

Branched and tubuloalveolar, Bowman's glands are located beneath the epithelium (in lamina propria). They send their ducts in between epithelial cells to pour their secretion on the surface of the epithelium,

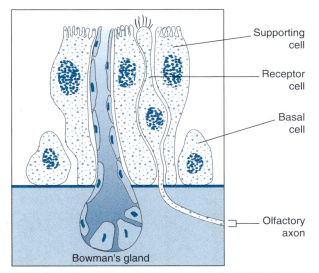

FIGURE 14–1. Olfactory mucosa, showing three types of epithelial cells: receptor, supporting, and basal. Ducts of Bowman's glands are interspersed with epithelial cells. Olfactory axons emerge from the basal part of receptor cells.

bathing the cilia of receptor cells and the microvilli of supporting cells. They contain serous and mucous cells. The secretion of Bowman's gland plays an important role in dissolving odorous substances and diffusing them to receptor cells.

Olfactory Mechanisms

Olfaction is a chemical sense. For a substance to be detected, it should have the following physical properties:

- Volatility, so that it can be sniffed
- Water solubility, so that it can diffuse through the olfactory epithelium
- Lipid solubility, so that it will interact with the lipids of the membranes of olfactory receptors

After an odorous substance is dissolved in the fluid bathing the surface of the olfactory mucosa, it interacts with receptors on the surface of the receptor cell. This interaction causes a change in membrane permeability. The ion flux that ensues gives rise to a slow surface negative wave (receptor or generator potential) that can be detected at the surface of the receptor cell. An all-or-none action potential, however, can be detected in the axons of receptor cells.

The olfactory receptors show a marked variability in sensitivity to different odors. They can detect methyl mercaptan (garlic odor) in a concentration of less than one millionth of a milligram per liter of air, but ethyl ether in a concentration of 5.8 mg per liter of air.

Olfactory receptors adapt rather quickly to a continuous stimulus. Although the olfactory mucosa can discriminate among a large number of different odors, its ability to detect changes in concentration of an odorous substance is rather poor. It is estimated that the concentration of an odorous substance must change by 30% before it can be detected by receptor cells. The mechanism of discrimination is poorly understood but is probably related to a spatial pattern of stimulation of the receptor cells.

The sense of olfaction is lost (anosmia) or diminished (hyposmia) in humans in connection with several conditions—common colds, trauma to the olfactory mucosa or nerve, and tumors in the base of the frontal lobe. Olfactory hallucinations occur in diseases of the temporal lobe, where the primary olfactory cortex is located.

TASTE

The gustatory (taste) sense organs in higher vertebrates are limited to the cavity of the mouth. The sensory organ of taste is the *taste bud* (Fig. 14–2), a pale ovoid structure within the stratified squamous epithelium. It is estimated that one vallate papilla of the tongue contains 200 taste buds on its sides and about 50 buds in the wall of the trench opposite the papilla. There are about 2000 taste buds in the human tongue. This number decreases progressively with age. In addi-

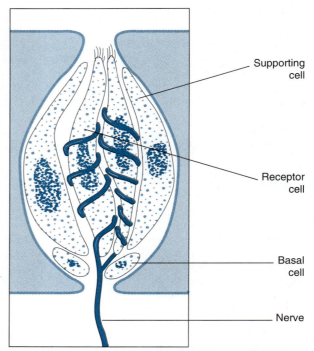

FIGURE 14–2. The cellular components of the taste bud, showing three types of epithelial cells: receptor (neuroepithelial), supporting, and basal. *The terminal nerve fibers wind themselves around receptor cells.*

tion to the vallate and fungiform papillae of the tongue, taste buds are found in the soft palate, oropharynx, and epiglottis.

Taste Buds

Each taste bud is composed of receptor (neuroepithelial), supporting, and basal cells, and nerve fibers.

Receptor Cells

Two types of receptor cells can be identified in taste buds, clear receptor cells and dense receptor cells. *Clear receptor cells* contain clear vesicles; *dense receptor cells* contain dense core vesicles that store glycosaminoglycans. Both cell types presumably function as receptors. They are believed to represent two stages in the development of receptor elements, the dense cell being the more mature. The apex of each receptor cell is modified into microvilli, which increase the receptor surface area and project into an opening, the taste pore. Approximately 4 to 20 receptor cells are located in the center of each taste bud. Receptor elements decrease in number with age. Receptor cells are stimulated by substances in solution.

Supporting Cells

Spindle-shaped cells surrounding the receptor cells, supporting cells are located at the periphery of the taste bud. They have both an insulating function and a secretory function. They are believed to secrete the substance that bathes the microvilli in the taste pore.

Basal Cells

Basal cells are located at the base of the taste bud and, by division, replenish the receptor cells that are continually lost.

Nerve Fibers

The nerve fibers in the taste bud are terminal nerve fibers of the facial, glossopharyngeal, and vagus nerves. They are peripheral processes of sensory neurons in the geniculate ganglion of the facial nerve and in the inferior ganglia of the glossopharyngeal and vagus nerves. They enter the taste bud at its base and wind themselves around the receptor cells in close apposition to receptor cell membranes. Synaptic vesicles cluster on the inner surfaces of receptor cell membranes at sites of apposition to nerve terminals.

Physiology of Taste

Although all taste buds look histologically alike, sensitivity to the four basic taste modalities is different in different regions of the tongue. Like olfaction, the sense of taste is a chemical sense. Although humans can taste a large number of substances, only four primary taste sensations are identified:

- Sour
- Salty
- Sweet
- Bitter

Most taste receptors respond to all four primary taste modalities at varying thresholds but respond preferentially at a very low threshold to only one or two. Thus, taste buds at the tip of the tongue respond best to sweet and salty substances, and those at the lateral margins and posterior part of the tongue respond best to sour and bitter substances, respectively.

The ability of taste buds to detect changes in concentration of a substance is poor, similar to the response of olfactory receptors. A difference in taste intensity remains undetected until the concentration of a substance has changed by 30%. The mechanism by which a substance is tasted is not well understood. Substances in solution enter the pore of the taste bud and come in contact with the surface of taste receptors. This contact induces a change in the electrical potential of the membrane of the receptor cells (receptor or generator potential). The receptor potential in turn generates an action potential in nerve terminals in opposition to the receptor cell surface.

Central Transmission of Taste Sensations

Taste sensations from the anterior two thirds of the tongue are mediated to the central nervous system via the chorda tympani of the seventh (facial) cranial nerve, those from the posterior one third of the tongue via the ninth (glossopharyngeal) cranial nerve, and those from the epiglottis and lower pharynx via the tenth (vagus) nerve. These nerves contain the peripheral processes of pseudo-unipolar sensory nerve cells located in the geniculate ganglion (seventh nerve), petrous ganglion (ninth nerve), and nodose ganglion (tenth nerve). These peripheral processes enter the deep ends of the taste buds and establish intimate contact with the neuroepithelial cells of the buds.

The central processes of these sensory neurons project to the nucleus of the tractus solitarius in the brain stem. Axons of neurons in the nucleus solitarius project upon a number of reticular nuclei before crossing the midline to reach the ventral posteromedial (VPM) nucleus of the thalamus, giving on their way collateral branches to such nuclei as the nucleus ambiguus and salivatory nuclei for reflex activity. From the VPM nucleus, axons project to the cerebral cortex to terminate upon neurons in the inferior part of the somesthetic cortex, just anterior to the face area.

VISION

Vision is by far the most important of the human senses. Most of our perception of the environment around us comes through our eyes. Our visual system is capable of adapting to extreme changes in light intensity to allow us to see clearly; it is also capable of color discrimination and depth perception. The organ of vision is the eye; accessory structures are the eyelids, lacrimal glands, and extrinsic eye muscles.

The eye has been compared to a camera. Although structurally the two are similar, the camera lacks the intricate automatic control mechanism involved in vision. As an optical instrument, the eye has four functional components: a protective coat, a nourishing lightproof coat, a dioptric system, and a receptive integrating layer. The *protective coat* is the tough, opaque sclera, which covers the posterior five sixths of the eyeball; it is continuous with the dura mater around the optic nerve. The anterior one sixth is covered by transparent cornea, which belongs to the dioptric system. The *nourishing coat* is made up of the vascular choroid, which supplies nutrients to the retina and, because of its rich content of melanocytes, acts as a *light-absorbing layer.* It corresponds to the pia-arachnoid layer of the nervous system. Anteriorly, this coat becomes the ciliary body and iris. The iris ends at a circular opening, the pupil.

The *dioptric system* comprises the cornea, the lens, the aqueous humor within the anterior eye chamber, and the vitreous body. The dioptric system helps focus the image on the retina. The greatest refraction of incoming light takes place at the air-cornea interface. The lens is supported by the suspensory ligament from the ciliary body, and changes in its shape permit change of focus. This is a function of the ciliary muscle, which is supplied by the parasympathetic nervous system. In late middle age, the lens loses its elastic properties and a condition known as presbyopia results, wherein accommodative power is diminished, especially for near vision. The amount of light entering the eye is regulated by the size of the pupil. Pupillary size is controlled by the action of the constrictor and dilator smooth muscles of the iris. The constrictor muscle is supplied by the parasympathetic nervous system, and the dilator muscle by the sympathetic nervous system.

The *receptive integrating layer* of the eye is the retina, which is an extension of the brain, to which it is connected by the optic nerve. The *rods and cones* are the sensory retinal receptors. The rods are about 20 times as numerous as the cones. The rods and cones differ in their distribution along the retina. In humans, a modified region of the retina, the fovea, contains only cones and is adapted for high visual acuity. At all other points along the retina, rods greatly outnumber cones. Rods function best for peripheral vision and during dim-light vision; cones function for central vision, during bright-light vision, and in color discrimination. The outer segments of rods and cones contain the visual pigments rhodopsin and iodopsin (cone opsin), respectively. Light falling on these pigments results in a series of chemical changes leading to depolarization of the receptor cell membrane (receptor or generator potential) and the formation of an action potential, which is then conducted to the brain.

The Sclera

The sclera is a dense fibrous tissue in which collagen bundles are intermixed with ground substance and fibroblasts. The anterior portion of the sclera constitutes the "white" of the eye. In infancy, the sclera is thin and relatively translucent, and it may look bluish because underlying pigmented structures are visible through it. The sclera is perforated posteriorly to allow passage of optic nerve fibers. The perforated area forms the *scleral foramen*. Short posterior ciliary arteries penetrate the area around the scleral foramen. Long posterior ciliary arteries pierce the sclera on the medial and lateral aspects of the scleral foramen and pass anteriorly to supply the anterior uveal tract. Thickness of the sclera varies; it is approximately 1 mm posteriorly and gradually thins to about 0.3 mm just posterior to the insertion of the rectus muscles. The *episclera* is a vascularized connective tissue that covers the sclera and merges with the conjunctiva at the junction of the sclera and cornea, an area called the limbus.

The Conjunctiva

The conjunctiva is a thin, transparent mucous membrane that lines the posterior surface of the lids *(palpebral conjunctiva)* and covers the eyeball *(bulbar conjunctiva)* except for the cornea. The area where the bulbar and palpebral conjunctivae meet is the *fornix*. The conjunctiva is made up of stratified columnar epithelium, about four layers thick, and a lamina propria of loose connective tissue rich in blood vessels. The lamina propria increases in density at deeper levels. Scattered among the epithelial cells are mucus-secreting goblet cells, which increase in number near the cornea. At the medial angle of each eye, there are two specialized structures formed, in part, of conjunctiva: the semilunar fold and the lacrimal caruncle. The *semilunar fold (plica semilunaris)* is a vertical crescent of conjunctiva with its free edges concave to the corneal margin. The *lacrimal caruncle* is modified skin containing sweat and oil glands.

The Cornea

The cornea, the "window" of the eye, is a colorless, nonvascular, transparent structure. Major refraction of light rays occurs at the air-corneal interface. The surface of the cornea is convex. Changes in surface convexity affect refraction and the clarity of the image. The transverse diameter of the cornea is about 10 mm at birth. The cornea attains its adult size of 12 mm during the first 2 years of life. It is composed of five distinct layers (Fig. 14–3):

- Corneal epithelium
- Anterior limiting membrane
- Substantia propria
- Posterior limiting membrane
- Corneal endothelium

The *corneal epithelium* is of the nonkeratinized

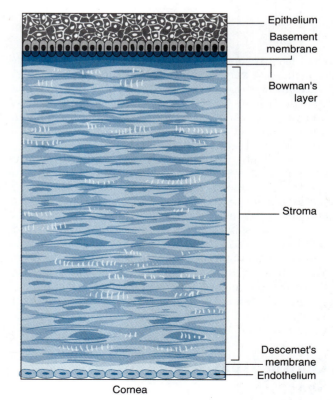

FIGURE 14–3. The five layers of the cornea. *Superficial to the deep corneal epithelium, Bowman's layer, the substantia propria (stroma), Descemet's membrane, and corneal endothelium are shown.*

stratified squamous type. The basal layer of cells is columnar, and the most superficial are flattened.

The second layer of the cornea, the *anterior limiting membrane*, was described by Sir William Bowman, an English surgeon, and therefore is also called *Bowman's membrane*. This membrane appears homogeneous and structureless on light microscopy. Electron microscopy, however, shows it to be composed of fine collagenous fibrils and intercellular substance. It measures 7 to 12 μm in thickness.

The *substantia propria* constitutes nine tenths of the thickness of the cornea and is composed of collagen fibrils, fibroblasts, and cementing substance. The fibrils are arranged in lamellae that run parallel to the surface of the cornea. The fibroblasts are flattened and lie between the fibrous lamellae. A mucopolysaccharide rich in chondroitin sulfate cements the different lamellae and the collagenous fibrils within lamellae together. The metachromatic protein polysaccharide ground substance and the arrangement of fibrils within the substantia propria contribute to the transparency of the cornea.

The *posterior limiting membrane* of the cornea was described by the French surgeon Descemet in 1758 and hence is also known by his name (Descemet's membrane). English anatomists state that it was first described by Benedict Duddell, an English oculist. The membrane appears homogeneous with the light microscope. Electron microscopy reveals a wide basement membrane made of atypical collagen. It is 5 to 10 μm in thickness.

The *corneal endothelium* consists of low cuboidal epithelium. The term *endothelium* is a misnomer, because this epithelium is bathed by aqueous humor of the anterior chamber, and not by blood or lymph.

A 7-μm-thick tear film covers the cornea. The film has three layers. The *oily superficial layer* is secreted by meibomian glands. It serves to reduce evaporation of the *middle aqueous layer*, which is derived from accessory lacrimal glands. The third layer is a very *thin mucous layer* that covers the superficial epithelial layer of the cornea.

Superficial abrasions of corneal epithelium heal rapidly without a scar. Regeneration of injured corneal epithelium is effected by the basal part of the epithelium, which has a turnover time of approximately 7 days. Injury to deeper layers of cornea, however, often results in a permanent corneal scar.

The Uvea

The uveal tract consists of three structures:

- Iris
- Ciliary body
- Choroid

The Iris

The iris, an extension of the choroid, is the most anterior structure of the uveal tract. It is a diaphragm that lies in front of the lens and divides the aqueous compartment into an anterior and a posterior chamber. The anterior surface of the iris has many ridges and furrows. The center of the iris is perforated by an aperture, the *pupil*. Pupillary constriction, as occurs when light is shone on the eye, is accomplished by activation of the sphincter pupillae muscle, which is innervated by the parasympathetic fibers within the oculomotor nerve (third cranial nerve). Dilatation of the pupil is facilitated by relaxation of the sphincter pupillae muscle and by stimulation of the dilator pupillae muscle, which is innervated by the sympathetic nervous system.

The color of the iris depends on the amount of pigment in its stroma. The pigmentation in a brown iris is more dense and diffuse than that in a blue iris. The iris is usually blue at birth in Caucasians, because of the relatively small amount of pigment in melanocytes. During the first few months of life, pigment increases, and by 6 months, one can determine whether the iris will become brown or will remain blue. The iris stroma in blacks is usually denser and contains more pigmented melanocytes at birth. Albinos have almost no pigment in their eyes. The pink color of their irises is due to the reflection of light from blood vessels of the iris.

The iris is made up of the following layers, arranged from anterior to posterior: anterior border layer, stroma, and pigment epithelium.

The *anterior border layer* is a condensation of iris stroma formed principally of pigment cells. The thickness of this layer determines the color of the iris. It is thin in blue-eyed individuals and thick in brown-eyed individuals.

The *stroma* consists of loose connective tissue, a large number of blood vessels, and scattered pigment connective tissue cells. The number of pigment cells varies with the complexion of the individual. The stroma also contains the circumferentially arranged smooth muscle fibers of the sphincter pupillae muscle at the margin of the pupil. The sphincter pupillae muscle is supplied by parasympathetic postganglionic fibers of the oculomotor nerve (third cranial nerve), whose neurons are located in the ciliary ganglion. Contraction of the sphincter pupillae muscle constricts the pupil. Blood vessels in the stromal layer run radially in a spiral fashion, permitting them to accommodate to changes in length with changes in pupillary diameter.

The *pigment epithelium* is a continuation of the ciliary epithelium on the posterior surface of the iris. It is formed of two layers of heavily pigmented cells. The anterior layer is made up of overlapping myoepithelial cells that constitute the dilator pupillae muscle. The dilator pupillae muscle is supplied by the sympathetic nervous system.

Ciliary Body

The ciliary body is a 6-mm-wide ring of muscle and vascular tissue located at the posterior aspect of the iris root and the choroid. Loose connective tissue surrounds the ciliary muscles. The ciliary muscles run in circular, radial, and meridional directions. The circular fibers lie at the inner edge of the ciliary body. Scattered among the muscle fibers are melanocytes.

As the ciliary body approaches the lens, it is thrown into numerous folds, the *ciliary processes*. Ciliary processes are lined by columnar or cuboidal epithelium overlying a core of loose connective tissue. The ciliary processes provide an anchor to the suspensory ligament of the lens. Delicate collagenous fibers *(zonular fibers)* of the suspensory ligament stretch between the lens capsule and the ciliary processes. When the eye is at rest, zonular fibers, under tension from elastic fibers in the choroid, stretch the lens. Contraction of the ciliary muscles within the ciliary body releases tension in the zonular fibers; the lens becomes more spherical, increasing its accommodating power, as in near vision.

The epithelium of ciliary processes contributes to the formation and diffusion of *aqueous humor* in the posterior chamber. Aqueous humor flows between the iris and the lens into the anterior chamber. In the anterior chamber, it flows to the angle formed by the cornea with the basal part of the iris. It penetrates the trabecular meshwork of the limbus to reach the canal of Schlemm, and into the veins of the sclera. Obstruction of the flow of the aqueous humor increases intraocular pressure, a condition known as glaucoma.

The Choroid

The choroid is a highly vascular coat situated between the retina and the sclera. It merges with the ciliary body just posterior to the corneoscleral junction. Its primary function is to provide nourishment to the outer layers of the retina. Between blood vessels, the choroid contains loose connective tissue rich in melanocytes. The larger choroidal arteries and veins are located next to the sclera. The inner layer of the choroid is rich in capillaries and is termed the *choriocapillary layer*. A thin homogeneous membrane, *Bruch's membrane*, separates the choriopapillary layer from the pigment epithelium of the retina.

The Lens

The lens is a biconvex, transparent disk located behind the iris. The narrow space between the lens and the iris is the *posterior chamber*. A homogeneous elastic capsule, 10 to 20 μm thick, surrounds the lens core. The capsule is rich in carbohydrates and consists of type IV collagen and glycoprotein. Beneath the lens capsule anteriorly is a single layer of simple cuboidal epithelial cells *(subcapsular epithelium)* that continue to form new lens fibers throughout a person's life. The *lens fibers* are nucleated, elongated, concentrically arranged, flattened cells that are closely packed. They eventually lose their nuclei, become compressed centrally, and create well-defined zones.

The lens is attached to the ciliary processes by the *zonules* of the *suspensory ligament*. At rest, the zonules are taut and exert a pull on the lens capsule, resulting in flattening of its surface. When the ciliary muscle contracts, the zonules relax, and the lens becomes more spherical, allowing more accommodating (focusing) power. Absence of zonules leads to a notch in the area of the lens in which the zonules are missing (coloboma). Pronounced absence of zonules leads to lens displacement toward the opposite side (subluxation of lens). With advancing age, lens elasticity decreases, rendering accommodation for near vision difficult. This condition, known as presbyopia, is corrected by use of glasses with convex lenses. Lens opacities may occur at any age; they are referred to as *cataracts*.

The Vitreous Body

The vitreous compartment is the largest cavity of the eye, occupying roughly two thirds of its volume. It is composed of a gel of water, a network of collagen fibers, and hyaluronic acid. The vitreous body is bounded anteriorly by the lens, zonules, and ciliary body and posteriorly by the retina and optic nerve. It is firmly attached to the retinal surface, especially at the ora serrata, the fovea, and the optic nerve head. The vitreous body, lens, aqueous humor, and cornea constitute a series of refractive media through which light passes to reach the retina.

The Retina

Light rays falling on the eye pass through its refractive media (cornea, lens, and anterior and posterior chambers) before reaching the visual receptor cells (the rods and cones) in the retina. The refractive media help focus the image on the retina.

The retina (Fig. 14–4), an ectodermal derivative, is an outward extension of the brain, to which it is connected by the optic nerve. The human retina is made up of the following layers, starting with the outermost:

- Layer of pigment epithelium
- Layer of rods and cones
- External limiting membrane
- Outer nuclear layer
- Outer plexiform layer
- Inner nuclear layer
- Inner plexiform layer
- Layer of ganglion cells
- Optic nerve layer
- Internal limiting membrane

LAYER OF PIGMENT EPITHELIUM. The pigment epithelium is a single layer of melanin-containing, pigmented cuboidal cells firmly bound at their bases to the choroid layer. The cell membrane at the apices of these epithelial cells is specialized into slender microvilli that interdigitate with the outer segments of photoreceptor cells. The lateral walls show conspicuous zonulae occludentes and zonulae adherentes as well as desmosomes and gap junctions. Retinal detachment, essentially a splitting of this layer from the other retinal layers, is nowadays treated with laser surgery.

LAYER OF RODS AND CONES. The rods and cones are the light-sensitive parts of the photoreceptors. The human

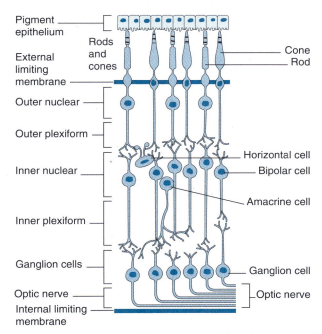

FIGURE 14–4. *The ten layers of the retina, arranged from the outermost (the layer of pigment epithelium) to the innermost (the internal limiting membrane).* Axons of ganglion cells compose the optic nerve. The retinal cells may be grouped into input (receptive) elements (rods and cones), intrinsic elements (bipolar, horizontal, and amacrine cells), and output elements (ganglion cells).

retina contains approximately 100 million rods and 6 to 7 million cones. The rods and cones differ in their distribution along the retina. In humans, a modified region called the *fovea* contains only cones and is adapted for high visual acuity. At all other points along the retina, rods greatly outnumber cones.

Rods. The rod photoreceptor cell is a modified neuron (50 by 3 μm), having as components the cell body, axonal process, and photosensitive process.

The *cell body* contains the nucleus. This part of the rod is located in the outer nuclear layer. The *axonal process* is located in the outer plexiform layer.

The *photosensitive process* is located in the layer of rods and cones. The photosensitive process of the rod is made up of two segments, outer and inner, connected by a narrow neck containing cilia. The outer segment has been shown by electron microscopy to be filled with stacks of double membrane disks (600 to 1000) containing the visual pigment *rhodopsin*. The disks are not continuous with the cell membrane. The function of the outer segment is to trap the light that reaches the retina. The visual pigment molecules are positioned within the disk membranes in such a way as to maximize the probability of their interacting with the path of incident light. The extensive invagination of the disk membranes increases the total surface area available for visual pigment. Rhodopsin is composed of a vitamin A aldehyde *(retinal)* combined with the protein scotopsin. Exposure to light breaks the bond between retinal and the protein. This chemical change triggers a change in the electrical potential and produces a generator (receptor) potential. The stacked disks in the outer segment are shed continually and are replaced by the infolding of the cell membrane. The outer segments are separated and supported by processes from the layer of pigment epithelium.

The inner segment of the rod's photosensitive process contains mitochondria, glycogen, endoplasmic reticulum, and Golgi apparatus. It is the site of formation of the protein scotopsin, which subsequently moves to the outer segment. The inner segment is connected to the cell body of the rod fiber, which traverses the external limiting membrane. The outer segment of rods is the photosensitive part of the rod, where the receptor potential is generated, whereas the inner segment is the site of metabolic activity, where protein and phospholipids are synthesized and energy is produced. Extremely sensitive to light, rods are the receptors used when low levels of light are available such as at night.

Cones. Cones have the same structural components as the rods (cell body, axonal process, and photosensitive process). They measure 16 by 1.5 μm.

The photosensitive processes of cones, like those of rods, contain outer and inner segments. The disks in the outer segments are attached to the cell membrane and are not shed. They are 0.014 μm thick and contain *iodopsin*, an unstable, light-sensitive visual pigment composed of vitamin A aldehyde conjugated to a specific protein (cone opsin). Cones are sensitive to light of higher intensity than that required for rod vision.

EXTERNAL LIMITING MEMBRANE. A sievelike sheet, the external limiting membrane is fenestrated to allow the passage of processes that connect the photosensitive processes of rods and cones with their cell bodies. It also contains the outer processes of Müller's (supporting) cells.

OUTER NUCLEAR LAYER. The outer nuclear layer of the retina contains the cell bodies of rods and cones with their nuclei. Cone nuclei are ovoid and limited to a single row close to the external limiting membrane. Rod nuclei are rounded and distributed in several layers.

OUTER PLEXIFORM LAYER. Also known as the outer synaptic layer, the outer plexiform layer contains axonal processes of rods and cones, as well as dendrites of bipolar cells and processes of horizontal cells.

INNER NUCLEAR LAYER. The inner nuclear layer contains cell bodies and nuclei of bipolar cells and association cells (horizontal and amacrine) as well as supporting (Müller's) cells. The layer has three zones: an outer zone containing horizontal cells, an intermediate zone containing bipolar cells, and an inner zone containing amacrine cells.

Three types of *bipolar cells* are recognized. Rod bipolar cells are related to several rod axons, midget bipolar cells are related to one cone axon, and flat bipolar cells are related to several cone axons.

The *horizontal association cells* are larger than bipolar cells. Their axons and dendrites are located in the outer plexiform layer. Their axons establish synapses with rod and cone axons, whereas their dendrites establish relationships with cone axons. Thus, they connect cones of one area with cones and rods of another area.

The *amacrine association cells* are pear-shaped.

Each has a single process that terminates on a bipolar or ganglion cell process in the inner plexiform layer.

Müller's supporting cells send their processes to the outer plexiform layer.

INNER PLEXIFORM LAYER. The inner plexiform, also called synaptic, layer contains axons of bipolar cells, dendrites of ganglion cells, and processes of the association (amacrine) cells.

LAYER OF GANGLION CELLS. The perikarya of multipolar ganglion cells constitute the eighth layer of the retina. Two types of ganglion cells are recognized on the basis of their dendritic connections: a *monosynaptic (midget) ganglion cell* related to a single bipolar midget cell and a *diffuse (polysynaptic) ganglion cell* related to several bipolar cells. The axons of ganglion cells form the optic nerve. This part of the retina is called the *blind spot*. In humans, the number of ganglion cells is estimated to be 1 million.

OPTIC NERVE LAYER. The optic nerve layer is composed of axons of ganglion cells that form the optic nerve, as well as some Müller's fibers and neuroglial cells. Axons of ganglion cells in this layer are unmyelinated but have a glial sheath around them. They run toward the posterior pole of the eye, where they form the optic disk and penetrate the sclera to form the optic nerve.

INTERNAL LIMITING MEMBRANE. The expanded inner ends of the processes of Müller's cells form the internal limiting membrane. Müller's cells, the cell bodies of which are located in the inner nuclear layer, send processes both outward to the external limiting membrane and inward to the internal limiting membrane. They are thus homologous to glial cells of the central nervous system.

Retinal Structure and Blood Supply

The retinal structure just described is maintained throughout the retina except at two sites, the fovea centralis in the central area of the retina and ora serrata at the periphery of the retina. In both sites, ganglion cell layer, inner plexiform layer, and bipolar cell layer are absent.

The *fovea centralis* represents the area of greatest visual acuity, and its center contains only cones arranged in multiple rows. The cones of the fovea are slender and resemble rods. The thinning of the retina at the fovea centralis reduces to a minimum tissue through which light passes, hence improving visual acuity. Cones in this area function for sharp vision and color perception.

Near the *ora serrata*, at the periphery of the retina, rods predominate, increase in thickness, and become shorter. The cones decrease in number and also become shorter.

The retina receives its vascular supply from two sources. The outer retina is vascularized by the choriocapillaris layer of the choroid. The inner retina receives its blood supply from the central artery of the retina and its branches. The foveal area, the area of most acute vision, is vascularized mostly by the underlying choriocapillaries of the choroid. If the retina surrounding the fovea becomes semiopaque, as in occlusion of the central retinal artery or in some of the lipid storage diseases (e.g., Tay-Sachs disease), the choroid underlying the thin avascular fovea appears as a bright red circle called a cherry-red spot.

Synaptic Organization of the Retina
(Fig. 14–5)

The human retina is considered to be a simple retina in which there is relatively little processing of information, compared with complex retinas, such as the frog's, in which information processing is more extensive.

The different types of cells encountered in the retina can be divided into three categories:

- Input elements (rods and cones)
- Output elements (ganglion cells)
- Intrinsic elements (bipolar, horizontal, and amacrine cells)

It is estimated that the human retina contains 100 million rods, 6 to 7 million cones, and 1 million ganglion cells. This provides input-to-output ratios of 100:1 for rods and 5:1 for cones. This difference correlates well with the function of cones, namely high acuity vision. The input-to-output ratio is lowest (approximately 1:1) in the fovea centralis, where visual acuity is highest.

Synaptic interaction in the retina takes place in two layers, the outer plexiform layer and the inner plexiform layer.

SYNAPTIC INTERACTION IN THE OUTER PLEXIFORM LAYER. In the outer plexiform layer, synaptic interaction occurs both vertically and horizontally. The vertical interaction is represented by the rod and cone terminals on bipolar cell dendrites. The horizontal interaction is represented by the interaction of horizontal cell processes with both

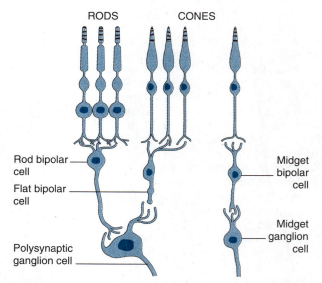

FIGURE 14–5. The types of synaptic activity within the retina. Synaptic interaction takes place in outer and inner plexiform layers. Synaptic interactions in the outer plexiform layer are between rods, cones, and bipolar cells. Interactions in the inner plexiform layer are between bipolar cells and ganglion cells.

rod and cone axons. Axon terminals of rods *(rod spherules)* are smaller than cone terminals; the latter are flat or pyramidal and large *(cone pedicles)*.

RECEPTOR–BIPOLAR CELL INTERACTION. As stated previously, there are three varieties of bipolar cells. A rod bipolar cell forms synapses with several rod spherules. A midget bipolar cell forms synapses with one cone pedicle. A flat bipolar cell forms synapses with several cone pedicles.

HORIZONTAL CELL–RECEPTOR INTERACTION. Horizontal cell processes form synapses with several cones or rods, relating cones of one area to rods and cones of another area. Processes of horizontal cells are not classified as either axons or dendrites and possibly transmit bidirectionally.

SYNAPTIC INTERACTION IN THE INNER PLEXIFORM LAYER. In the inner plexiform layer, synaptic interaction occurs vertically, between bipolar and ganglion cells, as well as horizontally, among amacrine, bipolar, and ganglion cells.

BIPOLAR CELL–GANGLION CELL INTERACTION. Rod bipolar cells project upon several ganglion cells. Midget bipolar cells relate to one ganglion cell (midget ganglion cell). Flat bipolar cells relate to several ganglion cells.

AMACRINE, BIPOLAR, AND GANGLION CELL INTERACTION. Amacrine cells relate to axons of bipolar cells as well as to dendrites and perikarya of ganglion cells. Amacrine cell processes, like horizontal cell processes, probably conduct bidirectionally.

CHARACTERISTICS OF SYNAPTIC INTERACTION. It is apparent, from the preceding description, that synaptic activity in the retina has the following characteristics:

- It is oriented both vertically (receptor-bipolar-ganglion cell axis) and horizontally (via horizontal and amacrine cell connections)
- It is carried out by both diffuse (flat bipolar– or rod bipolar–polysynaptic ganglion cell) and oligosynaptic (midget bipolar–midget ganglion cell) pathways.

Photochemistry and Physiology of the Retina

The retina contains two types of photoreceptors, the rods and the cones. The rods are highly sensitive to light, have a low threshold of stimulation, and are thus best suited for dim-light vision. Such vision, however, is poor in detail and does not differentiate colors *(achromatic)*. The cones, however, have a high threshold of stimulation and function best in strong illumination (daylight). They provide the substrate for acute vision as well as color vision.

Upon exposure to light, the visual pigments in the outer segments of the rods and cones (rhodopsin and cone opsin, respectively) break down into two components, retinal (colorless pigment) and the protein opsin. The degradation of visual pigment triggers a change in the electrical potential of the photoreceptors (receptor or generator potential). The generator potential of rods and cones (unlike similar potentials in other receptors) is in the hyperpolarizing direction. This unique response of the photoreceptors has been attributed to the fact that the photoreceptor membrane is depolarized in the resting state (darkness) by a constant leak of electrical current (sodium ion permeability) in the outer segment. Exposure to light reduces the permeability of the membrane to sodium ions, lowers the electrical current, and hyperpolarizes the membrane. Thus, hyperpolarizing currents in photoreceptors are produced by turning off depolarizing sodium ion conductance, whereas the orthodox hyperpolarization—inhibitory postsynaptic potential (IPSP)—seen in other neurons is produced by turning on hyperpolarizing potassium ion conductance in the neuronal membrane.

The generator potential of photoreceptors leads to hyperpolarization or depolarization of the bipolar and horizontal cells. Neither of these cell types, however, is capable of triggering a propagated action potential.

On the basis of their hyperpolarizing or depolarizing response, two types of bipolar cells are identified. One type responds by hyperpolarization to a light spot in the center of its receptive field and by depolarization to a light spot in the area surrounding the center *(the surround)*. The other type responds in a reverse fashion by depolarization to a light spot in the center of its receptive field and by hyperpolarization to the surround. The bipolar cell is the first of the retinal elements to show this variation of response in relation to the spatial position of the stimulus in its receptive field.

The amacrine cell responds to a light stimulus by a propagated, all-or-none action potential. It is the first cell of the retinal elements to generate a propagated action potential.

Ganglion cells discharge continuously at a slow rate in the absence of any stimulus. Upon superimposition of a circular beam of light, ganglion cells may behave in a variety of ways. Some cells increase their discharge in response to the superimposed stimulus ("on" cells). Others inhibit their discharge in response to the superimposed stimulus, but discharge again with a burst when the stimulus is turned off ("off" cells). Still others increase their discharge when the stimulus is turned both on and off ("on-off" cells). Furthermore, the behavior of ganglion cells, like that of bipolar cells, is regulated by the spatial position of the stimulus in their receptive field. "On" cells, which increase their discharge in response to a spot of light in the center of their receptive field, inhibit their discharge when light is shone in the area surrounding the center. The same principle applies to "off" cells, which inhibit their discharge in response to a light stimulus in the center of the receptive field, but increase their discharge when the stimulus is shone in the surround.

Furthermore, some ganglion cells respond only to a steady stimulus of light in their receptive field, whereas others respond only to a change in intensity of illumination; still others respond only to a stimulus moving in a particular direction.

Dark and Light Adaptation

When an individual moves from an environment of bright light to dim light or darkness, the retina adapts and becomes more sensitive to light. This process, called *dark adaptation*, takes about 20 minutes to become maximally effective. The time required for maximal adaptation to darkness can be shortened by wearing red glasses. Light waves in the red end of the spectrum do not effectively stimulate the rods, which remain dark-adapted. Nor do red light waves interfere with cone stimulation, so the individual can still see in bright light. The process of dark adaptation has two components, a fast one attributed to adaptation of cones and a slower one attributed to adaptation of rods.

Conversely, when an individual moves from a dark environment to a bright one, it takes time to adapt to the bright environment. This process, called *light adaptation*, takes about 5 minutes to be effective.

NIGHT BLINDNESS. Night blindness *(nyctalopia)* is encountered in individuals with vitamin A deficiency. As mentioned previously, photoreceptor pigment is formed of two substances, vitamin A aldehyde (retinal) and the protein opsin. In vitamin A deficiency, the total amount of visual pigment is reduced, thus decreasing the sensitivity to light of both rods and cones. Although this reduction does not interfere with bright-light (daylight) vision, it does significantly affect dark-light (night) vision, because the amount of light is not enough to excite the depleted visual pigment. This condition is treatable by administration of vitamin A.

Color Vision

Color vision is a function of the retina, lateral geniculate nucleus, and cerebral cortex.

In the retina, the cone receptors and the horizontal cells as well as ganglion cells take part in the integration of color vision. According to the Young-Helmholtz theory of color vision, there are three varieties of retinal cone receptors: those that respond maximally to wavelengths in the red end of the spectrum, those that respond maximally to wavelengths in the green end of the spectrum, and those that respond maximally to wavelengths in the blue range of the spectrum. A monochromatic color (red, green, or blue) stimulates one variety of cones maximally and the other varieties of cones to a variable but lesser degree. Blue light, for example, stimulates blue cones maximally, green cones much less so, and red cones not at all. This pattern is interpreted centrally as blue color. Two monochromatic colors stimulating two types of cones equally and simultaneously are interpreted as a different color; thus, if green and red lights stimulate green and red cones simultaneously and equally, they are interpreted as yellow. Simultaneous and equal stimulation by red, green, and blue lights is interpreted as white.

The horizontal cells respond to a particular monochromatic color by either depolarization or hyperpolarization. A red-green horizontal cell responds by depolarization to red light and by hyperpolarization to green light. Such a cell is turned off by equal and simultaneous stimulation by red and green. There are also yellow-blue horizontal cells, accounting for the four hues—red, green, blue, and yellow. The depolarization and hyperpolarization responses of horizontal cells also explain why red with green and blue with yellow are complementary colors, which, when mixed together in proper amounts, result in the cancellation of color.

Ganglion cells of the retina respond in an "on-off" manner to monochromatic light. Thus, there are green "on" and red "off" ganglion cells, blue "on" and yellow "off" ganglion cells, and so on.

Furthermore, there are color-sensitive neurons in the lateral geniculate nucleus and occipital cortex that respond maximally to color in one part of the spectrum. They also play a role in color discrimination. The color-contrast cells in the striate cortex form a distinct population separate from cells concerned with brightness contrast. As with cells concerned with brightness discrimination, the color-contrast cells can be divided into simple, complex, and hypercomplex cells.

COLOR BLINDNESS. Some people have a deficiency in or lack of a particular color cone. Such people have color weakness or color blindness, respectively. Most color-blind persons are red-green blind; a minority are blue blind. Among the group blind to red-green, there is a preponderance of green color blindness.

Color blindness for red and green is inherited by an X-linked recessive gene; thus, there are more males with red-green color blindness than females. Color blindness for blue is inherited through an autosomal gene.

Visual Pathways

Axons of ganglion cells in the retina gather together at the optic disk in the posterior pole of the eye, penetrate the sclera, and form the optic nerve. The point of exit of ganglion cell axons from the retina, the optic disk is devoid of receptor elements (blind spot). There are approximately 1 million axons in the optic nerve. Outside the sclera, the optic nerve is covered by extensions of the meninges that ensheathe the brain. Marked increase in intracranial pressure from tumors or bleeding inside the cranial cavity or increase in cerebrospinal fluid pressure around the nerve sufficient to interfere with venous return from the retina results in swelling of the optic disk (papilledema). This swelling can be seen using a special instrument, an ophthalmoscope, which views the retina through the pupil.

The optic nerve enters the cranial cavity through the optic foramen. Thus, tumors of the optic nerve (optic glioma) may be diagnosed by taking radiographs of the optic foramen, which appears enlarged in such conditions. Lesions of the optic nerve produce unilateral blindness on the side of the lesion (Fig. 14–6A).

The two optic nerves come together at the optic chiasma, where partial crossing of optic nerve fibers takes place. Optic nerve fibers from the nasal half of each retina cross at the optic chiasma. Fibers from the temporal halves remain uncrossed. The optic chiasma is related to the hypothalamus above and pituitary gland below. Thus, tumors in the pituitary gland encroaching (as they do initially) on the crossing fibers of the optic nerve cause degeneration of optic nerve fibers arising in the nasal halves of both retinae. This

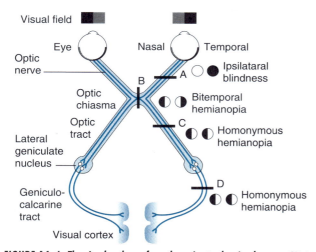

FIGURE 14–6. The visual pathway from the retina to the visual cortex. *Clinical manifestations of lesions in the optic nerve (A), optic chiasma (B), optic tract (C), and geniculocalcarine tract (optic radiation) (D) are shown.*

results in loss of vision in both temporal fields of vision (bitemporal hemianopia) (Fig. 14–6B).

The crossed and uncrossed fibers from both optic nerves join caudal to the optic chiasma to form the optic tract. Lesions of the optic tracts, therefore, cause degeneration of optic nerve fibers from the temporal half of the ipsilateral retina and nasal half of the contralateral retina. This produces loss of vision in the contralateral half of the visual field (homonymous hemianopia) (Fig. 14–6C).

The lateral geniculate nucleus is laminated into six layers. Not all parts of the retina are represented equally in the lateral geniculate nucleus. Proportionally much more of the nucleus is devoted to the representation of the central area than of the periphery of the retina.

Axons of neurons in the lateral geniculate nucleus project to the visual cortex in the occipital lobe via the geniculocalcarine tract (optic radiation). Lesions of the geniculocalcarine tract give rise to a contralateral homonymous hemianopia similar to that occurring with lesions of the optic tract (Fig. 14–6D).

Accessory Structures of the Eye

Eyelid

The eyelids are folds of skin that serve to protect the eye. A row of short, stout hairs are found at the free margin of the lid. Superficially, keratinized epidermis blends internally with the conjunctival mucous membrane. Underneath the epidermis is a connective tissue core in which striated and smooth muscles, glands, and hair follicles are located. The hair follicles are similar to those found elsewhere in the body, except for the absence, in lid follicles, of arrector pili smooth muscle. *Meibomian glands (tarsal glands)* are simple, branched alveolar sebaceous glands. The alveoli are connected to a long central excretory duct lined with stratified squamous epithelium. The glands open at the inner free margin of the lid at the junction of the skin and conjunctiva. Secretion of the glands serves to lubricate the lid surface. The meibomian glands were first noted by Casserius in 1609 and were described by Heinrich Meibom, a German anatomist, in 1666.

Lacrimal Gland

The lacrimal gland (located in the anterosuperior temporal portion of the orbit) is composed of a number of compound tubuloalveolar serous glands. The *serous acini* are made up of tall cells with basal nuclei. The secretory product fills the apical cytoplasm. The acini are separated by a thin connective tissue stroma. Myoepithelial cells surround the secretory elements of the gland. The aqueous secretion (tears), after flushing the conjunctival and corneal surfaces, drains into ducts that carry it, via the nasolacrimal duct, to the anterior portion of the inferior meatus of the nose.

HEARING

The Ear

The ear has three compartments: external, middle, and internal. The organs of hearing and equilibrium are located within the internal compartment of the ear.

External Ear

The external ear is formed of the auricle or pinna, external auditory canal, and tympanic membrane. The *auricle* has a core of elastic cartilage covered by skin.

The wall of the *external auditory canal* is made of elastic cartilage in its outer third and bone in the inner two thirds. The canal is lined by stratified squamous epithelium. Beneath the lining epithelium are sebaceous glands, hair follicles, and modified coiled tubular sweat glands *(ceruminous glands)*. The ceruminous glands secrete the cerumen (ear wax).

The *tympanic membrane* (ear drum) delimits the external auditory canal medially. The core of the tympanic membrane is tough connective tissue made up of collagen and elastic fibers and fibroblasts. The connective tissue core is lined externally (toward the external auditory canal) by thin skin and internally (toward the middle ear) by simple cuboidal epithelium continuous with the lining of the tympanic cavity (middle ear).

Middle Ear

The middle ear (tympanic cavity) is located within the temporal bone. It communicates with the nasopharynx anteriorly via the *eustachian (auditory) tube*, and with the mastoid air cells posteriorly. The *tympanic membrane* separates the middle ear from the external ear. The bony surface of the internal ear, with two windows (oval and round), separates the middle ear from the inner ear. The cavity of the middle ear is lined with simple squamous epithelium. Near the auditory tube, the simple epithelium is transformed into pseudostratified ciliated columnar epithelium. The middle ear cavity is traversed by three bony ossicles. The *malleus* is attached to the tympanic membrane, the *stapes* fits into the foramen ovale (oval window), and the *incus* is in between. The three ossicles transmit sound vibrations from the tympanic membrane to the oval window. The cavity also contains two muscles, the tensor tympani and stapedius. The tensor tympani inserts into the malleus, and the stapedius into the stapes.

Inner Ear

The inner ear, located within the petrous portion of the temporal bone, contains two systems of canals or cavities, the osseous labyrinth and the membranous labyrinth. Both systems contain fluids, *perilymph* in the osseous labyrinth and *endolymph* in the membranous labyrinth. The *osseous labyrinth* has a large central cavity, the vestibule, located medial to the tympanic cavity. Three semicircular canals open into the vestibule posteriorly, and a coiled winding tube, the *cochlea*, communicates with the vestibule anteriorly.

The *membranous labyrinth*, located within the osseous labyrinth, maintains a similar configuration. The central cavity of the membranous labyrinth (within the vestibule of the osseous labyrinth) contains two cavities. The *utricle*, the posterior cavity, communicates with the membranous labyrinth of the semicircular canals (semicircular ducts). The *saccule*, the anterior cavity, communicates with the membranous labyrinth of the cochlea (cochlear duct). At the junction of the membranous semicircular canals (semicircular ducts) with the utricle, the epithelium of the semicircular ducts becomes specialized to form a receptive sensory area (neuroepithelium) for equilibrium, the *crista ampullaris*. Similar sensory receptive areas in the utricle and saccule are the *macula utriculi* and the *macula sacculi*. The macula sacculi is located in the floor of the saccule, whereas the macula utriculi is in the lateral wall of the utricle at right angles to the saccule. The sensory receptive organ for hearing is the *organ of Corti* within the cochlear duct.

Mechanics of Audition

Sound waves traverse the external ear and middle ear before reaching the inner ear, where the auditory end organ (organ of Corti) is located.

The tympanic membrane between the external ear and middle ear vibrates in response to pressure changes produced by the incoming sound waves. Vibrations of the tympanic membrane are transmitted to the bony ossicles of the middle ear (malleus, incus, and stapes). The handle of the malleus is attached to the tympanic membrane, and the footplate of the stapes is attached to the oval window between the middle ear and inner ear. Vibrations of the footplate of the stapes are then transmitted to the membrane of the oval window and subsequently to the fluid medium (perilymph) of the inner ear.

The *tensor tympani muscle*, attached to the handle of the malleus, and the *stapedius muscle*, attached to the neck of the stapes, have a damping effect on sound waves. Loud sounds cause these muscles to contract reflexively, to prevent strong sound waves from excessively stimulating the hair cells of the organ of Corti; this is the *tympanic reflex*. When this damping effect is lost, as in lesions of the facial nerve (which supplies the stapedius muscle), sound stimuli are augmented unpleasantly (hyperacusis).

Because of the marked difference in elasticity and density between air and fluid, almost 99% of acoustic energy is reflected back at the air-fluid interface between the middle ear and inner ear. This is, however, counteracted by two mechanisms. First, the ratio between the surface areas of the tympanic membrane and the footplate of the stapes is approximately 25:1. However, because the tympanic membrane is not a piston but a stretched membrane attached around its edge, its effective area is 60% to 75% of its actual area. Thus, the ratio between the effective area of the tympanic membrane and the area of the footplate of the stapes is only 14:1. Second, the *lever effect* counteracts energy lost at the air-fluid interface. The movements of the tympanic membrane are transmitted to the malleus and incus, which move as one unit. The manubrium of the malleus is a longer lever than the long process of the incus. The force exerted at the footplate of the stapes is thus greater than that at the tympanic membrane by a ratio of 1.3:1.

The total pressure amplification via the two mechanisms just described thus counteracts the energy lost at the air-fluid interface. The total gain in force per unit area achieved by conductance in the middle ear is a factor of about 18.

Cochlea

The cochlea is a snail-shaped structure consisting of two and one-half spirals filled with fluid. It has three compartments, the scala vestibuli, scala tympani, and scala media (cochlear duct). The *scala vestibuli* and *scala tympani* are separated by a bony shelf (osseous spiral lamina) projecting from the modiolus across the osseous canal of the cochlea.

The *scala media*, lying between the scala vestibuli (above) and the scala tympani (below), contains the auditory end organ (organ of Corti). The scala vestibuli and scala tympani are continuous through the helicotrema at the apex of the coil. The *oval window* and *round window* separate, respectively, the scala vestibuli and scala tympani from the middle ear (Fig. 14–7).

Vibrations of the oval window are transmitted to the perilymph in the scala vestibuli and, subsequently, via *Reissner's membrane* (which separates the scala vestibuli from the scala media) to the endolymph of the scala media. Vibrations in the endolymph are then transmitted via the basilar membrane (which separates the scala media from the scala tympani) to the perilymph of the scala tympani and out through the round window.

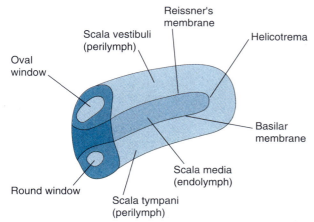

FIGURE 14–7. *The three compartments of the cochlea: the scala vestibuli and scala tympani, containing perilymph, and the scala media, containing endolymph. The scala vestibuli and scala tympani are continuous at the helicotrema. The oval and round windows separate the scala vestibuli and scala tympani from the middle ear.*

Auditory End Organ (Organ of Corti)

The organ of Corti (Fig. 14–8) is located in the scala media *(cochlear duct)*, which is separated from the underlying scala tympani by the basilar membrane and from the scala vestibuli by Reissner's (vestibular) membrane. The cochlear duct is part of the endolymphatic system and contains endolymph. The *basilar membrane* forms the base of the cochlear duct and gives support to the organ of Corti (Fig. 14–9). The outer wall of the cochlear duct is made up of the spiral ligament, which is a thickening of the periosteum. The crest of the spiral ligament forms the spiral prominence (Fig. 14–10).

The part of the spiral ligament between the spiral prominence and the vestibular (Reissner's) membrane is the *stria vascularis*. The epithelium here is thick and pseudostratified. The subepithelial connective tissue is rich in capillaries. The stria vascularis is believed to be

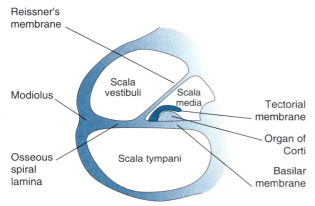

FIGURE 14–8. *The cochlear compartments, showing the organ of Corti in the scala media. The basilar membrane separates the scala media and scala tympani and provides the base for the organ of Corti. Reissner's membrane separates the scala media and scala vestibuli. The tectorial membrane extends over the free surface of the organ of Corti.*

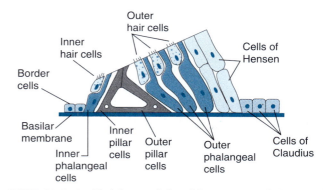

FIGURE 14–9. *Simplified diagram of the cellular components of the organ of Corti. The outer and inner hair cells and supporting cells are shown. The latter includes pillar cells, phalangeal cells, cells of Hensen, and cells of Claudius.*

active in the production of endolymph and the regulation of its ion content. The epithelium of the spiral prominence continues onto the basilar membrane. Cells here become cuboidal. Those cells continuing onto the pars pectinata of the basilar membrane are known as *cells of Claudius* (see Figs. 14–9 and 14–10). In parts of the cochlea, polyhedral cells separating the cells of Claudius and the basilar membrane are known as *cells of Boettcher* (Fig. 14–10).

HAIR CELLS. The auditory receptor cells, the *hair cells*, are of two types: inner hair cells, which number approximately 3,500 arranged in a single row, and outer hair cells, which number approximately 20,000 arranged in three to four rows.

The "hairs" of the hair cells are in contact with the *tectorial membrane*, which transmits to them vibrations from the endolymph. The hair cells are columnar or flask-shaped, with a basally located nucleus and about 50 to 100 hairlike projections (microvilli) emanating from their apical surfaces. Cochlear nerve fibers establish synapses with their basal membranes.

SUPPORTING CELLS. Supporting cells are tall, slender cells extending from the basilar membrane to the free surface of the organ of Corti. They include the following cell types: pillar or rod cells (outer and inner), phalangeal (Deiters's) cells (outer and inner), and cells of Hensen.

Pillar Cells. Pillar cells are filled with tonofibrils. The apices of the inner and outer pillar cells converge at the free surface of the organ of Corti and fan out as a cuticle to form, along with a similar formation of Deiters's cells, a thin plate through which the apices of the inner and outer hair cells pass.

Phalangeal (Deiters's) Cells. Arranged in three to four outer rows and one inner row, Deiters's cells give support to the outer and inner hair cells, respectively. They extend from the basilar membrane, like all supporting cells, to the free surface of the organ of Corti, where they contribute to the formation of the cuticular plate through which the hairs of the hair cells pass. Phalangeal cells are flask-shaped and contain tonofibrils. Some of the tonofibrils support the base of the hair cells; others extend along their sides to the free surface of the organ.

Cells of Hensen. Cells of Hensen are columnar cells

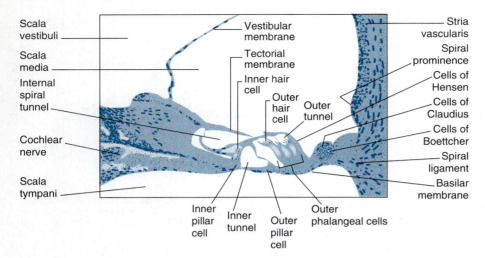

FIGURE 14–10. *The cochlear duct between the scala vestibuli and scala tympani.* Within the cochlear duct is the organ of Corti. The outer wall of the cochlear duct is the spiral ligament. The part of the spiral ligament between the spiral prominence and the vestibular membrane is the stria vascularis, which is believed to be active in production of endolymph.

located adjacent to the outermost row of outer phalangeal cells. They constitute the outer border of the organ of Corti. They merge laterally with cuboidal cells (cells of Claudius). Similar (cuboidal) cells adjacent to the inner phalangeal cells, known as *border cells,* constitute the inner border of the organ.

TECTORIAL MEMBRANE. The tectorial membrane is a gelatinous structure in which filamentous elements are embedded. It extends over the free surface of the organ of Corti. The hairs of the hair cells are attached to the tectorial membrane. Vibrations in the endolymph are transmitted to the tectorial membrane, resulting in deformation of the hairs attached to it. Such deformation initiates an impulse in the afferent nerve fibers in contact with the basal part of the hair cells.

NERVE SUPPLY. The hair cells of the organ of Corti receive two types of nerve supply, afferent and efferent.

The afferent fibers are peripheral processes of bipolar neurons in the spiral ganglion located in the bony core of the cochlear spiral. There are about 30,000 bipolar neurons in the spiral ganglion, 90% of which innervate the inner hair cells. Each inner hair cell receives contacts from about ten fibers; each fiber contacts only one inner hair cell. The remaining 10% of the peripheral processes of bipolar neurons innervate the outer hair cells; each fiber diverges to innervate many outer hair cells.

The efferent fibers originate in the contralateral superior olive in the pons. These fibers form the *olivocochlear bundle of Rasmussen,* which leaves the brain stem via the vestibular component of the vestibulocochlear (eighth cranial) nerve, joins the cochlear componet (vestibulocochlear anastomosis), and terminates peripherally upon the outer hair cells and the afferent terminal boutons innervating inner hair cells. These fibers have an inhibitory effect upon auditory stimuli.

Auditory Physiology

Conduction of Sound Waves

Sound waves may reach the inner ear via three routes:

- Ossicular route
- Air route
- Bone route

OSSICULAR ROUTE. The ossicular route normally conducts sound. Sound waves entering the external auditory meatus produce vibrations in the tympanic membrane, which are transmitted to the bony ossicles of the middle ear and through them to the footplate of the stapes. The energy lost at the air-fluid interface in the oval window is counteracted by the factors outlined previously.

AIR ROUTE. An alternate route, the air route is used when the orthodox ossicular route is not operative owing to disease of the ossicles. In this situation, vibrations of the tympanic membrane are transmitted through air in the middle ear to the round window. This route is not effective in sound conduction.

BONE ROUTE. Sound waves may also be conducted via the bones of the skull directly to the perilymph of the inner ear. This route plays a minor role in sound conduction in normal individuals, but is utilized by deaf people who can use hearing aids.

Fluid Vibration

Vibrations of the footplate of the stapes are transmitted to the perilymph of the scala vestibuli. Pressure waves in the perilymph are transmitted via Reissner's membrane to the endolymph of the scala media and, through the helicotrema, to the perilymph of the scala tympani.

Vibrations of Basilar Membrane

Pressure waves in the endolymph of the scala media produce traveling waves in the basilar membrane of the organ of Corti. The basilar membrane varies in width and degree of stiffness in different regions. It is widest and stiffest at its apex and thinnest and least stiff at its base.

Pressure waves in the endolymph initiate a traveling wave in the basilar membrane that proceeds from the base toward the apex of the membrane. The amplitude of the traveling waves varies at different sites on the membrane, depending on the frequency of sound waves. High-frequency sounds elicit waves with highest amplitude toward the base of the membrane. With low-frequency sounds, the waves with highest amplitude occur toward the apex of the membrane. Similarly, each sound frequency has a site of maximum amplitude wave on the basilar membrane. The frequency of the wave, measured in cycles per second (cps) or hertz (Hz), determines its pitch. The amplitude of the wave is correlated with its loudness; a special scale, the decibel (dB) scale, is used to measure this aspect of sound. Thus, the basilar membrane exhibits the phenomenon of tonotopic localization seen along the central auditory pathways all the way to the cortex.

Receptor Potential

Vibrations of the basilar membrane produce displacement of the hair cells, the hairs of which are attached to the tectorial membrane. The shearing force produced on the hairs by the displacement of hair cells is the adequate stimulus for the receptor nonpropagated potential of the hair cells. This receptor potential is also known as the *cochlear microphonic potential*. It can be recorded from the hair cells and their immediate neighborhood and is a faithful replica of the mechanical events of sound waves previously described. The genesis of receptor potentials is not fully understood. It is believed, however, to be due to a change in membrane potential between the hair cells and the surrounding endolymph induced by the bending of the hairs of hair cells.

Action Potential

The receptor potential initiates an action potential in the afferent nerves in contact with hair cells. The exact mechanism by which receptor potentials initiate action potentials is not fully understood. Records of afferent nerve activity reveal that the afferent nerves have a constant background activity (background noise) that is modified by an incoming sound stimulus.

Increasing the intensity of sound of a particular frequency raises the number of hair cells stimulated, the number of afferent nerve fibers activated, and the rate of discharge of impulses. A single nerve fiber responds to a range of frequencies but is most sensitive to a particular frequency, called its *characteristic frequency*; this is related to the region of the basilar membrane that the fiber innervates. Fibers innervating the part of the basilar membrane near the oval window have high characteristic frequencies, whereas those innervating the part of the basilar membrane near the apex of the cochlea have low characteristic frequencies.

Audiometry

The quantitative clinical assessment of hearing acuity is known as *audiometry*; the resulting record is the audiogram. In audiometry, pure tones of known frequency and varying intensity are presented via earphones to the individual, who is asked to signal a response when he or she hears a tone. The examiner records the audible frequencies and intensities on a chart. The record is then examined to compare the audible range of the individual with that of normal individuals.

Deafness

The range of audible frequencies in the normal adult is 20 to 20,000 Hz. With advancing age, there is a decrease in perception of high frequencies (high-frequency deafness). This loss correlates with the loss of hair cells in the basal turns of the cochlea. Similar high-frequency deafness is encountered in individuals intoxicated by the antibiotic streptomycin. Rock band performers, on the other hand, develop middle-frequency deafness.

Deafness disorders are generally separated into two groups, *conductive deafness* and *sensorineural deafness*. The first group includes deafness due to obstruction of the external auditory meatus by wax, as well as middle ear diseases, such as chronic otitis media, and ossicle sclerosis. The second group includes conditions in which hair cells are affected (advancing age, streptomycin toxicity) as well as diseases of the auditory nerve, such as nerve tumors (acoustic neuroma).

The two types of deafness can be identified clinically by use of the tuning fork. A vibrating tuning fork is placed in front of the ear and then on a bony prominence over the skull. A person with normal hearing can hear the tuning fork better when it is placed in front of the ear. A subject with conductive deafness hears the tuning fork better when it is placed over a bony prominence, because sound waves bypass the site of obstruction in the external auditory meatus or the middle ear and reach the auditory end organ via the round window or directly through skull bones to the perilymph.

In patients with unilateral sensorineural deafness, a tuning fork placed over the forehead will be heard best in the healthy ear, since air conduction in such patients is better than bone conduction.

VESTIBULAR SENSATION

The receptors of the vestibular sense organ are located in the semicircular canals, utricle, and saccule in the inner ear. The utricle and saccule are located in the main cavity of the bony labyrinth, the vestibule; the semicircular canals, three in number, are extensions of the utricle (Fig. 14–11). Vestibular sensory receptors are located in the floor of the utricle, wall of the saccule, and dilated portions (ampullae) of each of the three semicircular canals. The optimal stimulus for receptors in the utricle and saccule is linear acceleration of the body, whereas receptors in the semicircular canals respond to angular acceleration.

The vestibular receptor in the semicircular canal

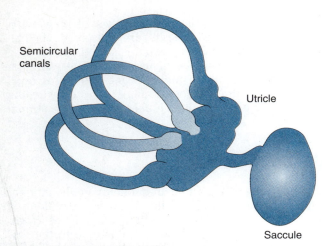

FIGURE 14–11. The vestibular end organ. *The three semicircular canals, the utricle, and the saccule are shown. Sensory receptors are located in the floor of the utricle, the wall of the saccule, and dilated portions of the semicircular canals.*

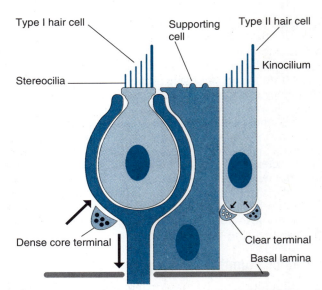

FIGURE 14–12. The vestibular sensory receptor, showing receptor hair cells (types I and II) and a supporting cell. *Each type of hair cell has stereocilia and a kinocilium on the free surface and establishes contact with nerve terminals on its basal surface.*

(crista ampullaris) is composed of hair cells and supporting cells (Fig. 14–12). The hair cells are of two types. The *type I hair cell* is flask-shaped and is surrounded by a nerve terminal *(calyx)*. The *type II hair cell* is cylindrical and is not surrounded by a calyx. Both types of hair cells show on their free surfaces about 40 to 100 short *stereocilia* (modified microvilli) and one long *kinocilium* attached to one border of the cell. The short stereocilia increase progressively in length toward the kinocilium. The stereocilia are nonmotile; the kinocilium is motile.

Supporting cells are slender columnar cells that reach the basal lamina; their free surfaces are specialized into microvilli. The subapical parts of supporting cells are related to adjacent hair cells by junctional complexes.

The apical processes of hair and supporting cells are embedded in a dome-shaped, gelatinous protein-polysaccharide mass, the *cupula*. The cupula swings from side to side in response to currents in the endolymph that bathes it.

The vestibular receptor organ of the utricle and saccule *(macula)* is similar in structure to that of the semicircular canals. The gelatinous mass into which the apical processes of hair and supporting cells project is the *otolithic membrane*. It is flat and contains numerous small crystalline bodies, the otoliths or otoconia, composed of calcium carbonate and protein.

The hair cells of the semicircular canals, utricle, and saccule receive both afferent and efferent nerve terminals (see Fig. 14–12). The afferent terminals contain clear vesicles, whereas efferent terminals contain dense core vesicles. In type II hair cells, both afferent and efferent terminals are related to the cell body and are sites of neurochemical transmission. In type I hair cells, the calyx that surrounds the hair cell is regarded as the afferent nerve terminal; it has not been established whether transmission in the calyx is chemical or electrical. The efferent terminals in the type I hair cell are applied to the external surface of the calyx.

Type I hair cells receive vestibular nerve fibers that are large in diameter and fast-conducting. Each vestibular nerve fiber innervates a small number of type I hair cells. Thus, type I hair cells are regarded as more

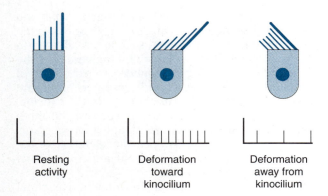

FIGURE 14–13. The effect of deformation of stereocilia on rate of impulse discharge from the vestibular sense organ. *Deformation toward the kinocilium increases the frequency of discharge, and discharge away from the kinocilium decreases the frequency of discharge of impulses.*

discriminative than type II hair cells, which receive small-diameter, slow-conducting vestibular nerve fibers projecting upon a large number of hair cells.

The stimulus adequate to discharge hair cells is movement of the cupula or otolithic membrane, which bends or deforms the stereocilia. The manner in which this deformation triggers ionic conductance in hair cells is uncertain. It is now well established that the resting vestibular end organ has a constant discharge of impulses detected in afferent vestibular nerve fibers. This resting activity is modified by mechanical deformation of the stereocilia. Bending the stereocilia toward the kinocilium increases the frequency of resting discharge, whereas bending the stereocilia away from the kinocilium lowers the frequency (Fig. 14–13). The signals emitted by hair cells of the vestibular end organ are transmitted to the central nervous system via processes of bipolar cells in Scarpa's ganglion.

Although we are normally not aware of the vestibular component of our sensory experience, this component is essential for the coordination of motor responses, eye movements, and posture.

CHAPTER FIFTEEN

Endocrine System

Neuroendocrine System 260
    Adenohypophysis 260
    Neurohypophysis 265
    Blood Supply of the Hypophysis 265

Pineal Gland 267
    Blood Vessels and Nerves 267
    Functions of the Pineal Gland 267

Thyroid Gland 267
    Thyroid Follicular Cells 269
    Parafollicular (Clear or C) Cells 270

Parathyroid Glands 270

Suprarenal Glands 272
    Histologic Features 272
    Suprarenal Cortex 273
    Hormones of the Suprarenal Cortical Cells 274
    Suprarenal Gland Medulla 274
    Blood Supply 275

Pancreatic Islets 276
    Blood and Nerve Supply 278

Gastroenteropancreatic Endocrine (GEP) System 278

Diffuse Neuroendocrine System 279

The development of multicellular organisms required the organization of the component cells into tissues of different types capable of carrying out specific functions. The control and integration of cellular and tissue functions were adopted by the nervous system. The nervous system, acting through the chemical messenger hormones of increasing complexity, brings about coordinated control of the internal environment, in which cells and tissues function.

This chapter is concerned with the organs of the endocrine system, with the exception of those present in the female and male reproductive systems, which are treated in Chapters 16 and 17, respectively. Figure 15–1 shows the locations of the major endocrine glands; Table 15–1 summarizes their functions.

A *hormone* is a chemical that is released by a cell or cells, at a specific time or under specific circumstances, into either the extracellular space or the vascular or lymphatic system to affect the function of other cells at various distances from the source. Chemically, there are three kinds of hormones: steroids, proteins, and amines. There are at least 20 steroid hormones in humans, including cortisol, cortisone, estrogen, progesterone, and testosterone. Adrenal cortical and sex hormones are steroids. Protein hormones are composed of amino acids linked together in peptide chains; the hormones of the hypophysis, pancreas, and parathyroid glands are examples. Amines are composed of amino acids but are not linked by peptide bonds. Hormones of this kind are: thyroxine from the thyroid gland, epinephrine (adrenaline) and norepinephrine (noradrenaline) from the adrenal medulla, and melatonin from the pineal gland (Table 15–2).

The cells and organs acted upon are known as the *target organ(s)*. The effective control of the cellular environment by the neuroendocrine system is directly responsible for the success and longevity of the organism. The neural component utilizes nerve fibers for conduction and neurotransmitters to transmit the mes-

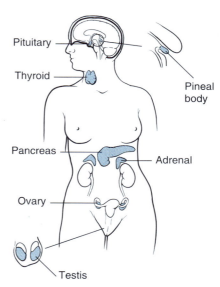

FIGURE 15–1. *Major endocrine glands. The location of the major endocrine organs is shown here, but many others are discussed in the text.*

sage into functional activity. This method is fast and highly specific. On the other hand, the diffuse neuroendocrine system is slower, and responses are less specific because the neuroendocrine transmitter is secreted and reaches the target cells by diffusion (so-called paracrine secretion) or, more widely, via the blood stream or lymphatics like a hormone of the endocrine system proper. The endocrine system proper is composed of a group or cluster of cells that secrete hormones into the blood stream to exert their effect at some distance from the source. This method is found to be less localized and slower, but the effect usually lasts considerably longer. This last method controls functions of great importance for survival of the organism. The two regulatory systems are interrelated and essential for satisfac-

TABLE 15-1. The Major Endocrine Glands

Endocrine Gland	Major Hormones	Primary Target Organs	Primary Effects
Adrenal cortex	Cortisol	Liver, muscles	Glucose metabolism
	Aldosterone	Kidney	Na^+ retention, K^+ excretion
Adrenal medulla	Epinephrine	Heart, bronchioles, blood vessels	Adrenergic stimulation
Hypothalamus	Releasing and inhibiting hormones	Anterior pituitary	Regulates secretion of anterior pituitary hormones
Intestine	Secretin and cholecystokinin	Stomach, liver, pancreas	Inhibits gastric motility; stimulates bile and pancreatic juice secretion
Islets of Langerhans (pancreas)	Insulin	Many organs	Promotes cellular uptake of glucose and formation of glycogen and fat
	Glucagon	Liver and adipose tissue	Stimulates hydrolysis of glycogen and fat
Parathyroids	Parathyroid hormone	Bone, intestine, kidneys	Increases Ca^{++} concentration in blood
Pineal	Melatonin	Hypothalamus, anterior pituitary	Affects secretion of gonadotrophic hormones
Pituitary			
Anterior	Trophic hormones	Endocrine glands, other organs	Stimulates growth and development of target organs, and secretion of other hormones
Posterior	Antidiuretic hormone	Kidneys, blood vessels	Promotes water retention and vasoconstriction
	Oxytocin	Uterus, mammary glands	Stimulates contraction of uterus and mammary secretory units
Thyroid	Thyroxine (T_4), triiodothyronine (T_3)	Most organs, blood	Growth and development; stimulates basal rate of cell respiration (basal metabolic rate, or BMR)
	Calcitonin		Regulates Ca^{++} levels within blood by inhibiting bone decalcification

TABLE 15-2. Types of Hormones

Type of Hormone	Composition	Examples
Steroid	Lipid with a cholesterol-type nucleus	Sex hormones, hormones from adrenal cortex
Protein	Amino acids bonded by peptide chains	Pituitary hormones, pancreatic hormones, parathyroid hormones, calcitonin from thyroid gland
Amine	Amino acids with no peptide bonds; molecule contains —NH_2 group	Thyroxine from thyroid gland, epinephrine from adrenal gland, melatonin from the pineal gland

tory existence in and freedom from the external environment. The three mechanisms of action are seen in Figures 15–2 to 15–4.

NEUROENDOCRINE SYSTEM

The hypophysis cerebri (pituitary gland) is an ovoid gland roughly 12 mm in the axial plane and 8 mm in the sagittal plane. It weighs about 0.5 gm. The gland is continuous with the central nervous system via the infundibulum, which is a hollow conical process joined to the tuber cinereum of the hypothalamus.

The hypophysis is divided into two major regions: one from the diencephalon, a downgrowth of the hypothalamus, and the other an ectodermal derivative from the stomatodeum. These are known as the *neurohypophysis* and the *adenohypophysis*, respectively. Both divisions include part of the infundibulum. The neurohypophysis includes the median eminence, infundibular stem, and the neural lobe, or pars posterior; an extension of the adenohypophysis, the pars tuberalis or infundibularis, is also included in the neurohypophysis. The bulk of the adenohypophysis is divided into the pars anterior or pars distalis and the pars intermedia. These two parts are separated in fetal and early postnatal life by a cleft, a vestige of Rathke's pouch. The pars intermedia is considered rudimentary in humans. Finally, the adenohypophysis also includes the pars tuberalis (Fig. 15–5).

Adenohypophysis

The adenohypophysis is highly vascular and consists of epithelial cells in cords separated by vascular sinusoids supported by reticular fibers.

Seven hormones are known to be secreted and released by the adenohypophysis: somatotropin, or somatotropic hormone (STH), in control of body growth; mammotropin or lactogenic hormone (LTH), stimulating growth and secretion by the female breast; adrenocorticotropin or adrenocorticotropic hormone (ACTH), governing the secretion of the suprarenal cortical hormones; thyrotropin or thyroid-stimulating hormone (TSH), controlling thyroid function; follicle-stimulating hormone (FSH), influencing growth and estrogen secretion in ovarian follicles and spermatogenesis in the testis; interstitial cell–stimulating hormone (ICSH) or luteinizing hormone (LH), effecting secretion of androgen by the testis and secretion of progesterone by the corpus luteum; and from the pars intermedia, melanocyte-stimulating hormone (MSH), increasing pigmentation of the skin. Although only summary descriptions of the functions of these seven hormones are given here, most have other important metabolic effects (Table 15–3).

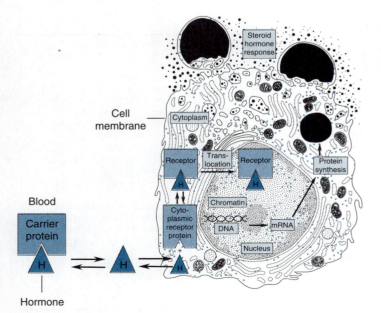

FIGURE 15–2. Hormonally induced cellular response. Circulating hormones that reach their target cells induce nuclear responses, which become translated into overall cellular function. These are the steps involved in steroid hormone–induced cellular synthetic activity.

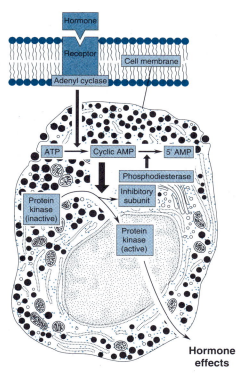

FIGURE 15–3. *Protein hormones and cellular activation. When circulating protein hormones reach their target cells, they attach to specific receptor sites on the cell membrane. This causes a chain reaction when adenyl cyclase enters the cell. ATP is changed into cyclic AMP, which brings about cellular synthetic activity.*

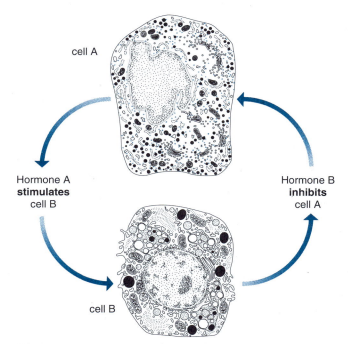

FIGURE 15–4. *Negative feedback. In the system seen here, the hypophysis secretes a stimulating hormone (e.g., pituitary corticotropin) that activates synthetic activity in its target cell (e.g., adrenal cell of zona fasciculata) (hormone from cell A stimulates cell B). The secreted hormone from cell B then inhibits secretion of additional stimulating hormone (hormone B inhibits cell A).*

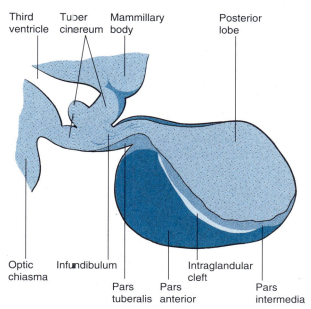

FIGURE 15–5. *Hypophysis cerebri (pituitary gland). Diagram of median section through the hypophysis, identifying its component parts.*

Composition of the Adenohypophysis

The seven hormones released by the adenohypophyis are secreted by three basic types of cells, the acidophils, basophils, and chromophobes (Fig. 15–6). The pars anterior is composed of five different kinds of cells, classified as two kinds of acidophils and three kinds of basophils.

Acidophils (α Cells)

SOMATOTROPHS. Somatotrophs tend to be ovoid (Fig. 15–7). The largest and most abundant adenohypophysial cells, they are usually found in clusters around sinusoids. They are stained by acid dyes such as orange G for light microscopy. The electron microscope reveals numerous electron-dense, round secretory granules about 350 to 500 nm in diameter and well-developed Golgi apparatuses (complexes). Somatotrophs have relatively small amounts of granular endoplasmic reticulum, particularly in the secretory phase. The nucleus is centrally located within the cells. Cells of eosinophilic (acidophilic) adenomas associated with acromegaly in adults or giantism in children are similar in ultrastructure to the description just given. If somatotropin is deficient, dwarfism occurs. The hormone is a protein with 191 amino acids and a molecular weight of 21,500.

MAMMOTROPHS. Mammotrophs (Fig. 15–8) secrete the polypeptide hormone prolactin (mammotropin, lactogenic hormone). They are particularly abundant during pregnancy and they hypertrophy during lactation. They are distinguished by their selective affinity for erythrosin and azocarmine. The secretory granules are the largest in the hypophysis, over 600 nm in diameter in pregnant and lactating females, but average about 200 nm and are fewer in number in nonpregnant females and in males. The granules are uniformly dense and may be

TABLE 15-3. Hormones of the Adenohypophysis and Their Regulatory Source(s)

Hormone	Action	Regulation
Growth hormone (GH) or somatotropin	Regulates mitotic activity and growth of body cells; promotes movement of amino acids through plasma membranes	Growth hormone–releasing factor (GH-RF) and growth hormone release inhibiting factor (GH-RIH) from the hypothalamus
Thyroid-stimulating hormone (TSH) or thyrotropin	Regulates hormonal activity of thyroid gland	Thyrotropin-releasing factor (TRF) from the hypothalamus
Adrenocorticotropic hormone (ACTH)	Controls secretion of certain hormones from the adrenal cortex; assists in breakdown of fats	Corticotropin-releasing factor (CRF) from the hypothalamus
Follicle-stimulating hormone (FSH)	In males, stimulates production of sperm cells; in females, regulates follicle development in ovary and stimulates secretion of estrogen	Gonadotrophin-releasing factor (GRF) from the hypothalamus
Luteinizing hormone (LH) or (in males) interstitial cell–stimulating hormone (ICSH)	Promotes secretion of sex hormones; in females, plays role in release of ovum, stimulates formation of corpus luteum and production of progesterone; in males, stimulates testosterone secretion	Gonadotrophin-releasing factor (GRF) from the hypothalamus
Prolactin	Promotes secretion of milk from mammary glands (lactation)	Hypothalamus through production of prolactin release inhibiting factor (PR-IF)
Melanocyte-stimulating hormone (MSH)	Stimulates pigmentation within the melanocytes of the skin	Melanocyte-stimulating hormone–releasing factor (MRF) and melanocyte-stimulating hormone inhibiting factor (MIF), both from the hypothalamus

ovoid or irregularly shaped as a result of the fusion of granules. The cells possess lysosomes, which presumably form autophagic vacuoles, which degrade excessive numbers of granules. As might be anticipated, active cells possess a significant granular endoplasmic reticulum and a prominent Golgi apparatus. Together with other female hormones, estrogen and progesterone, prolactin stimulates breast development during pregnancy. Subsequent to parturition, estrogen and progesterone levels decline, and then prolactin induces milk production.

Basophils (β Cells)

CORTICOTROPHS. Corticotrophs secrete adrenocorticotrophic hormone (ACTH) and two others of obscure function, lipotropin and an endorphin (Fig. 15–9). ACTH is composed of 39 amino acids and has a molecular weight of 4500. The precursor molecule for these is pro-opio-melanocorticotropin. The precursor molecule in humans is glycosylated, rendering granules containing the precursor PAS positive (take up periodic acid–Schiff stain); they are also slightly basophilic. The corticotrophs are not uniformly shaped and possess short dendritic processes. Because the secretory granules are about 500 nm in diameter, they are not difficult to identify by light microscopy. ACTH stimulates the adrenal cortex to synthesize and secrete glucocorticoids and adrenal androgen. It also effects synthesis and secretion of aldosterone by the zona glomerulosa.

THYROTROPHS (β BASOPHILS). Thyrotrophs secrete thyroid-

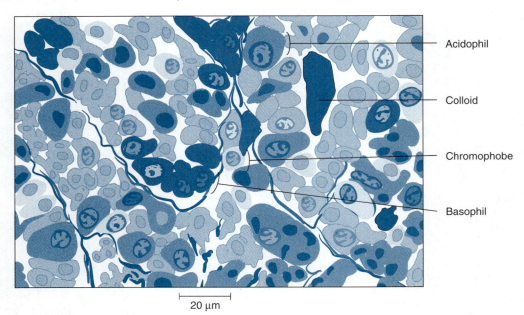

FIGURE 15–6. Adenohypophysis. The three basic cell types: acidophils, basophils, and chromophobes.

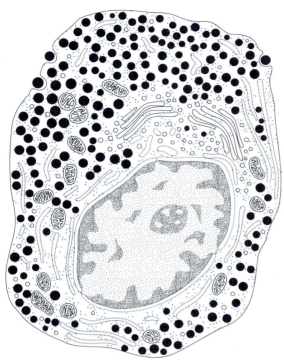

FIGURE 15–7. Somatotroph of adenohypophysis. Diagram of the typical somatroph, containing numerous secretory granules 500 to 550 nm in diameter. The somatotrophs are acidophilic; hence, they are designated as α cells. Somatotrophic hormone is a protein and has a molecular weight of 21,000. This hormone stimulates body growth.

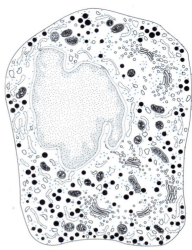

FIGURE 15–9. Corticotroph of adenohypophysis. This cell produces adrenocorticotropic hormone (ACTH). Its granules are about 500 nm in diameter and are not particularly abundant. ACTH is a polypeptide containing 39 amino acids and has a molecular weight of 4500. This hormone affects the cells of the zona fasciculata and zona reticularis, resulting primarily in the synthesis and secretion of glucocorticoids (also see text). These cells are classified as basophils (β cells).

stimulating hormone (Fig. 15–10). The hormone is composed of 201 amino acids and has a molecular weight of 28,000. The cells are usually elongated and polygonal, and they tend to be grouped together, in the middle of the adenohypophysis. Normally thyrotrophs are found as cords of cells, but they do not line the sinusoids. These cells stain selectively with the aldehyde-fuchsin stain. The thyrotrophs have the smallest granules (120 to 200 nm) in the adenohypophysis, are irregularly shaped, and are more electron lucent than those of the other basophils. Thyrotropin stimulates the thyroid gland to synthesize and excrete the thyroid hormones thyroxine (T_4) and triiodothyronine (T_3).

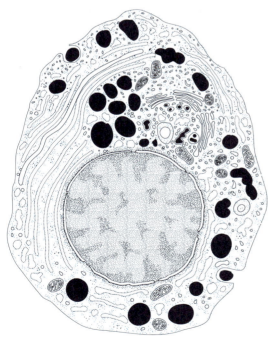

FIGURE 15–8. Mammotroph of the adenohypophysis. Mammotrophs have large secretory granules that vary in size from 600 to 900 nm and in shape from round to polymorphic. The mammotroph secretes lactogenic hormone (also known as prolactin), a protein with a molecular weight of 25,000. Lactogenic hormone stimulates lactation; hence, the number and size of mammotrophs increase during pregnancy and lactation. The mammotrophs are classified as acidophils (α cells).

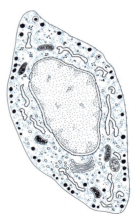

FIGURE 15–10. Thyrotroph of adenohypophysis. Thyrotrophs produce thyroid-stimulating hormone (TSH). They tend to be smaller and more angular than other cells of the adenohypophysis. Their granules are small, 120 to 200 nm in diameter, and are typically arranged one granule deep around the periphery of the cell. TSH is a glycoprotein, and thyrotrophs are classified with the basophils. The hormone has a molecular weight of about 20,000. The thyrotroph stimulates secretory activity of the thyroid follicular cells.

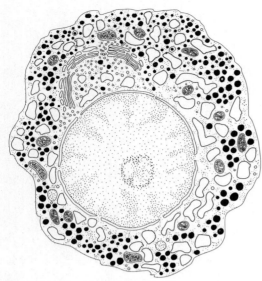

FIGURE 15-11. *Gonadotroph (producing the follicle-stimulating hormone) of the adenohypophysis. The follicle-stimulating hormone (FSH) from this gonadotroph has numerous granules about 300 nm in diameter. FSH is a glycoprotein, and the cells that synthesize it are classified with the basophils (β). In females, FSH stimulates the growth of ovarian follicles. In the male, it stimulates the seminiferous epithelium of the testis.*

GONADOTROPHS (δ BASOPHILS). Larger than thyrotrophs, gonadotrophs are generally rounded and line the sinusoids (Figs. 15-11 and 15-12). The secretory granules of these cells are PAS-positive. These cells may actually be of two subtypes: one type is more purple staining and generally peripherally located, and it may secrete follicle-stimulating hormone (FSH); the other type is more centrally located in the gland and stains a redder hue. The second type may secrete luteinizing hormone (LH) in women or interstitial cell–stimulating hormone (ICSH) in males. FSH stimulates early follicular development in the ovary in females and spermatogenesis in males. LH is responsible for the final maturation process of the oocyte and ovulation. LH also stimulates the interstitial cells of the testis (Leydig's cells) to synthesize and secrete testosterone.

Gonadotrophs have pleiomorphic nuclei, a well-developed granular endoplasmic reticulum and Golgi apparatus. The secretory granules are small (~300 nm) and tend to gather in rows near the apical cell membrane during secretory activity.

Chromophobes

About half the epithelial cells forming the adenohypophysis are chromophobes. These poorly staining cells appear to be of several types. They may include degranulated chromophil cells as well as stem cells that differentiate into chromophils and follicular cells surrounding cysts. Other obscure types have been reported, but they are of unknown function.

Pars Intermedia

The pars intermedia is composed of many β cells and follicles of chromophobe cells containing a colloidal product that is PAS positive. The secretory cells of the pars intermedia have α-endorphin– or β-endorphin–containing secretory granules. These cells have been found to contain a variety of peptide hormones, including ACTH and α-MSH (melanocyte-stimulating hormone) (Fig. 15-13).

Pars Tuberalis

The pars tuberalis is richly supplied with blood vessels that are surrounded by cords of undifferentiated cells interspersed with α and β cells.

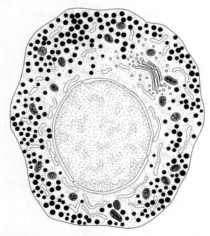

FIGURE 15-12. *Gonadotroph (producing luteinizing hormone [LH]) of the adenohypophysis. This gonadotroph also produces interstitial cell–stimulating hormone (ICSH) in males. The dense granules of this cell, containing the hormone (either LH or ICSH), are about 300 nm. The hormone of this cell type is a glycoprotein having a molecular weight of 26,000. The cell is classified as a basophil (β). In females, LH is necessary to produce a corpus luteum after the follicle has ruptured and released its ovum. In males, ICSH is responsible for the stimulation of the interstitial cells of the testis to produce and secret androgen.*

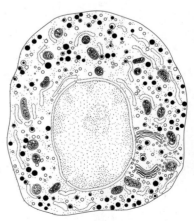

FIGURE 15-13. *Basophil of the pars intermedia of the hypophysis. These basophils are found lying between the pars distalis and the pars nervosa of the hypophysis. These cells are thought to produce melanocyte-stimulating hormone (MSH). MSH is a polypeptide, chemically similar to ACTH. The function of this basophil is to produce MSH, which stimulates melanin production in melanocytes, resulting in darkening of the skin. It may also have other important functions.*

Secretion Mechanism of Adenohypophysial Hormones

The release of adenohypophysial hormones into the sinusoids occurs by *exocytosis*. The cellular vesicles, containing "hormonal" granules, empty their granules into the perivascular spaces near sinusoids, which are formed of a fenestrated endothelium. The secretory product enters the circulation, apparently by diffusion.

The signal for secretory activity is the deliverance of releasing factors from neurons in the median eminence, nucleus infundibularis (arcuate nucleus), and other hypothalamic nuclei into the superior capillary bed of the venous hypophysial portal system, then subsequently to the adenohypophysis, to act on the endocrine cells. The neurosecretory cells are neuroendocrine transducers. They receive neural and hormonal signals and respond by secreting hormones. The neurons that produce releasing factors are peptidergic, and the neurons that modulate endocrine activity are monoaminergic, making synaptic contact with them. Tanycytes may also play a role in the control secretion of hormones.

Neurohypophysis

The neurohypophysis is a downgrowth of the diencephalic floor. The posterior lobe, infundibulum, and median eminence are usually grouped together and regarded as the neurohypophysis.

Axons originating from groups of hypothalamic neurons located in the supraoptic, paraventricular, and other nuclei terminate in the neurohypophysis. The axons are "short" and "long." The short axons end in the superior capillary beds of the venous portal system in the median eminence and infundibular stem; these may have a role in the neural control of adenohypophysial activity. The long axons are from the hypothalamohypophysial tract and terminate in the posterior lobe adjacent to sinusoids. These axons synthesize and release antidiuretic hormone (ADH) and oxytocin or vasopressin.

Neurohypophysial Hormones

The hormones released from the posterior lobe are vasopressin (antidiuretic hormone, ADH), which controls the renal tubular reabsorption of water, and oxytocin, which triggers contraction of uterine and other smooth (nonstriated) muscle. The active hormones are uncomplicated polypeptides, elaborated and carried within cells by a glycoprotein, neurophysin.

When the hormone is secreted into the circulation, a specific binding protein, the neurophysin polypeptide complex, is broken, and the hormone is subsequently complexed with plasma glycoproteins and carried to its target organs (Table 15–4).

The most common cell type, other than axons in the neurohypophysis, is the pituicyte. The cytoplasmic processes of pituicytes extend onto or near the walls of the adjacent fenestrated capillaries and sinusoids between nerve terminals. The axons terminate in perivascular spaces. The secretion of hormones from nerve endings must pass through two basal laminae: one surrounding the nerve terminal, the other surrounding the external surface of the extremely attenuated endothelium of capillaries. The hormones are released by exocytosis from axons with large, dense, hormone-containing endings. It is believed that hormone release is determined by excitation of nerve endings by action potentials (nerve impulses) carried along axons from the hypothalamus (Figs. 15–14 and 15–15).

Blood Supply of the Hypophysis

The arterial supply, from the internal carotids, arises as several superior hypophysial arteries and a single inferior hypophysial artery, bilaterally. The superior hypophysial arteries supply the median eminence, upper infundibulum and, via arteries of the trabeculae, the lower part of the infundibulum. The inferior hypophysial arteries branch into medial and lateral limbs, which anastomose across the midline to form an infundibular arterial ring. From the ring, small branches enter the neurohypophysis to supply its capillary bed. This capillary network extends throughout the entire neurohypophysis and is supplied bilaterally by both sets of hypophysial vessels. The arterial supply ends in long and short portal vessels. The portal vessels run to the pars anterior and both types of portal vessels become continuous with vascular sinusoids located between the secretory cords in the adenohypophysis, thus providing most of the blood for the adenohypophysis. The portal system carries hormone-releasing factors from the paracellular neurons of the hypothalamus to control the secretory activity of cells in the pars anterior. The portal system drains into the inferior hypophysial veins. The venous drainage from the neurohypophysis has not been finally determined, but several possible routes, all with far-reaching implications, are possible: the drainage may be via the adenohypophysis via the long and short portal vessels, via the inferior hypophysial vessels to the dural venous sinuses, or to the hypothalamus via venules in the median eminence.

TABLE 15–4. Hormones of the Neurohypophysis and Their Regulatory Source

Hormone	Action	Regulation
Oxytocin	Stimulates contractions of muscles in uterine wall; causes contraction of muscles in mammary glands	Hypothalamus in response to stretch in uterine walls and stimulation of breasts
Antidiuretic hormone	Reduces water loss from kidneys; elevates blood pressure	Hypothalamus in response to changes in blood-water concentration

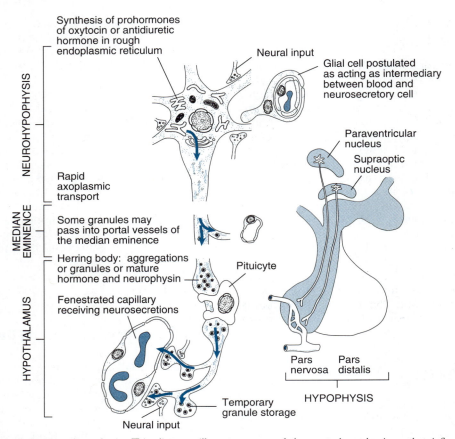

FIGURE 15-14. *Control of the neurohypophysis. This diagram illustrates some of the control mechanisms that influence the production of neurohypophysial hormones.*

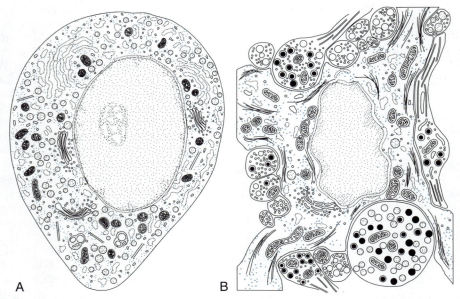

FIGURE 15-15. *Neurosecretory cell and pituicyte of neurohypophysis. A, Neurosecretory cells are nerve cells highly specialized for the synthesis and secretion of hormones. These neurons have numerous secretory granules, which vary in size from 120 to 200 nm in diameter and are thought to contain vasopressin (antidiuretic hormone, ADH) and oxytocin. The granules are carried down the axons from the hypothalamus and stored in axon terminals in the pars nervosa via the hypothalamohypophysial tract. The hormones, when released, are carried into an extensive capillary plexus. Other neurosecretory cells, located in the hypothalamus and terminating in the median eminence of the hypophysis, synthesize and secrete releasing factors that affect the cells of the anterior hypophysis. Five of the releasing factors stimulate secretion of hormones from five specific adenohypophysial cells, and one of the releasing factors inhibits secretion (of prolactin). B, Pituicytes are cells that have long processes. These cells partially enfold axons of the hypothalamohypophysial tract, containing secretory granules that carry the hormones vasopressin and oxytocin. The pituicyte is thought to be a specialized neuroglial cell. Note the variety of secretory granules and vesicles in the axons.*

PINEAL GLAND

The pineal gland is composed of cords and follicles of pinealocytes and neuroglial cells that intermingle with nerves and blood vessels.

The pinealocytes form the parenchyma of the gland (Fig. 15–16A). Each cell may contain a spherical, oval, or lobulated nucleus. Pinealocytes possess basophilic processes, of irregular configuration, containing numerous microtubules in parallel arrays. The processes terminate in swellings near capillaries and ependymal cells of the pineal recess. The terminal swellings or buds contain granular endoplasmic reticulum, mitochondria, and electron-dense–cored vesicles containing monoamines and polypeptide hormones. The release of these hormones is thought to require the sympathetic nervous system. The mechanism of release of these hormones from the cells by exocytosis includes debris of fragments of cell membrane and other substances complexed with hormone granules. When the hormone-debris complex is dissociated, the debris attracts calcium ions and forms "brain sand," or corpora arenacea. Contrary to popular belief, the "brain sand" may indicate secretory activity rather than some process of pineal atrophy.

Pinealocytes contain both granular and agranular endoplasmic reticula, an extensive Golgi apparatus, numerous mitochondria, and lipid droplets. An unusual organelle is also found, composed of perforated lamellae and bundles of microtubules; several names have been suggested for the organelle, including *canaliculate lamellar bodies* and *annulate lamellae*, but their function remains obscure.

Neuroglial cells are similar to astrocytes and partially separate pinealocytes. In the pineal stalk, many neuroglial cells have extensive elongated processes. Numerous filaments extend throughout their processes (Fig. 15–16B).

Blood Vessels and Nerves

Pineal capillaries possess thin, often fenestrated endothelial cells and thin and sometimes incomplete basal laminae.

The nonmyelinated autonomic nerve fibers are primarily noradrenergic and contain dense-cored vessels in their terminal swellings. The sympathetic fibers arise in the superior cervical ganglion. The fibers terminate in perivascular spaces between pinealocytes or synapse with them.

Functions of the Pineal Gland

Formerly considered a phylogenetic relic, the mammalian pineal is now known to be an endocrine gland that modifies the activity of the adenohypophysis, neurohypophysis, pancreatic islets, parathyroids, adrenal cortex, adrenal medulla, and the gonads. It is believed that inhibitory, indolamine, and polypeptide hormones secreted by pinealocytes reduce synthesis and release of hormones of the pars anterior of the hypophysis. The activity is directly on the secretory cells and indirectly on the hypothalamus.

Evidence has been given for a circadian rhythm in human pineal function. Plasma melatonin levels rise during darkness and fall during daylight.

THYROID GLAND

The thyroid gland is located in the lower part of the neck at the level of the fifth cervical vertebra to the first thoracic vertebra. It is composed of two "conical" pyramidal lobes joined by a narrow bridge of glandular tissue called the *isthmus* (Fig. 15–17).

The gland's weight varies but is approximately 25 grams. The thyroid is somewhat heavier in females and enlarges slightly during menstruation and pregnancy.

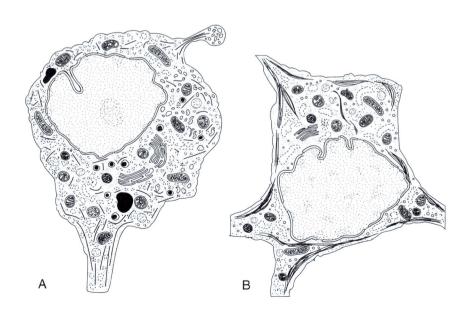

FIGURE 15–16. Pinealocyte and interstitial (neuroglial) cells. The pineal gland contains two types of cells. A, Pinealocytes are stellate cells with processes that end in a globular enlargement. The granules of these cells are small and dense and are surrounded by a membrane. Melatonin has been identified in the pineal gland. The influence of this gland is thought to be widespread, but hard evidence is still lacking. B, The interstitial cells, or neuroglial cells, tend to separate the parenchymal cells or pinealocytes. The role of these cells is uncertain.

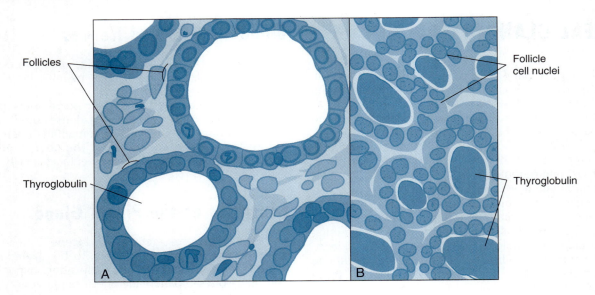

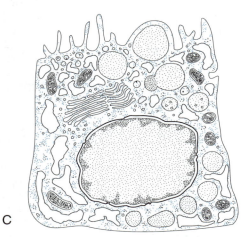

FIGURE 15-17. *Thyroid follicles and the follicular cell. A, Note the cuboidal cells that line the follicles. B, The follicles contain thyroglobulin, a glycoprotein that stains positively with the PAS stain. Thyroid hormones are released when stored follicular colloid is reabsorbed by the follicular cells, and are degraded to thyroxin and triiodothyronine before their release to the surrounding capillary bed. C, Diagram of electron-micrographic structure of a follicular cell.*

Small masses of thyroid—*accessory thyroid glands*—may be vestiges of the embryologic thyroglossal duct that persist and extend from the isthmus to the lingual foramen cecum. Persistent normal and pathologic thyroid glandular tissue has been reported along the neck and in the back of the tongue. The gland has a thin connective tissue capsule that also divides the gland into masses irregular in size and form. The substance or parenchyma of the gland arises mainly from the endoderm of the thyroglossal duct. The thyroglossal duct is usually, but not always, a transient embryonic structure extending between the gland and tongue. In development, the solid distal end of the duct, composed of epithelial cords of cells, begins to branch, and the spaces formed between cells become filled with a viscid, yellow colloid. The thyroid colloid is composed of a glycoprotein, thyroglobulin, with a molecular weight of 660,000. Observations of sections of the thyroid gland suggest that the endodermal epithelium develops separate, spherical follicles about 0.02 to 0.9 mm in diameter. Each follicle has a central core of the colloidal material surrounded by a simple epithelium of variable height and, overall, a basal lamina. This concept of completely isolated mature follicles may not be accurate, because three-dimensional reconstructions reveal that follicles typically have a common, continuous epithelium bordering them and linking them together. It is thought that, in humans, the follicles of the entire thyroid gland contain about a 2.5-month supply of hormone (Table 15–5).

The colloid stains with the eosin of the hematoxylin and eosin stain (H&E) and is composed of an iodinated glycoprotein, iodothyroglobulin, a precursor of thyroid hormones. Thyroglobulin is also PAS positive owing to its glycoprotein nature. The hormones of the thyroid gland are triiodothyronine (T_3) and tetraiodothyronine or thyroxine (T_4). The follicles are surrounded by a connective tissue stroma infiltrated with dense

TABLE 15-5. Hormones of the Thyroid Gland

Hormone	Action	Regulation
Thyroxine (T_4)	Increases rate of protein synthesis and rate of energy release from carbohydrates; regulates rate of growth; stimulates maturity of nervous system	Hypothalamus and release of TSH from adenohypophysis of the pituitary gland
Triiodothyronine (T_3)	Same as action of T_4	Same as for T_4
Calcitonin (thyrocalcitonin)	Lowers blood calcium by inhibiting the release of calcium from bone tissue	Calcium levels in blood

plexuses of fenestrated capillaries of the blood vascular and lymphatic systems, and sympathetic nerve fibers that accompany and regulate the arterial supply.

The thyroid gland parenchyma contains a second parafollicular endocrine cell type, the so-called clear or light (C) cells. These produce thyrocalcitonin, a peptide hormone composed of 32 amino acids and with a molecular weight of 3500. These C cells come from the ultimobranchial bodies in development. The *ultimobranchial body* is an endodermal diverticular portion of the caudal pharyngeal complex. It loses its connection with the pharynx, becomes closely associated with the expanding lateral lobe of the thyroid gland, and is enveloped by the thyroid gland (Fig. 15–18).

Thyroid Follicular Cells

Follicular cells vary from cuboidal to columnar, according to their functional state. The activity of follicular cells depends on circulating thyrotropin or thyroid-stimulating hormone (TSH) from the hypophysis (pituitary gland). In the absence of TSH, follicular cells become squat, cuboidal, or even squamous and are in the "resting" metabolic state. The follicular lumen is filled with colloid, an iodinated thyroglobulin. When TSH is circulating at normally high levels, the cells show endocytosis of colloid at the luminal (apical) aspects of follicular cells, and cavities appear in the colloid near the active epithelium. Prolonged (abnormal) high secretion levels of TSH induces follicular hypertrophy, hyperplasia, marked reabsorption of colloid, and increased vascularity.

Follicular cells are polarized both ultrastructurally and functionally. Follicular cells activated by TSH begin apical synthesis and luminal exocytosis of thyroglobulin. At the same time, with thyroglobulin directed in a basal direction, endocytosis, degradation, and release of thyroid hormones occurs, with both T_3 and T_4 entering the capillary network (both blood and lymphatic) that surrounds the follicles. The functional duality is shown by the arrangement of their organelles. Follicular cells form a continuous sheet by being linked together by junctional complexes surrounding the colloid they secrete. The bases of the cells rest on a basal lamina (basement membrane). Each cell has a basal nucleus, extensive endoplasmic reticulum, and supranuclear Golgi apparatus (complex). The Golgi apparatus is particularly prominent in TSH-activated cells. Apical to the Golgi apparatus are secretory vesicles derived from it, which carry glycoprotein. The glycoprotein is assembled by the activity of the granular endoplasmic reticulum (GER) and Golgi complex (apparatus). The secretory vesicles are carried to the apical plasmalemma and released by exocytosis.

Iodine, which completes the formation of thyroglobulin, is derived from the blood and enters the basal plasmalemma of follicular cells through an active transport mechanism. Iodide, normally carried in the body, is oxidized to iodine by thyroid peroxidase located in the apical plasmalemma. Iodine is attached to the tyrosyl groups of the glycoprotein synthesized by follicular cells, forming mono- and di-iodotyrosyls. The iodinated compounds are coupled into iodothyronyl groups. These thyroid hormones in peptide linkage complete the formation of iodinated thyroglobulin, which is the precursor of thyroid hormones. The source of iodine for many humans is iodized table salt. With the effort to reduce sodium intake because of its effect on blood pressure, goiter (thyroid enlargement due to iodine deficiency) may once again become more common.

The follicular cells have apical microvilli, which are numerous and short in resting cells. TSH-stimulated cells have elongate and branched microvilli and cytoplasmic extensions that extend into the adjacent laminal colloid. The elongate cytoplasmic processes surround small portions of the colloid and take them into the cell. Following endocytosis, lysosomes migrate from their typical basal position in the resting state toward the apex, where they fuse with intracellular droplets of colloid to form secondary lysosomes (phagolysosomes), which then return to the base of the cell. The colloid with iodinated thyroglobulin is degraded by acid proteases and peptidases in the secondary lysosome, releasing the thyroid hormones T_3 and T_4, which are then released from the basal plasmalemma and carried away in blood and lymph capillaries (Fig. 15–19).

Triiodothyronine is the primary stimulator of the cellular metabolic rate. Its action is very strong and immediate, whereas tetraiodothyronine (thyroxine) is also powerful but does not act as quickly.

Overproduction of T_3 and T_4 produces thyrotoxicosis and exophthalmic goiter, and hyposecretion results in myxedema in adults and cretinism in infants. The synthesis, secretion, and release of T_3 and T_4 are controlled primarily by the adenohypophysial thyrotropic hormone (TSH). In Graves' disease, however, antibodies to human thyroid–stimulating immunoglobulin (HTSI) bind to TSH receptors in the follicular cells, resulting in loss of control and excessive hormone production. Increased sensitivity of tissues to epinephrine and norepinephrine is caused by thyroid hormones.

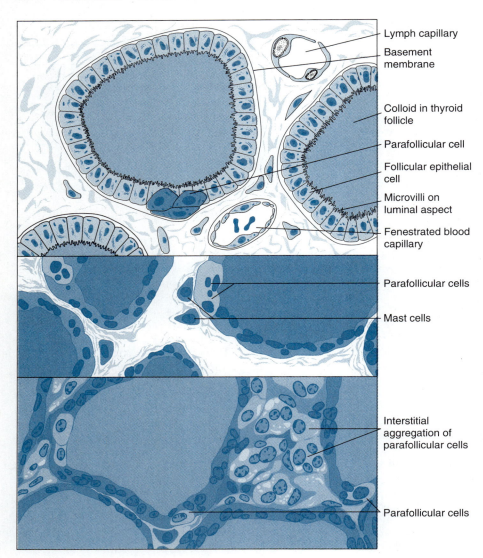

FIGURE 15–18. *Parafollicular cells by light microscopy. Note the parafollicular cells associated with the thyroid follicle and also in their interstitial location. These cells do not stain heavily with most stains; hence, they are also known as C or clear cells. These cells produce thyrocalcitonin and release the hormone into the interstitial space. Note that C cells do not contact the colloid in the thyroid follicle when they are associated with thyroid follicular cells. However, they reside within the basal lamina of the follicle. Thyrocalcitonin increases the storage of calcium ions, but its exact role in humans is uncertain.*

Although the function of follicles is primarily controlled by TSH, they also receive a sympathetic nerve supply. The exact role of the sympathetic nerve supply is uncertain; it may effect short-term, transient, and rapid responses of the gland, and the greater role of TSH may serve sustained glandular control.

Parafollicular (Clear or C) Cells

The parafollicular cells appear to belong to the amine precursor uptake and decarboxylation (APUD) activity of numerous cells found in various regions of the body (discussed later in this chapter). The parafollicular or C cells are of neural crest origin. They lie singly or in small groups (Fig. 15–18), in relation to follicles and always within the basal lamina (basement membrane) of the follicle. They often insinuate themselves between follicular cells, but their apices (actually bases) never reach the follicular lumen. The true apex of the C cell faces away from the lumen of the follicle, and its secretory product is released into the extracellular space.

The C cell is oval or polyhedral and is larger than thyroid hormone–secreting follicular cells. Unlike their companions, parafollicular cells have no nerve supply. The cytoplasm contains some storage form of thyrocalcitonin. The cytoplasm therefore also contains granular endoplasmic reticulum, Golgi apparatus, numerous mitochondria, and free ribosomes (Fig. 15–20).

It is thought that the primary factor in thyrocalcitonin release is the blood serum concentration of calcium. If the blood circulating through the thyroid gland has a "high" calcium level, thyrocalcitonin is released, whereas with a "low" concentration of calcium (hypocalcemia), thyrocalcitonin is not released. The exact opposite effect is seen in parathyroid hormone release when serum calcium levels are low (Fig. 15–18).

The role of thyrocalcitonin in humans is not certain.

PARATHYROID GLANDS

The parathyroid glands are small, slightly yellowish, and ovoid. They are usually formed in the posterior

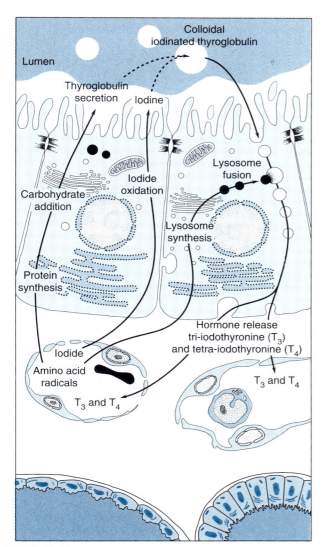

FIGURE 15-19. *Diagram of thyroid cell function. In this diagram, the elaboration, storage, and release of thyroid hormones are depicted. Note that when the thyroid hormones are released, they may enter both the capillary and lymphatic (capillary) systems. Inactive follicular cells may be almost squamous, and highly active follicular cells, columnar; they tend to be cuboidal.*

to secretory activity. Active cells have significant Golgi profiles, membrane-bound granules, and an extensive granular endoplasmic reticulum. Inactive chief cells have much smaller Golgi apparatuses, granular endoplasmic reticulum, glycogen accumulation, and lipofucsin granules. Active chief cells are fewer in number than inactive chief cells. In the thyroid gland, functional activity of follicular cells is synchronized; chief cells, on the other hand, appear to undergo secretory cycles independently from their neighbors.

A second cell type is also found in the parathyroid gland, and its role is uncertain. The oxyphil or eosinophil cells appear before puberty and increase in number with age. The oxyphil cell is larger than the chief cell, its cytoplasm stains deeply with eosin, and its nucleus appears smaller and more deeply stained (more heterochromatic) than that of the chief cell. Ultrastructural observations confirm the presence of extremely numerous mitochondria that are tightly packed and often of unusual shape. The cytoplasm also contains a sparse endoplasmic reticulum, some glycogen, and occasionally a small Golgi apparatus. No secretory granules have been reported.

Parathyroid hormone (PTH), secreted by the chief cells, is a single chain polypeptide with 84 amino acid residues. It is responsible for the level of calcium and phosphorus in the blood serum. Two other hormones, thyrocalcitonin (already discussed) and hydroxycholecalciferol, are also involved. Hydroxycholecalciferol is a product of the successive action of hepatic and renal cells on vitamin D.

The secretion of parathyroid hormone (PTH) is controlled by the level of calcium in the blood perfusing the parathyroid glands. PTH acts upon osteoclasts and osteocytes. The rapid response of PTH acts upon osteocytes to increase the release of calcium ions into the blood at the expense of bone, through osteocytic

border in the middle and inferior parts as well as within the capsule of the thyroid gland. They are about 5.5 mm long, 2 mm wide, and 1.5 mm thick. They vary from two to six or more in number.

The parathyroid gland has a thin connective tissue capsule that provides intraglandular septa (Fig. 15–21).

Before puberty, the gland is composed primarily of chief or principal cells arranged in wide, irregular interconnecting columns. The chief or principal cells synthesize and secrete parathyroid hormone or parathormone. The chief cells are seen in three forms, so-called light, dark, and clear. With routine light-microscopic staining procedures, their appearance reflects the degree of cytoplasmic staining capacity (ability to concentrate stain). The cytoplasm appears homogeneous.

Human chief cells vary in appearance according

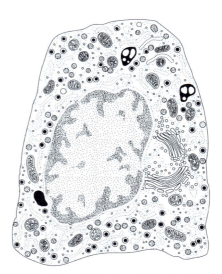

FIGURE 15-20. *Thyroid parafollicular cell. Located singly or together within the basal lamina of the thyroid follicle or in the interstitial space, these cells are thought to produce the hormone thyrocalcitonin. The specific granules carrying the hormone are dense and small (100 to 200 nm), and they are membrane bound. The cells vary in shape from cuboidal to oval.*

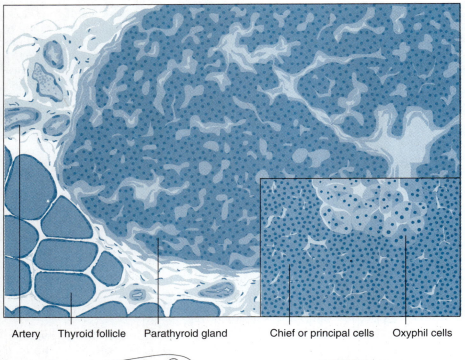

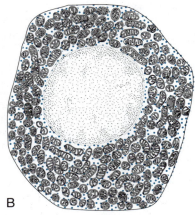

FIGURE 15-21. *Parathyroid gland and its cells. The number of parathyroid glands vary from two to six and they are essential for life. Two types of cells constitute the parathyroid gland: A, chief (principal) and oxyphil. It is believed that the granules of the chief cells carry the parathyroid hormone. B, The oxyphil cell is filled with mitochondria but their function is unknown. This cell type is probably not engaged in hormone synthesis. Oxyphil cells are typically larger than chief cells. The main illustration is at low magnification. Inset shows differences between the two cell types at intermediate magnification.*

osteolysis. PTH has a delayed or slow effect if a high level of PTH secretion is maintained. Osteoclasts are stimulated to begin internal bone remodeling. PTH affects renal ion transport by increasing the excretion of phosphate, potassium, and sodium and by decreasing the loss of calcium.

Unlike the thyroid, the parathyroid glands are essential for life. If all parathyroid tissue is removed, *tetany* (convulsive muscular spasms) occurs. Tetany results from the fall in blood calcium. Excessive parathormone secretion results in the removal of calcium ions from bones, a disease known as *generalized osteitis fibrosa*. Excess release of calcium ions into the blood causes hypercalcemia, which may lead to fatal kidney disease (renal tubule calcification).

SUPRARENAL GLANDS

The suprarenal glands, essential for life, are flat, small yellowish bodies, each weighing about 6 grams and surrounded by renal fatty fascia. They are located anteromedial to the superior renal poles. Accessory adrenal glands usually are small and composed of adrenal cortical cells. If present, they may be located near the main gland, but they may also be distributed at some distance, e.g., spermatic cord or broad ligament of the uterus.

Histologic Features

A sectioned adrenal gland shows a yellowish outer cortex forming most of the mass of the gland. The medulla, which tends to be red, constitutes only about one tenth or less of the mature gland. The medulla is almost completely covered by cortex except at the hilus, which contains the suprarenal vein, the vessel that drains the gland of blood and hormones. The gland has a thick, tough connective tissue capsule, composed primarily of collagenous fibers. From the capsule, trabeculae enter the parenchyma of the cortex of the gland. The capsule contains an arterial plexus of blood vessels that supplies the gland (Fig. 15–22).

Suprarenal Cortex

The cortex of the gland has three distinct morphologic areas. Because of their appearance in histologic sections, these areas or zones are named zona glomerulosa, zona fasciculata, and zona reticularis.

Zona Glomerulosa

The outermost functional part of the gland, the zona glomerulosa, is subcapsular and composed of polyhedral cells arranged in rounded groupings. The cells possess deeply staining nuclear chromatin; the cytoplasm tends to be basophilic and contains a small scattering of lipid droplets. The ultrastructural appearance includes the presence of numerous microtubules, elongate mitochondria, and abundant agranular endoplasmic reticulum, and, as suggested by light microscopy, little granular endoplasmic reticulum. These cells

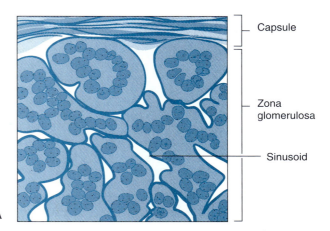

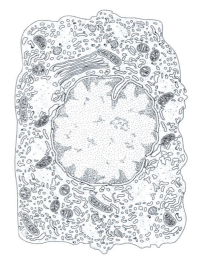

FIGURE 15–23. *Suprarenal gland, cells of zona glomerulosa. The cells of the zona glomerulosa are peripherally located beneath the capsule of the suprarenal gland. The cells form clusters without a significant lumen. The cells are low columnar, with spherical, deeply staining nuclei. The zona glomerulosa secretes hormones concerned primarily with mineral metabolism, i.e., deoxycorticosterone and aldosterone.*

are typical of steroid synthesizing cells. The zona glomerulosa is not well-developed in humans (Fig. 15–23).

Zona Fasciculata

The zona fasciculata, subjacent to zona glomerulosa, consists of large cells arranged, as their name suggests, in columns two cells wide. Between the parallel columns, fenestrated venous sinusoids are positioned. The nuclei are seen in marked contrast to the eosinophilic cytoplasm. These cells contain numerous lipid droplets composed of cholesterol, fats, fatty acids, and phospholipids. The lipid droplets are scattered between elements of the most abundant organelle, the agranular endoplasmic reticulum. The Golgi apparatus is highly developed. Mitochondria are usually spherical and are filled with tubular cristae (Fig. 15–24).

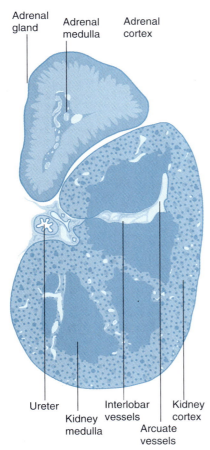

FIGURE 15–22. *Suprarenal gland. This is a macroscopic diagram of a fetal adrenal gland and kidney. The suprarenal gland can be seen to be composed of two regions: cortex and medulla. The zona glomerulosa and zona fasciculata (the outer and middle parts of the gland) are easily recognizable.*

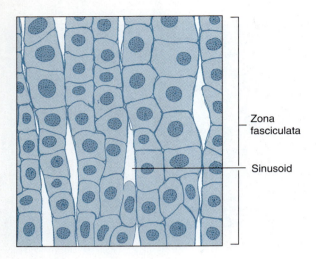

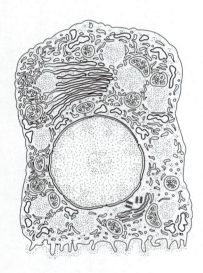

FIGURE 15–24. *Suprarenal gland, cells of zona fasciculata. The zona fasciculata is the middle zone and the broadest zone of the adrenal cortex. The cells are arranged in parallel cords one to two cells thick. The cells are cuboidal and frequently contain two nuclei. Vacuoles seen in these cells represent dissolved lipid droplets. Cholesterol is synthesized in the zona fasciculata. Cells also synthesize and secrete glucocorticoids, cortisone, and cortisol.*

Zona Reticularis

The third and innermost layer of the suprarenal cortex consists of branching, interconnecting columns of cells. The cytoplasm of these cells is filled with agranular endoplasmic reticulum, numerous lysosomes, and lipochrome pigment bodies, suggesting degradatory activity in the cell. It has been suggested that exaggerated cell death is occurring; however, electron microscopy studies do not support the suggestion. Autoradiographic studies have indicated the most intense cellular proliferation in the zona glomerulosa and peripheral parts of the zona reticularis and, less intensely, divisional figures (mitoses) in all parts of the cortex (Fig. 15–25).

Hormones of the Suprarenal Cortical Cells

The cortices of the suprarenal glands are essential for life. Their removal, without replacement therapy, results in death.

The cortical cells produce several hormones. Cells of the zona glomerulosa produce aldosterone, which has its effect on electrolyte and water balance. Cells of the zona fasciculata produce hormones that control carbohydrate balance, the glucocorticoids (e.g., cortisol). Cells in the zona reticularis probably produce sex hormones, including androgens, estrogen, and progesterone (Table 15–6).

Suprarenal Gland Medulla

The medulla of the suprarenal gland is fundamentally different from the cortex. It is composed of groups of chromaffin cells separated by wide venous sinusoids. The chromaffin cells synthesize and release norepinephrine and epinephrine into the venous sinusoids after stimulation by preganglionic sympathetic nerve fibers, which control the medulla (Table 15–7).

Although some mammals appear to have separate cells synthesizing and releasing epinephrine and norepinephrine, these functions are apparently carried out by a single cell type in humans. The secretory cells are

TABLE 15-6. Hormones of the Adrenal Cortex

Hormone	Action	Regulation
Mineralocorticoids	Regulate the concentration of extracellular electrolytes, especially sodium and potassium	Electrolyte concentration in blood
Glucocorticoids	Influence the metabolism of carbohydrates, proteins, and fats; promote vasoconstriction; anti-inflammatory compounds	ACTH from the adenohypophysis of the pituitary gland in response to stress
Gonadocorticoids	Supplement the sex hormones from the gonads	

large and columnar and form single cell rows adjacent to fenestrated venous sinusoids. The nuclei are located in the basal part of the cell distal to the sinusoids. In the adjacent extracellular space, the nerve terminals of preganglionic sympathetic nerve fibers synapse with the chromaffin cells.

The cytoplasm of the chromaffin cell is basophilic; hence, it contains abundant granular endoplasmic reticulum, mitochondria, Golgi apparatus, and agranular vesicles. This is typical of cells of high metabolic, synthetic activity. The norepinephrine-producing cells have rounded or elliptical vesicles, which become very electron dense after aldehyde and osmium tetroxide fixation. On the other hand, in the epinephrine-producing cells, the vesicles contain granules that appear pale with identical fixation treatment. The granules of epinephrine-producing cells often appear with a clear area between the granular contents (epinephrine) and the membrane of the agranular reticulum surrounding them. The contents of the packaging membrane are emptied into the apical extracellular space, where the hormone enters the fenestrated endothelium of venous sinusoids, and then into the hilar suprarenal vein (Fig. 15-26).

Normally, only small amounts of epinephrine or norepinephrine are released; however, in situations of fear, anger, and stress, their secretion is significantly increased. Norepinephrine increases heart rate, vasoconstriction, and blood pressure. Epinephrine increases carbohydrate metabolism.

The suprarenal gland medulla is not essential for life, and its removal is not accompanied by significant physiologic changes. As noted earlier, the opposite is true if the cortex is removed.

The medullary chromaffin cells are of neural crest origin. When the fixative contains potassium dichromate, epinephrine and norepinephrine are oxidized, resulting in a characteristic brown appearance of granules containing these two hormones; this is called the *chromaffin reaction*.

Blood Supply

The suprarenal gland is highly vascular, having three arterial sources: inferior phrenic arteries, abdomi-

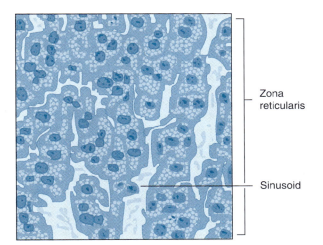

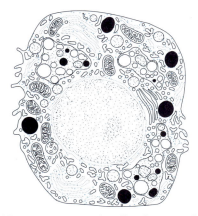

FIGURE 15-25. *Suprarenal gland, cells of zona reticularis. In the innermost layer of the adrenal cortex, the cells are arranged in irregular cords, are smaller than those of the zona fasciculata, and stain darker. Sinusoids separate cords of cells. The cells synthesize and secrete the same hormones as the zona fasciculata, i.e., glucocorticoids, cortisone, and cortisol. These hormones participate in carbohydrate, protein, and fat metabolism.*

TABLE 15-7. Comparison of the Hormones from the Adrenal Medulla

Epinephrine	Norepinephrine
Elevates blood pressure because of increased cardiac output and peripheral vasoconstriction	Elevates blood pressure because of generalized vasoconstriction
Accelerates respiratory rate and dilates respiratory passageways	Similar effect but to a lesser degree
Increases efficiency of muscular contraction	Similar effect but to a lesser degree
Increases rate of glycogen breakdown into glucose, so blood glucose rises	Similar effect but to a lesser degree
Increases rate of fatty acid released from fat, so blood fatty acids rise	Similar effect but to a lesser degree
Increases release of ACTH and TSH from the adenohypophysis of the pituitary gland	No such effect

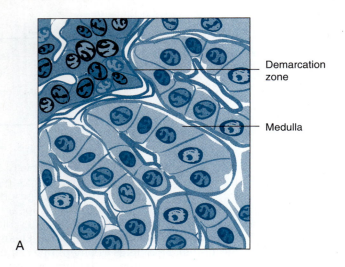

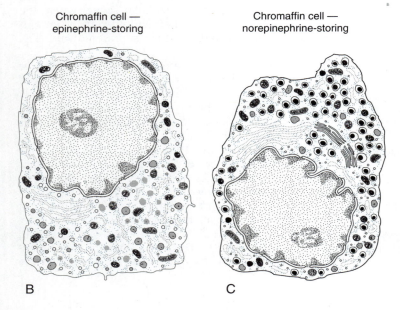

FIGURE 15–26. Suprarenal gland, cells of the medulla. Not essential for life, the hormones secreted by the adrenal medulla influence metabolic rate and cardiovascular function, and induce lipolysis and the release of fatty acids from adipose tissue. A, The cells are polyhedral and arranged in anastomosing cords. They have prominent nuclei and possess numerous chromaffin granules, which are precursors of epinephrine and norepinephrine. It is thought that these two hormones are secreted by two different cells as depicted in B and C.

nal aorta, and renal arteries. The arteries and arterioles ramify throughout the capsule, forming a capsular plexus of sinusoids before entering the gland. The vascular plexus of fenestrated sinusoids continues through the outer cortical region (zona glomerulosa); these re-form long, relatively unbranched vessels (zona fasciculata), only to become plexiform once again in the inner region (zona reticularis). The vessels remain plexiform and enter the adrenal medulla. After emerging from the medulla, the fenestrated sinusoidal plexuses re-form, becoming veins that drain into the central or medullary vein. The adrenal medulla also receives direct or bypass arteriolar supply from the capsular arteries. These medullary arterioles become plexiform capillary beds, then re-form as veins that join the central medullary vein. The medullary veins usually drain into the inferior vena cava (right side) and renal vein (left side) (Fig. 15–27).

PANCREATIC ISLETS

The pancreatic islets (islets of Langerhans) are composed of semispherical clusters of cells distributed throughout the exocrine tissue of the pancreas. The human pancreas may have as many as 10^6 islets. The islets are roughly 150 μm in diameter and are most common in the pancreatic tail. Not uncommonly, isolated cells are found in aberrant locations such as exocrine glands and ducts. The primary cell types that make up the islets are four in number, α (alpha), β (beta), δ (delta), and PP (polypeptide) cells.

The most numerous cells are types α and β. Confirmed by immunofluorescence microscopy and by immunoelectron microscopy, the α cell synthesizes glucagon, and the β cell, insulin. Human α cells tend to be peripherally located, and β cells more centrally.

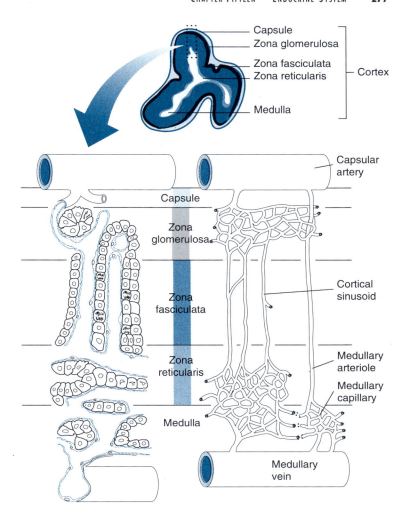

FIGURE 15–27. *Diagram of suprarenal histology. Note the arrangement of the extensive blood vessels and sinusoids within the adrenal gland and the secretory products of each of the different cell types.*

Recognition of specific pancreatic islet cells by light microscopy involves the visualization of specific granules within the cytoplasm. In α cells (glucagon synthesizing), granules (300 mm) are fixed by alcohol and become a brilliant orange or red when stained with orange G or Mallory-Azan stain but are unstained with aldehyde-fucsin. Beta cell (insulin synthesizing) granules (300 nm) are alcohol soluble, but when appropriately fixed (Bouin's solution or SUSA), they stain with aldehyde-fucsin. The δ cell, thought to synthesize gastrin, also contains somatostatin or another similar peptide. Human δ cells are located with α cells, peripherally in the islet (Fig. 15–28 and Table 15–8).

The distribution of α cells and δ cells peripherally and β cells centrally suggests functional segregation. The medulla (β cells) produces insulin, which is secreted at a rate determined by the blood concentration of glucose and a mixed cortical function in which all three cells participate. Impairment of insulin secretion results in hyperglycemia and the clinical condition of diabetes mellitus. The periphery is rich in neurovascular elements and is though to mediate rapid responses to changes in the internal environment. In the periphery, somatostatin released by δ cells may serve to inhibit the secretory activity of α or β cells. In humans, δ cells appear to be in intimate contact with α cells; hence, it is possible that δ cells have regulatory (inhibitory) control over glucagon-releasing α cells. It is known that α and δ cells are joined by gap junctions.

Autonomic neurotransmitters (hormones) such as

TABLE 15–8. Hormones of the Pancreas

Hormone	Action	Regulation
Glucagon	Stimulates the liver to convert glycogen into glucose, so blood glucose levels rise	Blood glucose level through negative feedback in pancreas
Insulin	Promotes movement of glucose through cell membranes; stimulates liver to convert glucose into glycogen; promotes the transport of amino acids into cells; assists in synthesis of proteins and fats	Blood glucose level through negative feedback in pancreas

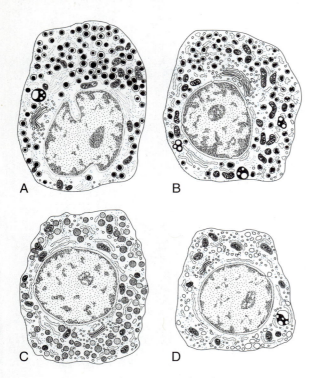

FIGURE 15-28. Islet of Langerhans, four cell types. Note the four cell types of the islet of Langerhans. The granules differ significantly in the α, β, and δ cells. The chromophobe is almost devoid of granules. The α cell (A) is thought to synthesize and release glucagon, the hormone that has a glycogenolytic effect, which raises blood glucose. The β cells (B) are the source of insulin, the hormone that lowers blood glucose and increases formation of glycogen, the storage form of glucose. The δ cell (C) is an enigma, as there is no physiologic evidence for a third hormone-secreting cell type in the islet. It may be related to α cells. The chromophobe (D) is also without known function and may also be related to α cells.

acetylcholine and norepinephrine also effect secretion by α and β cells. Acetycholine enhances the secretion of insulin and glucagon. Norepinephrine, on the other hand, prevents glucose-induced insulin release.

In addition to the α, β, and δ cells, peptide-secreting cells are found in the human pancreas. There are probably two types, one of which produces pancreatic polypeptide (PP). The granules in this small cell are about 140 nm in diameter. The other cell type has an ultrastructure like that of the D_1 cells of the gastric mucosa and may produce vasoactive intestinal polypeptide (VIP). The secretory product of the pancreatic D_1 cell is not certain.

It is of some interest that the D_1 and PP cells are not limited in location to the pancreatic islet but are found in the exocrine part of the pancreas as well.

Blood and Nerve Supply

Each pancreatic islet has a capillary bed as dense as in a renal glomerulus, and each islet is drained by one to three venules, which join to form an intralobular vein that is continuous with the portal circulation. The capillaries are fenestrated.

The pancreatic nerve supply is from the celiac plexus and enters the gland with the arteries of supply. The efferent supply is better understood than the afferent supply. The efferents consist of sympathetic postganglionic fibers from the celiac ganglion and parasympathetic preganglionics from the right vagus. These nonmyelinated nerve fibers are vasomotor (sympathetic) and parenchymal (both sympathetic and parasympathetic). Although several types of nerve terminals are known (cholinergic, adrenergic, and a third, uncertain type), their cellular specificity has not been established. In addition to chemical synapses, some electrical or gap junctions may also occur between nerve and islet cells, just as they have been shown to occur between islet cells.

GASTROENTEROPANCREATIC ENDOCRINE (GEP) SYSTEM

The gastroenteropancreatic endocrine system is composed of scattered, often single, hormone-producing cells in the gastrointestinal mucosa and pancreas. Electron microscopy techniques and immunocytochemistry have been instrumental in identifying the cells of this system of endocrine cells. At least 15 types of cells have been found in humans, and they are not easily located. Type B (β) cells are found only in the pancreas, but at least three other types are found not only in the pancreas but also in the gastrointestinal mucosa.

The endocrine cells of the GEP system have certain common features. They all produce peptides or amines that are active as hormones or neurotransmitters, and they all contain neuron-specific isoenzymes of the glycolytic enzyme enolase. The cells all belong to the APUD (amine precursor uptake and decarboxylation) system of cells that apparently modulate autonomic activity and also one another. The mode of action of the GEP system is unclear, but the regions served may be considered places where neural, paracrine, and endocrine controls of activity are closely tied together.

TABLE 15-9. The APUD Cells of the Diffuse Neuroendocrine System

Location	Type	Main Secretion Peptide	Main Secretion Amine
Cells of neural crest origin			
Thyroid	Parafollicular (C)	Calcitonin	5-HT, dopamine
Ultimobranchial body	C	Calcitonin	5-HT, dopamine
	Type I gliomus	—	Dopamine, norepinephrine
Carotid body	Small, intensely fluorescent	—	
Sympathetic ganglia	Chromaffin	—	Norepinephrine
Adrenal medulla	Chromaffin	—	Epinephrine Norepinephrine
Skin	Melanoblast	—	Promelanin
Urogenital tract	EC	—	5-HT
	C	—	—
Cells of placodal or specialized ectodermal origin			
Hypothalamus	Nucleus paraventricularis	Oxytocin, CRF	—
	Nucleus supraopticus	Vasopressin	—
	Nucleus suprachiasmaticus	—	—
	Nucleus dorsomedialis/ventromedialis	TRF	—
	Nucleus arcuatus (nucleus infundibularis)	LHRF	Dopamine
	Anterior and posterior nuclear "zones" of hypothalamus	SRF, CRF	—
	Nucleus periventricularis	Somatostatin	—
Pineal gland	P	LHRF	5-HT, melatonin
Parathyroid	Chief	PTH	—
Pituitary	Somatotroph	Somatotropin	Dopamine
	Mammatroph	Prolactin	Dopamine
	Gonadotroph	Follitropin	Dopamine
	Gonadotroph	Luteotropin	Dopamine
	Corticotroph	Coticotropin	—
	M	Melanotropin	Tryptamine
	Thyrotroph	Thyrotropin	Dopamine
Placenta	Endocrine	Gonadotropin	—
	Endocrine	Somatomammotropin	—
	Endocrine	Corticotropin	—
Cells of uncertain origin			
Pancreas	A	Glucagon	5-HT
	B	Insulin	5-HT
	D	Somatostatin	Dopamine
	D_1	VIP-like	Dopamine
	P	Bombesin-like	—
	PP	Pancreatic polypeptide	Dopamine
Stomach	A	Glucagon	—
	D	Somatostatin	—
	ECL	—	Histamine?
	EC_1	Substance P	5-HT
	G	Gastrin, enkephalin	—
	X	—	—
Intestine	D	Somatostatin	—
	$D_1(H)$	VIP	—
	EC_1	Substance P	5-HT
	EC_2	Motilin	5-HT
	EC_n	—	5-HT
	I	Cholecystokinin	—
	K	GIP	—
	L	Enteroglucagon	—
	N	Neurotensin	—
	S	Secretin	—
Lung	Kulchitsky (P_a)	—	—
Heart	Myoendocrine	Cardiodilation, atrial natriuretic factor	—

*A dash (—) indicates substance has not been identified, *CRF*, corticotropin-releasing factor; *GIP*, gastric-inhibitory peptide; *5-HT*, 5-hydroxytryptamine; *LHRF*, luteotropin-releasing (luteinizing hormone-releasing factor); *PTH*, parathyroid hormone; *SRF*, somatotropin-releasing factor; *TRF*, thyrotropin-releasing factor; *VIP*, vasoactive intestinal peptide.

DIFFUSE NEUROENDOCRINE SYSTEM

At least 40 different cell types have been characterized as APUD cells and are included in what has been described as the diffuse neuroendocrine system. These include the GEP cells just described. A list of these cells and their secretions is given in Table 15–9. Although the reader may not see many of these specific cell types, except through research methods, they are listed here because of their emerging importance. Some investigators consider APUD cells to be a third division of the nervous system. It is believed that these cells support, modify, and amplify the activities of neurons in both the autonomic and somatic divisions.

CHAPTER SIXTEEN

Female Reproductive System

Ovaries	282
Oviduct (Fallopian Tube)	287
Fertilization	289
Endocrine Regulation of the Ovarian Cycle	289
Uterus	291
Menstrual Cycle	292
Implantation and Formation of the Placenta	295
Uterine Cervix	297
Vagina	298
External Genitalia	300
Mammary Glands	300

The female reproductive system comprises paired gonads, the *ovaries*, in which the early stages of maturation of the female haploid gamete, the *ovum*, occur. The *gonads*, or primary sex organs of the male and female, serve as both *endocrine* and *exocrine* glands. The principal steroid sex hormones of ovarian origin in the human female are *estradiol*, which is a product of the functional units of the ovary, the *ovarian follicles*, and *progesterone*, which is a secretion of the modified post-ovulatory follicle, the *corpus luteum*. The exocrine (cytocrine) product of the ovary is the developing ovum, which is shed from the ovarian surface in the human in an immature (*oocyte*) stage. The *genitalia* of the female reside both externally and internally (Fig. 16–1). The external structures include the *mons pubis*, the perineal structures comprising the *vulva* (the *labia majora* and *minora*), together with the *bulbourethral glands* and the *clitoris*. Internal organs of reproduction are the *ovaries, oviducts, uterus*, and *vagina* (Figs. 16–1 and 16–2). Because of the intimate physiologic regulatory feedback mechanisms that unify the ovaries, uterus, adenohypophysis, and hypothalamus, a *gonadal-hypothalamic* or *gonadal-hypophysial axis* is often cited as the unified functional reproductive unit in both male and female.

The ovary and uterus undergo cyclical morphologic and profound physiologic changes in response to hypophysial secretions during the *menstrual cycle*—the roughly 28-day cycle of maturation of ovarian follicles that commences at *puberty* with the first menstrual flow (the *menses*) and continues until cessation at age 45 to 50 years of regular ovulation and menstruation—and the onset of *menopause*. Although they are most closely related structurally and developmentally to the integument, the mammary glands are regarded as functional accessories to the reproductive system and thus are considered in this chapter as well.

OVARIES

The paired ovaries lie in relation to the lateral wall of the pelvis, on either side of the uterus, and are suspended by a fold of peritoneum, the ovarian suspensory ligament, which contains the ovarian vessels. The ovaries are in intimate relationship laterally with the terminal, fimbriated portion of the oviduct. Prior to puberty, the surface of the ovaries is smooth and pink; following the menarche and the initiation of ovulation, the surface typically exhibits rough contours and bulges, and is grayish pink. The gonad is frequently described as almond-shaped, some 3 cm in length, 1

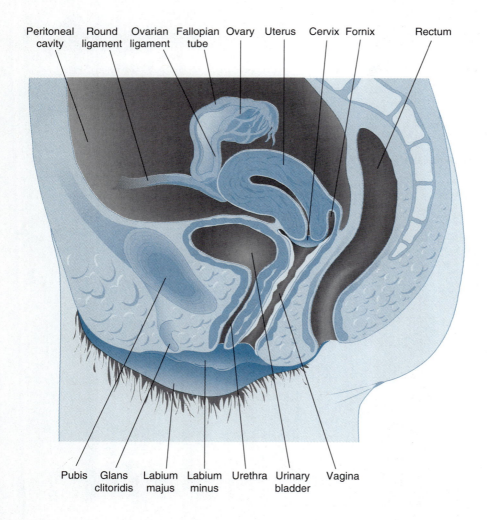

FIGURE 16–1. Diagrammatic representation of a midsagittal section through the female pelvis. Note the relationships of the reproductive organs to one another and to other pelvic structures.

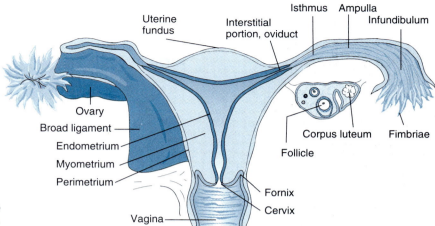

FIGURE 16–2. Organs of the reproductive system of the human female. Note the relationships of the ovary, oviduct, uterus, and vagina.

cm in thickness, and 1.5 cm in width. Vasculature and nerves enter and leave the ovary at its hilum, situated on its medial surface.

A section through the ovary of a woman of reproductive age examined with a hand lens reveals an outer, cortical region that contains empty vesicles of various sizes, the *ovarian follicles,* as well as yellow and white accumulations of tissue, each of which is termed a *corpus luteum* and *corpus albicans,* respectively. These all represent different stages in follicular maturation, as discussed in the following section. These cortical structures are absent from an ill-defined ovarian medulla, which contains a plexus of arteries and veins, and ovarian stroma. Radial branches of the medullary arteries supply the ovarian cortex and developing follicles. The ovary is encapsulated by white fibrous connective tissue, the *tunica albuginea,* which gives the grayish-white color to the ovary in the living state. A cellular continuation of the peritoneum forms the outermost covering of the ovarian surface; this single mesothelial layer is termed the *germinal epithelium,* a holdover from an erroneous, earlier interpretation of this cell layer as the source of the germ cells of the gonad.

During the embryogenesis of the ovary, primordial germ cells migrate from their endodermal site of origin within the embryonic yolk sac to the presumptive ovary, divide, and populate its cortical region. These cells, the *oogonia,* are analogous to the spermatogonia of the male gonad (see Chapter 17). In the human, the oogonia cease mitotic division during fetal development and, in fact, decrease in number from several million per ovary early in fetal development to several hundred thousand per ovary at birth. Beginning at 3 months, the oogonia begin to enter *meiotic prophase*; they arrest there in the diplotene stage. By definition, a developing germ cell undergoing first meiotic division is classified as a primary gametocyte, and in the female, therefore, as a *primary oocyte.* The oocytes become surrounded by epithelial follicular cells and a basal lamina; this unit of germ cell plus investments is termed a *primordial follicle.* Remarkably, primordial follicles remain quiescent until they may be stimulated to initiate growth and maturation at some time during the four-decade reproductive lifetime of the human female. Only some 400 to 500 such follicles will mature to ovulation (one per menstrual cycle), although many more follicles will initiate the growth process and involute prior to ovulation. This process of involution, follicular degeneration, and oocyte loss is termed *follicular atresia,* and the follicles, *atretic follicles.* The mechanisms controlling which follicles begin growth, which mature to ovulatory follicles, and which undergo atresia are currently unknown.

Ovarian Follicles

Thus, from the preceding description, it is seen that the ovarian follicle is both the structural and functional unit of the ovary. The growth and development of ovarian follicles occur in an orderly sequence of progressive increase in size and morphologic complexity that forms the basis of identifying stages in this continuous process, as summarized in Figure 16–3.

Primordial Follicles

As would be expected of the quiescent reserve units within the adult ovary, the primary follicles are both the smallest and most numerous of the ovarian follicles. They are located immediately deep to the tunica albuginea, frequently in loosely arranged groups. Each consists of a spherical oocyte, surrounded by a single layer of squamous follicular epithelial cells (Fig. 16–4A). The nucleus of the oocyte is round, is eccentrically placed within the cytoplasm, and exhibits a prominent nucleolus. At the diplotene stage of meiotic prophase, the chromosomes are not particularly distinct, and the nucleus is pale staining. Cytoplasmic organelles are sparse, with the exception of many mitochondria that tend to cluster near the nucleus. Occasional annulate lamellae, a small Golgi apparatus, and scattered profiles of endoplasmic reticulum bearing few ribosomes can be found. An unremarkable basement membrane demarcates the peripheral boundary of the

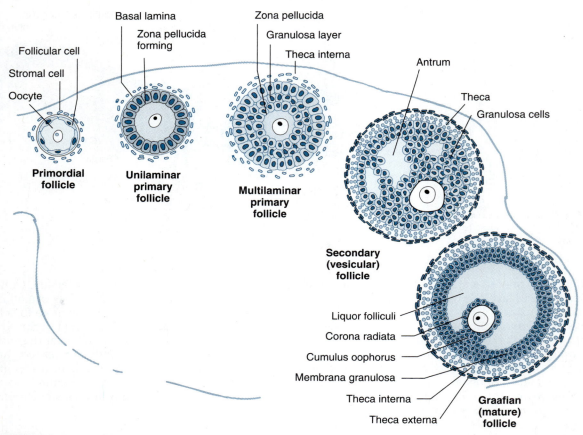

FIGURE 16–3. *Diagrammatic representation of the sequence of maturation of an ovarian follicle, from primordial to graafian follicle.*

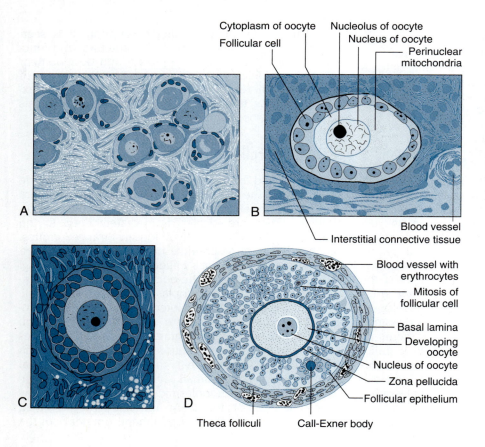

FIGURE 16–4. Progressive stages in the development of an ovarian follicle. A, *Primordial follicles.* Note the large oocyte surrounded by a squamous layer of ovarian follicular cells. B, *Primary (unilaminar) follicle.* At an early stage of growth, the follicle enlarges and the epithelium becomes cuboidal. C, *Primary (bilaminar) follicle.* Note the stratification of the cuboidal epithelium surrounding the oocyte. D, *Late primary (multilaminar) follicle.* Such follicles exhibit a multilayered follicular epithelium (granulosa), a well-defined thecal layer, and a large oocyte with prominent zona pellucida.

follicle from the surrounding interstitial connective tissue.

Primary (Growing) Follicle

The entrance of an ovarian follicle into the growth cycle is marked by morphologic changes in the oocyte, its surrounding follicular epithelial cells, and the stroma adjacent to the follicle (Fig. 16–4, B and C). The oocyte increases in diameter from its 25-μm size in the resting state. Its cytoplasmic organelles, such as the Golgi apparatus and endoplasmic reticulum, increase in number, size, and complexity; mitochondria increase in number and disperse from their perinuclear position; and ribosomes, both free and in association with the endoplasmic reticulum, are numerous. Together, these changes attest to the augmented synthetic capacity of the oocyte. Recent evidence suggests a primary role for the oocyte in the secretion of the PAS-positive (stains with periodic acid–Schiff stain) amorphous refractile layer of glycoprotein, the *zona pellucida*, which is secreted at the interface between the oocyte and the apices of the follicular epithelial cells. The squamous follicular epithelial cells assume a greater height in early growing follicles and send cytoplasmic processes through the zona pellucida, where gap junctions are formed between these processes and microvillous extensions of the oocyte cell surface. The periphery of the follicle becomes demarcated by a more conspicuous basal lamina, and the surrounding connective tissue more compactly and circumferentially disposed around the follicle. This mantel of connective tissue is termed the *theca folliculi*. Follicles at this phase of development are designated *unilaminar primary follicles* (see Fig. 16–3).

Progressive growth of the follicle results in the formation of a stratified follicular epithelium, designated the *granulosa*, and the follicle accordingly is designated a *multilaminar primary follicle* (Fig. 16–4D). In such follicles, the thecal layer is prominent. The oocyte continues to enlarge, reaching a diameter of approximately 125 to 150 μm. Its enlarged, vesicular nucleus is termed the *germinal vesicle*.

Secondary (Antral) Follicles

With the continued growth in diameter of the follicle, the follicular epithelium becomes progressively higher and begins to accumulate fluid in the intercellular spaces between the granulosa cells. These fluid-filled spaces, *antral spaces*, gradually coalesce to form a single, large space within the granulosa termed the *antrum* (Figs. 16–3 and 16–5A). The fluid filling the spaces is termed follicular fluid, or *liquor folliculi*. By convention, growing follicles exhibiting antral spaces or a single large antrum are termed *secondary* or *vesicular follicles*. The follicular fluid is rich in glycosaminoglycans, protein, steroids (progesterone and androgen, in addition to estradiol), as well as steroid-binding protein.

In sizable secondary follicles, the antrum has enlarged to such an extent that the granulosa and the oocyte are displaced to one side of the follicle (see Figs. 16–3 and 16–5). The pillow of granulosa cells that

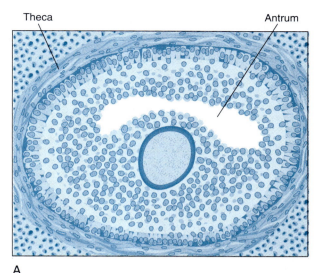

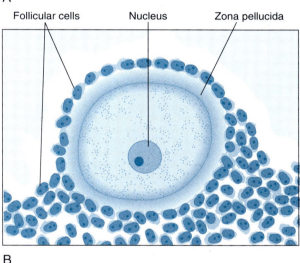

FIGURE 16–5. Secondary follicle and detail of oocyte. A, *Secondary follicles differ from primary follicles in that a fluid-filled space, the antrum, is present. The oocyte is displaced toward one side of the follicle as the antrum enlarges.* B, *Note the large oocyte, its nucleus with prominent nucleolus, and its distinctive zona pellucida. The layer of follicular cells surrounding the oocyte is termed the* corona radiata. *The mass of follicular cells underlying the oocyte constitutes the* cumulus oophorus.

attaches the oocyte to the follicular wall is termed the *cumulus oophorus,* and that adherent layer of follicular cells subjacent to the zona pellucida is termed the *corona radiata* (see Fig. 16–5B).

The thecal layer surrounding the follicle continues to enlarge, and inner and outer layers may be discerned in secondary follicles; they are the *theca interna* and *theca externa,* respectively. The cells of the theca interna exhibit fine structural features consistent with steroid secretion, including many mitochondria with tubular cristae, lipid stores, and abundant smooth endoplasmic reticulum. They have been demonstrated to secrete *androstenediol,* an androgen precursor of estradiol that when transported into the follicle, is aromatized to estradiol by the granulosa cells. *Estradiol,* the principal estrogen of the human female, is subsequently transported back across the basal lamina to the extensive capillary plexus of the theca interna, from which it is distributed systemically. Estradiol within the follicular fluid rises in concentration and is considered essential to the ultimate growth and maturation of the follicle and oocyte.

Mature (Graafian) Follicle

Mature follicles immediately preceding ovulation are termed *graafian* or *tertiary follicles*. In marked contrast to other mammals, which give birth to litters and therefore mature many ova in any one reproductive (*estrus*) cycle, it is usual in the human that a single follicle ovulates one oocyte at midcycle every 28 days. The ovulatory event usually alternates in the right and left ovaries. Graafian follicles visibly bulge the surface of the ovary at the thinned site at the surface of the ovary at which ovulation will take place. Remarkably, a follicle a few micrometers in diameter at the beginning of the cycle may grow within 14 days to a diameter of 15 to 20 millimeters or greater by the time of ovulation at midcycle.

Atretic Follicles

Recent evidence suggests that the dominant follicle among the many that begin as primary follicles in any one cycle secretes a protein factor, *follicular regulatory protein*, which retards the growth of other follicles, possibly by inhibiting the follicular response to gonadotropins, and thus promoting *follicular atresia*. Atresia may at first seem a biologic extravagance, but the suggestion has been advanced that the several developing ovarian follicles at the beginning of each menstrual cycle contribute a substantial portion of circulating estrogen in the first half of the cycle, and that one follicle could not secrete sufficient estradiol to raise serum titers to the levels required to trigger the gonadal-hypophysial feedback mechanisms detailed in a later section. Follicular atresia may occur at any follicular stage.

Morphologically, atretic primary follicles are frequently recognized first by degeneration of the oocyte, and subsequently by disruption of the follicle. In the case of larger follicles undergoing atresia, alterations in the follicular epithelium—vascular invasion, loss of compactness, and shedding of cells into the antrum, for example—often precede visible alterations in the oocyte. Atresia of such larger follicles commonly includes a thickening and hyalinization of the basal lamina, resulting in the distinctive *glassy membrane* that is a hallmark of larger atretic follicles. Although the granulosa and oocyte of atretic follicles may degenerate, the cells of the theca interna frequently persist as a functional source of androgens and are recognized as *interstitial cells*.

Corpus Luteum

The *corpus luteum* (yellow body) is a temporary endocrine organ and the major source of ovarian steroid hormones in the latter half of the menstrual cycle as well as during the first few months of pregnancy if fertilization and successful implantation follow ovulation. If pregnancy is not established, the corpus luteum undergoes regression and degradation, to form a *corpus albicans* (white body), which persists as a distinctive hyaline collagenous formation within the interstitium until it is resolved by macrophagic activity. The corpus luteum that persists only through the immediate menstrual cycle is designated a *corpus luteum spurium*, or corpus luteum of menstruation; the corpus luteum maintained into pregnancy is termed a *corpus luteum verum*, or corpus luteum of pregnancy. The formation and maintenance of the corpus luteum depends on secretion of *luteinizing hormone (LH)* from the anterior pituitary. With reduced circulating LH toward the end of the menstrual cycle, the corpus luteum regresses, unless placental secretion of *human chorionic gonadotropin* (which mimics the action of LH) sustains its structure and secretory capacity during the early months of pregnancy. These relationships are discussed more fully in a later section.

The lumen of the postovulatory follicle may contain a clot of blood stemming from rupture of thecal capillaries at the time of ovulation. The cavity and clot are later invaded by connective tissue. An early alteration of the old follicular epithelium is the breakdown of the basal lamina and the invasion of thecal capillaries and connective tissue into the granulosa. This alteration sets the stage for the formation of a new, richly vascular endocrine organ, the corpus luteum.

The parenchyma of the corpus luteum is derived from the two major cell populations of the old follicle, i.e., the granulosa, and the secretory cells of the theca interna. Respectively, these differentiate into *granulosa lutein cells* and *theca lutein (paralutein) cells*. Granulosa lutein cells form by hypertrophy, rather than mitosis, of the follicular granulosa cells; they occupy the deeper, more central portions of the corpus luteum and constitute some 80% of the bulk of the parenchyma. These cells enlarge to 20 to 35 μm in diameter, are pale staining, and exhibit fine structural characteristics typical of steroid-secreting cells. Their principal secretion is *progesterone*, but they have been implicated by immunocytochemical studies to participate in the synthesis of the polypeptide hormone *relaxin* as well. The theca lutein cells are about half the diameter of granulosa lutein cells, are more intensely staining, and are clustered about the periphery of the corpus luteum as well as along the incursions of connective tissue and vasculature that have invaded the old follicle (Fig. 16–6). These cells also are specialized for steroid secretion and are considered to secrete estradiol and estrone in addition to progesterone.

Ovulation and First Meiotic Division

Ovulation is the release of the developing ovum from a graafian follicle onto the surface of the ovary.

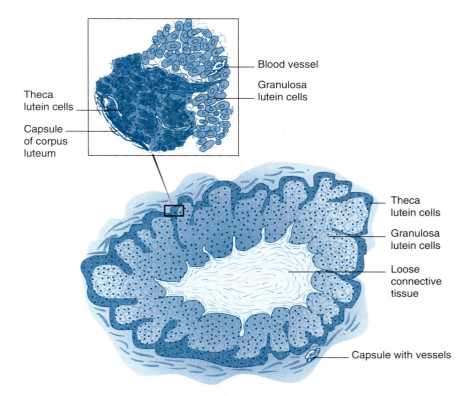

FIGURE 16-6. Diagrammatic representation of the human corpus luteum. *The corpus luteum forms from the ruptured ovarian follicle. Note the central lumen containing connective tissue, the remnants of the surrounding thecal layers, and the convoluted mass of tissue derived from both thecal and follicular cells of the follicle. Inset, Note the smaller darker cells arranged in cords derived from the theca (theca lutein cells) and the larger, pale-staining cells derived from the granulosa (granulosa lutein cells).*

Immediate postovulatory events include egg transport through the ostium of the oviduct to its interior. There, in the presence of spermatozoa, fertilization and final maturation division of the oocyte occur.

Ovulation typically occurs at midcycle (day 14 of an idealized menstrual cycle). The graafian follicle overgrows the ovarian cortex, where it bulges visibly beyond the ovarian surface; near the time of ovulation, such follicles may be observed via laparoscopic examination as translucent vesicles. The follicle bulges and is visible because the entire cortical region overlying the follicle, including the tunica albuginea and interstitial connective tissue, has become greatly reduced in thickness. Recent evidence has established that this attenuation is likely enzymatic; it is correlated with increased follicular levels of collagenase, which is thought to act on the tunica albuginea and collagen fibers of the interstitium. Furthermore, *plasminogen activator* from the granulosa cells activates *plasminogen* within the liquor folliculi to *plasmin*. Plasmin, in turn, is hypothesized to participate in the structural degradation of the basal lamina of the follicle as well as to convert procollagenase to its active molecular form.

The outwardmost portion of the bulging follicle blanches, owing to reduced blood flow to the theca interna, and is recognized as a white spot (*macula pellucida*) or the *stigma*, which marks the precise location at which follicular rupture will occur. The oocyte, together with an adherent retinue of granulosa cells of the cumulus oophorus, detaches from the follicular epithelium and floats free within the antrum. The oocyte and its surrounding cumulus mass are released from the ruptured follicle gradually and without apparent increase in fluid pressure, together with a copious amount of follicular fluid.

The events of oocyte maturation and meiotic division are intricately timed in relation to the events just described. A matter of hours prior to ovulation, the primary oocyte completes first meiotic division, giving rise to two daughter cells, a large *secondary oocyte,* and a diminutive *first polar body.* The secondary oocyte progresses within the follicle to metaphase of second meiotic division, in which stage it is ovulated. Final meiotic maturation in the human occurs only in the event of fertilization. The postovulatory oocytes remain viable only some 24 hours and then degenerate if fertilization has not occurred.

OVIDUCT (FALLOPIAN TUBE)

The muscular oviduct (fallopian tube, uterine tube) anatomically and functionally unites the ovary and the uterus. Its overall shape resembles a horn, with the flared proximal (ovarian) end open to the peritoneal cavity and the distal end open to the uterine cavity. The tube is 10 to 12 cm in length and is suspended by a fold of peritoneum, the mesosalpinx (from the Greek *salpinyx,* meaning horn) (Figs. 16-7 and 16-8). Its uterine portion, embedded within the wall of the uterus, is termed the *interstitial* or *intramural* portion. The narrowed medial third of the tube closest to the uterus is called the *isthmus,* and the somewhat expanded adjoining segment is designated the *ampulla.* The flared proximal portion of the ampulla, immediately subjacent to the ovary, is termed the *infundibulum.*

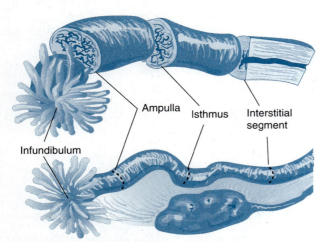

FIGURE 16–7. *Locations of histologic sections shown in Figure 16–8, through the various named portions of the human oviduct.* Note the fimbriae that project from the infundibulum toward the ovary.

Long fronds of the infundibular mucosa, the *fimbriae*, extend from the infundibulum (see Figs. 16–2 and 16–7). Each fimbria contains a core of smooth muscle and is covered by a heavily ciliated simple columnar epithelium. The wall of the oviduct consists of a complexly folded mucosa, a well-developed muscularis, and a serosal (peritoneal) outer lining. The tube is highly specialized for its roles in (1) capturing the ovulated oocyte within its cumulus mass and transporting it from the peritoneal surface of the ovary to the interior of the tube, (2) providing a suitable site for fertilization to occur, and (3) transporting the embryo to the uterine cavity.

Egg Capture and Transport

Ovulation occurs onto the peritoneal surface of the ovary. If the ovulated oocyte were to fall from the surface of the ovary, it would enter the peritoneal cavity and be lost. Because the ostium of the oviduct is open to the peritoneal cavity as well, spermatozoa may enter the cavity and fertilize the oocyte. An abortive attempt to implant upon the peritoneal surface or upon a pelvic or abdominal organ can induce massive intraabdominal bleeding. Such implantations at a site other than the endometrium are termed *ectopic pregnancies*. A common site for such ectopic implantation is the oviduct, resulting from faulty or delayed transport of the embryo to the uterus. Such an implantation is called a *tubal pregnancy*.

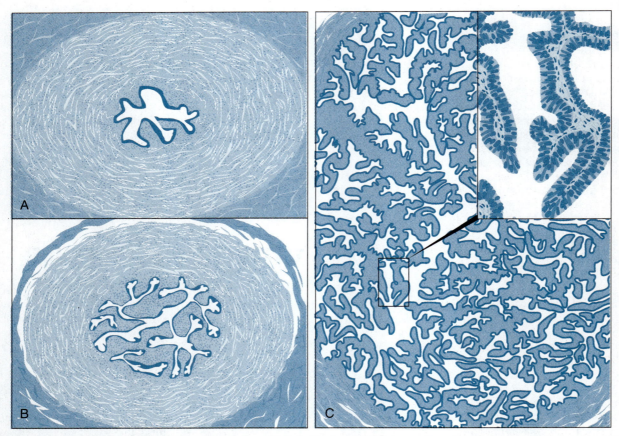

FIGURE 16–8. *Histologic sections from the locations shown in Figure 16–7.* A, The interstitial (intramural) portion passes through the uterine wall; it is surrounded by a thick muscular layer, and its lumen is small with few mucosal folds. B, The isthmus, a narrowed portion of the oviduct, exhibits a prominent muscular layer and mucosal folds. C, The ampulla is characterized by a thinner muscular wall and a mucosa in complex branching folds. Inset, Higher-magnification view of the region of the ampullary mucosa shown in C. Note the branching nature of the folds, the thin core of loose connective tissue, and the simple columnar epithelium consisting of columnar ciliated cells and nonciliated secretory cells.

Direct observation of egg transport into the oviduct shows conclusively that the sticky cumulus mass surrounding the oocyte provides the traction necessary for effective capture of the cumulus mass and oocyte and their transport toward the entrance, or abdominal *ostium,* of the oviduct. The fimbriae are stimulated to make caressing motions over the surface of the ovary at the time of ovulation, and the fluid currents induced by the ciliary action, together with direct transport of the cumulus mass upon the ciliated surface of the fimbriae, result in its passage to the ostium and into the ampulla of the oviduct.

Fertilization Site

Fertilization usually takes place within the oviduct, frequently within the ampulla. The mucosa of the ampulla is characterized by many complex longitudinal folds, which become less numerous and less extensive in the more distal regions of the oviduct (Fig. 16–8). The epithelium of the mucosa is simple columnar, with two subpopulations of cells, namely, ciliated cells and secretory cells (Fig. 16–8C, *inset*). They are considered to be functional variants of a single cell type; the relative proportions of the cell types are under hormonal control and vary with the menstrual cycle. In no other ciliary epithelium is ciliogenesis under steroid regulation. The number of ciliated cells and the vigor of ciliary beat are greatest at the time of ovulation and egg transport. The secretions of the oviduct and uterus are considered nutritive to the ovum, and they also serve in the biochemical activation (*capacitation*) of spermatozoa, rendering them optimally capable of fertilization. The secretions provide a viscous fluid interface on which the cumulus mass and its contained oocyte are moved distally through the oviduct toward the uterus, guided by the ciliated longitudinal folds of the mucosa.

Transport of the Embryo to Uterus

Transport within the ampulla and isthmus is greatly facilitated by strong, rhythmic, peristaltic contractions initiated by the muscularis, which is organized indistinctly into inner circular (spiral) and sparse outer longitudinal layers. One of the remarkable unexplained physiologic features of the fallopian tube is that transport of the early cleavage-stage embryo is arrested at the ampullary-isthmic junction for several days, until such time as the uterine mucosa is optimally favorable for implantation (see Fig. 16–12).

The oviduct is susceptible to several clinically significant pathologic conditions that can impair sperm and egg transport. Blockage of the oviduct may result from *congenital malformations* or from prolonged bacterial infection and inflammation of the mucosa (*chronic salpingitis*) such as may result from gonorrhea. *Scarring* and *stricture* of the tubal lumen resulting from such infection may impair egg transport, delaying arrival of the embryo at the uterus beyond the optimal time for implantation. Faulty egg transport may also dispose toward implantation within the tube itself, resulting in *tubal pregnancy.*

FERTILIZATION

Fertilization is defined as the incorporation of a spermatozoon into the egg cytoplasm (ooplasm). In the human, the oocyte is viable and fertilizable for approximately 24 hours after ovulation. If fertilization fails to occur, the oocyte degenerates within the fallopian tube.

Far from being a mere physical "torpedoing" of the egg by a sperm, fertilization has come to be appreciated as a complex process of receptor-mediated binding of the sperm to the egg surface and incorporation of the sperm into the ooplasm by fusion of the oolemma and sperm plasma membrane. Relatively few sperm of the several hundred thousand typically ejaculated are usually present at the site of fertilization, a factor which reduces the likelihood that multiple sperm enter the egg, a lethal condition termed *polyspermy.* Following dispersal of the cumulus mass of cells, sperm gain access to the outermost layer of the oocyte surface, the zona pellucida. The zona consists of three glycoproteins, ZP1, ZP2, and ZP3, ranging in molecular weight from 83 to 200 kD. Specific oligosaccharides of ZP3 serve as *sperm receptors* and bind to a specific protein in the sperm plasmalemma. This event triggers fusion of the sperm acrosomal membrane (see discussion of sperm morphology in Chapter 17) with the sperm plasmalemma at multiple points, thus creating channels for the release of acid hydrolases and other enzymes capable of degrading the underlying zona pellucida. Once a sperm has gained access to the oolemma, the egg and sperm plasma membranes fuse, triggering the *cortical reaction.* Peripherally located vesicles (*cortical granules*) within the ooplasm exocytose enzymes that act upon the glycoproteins of the zona, nullifying their sperm-binding capacity. This loss of sperm binding is another important block of entry of multiple sperm.

Sperm entry into the secondary oocyte also initiates (by some as yet unknown mechanism) the completion of second meiotic division and the formation of the mature, haploid egg, the *ovum*, together with a *second polar body.* Upon the fusion of the haploid pronucleus of the ovum with the decondensed haploid pronucleus of the sperm (an event termed *syngamy*), the diploid (2N) number of chromosomes and DNA is reestablished in the new single-cell individual, the *zygote.* The early cleavage stages of the embryo occur within the oviduct, during the first 5 days after fertilization (see Fig. 16–12).

ENDOCRINE REGULATION OF THE OVARIAN CYCLE

The maturation of ovarian follicles is under intricate hormonal control of the gonadal-hypophysial axis.

Two gonadotropins synthesized by the gonadotrophs of the adenohypophysis and essential to the maturation of the ovarian follicle are follicle-stimulating hormone (*FSH*) and luteinizing hormone (*LH*). Release of these hormones from the gonadotrophs of the pituitary is regulated by gonadotropin-releasing hormone (*GnRH*), synthesized by neurosecretory neurons of the hypothalamus (see Chapter 15). The ovary is itself a steroid-producing endocrine organ, as noted in previous sections, in that it elaborates estradiol within the ovarian follicle and estrogens and progesterone within the corpus luteum. These secretions participate in the dynamic feedback system involving the hypothalamo-hypophysial complex (Figs. 16–9 and 16–10).

FSH promotes the growth and differentiation of ovarian follicles beyond the formation of primary follicles. The initiating stimulus that regulates the progression from primordial follicle to primary follicle is yet to be defined. Interestingly, the FSH receptors of the follicle are localized exclusively on granulosa cells. Under FSH influence, the follicular epithelium proliferates, increases its number of FSH receptors, and activates the enzyme *aromatase*, which is necessary for the biochemical conversion of androgen (synthesized by the theca interna cells under stimulation of LH) to estradiol. The titer of estradiol within the liquor folliculi further stimulates the proliferation of the follicular epithelium (granulosa). Estradiol diffuses from the follicle and is delivered to the systemic circulation via the rich capillary plexus of the theca interna. Just prior to menstrual

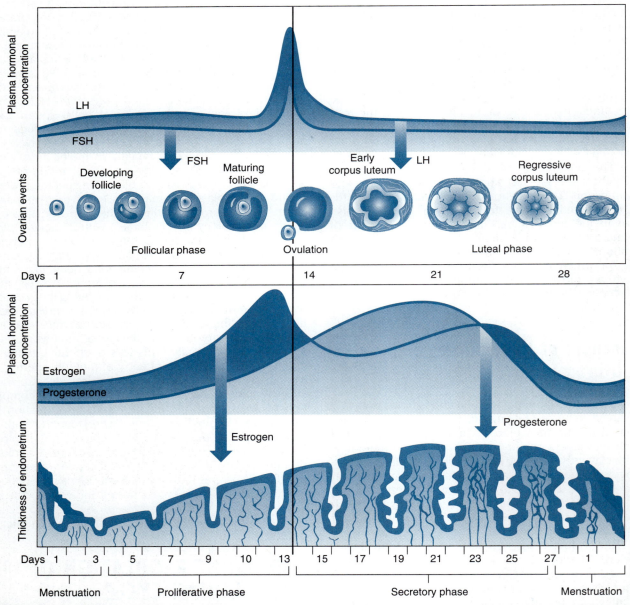

FIGURE 16–9. *Diagram showing the interrelationships during the menstrual cycle of ovarian and uterine structures, and plasma concentrations of pituitary gonadotropins, estrogen, and progesterone. Ovarian events are shown in the upper half of the figure, and correlated uterine development in the lower half.*

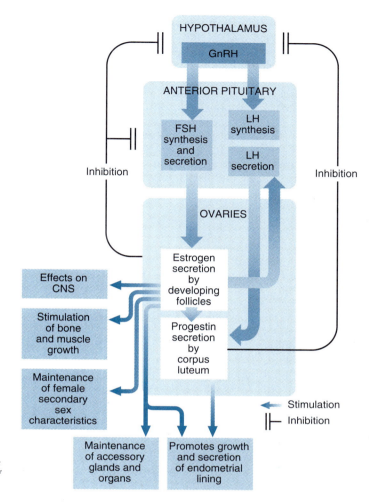

FIGURE 16-10. Diagram depicting hormonal feedback mechanisms regulating ovarian function. See text for explanation of abbreviations.

midcycle, the concentration of circulating estradiol in the blood exerts a positive feedback on the anterior pituitary, increasing its sensitivity to GnRH and thus enhancing a midcycle release of luteining hormone (the "LH surge"), which induces ovulation less than 20 hours following the LH serum peak (see Figs. 16–9 and 16–10). The same surge correlates with the stimulation of the primary oocyte within the graafian follicle to complete first meiotic division. Estrogen acts also in a negative feedback loop with the anterior pituitary to inhibit FSH release, thus inhibiting the maturation of additional ovarian follicles during the latter half of the menstrual cycle.

Analogously, the oral administration of ovarian steroid analogs to suppress hypothalamic GnRH serves clinically as the basis for several variant means of *oral contraception*. In most regimens, the goal of blocking ovulation is achieved by suppressing the LH surge critical to the induction of ovulation.

LH receptors, initially confined to the cells of the theca interna, are induced during the preovulatory period in the granulosa cells. Therefore, when circulating LH levels rise, the granulosa cells respond by secreting a new steroid, progesterone, as their secretion of estradiol declines. Progesterone, the dominant hormone of the second half of the menstrual cycle, is responsible, together with estrogens, for the buildup of the uterine endometrium in preparation for implantation and placenta formation. Under continued LH stimulation, the postovulatory follicle completes its redifferentiation into the corpus luteum. High circulating progesterone levels are inhibitory to LH, however, through hypothalamic inhibition of GnRH (see Fig. 16–10). Falling LH levels at the end of the menstrual cycle set the stage for regression of the corpus luteum and menstruation (see Fig. 16–9).

The secretion by the ovary of follicular regulatory hormone and relaxin has been noted in previous sections. Yet another hormone of ovarian (corpus luteum) origin is inhibin, which acts, together with estradiol, as an inhibitor of FSH and LH secretion.

UTERUS

The uterus, its shape frequently likened to an inverted pear, varies in size among nonpregnant women, but is on average 6.3 cm in length, 4.5 cm in breadth, and 2.5 cm in thickness. It exhibits several named anatomic parts (see Fig. 16–2), including an expanded *body* (corpus); a domed anterior portion, the uterine *fundus*, where implantation usually occurs and into which the oviducts (uterine tubes) insert; and a somewhat cylindrical *cervix*, which is coextensive with the vagina at the *fornix* (see Fig. 16–1). The opening of the cervix into the body is termed the *internal os*, and the opening of the cervix into the vagina the *external os*, of the uterus.

The uterine wall consists of three layers (see Fig. 16–2). Enumerated from the inside they are (1) the mucosa, termed in the uterus the *endometrium* (endo + Greek *metra*, meaning uterus), (2) the muscularis, termed the *myometrium*, and (3) the *perimetrium*, which is either serosa or adventitia, depending on the portion of the uterus examined.

Myometrium

The myometrium consists of interlacing bundles of smooth muscle, arranged in three or four indistinct layers separated by connective tissue. In the nongravid state, the myometrium is approximately 1.25 cm thick, but it undergoes dramatic alterations in response to hormonal stimulation. For example, the length of the smooth muscle cells varies during the menstrual cycle from 40 to 90 μm. The fibers are shortest during menstruation; uterine smooth muscle atrophies in the absence of estrogen. Likewise, during pregnancy, the great increase in size of the uterus results in a 24-fold overall increase in the mass of the uterus, with a 10-fold increase in the length of muscle fibers. Both hypertrophy and hyperplasia of muscle, as well as proliferation of connective tissue contribute to this increase in organ size. Myocytes purportedly secrete collagen during pregnancy, thus contributing to the proliferation of the connective tissue compartment. The myometrium is responsive to a variety of hormones, among them *oxytocin*, which stimulates uterine contraction and is frequently employed clinically to induce labor; *relaxin*, which, among other actions, relaxes the uterus during pregnancy and softens the uterine cervix prior to parturition; *progesterone*, which inhibits contraction of uterine smooth muscle during the secretory phase of the menstrual cycle to obviate interference with implantation; and *prostaglandins*, which have been implicated in the initiation of uterine contractions at the time of birth.

Endometrium

The endometrium comprises the mucosal lining of the uterus. It consists therefore of an epithelium and underlying tunica propria that are exquisitely responsive to steroid hormonal stimulation or deprivation. At its peak of development, the endometrium measures some 5 mm thick. Its epithelium is simple columnar and consists of both ciliated and secretory cells. The epithelium sends tubular glands into the tunica propria, which is termed the *endometrial stroma*. The stroma consists of loosely arranged connective tissue with abundant extracellular matrix.

Microscopically, two zones of the endometrium may be distinguished, a superficial stratum functionale (functionalis), and a basal portion, the stratum basale (basalis), which borders the myometrium and into which the bases of the endometrial glands project. During the menstrual phase of the endometrium, it is the functionalis that is sloughed. The epithelium lining the glands retained within the basalis migrates over the denuded basalis, and forms the basis for the eventual regeneration of the functionalis during the next menstrual cycle. The arterial supply to the mucosa is critical to the full development of the secretory potential of the endometrium. From arcuate arteries within the myometrium, straight arteries arise that supply the basalis and coiled arteries arise that contribute in the lower functionalis to an extensive capillary plexus underlying the surface epithelium.

MENSTRUAL CYCLE

Cyclical alterations in endometrial morphology and functional state occur that depend on the ovarian hormonal cycle discussed in a previous section and that are summarized in Figure 16–9. This cycle is called the *menstrual cycle* (from Latin *mensis*, for month), for its monthly occurrence in women of reproductive age. The cycle persists from the first menstrual period at age 12 to 15 (*menarche*) to the cessation of menstruation at age 45 to 50 (*menopause*). Cessation of the menstrual cycle at menopause marks the cessation of ovarian follicular development in the ovary and of the attendant cyclical hormonal states on which the menstrual cycle depends. Menopause therefore marks the end of the woman's fertile reproductive life.

The menstrual cycle is a progression of events that must be considered as a continuum. To understand the sequence, however, it is instructive to subdivide the cycle into preovulatory and postovulatory periods and to time the cycle on the basis of the easily determined first day of menstrual discharge. Using this convention, an idealized 28-day cycle may be divided into phases as follows: The *menstrual phase* is defined as days 1 through 4 of the cycle; the *proliferative phase*, as days 5 through 14; and the *secretory phase*, as days 15 through 28. It must be stressed that the cycle varies appreciably among women and also may vary from one month to another for any individual.

Proliferative (Follicular, Estrogenic) Phase (Fig. 16–11A)

Even prior to the complete cessation of menstruation, the restoration of the surface epithelium of the functionalis is begun. Epithelial cells from within the crypts of glands deep within the stratum basale migrate over the open ends of the glands and cover regions of denuded stroma with an epithelial lining. This process is accompanied by the regeneration of blood vessels and the proliferation of stromal cells, which lay down copious extracellular matrix and connective tissue fibers. Over the period of regeneration extending to the

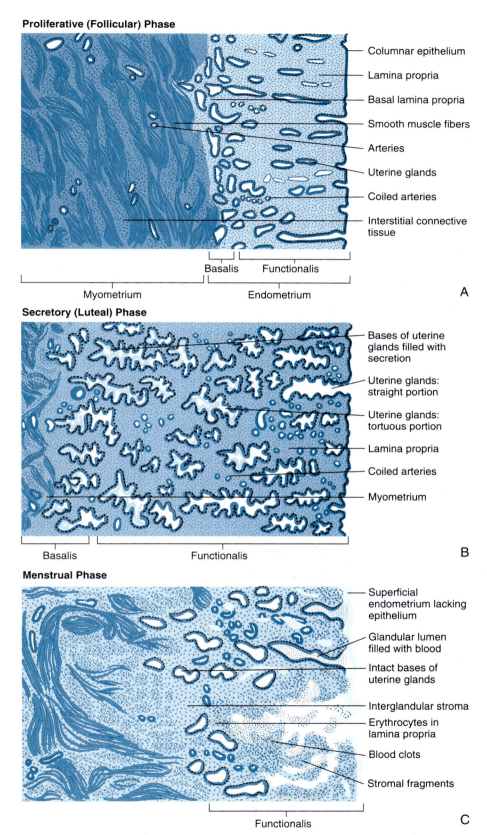

FIGURE 16–11. Histologic features of the uterine endometrium during various stages of the menstrual cycle. All are presented at the same magnification to facilitate comparison. A, Proliferative (follicular) phase. Note the relatively thin mucosa containing straight, unbranched glands. B, Secretory (luteal) phase. Note the greatly thickened endometrium containing tortuous, sacculated glands with enclosed secretory product. Numerous vascular profiles (coiled arteries) are also present. C, Menstrual phase. The endometrium undergoes necrosis owing to ischemia. Note the disorganization and breakdown of the glandular endometrium. Repair of the endometrium will occur from the intact bases of uterine glands in the stratum basalis.

time of ovulation, the endometrium will undergo a several-fold increase in height, to 2 to 3 mm. Within the endometrium, many mitotic figures are found in the epithelium, glands, and stoma. Spiral arteries, severed near the basalis at menstruation, regenerate into the functionalis and ramify within the stroma. Glands lengthen within the tunica propria, and their initial straight tubular profiles gradually give way to a more sinuous appearance late in the proliferative phase. Glycogen begins to accumulate within the glandular epithelium, and cytoplasmic organelles indicative of restored synthetic capacity, such as rough endoplasmic reticulum and Golgi apparatus, increase in size and complexity.

Secretory (Luteal, Progestational) Phase

(Fig. 16–11B)

The secretory phase extends from the time of ovulation and corpus luteum formation to menstruation and is dominated by progesterone. It is under stimulation by progesterone acting together with estrogen, which remains relatively high throughout this phase (see Fig. 16–9), that the endometrium reaches its maximal development and active secretory state. The glands during the secretory phase assume a highly coiled configuration; the lumens of the glands become dilated, sacculated, and filled with a glycoprotein secretory product that serves as a nutritive source for the embryo in the 2 days it typically spends within the uterine lumen prior to implantation (Fig. 16–12). Large stores of glycogen accumulate within the basal cytoplasm of the glandular cells, displacing the nuclei apically prior to the initiation of active secretion, after which this transitory feature is no longer observed. Stromal edema increases the height of the endometrium to approximately 5 mm, its maximum height during the cycle. Spiral arteries continue their process of elongation and convolution within the tunica propria and reach the subsurface stroma, which itself may appear highly cellular and compact. The timing and progression of these events are such that by approximately day 21, the endometrium reaches a fully secretory state and can support the implantation of the embryo, which occurs over 2 to 3 days after entry into the uterus. Given the usual appropriate arrest of transport within the fallopian tube, the multicellular embryo enters the uterus at precisely this time (see Fig. 16–12).

Menstrual Phase (Menses)

(Fig. 16–11C)

Rhythmic dilation of the coiled arteries occurs throughout most of the menstrual cycle, resulting in alternating suffusion and blanching of the functionalis. Near the time of menstruation, however, prostaglandin-mediated spasm of the coiled arteries occurs, compromising the blood supply to the upper two thirds of the functionalis for hours at a time. The endometrium assumes a compacted appearance owing to loss of interstitial fluid. Secretion ceases within the glands, and leukocytic infiltration of the stoma is initiated. Following about 2 days of intermittent interruption of blood flow, constriction of the coiled arteries becomes continuous, and severe ischemia of the functionalis results, followed by necrotic changes within both the vessel walls distal to the constriction and the tissues of the functionalis. Sudden release of the constriction within these vessels at the base of the functionalis causes rupture of the peripheral vessels and release of blood

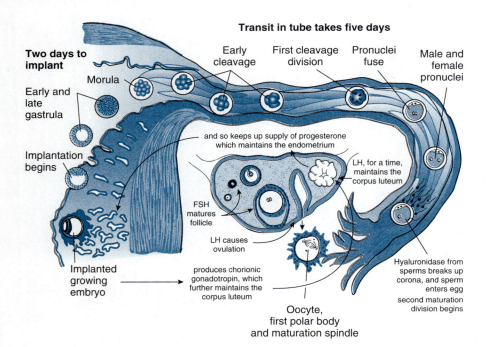

FIGURE 16–12. Diagram illustrating the transit of a fertilized ovum through the oviduct and into the uterine lumen, where the embryo implants. Note (in counterclockwise sequence) that fertilization normally occurs within the oviduct; that transit through the oviduct requires several days, during which the uterine endometrium enters its secretory phase; and that implantation of the embryo and the formation of the placenta result in the production of chorionic gonadotropin, which maintains the corpus luteum.

into the stroma and uterine lumen. Over a period of 3 to 4 days, the entire functionalis necrotizes and is sloughed. Epithelial and stromal rescue again occurs from the glandular reserve within the stratum basale, and the proliferative cycle resumes under estrogen stimulation from the next generation of growing ovarian follicles.

In the case of successful implantation of an embryo and establishment of the placenta, menstruation is prevented. A placental hormone, *human chorionic gonadotropin,* mimics the action of LH upon the corpus luteum, preventing collapse of the endometrial secretory phase by the continued viability of the corpus luteum and the secretion of luteal estrogen and progesterone (see Fig. 16–12).

IMPLANTATION AND FORMATION OF THE PLACENTA

Placenta

The placenta is of dual origin, with distinct fetal and maternal contributions. The overriding plan of the placenta is to bring maternal and fetal blood into close proximity, without actual mixing, to facilitate the exchange of gases, nutrients, and wastes. Normally, such substances as water, electrolytes, carbohydrates, proteins, lipid, hormones, vitamins, selected antibodies, and oxygen pass from the maternal circulation to the fetal. Water, hormones, carbon dioxide, and metabolic waste products pass from the fetal circulation to the maternal. Successful implantation of the embryo within the secretory endometrium is a critical event in the initial formation of the placenta.

Implantation

The embryo is transported to the uterine cavity in the *morula stage* of development (see Fig. 16–12). Divisions of the multicelled embryo continue within the uterus, where the embryo resides on the surface of the secretory endometrium, enveloped in its nutrient-rich secretions. At *blastocyst stage*, the embryonic *trophoblast* is differentiated. The zona pellucida is shed from the embryonic surface, exposing the highly invasive trophoblast cells directly to the maternal endometrial mucosa. Successful *implantation* or *nidation* involves the penetration of the embryo through the endometrial epithelium and into its richly vascular stroma, usually between days 7 and 9 postovulation. This penetration is initially via an intercellular route, as trophoblastic cells probe through the intercellular space between the endometrial epithelium to gain entrance to the stroma, where erosion of maternal capillaries ensures a source of nutrition for the growing embryo.

Functions of the Trophoblast

As the trophoblast continues to proliferate, it differentiates into two layers, an inner cytotrophoblast and an external syncytiotrophoblast. The *syncytiotrophoblast* is a syncytium derived from the cytotrophoblast. Its surface is studded with microvilli and exhibits many ectoplasmic smooth vesicles indicative of pinocytotic transport. Deeper within the cytoplasm are found both rough and smooth endoplasmic reticulum, a large Golgi complex, and numerous mitochondria. These features are consistent with immunocytochemical evidence implicating the syncytiotrophoblast in the secretion of the glycoprotein hormone *human chorionic gonadotropin* (HCG), the protein hormone *placental lactogen,* and the steroids *estrogen and progesterone.* HCG has been detected as early as 8 days postovulation and is crucial, as emphasized previously, to the successful continuation of progesterone secretion by the corpus luteum and the secretory phase of the endometrium.

The *cytotrophoblasts* retain an undifferentiated appearance even in the mature placenta. Their pale-staining cytoplasm exhibits few organelles, and they serve as a source of cells for the overlying syncytium. In the mature placenta, they are attached to the syncytiotrophoblast by desmosomes and continue to serve as a stem cell source for the syncytiotrophoblasts, but after the fifth month, cytotrophoblasts are not mitotically active and form only a discontinuous layer basal to the syncytiotrophoblast.

The Placental Blueprint

The successfully implanted blastocyst has sunk, by day 11, deeply within the endometrium, and the syncytiotrophoblast lines spaces, termed *lacunae,* which fill with nutritive, maternal blood from maternal arteries and veins that have been eroded in the process of lacuna formation. This establishes the basic theme for the future, fully developed human placenta, in which maternal blood bathes an epithelially lined fetal interface, allowing for the exchange of substances noted earlier.

The Endometrium of Pregnancy: The Decidua

The entire endometrium of pregnancy is known as the *decidua,* and it is characterized by an abundance of large, pale-staining cells of stomal cell origin known as *decidual cells* (Fig. 16–13A). The differentiation of decidual cells (decidualization of the endometrium) is stimulated by the implantation event. The function of these cells is not known with certainty, although they have been postulated to serve a nutritive function for the early embryo, and, at the time of parturition, to assist in the separation (dehiscence) of the placenta from the uterine wall. That region of the endometrium between the embryo and the myometrium is termed

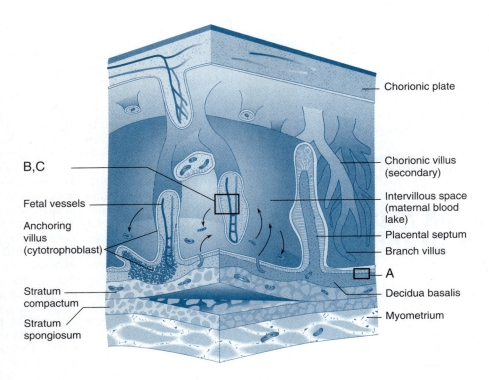
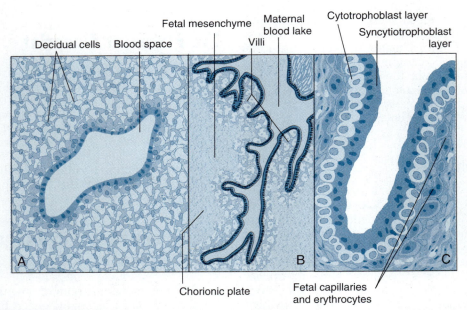

FIGURE 16–13. Schematic representation of human placental structures. *Note particularly the relationship of fetal chorionic villi to the maternal blood space. This compartment is supplied by arterial blood from decidual arterioles that drains through decidual veins. Some villi (anchoring villi) bridge the entire width of the maternal blood space and join the fetal and maternal portions of the placenta. Views A, B, and C are higher-magnification views of the regions indicated in top diagram. A, The endometrium of pregnancy is termed the* decidua. *Note the proliferation of endometrial stromal cells, the large decidual cells of pregnancy. B, The origin of chorionic villi from the chorionic plate. C, The epithelial covering of a chorionic villus consists of outer syncytial and underlying cellular layers termed, respectively, the* syncytiotrophoblast *and* cytotrophoblast.

the *decidua basalis*; the region that lies between the embryo and the uterine surface, the *decidua capsularis*; and the remainder, the *decidua parietalis*.

Formation of Placental Villi

The trophoblast, in association with the extraembryonic mesenchyme, is termed the *chorion*. Beginning at postovulation day 15, the trophoblast extends long cords from its surface, called *primary chorionic villi*. The invasion of these villi soon after their formation with a central core of mesenchyme converts the primary villi to *secondary chorionic villi*. The growth by the end of the third week of development of fetal blood vessels into the mesenchymal core of the secondary villi forms *tertiary* or *definitive chorionic villi*. Chorionic villi lie free within the intervillous space, the maternal blood space now greatly enlarged and lined with trophoblast that is derived from the trophoblastic lacunae formed at implantation.

The Definitive Placenta and Fetal/Maternal Placental Barrier

Figure 16–13 depicts the relationship of these free chorionic villi and the maternal blood space (intervillous space) with so-called anchoring villi, which unite the fetal chorionic plate and the maternal decidua basalis as a unified organ, the placenta. The chorionic villi are lined by the two layers of trophoblast already traced in their development, the external syncytiotrophoblast, now in direct contact with maternal blood, and its underlying cytotrophoblast layer (see Fig. 16–13B and C). These layers form a stratified epithelium underlaid by a basal lamina. Thus, the human placenta is classified as *hemochorial*; maternal blood (heme) within the intervillous space (maternal blood lake) is in direct contact with the chorionic villi. This architecture establishes a very efficient, yet totally separate exchange system between the blood vascular systems of the mother and fetus. The anatomic basis for the maternal/fetal placental barrier in the human therefore can be defined in terms of those structures that a molecule would pass in being transported from the fetal to the maternal circulation. In order, from fetus to mother, they are: (1) the fetal capillary endothelium, (2) the endothelial basal lamina, (3) the fetal mesenchyme of the villous core, (4) the basal lamina of the trophoblast epithelium, (5) the cytotrophoblast (in the first half of pregnancy when it forms a continuous layer), and (6) the syncytiotrophoblast layer. Specific molecules are transported across the barrier in a variety of ways. Oxygen, carbon dioxide, electrolytes, fatty acids, and steroids are considered to pass this barrier by passive diffusion. Facilitated diffusion is likely involved in the transport of glucose and certain other substances. Receptors for insulin, transferrin, and the F_c portion of immunoglobulins have been localized to the syncytiotrophoblast layer, and these substances are moved across the syncytium via receptor-mediated endocytosis.

Fetal/Placental Circulation

The fetal venous vessels within the chorionic villi drain to the single umbilical vein of the umbilical cord, which carries oxygenated blood and nutrients from the mother to the fetus. The paired umbilical arteries return CO_2-laden blood and metabolic waste to the capillaries of the chorionic villi for exchange across the placental barrier.

UTERINE CERVIX

The cervix forms a canal joining the body of the uterus to the external os and vagina (see Figs. 16–1, 16–2, and 16–14). It is about 3 cm in length and exhibits a mucosa and wall that differ markedly from those of the uterus proper. It is thrown into branching folds, the *plicae palmatae*, and its lining epithelium consists of a simple, tall columnar, mucus-secreting epithelium that does not demonstrate the marked cyclic response dur-

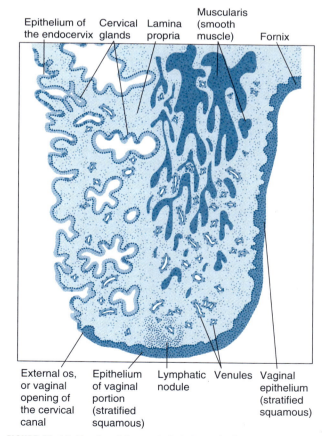

FIGURE 16–14. *Drawing of human cervix in longitudinal section (compare with Fig. 16–2). Note the transition of the stratified squamous epithelium lining the vaginal portion of the cervix, and the columnar epithelium lining the endocervix. The mucosa of the endocervix contains large mucous glands, the cervical glands.*

ing the menstrual cycle evidenced in the endometrium. Prominent features of the cervical mucosa are the cervical mucous glands, which deeply invaginate the mucosal surface (see Fig. 16–14), are extensively branched, and lie obliquely to the long axis of the cervical canal. The epithelium lining the glands resembles that of the surface epithelium of the canal. The wall of the cervix consists principally of connective tissue, with little smooth muscle. Softening of the robust connective tissue wall of the cervix occurs immediately prior to childbirth, in response to the hormone relaxin, enabling dilation of the canal to accommodate parturition.

The cervical mucus exhibits variation in consistency and volume during the phases of the menstrual cycle. At the time of ovulation, the mucus is copious, watery, and of low viscosity; spermatozoa pass through the cervical mucus with ease. Cervical mucus in the postovulatory period or during pregnancy is much more viscous and less copious, a probable response to progesterone secretion; the thick mucus forms a functional block to the passage of microorganisms or sperm. The mucus of the endocervix is reported to contain *lysozyme,* which is bacteriocidal and may serve to control bacterial flora of the lower female reproductive tract.

Blockage of the mucous glands may cause retention of secretion, dilation of the gland, and the formation of *nabothian cysts.* The columnar epithelium of the cervix changes abruptly near the external os to the nonkeratinized, stratified squamous epithelium typical of the vaginal canal. It is this region that is disposed to neoplastic transformation; *adenocarcinoma of the cervix* accounts for 10% of all cancer deaths in women, but early detection is facilitated by regular examination of the exfoliated squamous cells of the cervical epithelium for abnormal cells (*Papanicolaou's* test or *smear*).

VAGINA

The birth canal, or vagina (from the Latin for sheath), is a highly elastic fibromuscular tube some 7 to 9 cm in length that extends from the vulva to the cervix (see Figs. 16–1 and 16–2). It forms a cuff around the cervix and is reflected from its protruding surface at the fornix. The vaginal wall consists of three layers, the *mucosa* of stratified squamous, nonkeratinized epithelium, a *muscularis* that exhibits smooth muscle bundles arrayed both longitudinally and circularly with the longitudinal orientation most discernible in the outer half, and an *adventitia* of dense irregular connective tissue (Fig. 16–15). The mucosa exhibits anterior and posterior longitudinal folds and transverse rugae (see Fig. 16–2).

In the human, the thick (150 to 200 μm) epithelium does not respond markedly to hormonal changes with the menstrual cycle. It does increase in height with estrogenic stimulation during the follicular phase of the cycle and, consistent with this observation, thins appreciably at menopause. The cells of the more superficial layers of the epithelium accumulate glycogen at midcycle, and desquamation is most evident late in the luteal phase and at menstruation. The shedding of cells rich in glycogen disposes to breakdown of glycogen by lactobacilli, which promotes an acid pH within the vaginal lumen. The acid pH may pay an important role in preventing certain bacterial and fungal infections of the tube.

The epithelium rests on a thick tunica propria that exhibits many elastic fibers, small veins, and venules. No epithelial or subepithelial glands are present in the vagina. The secretions of the uterine cervix contribute to the lubrication of the vagina, and it is postulated as well that the vascularity of the tunica propria may dispose toward the exudation and movement of fluid from the vasculature through the epithelium, explaining in part the observation of increased vaginal fluid in response to sexual stimulation, although this explanation may require reevaluation in light of tracer studies establishing a permeability barrier across the epithelium.

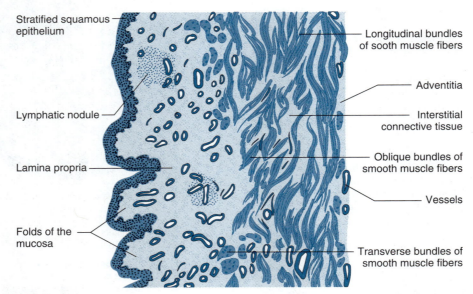

***FIGURE 16–15.** The vagina, longitudinal section. Observe the interlacing layers of smooth muscle underlying a thick lamina propria devoid of glands and covered by a stratified squamous (nonkeratinizing) epithelium.*

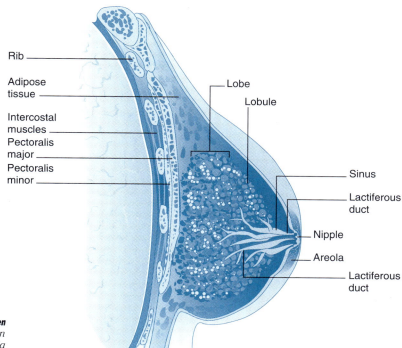

FIGURE 16–16. Diagram of human breast structure as seen in sagittal section. *Note the organization of the organ into lobes and lobules, which drain to the nipple via lactiferous ducts.*

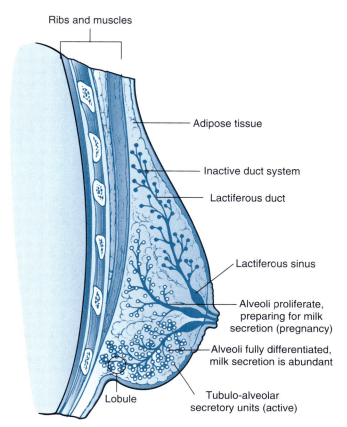

FIGURE 16–17. Histology of the mammary gland during various functional states. *Note the relationship of the terminal secretory alveoli to the lactiferous ducts, lactiferous sinuses, and the nipple. Secretory alveoli originate from the terminal branches of the ductal system.*

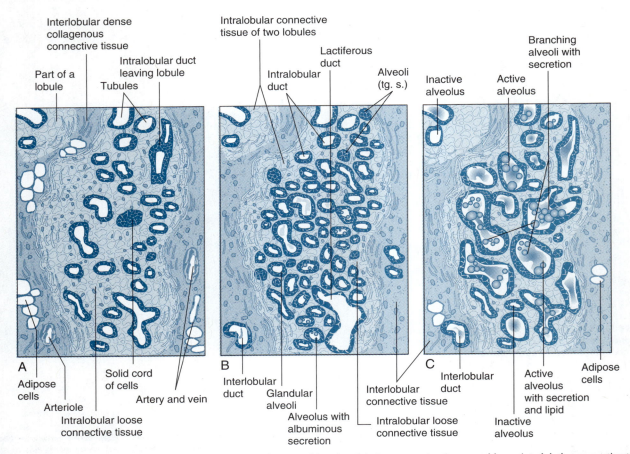

FIGURE 16–18. *A, Inactive mammary gland. Note the preponderance of fatty interlobular connective tissue, and loose intralobular connective tissue containing ductal structures but no secretory units. B, Mammary gland, first half of pregnancy. Both ducts and secretory alveoli have increased at the expense of the intralobular connective tissue. C, Lactating mammary gland. Large secretory units (alveoli) containing secretion characterize the lactating gland. Large ducts are present in the interlobular connective tissue.*

EXTERNAL GENITALIA

The female external genitalia (the *vulva*) comprise the *labia minora*, the *labia majora*, the *clitoris*, and numerous glands emptying into the *vestibule*, the area bounded by the labia minora (see Fig. 16–1). The *labia majora* are longitudinal folds covered by general body surface epithelium. They contain considerable subcutaneous fat, together with obliquely disposed hair follicles that impart the characteristic coarse, curly character to pubic hair. The *labia minora*, by contrast, exhibit a subcutaneous bed rich in elastic fibers but lacking in adipose tissue. Also lacking are hair follicles on the skin surface, but numerous sebaceous glands are present that open directly upon the surface of the skin. The clitoris, homologous to the penis in the male, is represented by two dorsal erectile bodies capped by a rudimentary glans clitoridis and shrouded with a prepuce (for comparison, see illustrations of the penis in Chapter 17). The thin covering epidermis lacks hair follicles or glandular units but is well endowed with nerve fibers and specialized sensory receptors. Sexual arousal results in its engorgement and tumescence. Glands of note within the perineal region include mucous glands of the vestibule, analogous to the glands of Littre in the male; the paraurethral glands of Skene, which are disposed around the meatus of the urethra; and the vulvovaginal glands of Bartholin, situated in the lateral walls of the vestibule. These secrete a lubricating mucus similar to that of the bulbourethral glands (Cowper's glands) in the male.

MAMMARY GLANDS

The paired mammary glands (*mammae*) arise as accessory structures of the integument but subserve the reproductive function of secretion of milk for the suckling infant. They arise embryologically as downgrowth derivatives of the epithelium, analogous to the origin of sweat glands, which they resemble in their microscopic anatomy in the quiescent state. Each gland consists of 15 to 25 *lobes,* each of which contains tubuloalveolar secretory units draining to a single *lactiferous duct* (Fig. 16–16). These ducts drain to the body surface at the *nipple* (mammary papilla), which is centrally located within a deeply pigmented region, the *areola*. Near the terminus deep to the areola, each lactiferous duct dilates into a *lactiferous sinus (ampulla)*, a site at which some secretion product, milk, may accumulate (Fig. 16–17). The glands are under complex hormonal and neuronal control of secretion, or *lactation*, and their morphology depends upon the hormonal status of the individual. In fact, fluid secretion from the breasts of neonates is not unusual, owing to the priming of the gland's secretory units by placental and maternal hormones. It is instructive to compare the histology of the gland in the inactive (resting) state, during pregnancy, and in active lactation.

Inactive (Resting) Mammary Gland

The general cytoarchitectural plan for breast development is that under appropriate hormonal stimulation, the ductal system increases in its complexity of branching and that secretory units form in relationship to the terminal ductal units. The prepubescent gland in both sexes is similar in morphology; the gland consists mainly of branching lactiferous ducts with no developed secretory units. Breast development in pubescent girls, however, occurs as a secondary sex characteristic under the influence of ovarian estrogen and progesterone. It is thought that ductal proliferation develops under the principal influence of estrogen, whereas development of secretory units is considered to be a function of both estrogen and progesterone. Other hormones, notably prolactin and growth hormone, play roles in these processes as well.

The lactiferous ducts proliferate, and the hallmark morphologic unit of the adult female gland, the *lobule*, develops in association with the tips of the smallest (terminal) *interlobular ducts*. These ducts consist of a simple cuboidal epithelium underlaid by a basal lamina and surrounded by a discontinuous layer of *myoepithelial cells*. Interlobular ducts are those to which *intralobular ducts* within the secretory unit will drain. A lobule, therefore, consists of a number of secretory units (acini) and their associated intralobular ducts together with supporting areolar connective tissue (see Figs. 16–16 and 16–17). Adjacent lobules are partitioned one from another by slightly more compact connective tissue. Histological features of the inactive gland are depicted in Fig. 16–18A. The bulk of the gland consists of fatty connective tissue, with ill-defined lobules consisting of loosely packed profiles of tubular or acinar secretory units in association with intralobular ducts.

Mammary Gland of Pregnancy

During pregnancy, the mammary glands undergo a considerable degree of development of both ductal and secretory structures (Fig. 16–18B). Lobular secretory units become more pronounced and expand at the expense of the fatty interlobular connective tissue. More secretory units are associated with the duct system, and alveoli appear more closely packed within lobules. By the latter half of pregnancy, the breast undergoes further development, increasing in size as well as complex-

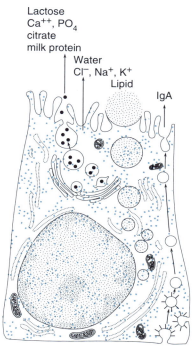

FIGURE 16–19. Diagrammatic representation of milk secretion. Note the secretion of casein, lactate, calcium, and citrate by exocytosis from secretory vesicles formed in the Golgi complex. The cell membrane allows free diffusion of water and ions, whereas lipid droplets are released from the cell by means of a form of apocrine secretion unique to the mammary gland. Immunoglobulin (IgA) undergoes receptor-mediated endocytosis at the basal and lateral aspects of the secretory cell, is transported to the apical plasma membrane, and is released into the alveolar lumen.

ity of the secretory units. Intralobular connective tissue is sparse, the secretory alveoli having grown larger and more numerous. Interlobular connective tissue separates adjacent, closely packed lobules.

Lactating Mammary Gland

Active postpartum lactation is accompanied by closely packed, large dilated secretory acini that contain secretory product within their lumens (Fig. 16–18C). The loose connective tissue may reveal plasma cells within it, reflecting the secretion of antibodies from these cells in the mother's milk. The epithelium of secreting acini is reduced in height to low cuboidal, and the cytoplasm of the acinar cells contains many lipid droplets secreted by means of a conservative apocrine mode of secretion, involving loss of a small margin of apical cytoplasm as the lipid droplets are packaged for exocytosis (see Fig. 16–19). Additional constituents of the milk, such as caseins and other milk proteins, are secreted via vacuoles arising in the Golgi apparatus and are exocytosed.

The first secretions from the breast following parturition constitute *colostrum*. Colostrum is rich in antibodies, especially secretory IgA, which conveys a degree of passive immunity from the mother to infant. In addition, colostrum is richer in protein and lower in fat than regular human milk. Even later in the breastfeeding process, it is estimated that the mother at the fourth or fifth month may be secreting up to 0.5 g of antibody per day, which in the infant's gut serves to combat enteric infections, a principal cause of perinatal death. Following the cessation of suckling, the mammary glands gradually revert to a histologic profile of the resting gland.

The human breast is highly susceptible to neoplastic transformation. It is estimated that in the United States, one of every nine women will develop a malignancy of the breast in her lifetime. Most such tumors are derived from the epithelial lining of the ducts and are thus classified as carcinomas. Metastasis through the extensive lymph vascular network of the breasts to regional nodes and beyond is not uncommon, and disseminated metastatic spread of the carcinoma unfortunately is a major cause of death from this disease. Better methods of early detection (e.g., alert self-examination, regular physical examinations, ultrasound, and mammography) have increased the chances of successful treatment of this widespread malignancy.

CHAPTER SEVENTEEN

MALE REPRODUCTIVE SYSTEM

TESTIS 304

SEMINIFEROUS TUBULES AND INTRATESTICULAR DUCTS 304
   Seminiferous (Germinal) Epithelium 305
     SERTOLI CELLS 305
     GERM CELLS 307
     SPERMATOZOON 309
     CYCLE AND WAVE OF THE SEMINIFEROUS EPITHELIUM 311
     SPERM PRODUCTION AND FERTILITY 312

INTERSTITIAL TISSUE AND CELLS OF LEYDIG 312

EXCURRENT DUCT SYSTEM 314
   Intratesticular Ducts 314
   Extratesticular Ducts 314
     EPIDIDYMIS 314
     VAS (DUCTUS) DEFERENS 315
     EJACULATORY DUCT 315

ACCESSORY GLANDS 315
   Seminal Vesicle 315
   Prostate Gland 317
   Bulbourethral Glands 318

PENIS 318

SEMEN 319

As is the case in the female, the male reproductive system comprises paired gonads, the *testes* (singular, testis), in which *gametogenesis* occurs, together with a complex system of ducts that nurture and transport the morphologically mature gametes, the *spermatozoa* (sperm). As in the female, the male gonad is both a *cytocrine and an endocrine organ*: its cellular product is sperm, and its principal endocrine secretion, the male androgen, testosterone. The *genitalia* of the male are both external and internal (Fig. 17–1). The external genitalia include the paired testes, contained within the scrotum, and the copulatory organ, the penis. Internal structures are the accessory sex glands: the prostate gland, the seminal vesicles, and the bulbourethral gland (Cowper's gland). The extratesticular *excurrent duct system* consists of the epididymis (plural, epididymides), the vas (ductus) deferens, ejaculatory ducts, and the several named portions of the urethra (described in Chapter 12). The testes, epididymides, and first portion of the vas deferens are contained within the pendulous scrotal pouch, into which the testes descend prenatally. In the scrotum, the testis lies within a serous sac, the *tunica vaginalis*, derived from the abdominal peritoneum. The formation of sperm cells (*spermatogenesis*) depends upon the lower temperature (2 to 3°F below deep body temperature) maintained within the scrotal chamber. Failure of the testes to descend, *cryptorchidism*, results in impaired spermatogenic, but not necessarily endocrine, function of the testis.

TESTIS

The male gonad, like the ovary, is protected by a tough, white fibrous connective tissue capsule, the *tunica albuginea*. Incomplete connective tissue septa course radially from the capsule, toward a posteriorly placed invagination of the capsule, the *mediastinum testis* (Fig. 17–2). These histologically indistinct lobules each contain one to four contorted tubules, the *seminif-*

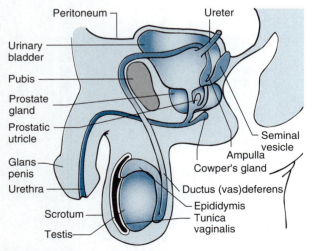

FIGURE 17–1. *Diagrammatic representation of a midsagittal section through the male pelvis. The relationships of the reproductive organs with the pelvis and scrotum are shown.*

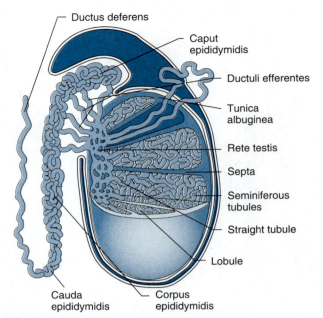

FIGURE 17–2. *Diagram of the testis and its ducts, with the apical portion of the testis cut away to reveal internal structures. Note the compartmentalization of the testis into lobules containing tortuous, U-shaped seminiferous tubules, which drain to the rete testis. The rete testis drains to the epididymis via the ductuli efferentes.*

erous tubules, which lie in a loose *interstitial connective tissue* containing the blood and lymph vascular supply of the tubules, and the *interstitial cells of Leydig*, the cells that secrete the androgen steroid testosterone.

SEMINIFEROUS TUBULES AND INTRATESTICULAR DUCTS

Each of the seminiferous tubules, some 30 to 70 cm in length and 150 μm in diameter, is U-shaped. The tubules are confluent with a canalicular meshwork within the posteriorly placed mediastinum, the *rete testis*. The terminal portions of the seminiferous tubules, where they empty into the rete, are straight rather than convoluted, and are termed *tubuli recti* (see Fig. 17–2). The anastomosing channels of the rete drain to ten or more *ductuli efferentes*, which pierce the tunica albuginea and form the major portion of the head of the *epididymis*, which lies in relation to the superior pole of the testis (see Fig. 17–2).

Microscopically, the tubules consist of a tunica propria and a lining epithelium, the *germinal* or *seminiferous epithelium*. The tunica propria consists of a variable number of circumferentially disposed layers of boundary tissue; the outer layers may include endothelium of labyrinthine intertubular lymphatics as well as fibroblasts. The flattened, polygonal layer of cells abutting the epithelial basal lamina in many mammalian species are epithelioid cells that exhibit certain fine structural features of smooth muscle. For these reasons, they are designated *myoid cells,* and they are most likely responsible for the shallow contractions observed to occur in the seminiferous tubules of some species. In monkeys and in humans, however, tubular contractions are not observed, and the cells of the boundary layers lack actin filaments.

Seminiferous (Germinal) Epithelium

The epithelium lining the tubules is a complex, stratified epithelium that defies classification according to the standard criteria cited in Chapter 2. The seminiferous epithelium consists of both supporting cells, the Sertoli cells, and germ cells undergoing meiosis and morphologic maturation in the complex process of *spermatogenesis* (from the Greek *sperma*, seed, and *genesis*, to form). The morphologically distinct cells of the germ line that reside within the epithelium are the spermatogonia, primary spermatocytes, secondary spermatocytes; and spermatids. Sperm lie free within the tubular lumen. The number of cell layers constituting the epithelium varies with the precise stage of the maturation process in any given segment of the tubule and is therefore highly variable; however, its height usually lies within the range of four to eight layers.

The general blueprint for the seminiferous epithelium is not unlike that of other proliferating or secreting epithelia, namely, a more basally placed population of dividing cells, the daughter cells of which are continuously moved toward the apical surface, where they differentiate and eventually are shed. In this case, however, the divisions within the epithelium are both mitotic divisions of the spermatogonia within the basal layer of the epithelium, and meiotic (reduction) divisions within the more apical regions of the epithelium. The differentiated cells that are shed from the apical free surface of the epithelium are morphologically mature, haploid gametes.

Sertoli Cells

Sertoli cells are the relative constants in an epithelium in continuous cellular flux. They do not divide during adult life, are (together with the spermatogonia) among the most resistant cells of the germinal epithelium to irradiation, and remain as the predominant cell type of the epithelium in the senescent gonad. Far from being static cells, however, they are dynamic participants in the secretory, transport, and endocrine functions of the epithelium.

In three dimensions, Sertoli cells may be visualized as elongated pyramids, with their bases lodged on the basal lamina and their apices reaching the tubular lumen. A euchromatic nucleus, often presenting a triangular profile in section, typically contains a large, distinct nucleolus with a substructure peculiar to its cell type. The location of the nucleus is frequently basal, but it is translocated more apically during defined stages in the process of spermatogenesis.

Fine Structural Features

The Sertoli cell cytoplasm contains a wealth of cytoplasmic organelles and inclusions, such as numerous long, vertically oriented mitochondria, commonly in association with abundant smooth endoplasmic reticulum (SER) and profiles of rough endoplasmic reticulum (RER). Cytoskeletal elements, including actin filaments and microtubules, are numerous, consistent with the changes in shape the cell must undergo in its sustentacular role of an apically migrating population of developing germ cells. Lysosomes are present in large numbers, as are residual bodies and accumulated lipochrome pigment, and in the human, distinctive, fusiform crystalloids (of Charcot-Böttcher) are present as well. The Golgi apparatus is prominent but lacks associated secretory granules.

Role in Mechanical Support for Germ Cells

Owing to the intimate physical proximity of the Sertoli cells to the germinal cells, the Sertoli cells have long been correctly regarded as *sustentacular cells*, lending mechanical support to the cells of the germ line. Fine structural studies have confirmed that each of the germ cells within the epithelium is enfolded by Sertoli cell processes. Because of these complex cytoplasmic relationships with germ cells, the cell boundaries of the Sertoli cells are indistinct, so much so that early microscopists considered that they consti-

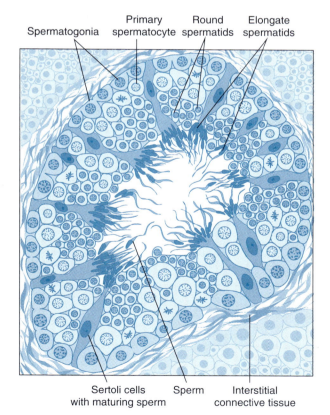

FIGURE 17–3. Histologic section of human testis. The complexity of the seminiferous epithelium is depicted in this actively spermatogenic tubule, sectioned transversely. Note the various populations of germ cells, intimately supported by Sertoli cells.

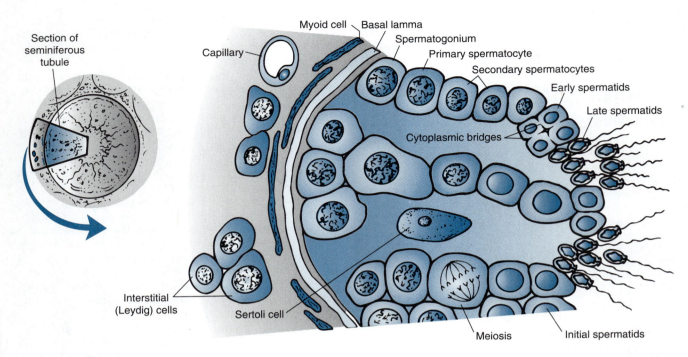

FIGURE 17–4. Diagram showing a wedge of a seminiferous tubule and its subjacent interstitial tissue. Note particularly the orderly progression of spermatogenesis that occurs from base to apex within the seminiferous epithelium lining the tubule.

tuted a syncytium. The lateral plasma membranes of adjacent Sertoli cells are coupled with zonular occluding junctions, gap junctions, and highly specialized non-occluding junctional complexes peculiar to Sertoli cells. The complexities of how these junctions are formed and then re-formed after passage of the migrating germ cells apically between them are not understood. As knowledge of the diverse physiologic roles played by the Sertoli cells within the seminiferous epithelium increases, however, the concept that the Sertoli cells serve as nurse cells within the epithelium has gained validity.

Secretory Functions

Neither the Sertoli cell's nutritive function for germ cells nor its secretory functions are well understood. Numerous proteins are secreted in vitro by Sertoli cell–

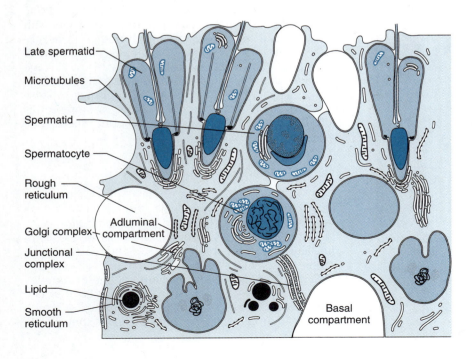

FIGURE 17–5. Diagrammatic representation of a segment of the seminiferous epithelium, as revealed by electron microscopy. Note particularly the intimate relationship of the Sertoli cell cytoplasm that encompasses all germinal cells. Tight junctions within the unique junctional complexes joining adjacent Sertoli cells compartmentalize the seminiferous epithelium into basal and adluminal compartments. These junctions thus form the principal morphologic basis of the blood-testis barrier. Spermatogonia lie within the basal compartment, and the meiotic germ cells differentiate within the apical compartment.

enriched cultures, but their roles in vivo have for the most part not been determined. One protein ascribed to the Sertoli cell with confidence is *androgen-binding protein,* which binds testosterone made in the testicular interstitium and transports it across the germinal epithelium, into the tubular lumen, and subsequently to the epididymis. High intraepithelial testosterone levels are thought to augment spermatogenesis in the presence of follicle-stimulating hormone (FSH). Another secretion of the Sertoli cell is *inhibin,* a glycoprotein heterodimer that acts as a negative feedback regulator to suppress FSH release by the anterior pituitary during periods when the normal complement of germ cells is present in the seminiferous epithelium. Depletion of the number of germ cells prompts FSH levels to rise together with spermatogenic activity. A final secretion of the Sertoli cell is water, which is transported in liter quantities daily across the germinal epithelium and into the tubular lumens of the seminiferous tubules. Given the lack of peristaltic activity of the seminiferous tubules, this fluid flux across the epithelium serves a crucial role in the transport of the sperm mass distally within the intratesticular ducts.

Phagocytosis

During the final stages of maturation of the spermatids to sperm, residual cytoplasm and organelles are relegated to a body of cytoplasm appended to the caudal portion of the developing sperm (see Figs. 17–7 and 17–8). These cytoplasmic remnants are termed *residual bodies,* and they are phagocytized by the Sertoli cell, where they are degraded in the cell's lysosomal system.

Role in Blood/Testis Barrier

In experimental studies of vascular permeability, it was noted that the seminiferous tubules failed to be penetrated by certain vital dyes and tracer molecules that were extravasated from the capillaries of the interstitium and that stained the interstitial compartment of the testis. Electron-microscopic tracer studies of this blood/epithelial (blood/testis) barrier subsequently demonstrated that the structural basis for this exclusion of even low-molecular-weight protein lies at the level of occluding junctions between basal processes of Sertoli cells. These junctions are located within the epithelium immediately above the most basally situated germ cells, the spermatogonia. Thus, two compartments are defined by the levels of the junctions, a basal compartment, which surrounds the premeiotic spermatogonia, and an *apical compartment,* in which the meiotic populations of germ cells divide and subsequently mature. Thus, passage across the barrier must occur transcellularly, through the Sertoli cell. The significance of this compartmentalization of premeiotic and postmeiotic cells is not known, although it may be postulated that unique hormonal or nutritive environments are maintained that nurture or regulate the divisions of the cells in their respective compartments. Conversely, the junctions provide a barrier against the intercellular backflow to the interstitium of proteins from the newly formed postmeiotic cell populations, molecules that would be recognized as nonself by the body's immune surveillance mechanisms.

Germ Cells

Unlike the human ovary, which contains no oogonia and therefore is endowed with a finite, determined number of germ cells (oocytes) at birth, the germinal epithelium of the male contains a mitotically active population of spermatogonia. Thus, the germinal epithelium is periodically replenished with spermatocytes, ensuring uninterrupted spermatogenesis. Several phases of this process of differentiation are recognized.

- *Spermatogenesis* refers to the entire process of sperm formation, from its inception to sperm release into the lumen of the tubule
- *Spermatocytogenesis* refers to the formation of spermatocytes, the daughter cells of designated (type B) spermatogonia
- *Meiosis,* or reduction division, is completed within the midportion of the epithelium, giving rise to spermatids that, although haploid in DNA and chromosome number, are morphologically immature
- *Spermiogenesis* describes the morphologic maturation of the round spermatids to spermatozoa
- *Spermiation* refers to the process of release of the mature spermatids as spermatozoa free within the tubular lumen.

Spermatogenesis and Meiosis

SPERMATOCYTOGENESIS. The onset of puberty and secretion of testosterone by the Leydig cells stimulates the undifferentiated stem cells of the germinal epithelium, the *spermatogonia,* to initiate mitotic division within the basal compartment. Subpopulations of spermatogonia are recognized on the basis of their morphology: type A dark (Ad), type A pale (Ap), and type B. The Ad cells are considered the stem cells, giving rise to other Ad cells and Ap cells. The Ap cells undergo multiple mitotic divisions with incomplete cytokinesis, such that successive generations of daughter cells are linked by cytoplasmic bridges (Fig. 17–6). They mature into type B cells, which also replicate by mitosis. Clusters of type B cells become committed by some undetermined mechanism to undergo meiosis. They undergo DNA synthesis, becoming tetraploid (4N) in nuclear DNA, and move out of the basal compartment and into the adluminal compartment of the seminiferous epithelium, where they are easily recognized as *primary spermatocytes.*

MEIOSIS. The primary spermatocytes enter the extended period of meiotic prophase, which consists of the leptotene, zygotene, pachytene, and diplotene phases. During *diplotene,* mixing of the parental genomes occurs between the paired diploid homologous chromosomes, during that process unique to meiosis termed crossing-over. The diploid sets of chromosomes

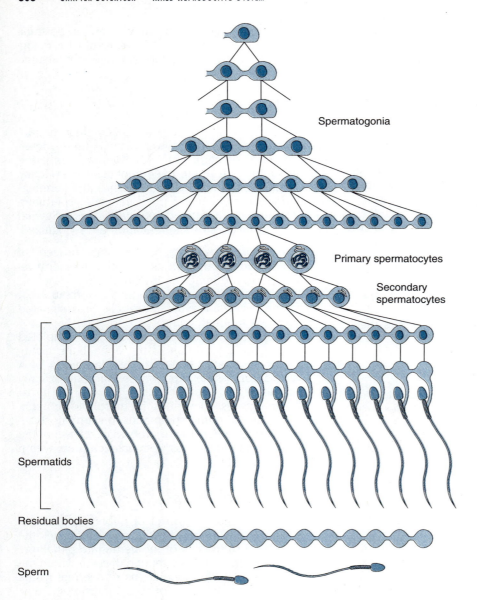

FIGURE 17-6. *Diagram depicting the cytoplasmic relationships persisting between developing germ cells. Incomplete cytokinesis of spermatogonia committed to differentiation of spermatocytes gives rise to a syncytial population of subsequent spermatogonia, spermatocytes, and spermatids. This relationship persists until the time of spermiation.*

separate one from another during the phase of diakinesis; they line up on the metaphase plate and are relegated randomly at anaphase to the daughter cells, called secondary spermatocytes. These cells are short-lived, and divide soon, without undergoing DNA synthesis, giving rise to haploid (N) daughter cells called *spermatids*.

SPERMIOGENESIS. The small, round spermatids occupy the apical portions of the seminiferous epithelium. They undergo cytodifferentiation, during the process of spermiogenesis, and become designated *elongated spermatids*, which when fully differentiated are shed from the apical Sertoli cell cytoplasm as mature sperm into the tubular lumen in the process of spermiation.

Histologic and Cytologic Features of the Germ Cells

The continuum of spermatogenesis is difficult to conceptualize from histologic sections of seminiferous tubules. Identification of the named cell types above is aided, however, by the fact that they reside within the seminiferous epithelium in groups, in order of their formation, from base to apex. Furthermore, each cell type exhibits distinguishing morphologic features that aid identification.

The most basally situated cells in the seminiferous epithelium are the spermatogonia, small cells (some 12 μm in diameter) that reside on the basal lamina. Their cytoplasm stains poorly and exhibits a fine granularity. Large cytoplasmic crystalloids (of Lubarsch) may be present. The type A spermatogonia are dome-shaped, with an ovoid nucleus containing a finely granular chromatin pattern and nucleoli that tend to be peripherally placed. The Ad nucleus stains more avidly than does that of the Ap cell. Cells of similar size and position within the epithelium, but having a more rounded nucleus, a single, centrally located nucleolus, and coursely clumped, marginated heterochromatin, are type B spermatogonia.

Primary spermatocytes arise from mitotic division of type B spermatogonia and reside just apical to the spermatogonial population. These cells are readily recognized as the largest round cells of the germinal epithelium; their nuclei exhibit the range of chromosomal condensation typical of meiotic prophase, from fine, thread-like nuclear inclusions in the leptotene phase to the thick, condensed chromosomal pairs evident in the zygotene and pachytene phases.

Secondary spermatocytes are considerably smaller than primaries (8 to 9 μm). In contrast to the meiotic nucleus of the primary spermatocytes, their nuclei are spherical and have a finely granular chromatin pattern; they reside just apical to the population of primaries. Because these cells are already programmed for second meiotic division, and *do not duplicate their DNA*, they reside within the epithelium only about 8 hours before giving rise to haploid daughter cells, spermatids.

Spermiogenesis

Newly formed *spermatids* are round cells with spherical nuclei that closely resemble secondary spermatocytes but are smaller in diameter (5 to 6 μm). They undergo a complex series of cytoplasmic and nuclear alterations during the process of spermiogenesis: dramatic chromatin condensation, nuclear elongation, and formation of the acrosome at the rostral pole of the cell and a flagellum at its caudal pole. These changes are accompanied by the shedding of much of the cell's cytoplasm and organelles in the cytoplasmic residual bodies, which are phagocytized by the Sertoli cells late in the process of spermiogenesis.

Spermiogenesis is a continuous process that is completed in the human over a 16-day period. It may for descriptive purposes be divided into four stages, the Golgi, cap, acrosomal, and maturation phases. Spermiogenesis proceeds within the spermatids nested in groups within the apical cytoplasm of the nurse cells. They remain joined by the intercellular bridges noted earlier that join all developing germ cells (see Fig. 17–6). Thus, groups of spermatids all mature in unison and undergo spermiation *en masse* in any given segment of the seminiferous tubule. This allows for the orderly progression and coordinated migration of the next generation of germ cells through the germinal epithelium.

THE GOLGI PHASE. The spermatids enter spermiogenesis endowed with a complement of cytoplasmic organelles that includes a prominent Golgi complex, mitochondria, centrioles, microtubules, and a centrally positioned, round nucleus. As in all differentiating systems, the establishment of cellular polarity sets the stage for subsequent events. The polarizing events in spermiogenesis are (1) the association of the Golgi complex with one side of the nucleus and (2) the migration of the centrioles to precisely the opposite pole of the cell. Within the Golgi complex, small PAS-positive (stain with periodic acid–Schiff stain) granules, the *proacrosomal granules*, form. These eventually coalesce within a membranous vesicle, the acrosomal vesicle, to form a single acrosomal granule. The acrosomal vesicle contacts the nuclear membrane, flattens, and begins to spread over the anterior pole of the nucleus. The centrioles, which migrate initially to the cellular periphery, move toward the nucleus and, while doing so, initiate formation of the microtubular *axoneme*, which forms the central core of the sperm flagellum. Nuclear chromatin begins its condensation, which will continue through spermiogenesis.

CAP PHASE. The acrosomal vesicle continues to flatten, migrate laterally, and encompass the entire rostral half of the nucleus as a hemispherical cap. The acrosomal granule remains associated with the rostral pole of the head. The nuclear membrane in relation to this acrosomal cap becomes dense and lacks nuclear pores.

ACROSOMAL PHASE. The nucleus continues its process of condensation and elongation, and the acrosomal vesicle and granule are fashioned over the anterior portion of the developing head of the sperm as the acrosome. The acrosome has been likened to a primary lysosome, in that it contains hydrolytic enzymes that function in the fertilization process, as detailed later. Nuclear elongation occurs in close relationship with a cylindrical sheath of microtubules, the manchette (Fig. 17–7), which is thought in some manner to guide and facilitate the rostrocaudal elongation and thinning of the nucleus to its definitive shape. The anterior pole of the cell becomes directed toward the base of the epithelium, whereas at the caudal pole, the displaced apical cytoplasm, together with the developing flagellum, extend toward the tubular lumen (see Fig. 17–7). Mitochondria come to be associated with the first portion of the sperm flagellum, the middle piece. They are arranged in a helical sheath around the axonemal core and the nine outer dense fibers (see Fig. 17–7), which are associated with the flagellum beginning in the middle piece. This association represents the establishment of a significant cytophysiologic relationship: The middle piece is the site of initiation of *flagellar contraction*, an ATP-dependent process in turn dependent upon mitochondrial oxidative phosphorylation. The flagellar middle piece and principal piece are demarcated by a ring of dense material, the annulus, to which the flagellar membrane is anchored. The flagellar principal piece runs distally from the annulus, enclosed in its fibrous sheath, a structure that also is differentiated and added to the flagellum during the later periods of spermiogenesis.

MATURATION PHASE. The excess cytoplasm of the developing sperm is displaced caudally and is shed as residual bodies; these, in turn, are phagocytized by the Sertoli cell. At the completion of this phase, the Sertoli cell releases its cache of mature spermatids into the tubular lumen, where the gametes are then properly designated spermatozoa (Fig. 17–8). The cellular mechanisms underlying this process of release (spermiation) are not clear but may involve cytoskeletal elements, particularly actin filaments, present within the Sertoli cell cytoplasm.

Spermatozoon
Light-Microscopic Appearance

At the time of spermiation, the sperm are morphologically mature but not motile (motility is gained

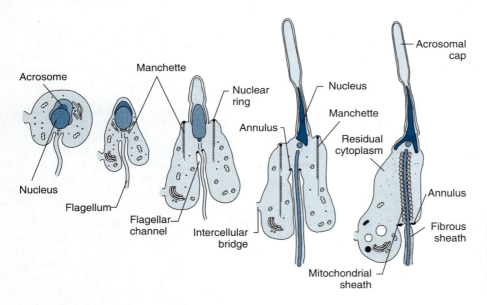

FIGURE 17-7. Diagram illustrating the progressive morphologic differentiation that occurs during spermiogenesis in the guinea pig. Note the formation and maturation of the acrosomal cap, the elements of the flagellum, and the formation of the residual cytoplasmic body.

within the epididymis). Using routine phase light microscopy (Fig. 17–9), little detail of cellular structure is gained, beyond (1) distinction of the head from flagellum (with its thickened middle piece usually being resolved), (2) the presence of a constricted neck portion at the origin of the flagellum, and (3) the persistence, also at the neck region in the human sperm, of a residual droplet of cytoplasm, a normal remnant of spermiogenesis. Light-microscopic evaluation of a semen sample is useful in the urology clinic for assessing sperm number and percent motility, and for screening for abnormally shaped sperm. A description of sperm morphology beyond these features, most of which had been remarked upon by Leeuwenhoek in his studies of the 1600s, awaited the advent of electron microscopy.

Fine Structure

The generalized fine-structural appearance of the mammalian sperm is depicted in Figure 17–10. In the normal human sperm, the *head* is approximately 4 to 5 μm in length and 2.5 to 3.5 μm in width, seen as a flat oval in frontal view. On edge, however, the head is revealed to be thicker at its base than its apex, and the cell appears piriform in profile. The condensed chromatin of the nucleus occupies most of the head region, with the condomform acrosome intimately applied to the anterior two thirds of the head.

The *acrosome* contains enzymes that facilitate the entry of the sperm into the ovum through the zona pellucida and perhaps the dispersal of the cumulus mass. Among the enzymes that have been documented in the lysosome are a trypsin-like protease acrosin, neuraminidase, hyaluronidase, acid phosphatase, and arylsulfatase. At fertilization, the cytoplasmic acrosomal membrane and the plasma membrane (removed in Fig. 17–10) fuse and release the acid hydrolases at the egg cell surface.

Electron microscopy of the *condensed chromatin*

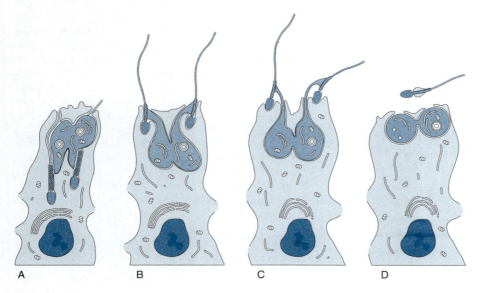

FIGURE 17-8. Diagram illustrating the progressive release of spermatids into the tubular lumen as spermatozoa. The syncytial mass of spermatid residual cytoplasm remains within the Sertoli cell, and only a small cytoplasmic droplet is retained by the released sperm.

A B C D

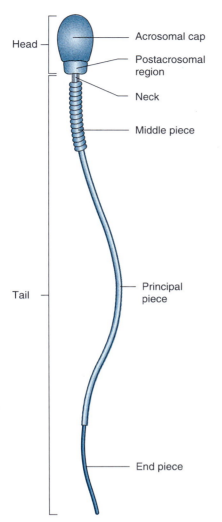

FIGURE 17–9. *Diagram of a mammalian spermatozoon, showing features visible with light microscopy.*

annulus, a dense, ringlike specialization adherent to the plasma membrane of the flagellum; a suggested function is to prevent distal slippage of the girdle of mitochondria during flagellar action.

By far the longest portion (45 μm) of the sperm flagellum, the *principal piece* is of smaller diameter than the middle piece. Its central 9 + 2 axoneme is surrounded by seven outer dense fibers (see Fig. 17–10), all being enclosed peripherally by the *fibrous sheath*.

The fibrous sheath and complement of outer dense fibers terminate abruptly some 5 to 7 μm before the termination of the flagellum, defining a thin terminal segment of the flagellum, the *end piece*, which somewhat resembles a cilium until even the 9 + 2 axonemal pattern is disrupted at the very distal portion of the end piece.

Cycle and Wave of the Seminiferous Epithelium

The process of spermatogenesis is continuous within the seminiferous tubules in the human. Therefore, during the time at which spermatids are undergoing spermiogenesis, for example, the spermatogonia continue to divide, and spermatocytes undergo meiosis, preparatory to giving rise to the next generation of spermatids. These simultaneous events generate an ex-

of the nucleus has yielded disappointingly little information concerning its substructure. Irregular, clear vacuolar defects in nuclear condensation, rarely seen except in the human sperm, are not uncommon. Their significance and relevance to fertilizing capacity are unknown.

The *neck region* of the human sperm contains a single, proximal centriole, the distal having undergone regression during spermiogenesis. The capitulum, or basal plate, lies within an indentation, the implantation fossa, at the base of the head; it gives rise to striated fibers continuous with the nine outer dense fibers of the flagellum. These nine fibers parallel the course of the microtubular axoneme through the midpiece, and seven fibers continue through the principal piece of the sperm tail. They are thought to be not contractile but rather resilient structural components of the flagellum.

The flagellar *middle piece* is that portion of the flagellum containing a cylindrical helically arranged *sheath of mitochondria* immediately beneath the plasmalemma. This portion of the flagellum is approximately 5 to 7 μm in length and terminates at the

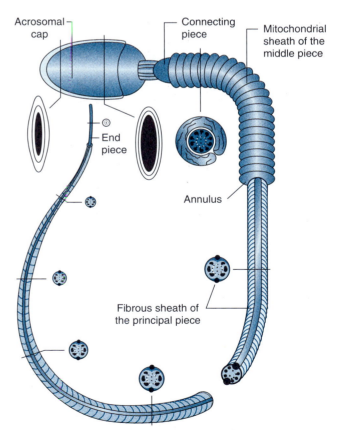

FIGURE 17–10. *Diagram of a mammalian spermatozoon, showing features revealed by electron microscopy.*

ceedingly complex series of cellular associations within the seminiferous epithelium. This series of cellular associations, however, occurs in an orderly, predictable progression over time. This periodicity permits definition of what is termed the *cycle of the seminiferous epithelium,* the interval of time between successive identical baso-apical associations of germ cells within the seminiferous epithelium. This period is species specific and has been determined from radiolabeled thymidine uptake studies to be 16 days in humans. It is calculated four cycles are needed to progress from a type B spermatogonium through spermiation, or about 64 days in humans for the entire process of spermatogenesis to take place.

If spermatogenesis were to proceed along the entire length of the tubules in this lock-step cyclical manner, then all histologic cross-sections of sections within a lobule would be expected to show identical cellular associations when examined at any given time. The histology student is painfully aware that such is not the case. Rather, the tubular profiles present a seemingly endless array of different cellular associations. This fact is explained on the basis that the seminiferous tubules, particularly in rodents in which the process has been best studied, are *functionally* partitioned into discrete regions, each of which cycles through the process of spermatogenesis, seemingly as though it were an independent germinal unit. The regions of the tubule are in fact exquisitely coordinated in their spermatogenic activity, however, perhaps through the ionic coupling afforded by the gap junctions formed between adjacent Sertoli cells. If histologic sections were taken serially along the whole length of a seminiferous tubule, it would be seen that the tubular epithelium faithfully repeats, in order, all the same cellular associations of spermatogenesis which would be observed over time at any one point in the tubule. This permits a *wave of the seminiferous epithelium* to be defined as that distance along the tubule between successive, identical cellular associations. Put differently, the cycle of the seminiferous epithelium is to time what the wave of the epithelium is to distance.

The wave and cycle of the seminiferous epithelium were defined first in rodents, in which the 12 or more successive cellular associations of spermatogenesis along the length of the tubule are very precisely demarcated. In humans, only six repeating associations are recognized, and they tend to overlap in adjacent regions of the tubule, rendering the study of the process more difficult. The six associations of germ cells found in the seminiferous epithelium in humans are illustrated in Figure 17–11. Because of the overlaps, single histologic cross-sections of human seminiferous tubules may be encountered in which two or more stages in the cycle are represented.

The organization of the seminiferous epithelium into waves and cycles permits the advantageous continuous maturation and release of spermatozoa. Were all tubules to be locked into synchronous sperm formation and spermiation, the distal ducts and storage capacity of the system would be overwhelmed by periodic superabundances of sperm, and the human male would experience alternating periods of fertility and infertility on a 64-day cycle.

Sperm Production and Fertility

It is instructive to examine the magnitude of the generative capacity of the seminiferous epithelium. Estimates place *daily* sperm production in humans at a remarkable mean value of 94.6×10^6, or some 5.6×10^6 per gram of testis; however, several rodent species outstrip this production per gram testis by a factor of four. Such productive capacity of an epithelium is understood only as surface area of the seminiferous epithelium is considered. If, in the human, both testes contain a total of 800 to 1200 seminiferous tubules, each 30 to 70 cm long, the aggregate productive length of the tubules approaches a third of a mile. Normally, ejaculate volume in humans is in the order of 2 to 5 ml, containing 40 to 100×10^6 sperm per ml. The fertility threshold in humans approximates 20×10^6 per ml. Storage reserves amount to sperm sufficient for two fertile ejaculates.

Testicular tubular fluid is an often overlooked component of the exocrine secretion of the testis. Its volume in not known in humans, but has been collected in liter quantities per 24 hours from the rete testis of rams. This fluid is instrumental in wafting the sperm through the intratesticular seminiferous tubules and intratesticular duct system, which lacks cilia and effective peristaltic contractility.

Tumors of the testis include neoplasms arising from germinal cells, Sertoli cells, and interstitial cells. Testicular tumors of germ cell origin (seminomas) are not uncommon in young adult males.

INTERSTITIAL TISSUE AND CELLS OF LEYDIG

The connective tissue of the interstitial (intertubular) space of the human testis (see Figs. 17–3 and 17–4) exhibits a paucity of fibrous elements and conspicuous accumulations of extravasated fluid. The interstitial cells of Leydig may form clusters of cells perivascularly or throughout the interstitium. The steroid hormone they secrete, testosterone, apparently reaches the interstitial venous and lymphatic channels, as well as the base of adjacent seminiferous tubules, by diffusion through the copious interstitial fluid. Leydig's cells are polygonal with a prominent, round euchromatic nucleus. Their cytoplasm is rich in those hallmark cytologic features of steroid-secreting cells, namely, many mitochondria (in certain species, bearing tubular cristae), abundant smooth endoplasmic reticulum, and lipid stores. Unique features of the human Leydig cell are the conspicuous crystals of Reinke, thought to be protein in nature; their significance is unknown.

The Leydig cells secrete testosterone in response to interstitial cell–stimulating hormone (ICSH). Systemically, testosterone promotes the development and maintenance of male secondary sexual characteristics.

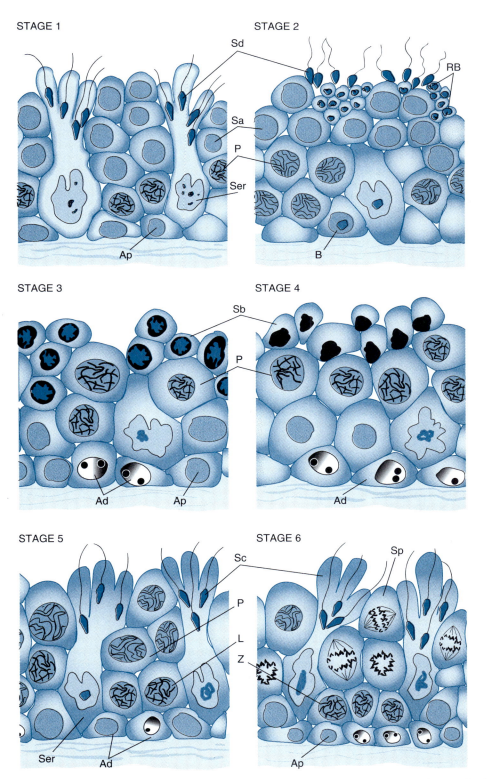

FIGURE 17-11. *Diagrammatic representation of the six recognizable stages of the seminiferous epithelium in the human.* Ser, *Sertoli cell;* Ad *and* Ap, *dark and pale, respectively, type A spermatogonia;* B, *type B spermatogonia;* L, *leptotene spermatocyte;* Z, *zygotene spermatocyte;* P, *pachytene spermatocyte;* Sa, Sb, Sc, Sd, *spermatids in various stages of differentiation;* RB, *residual bodies (of Regnaud).*

Within the testis, testosterone is essential, together with FSH, for spermatogenesis, and is found within the seminiferous epithelium bound to androgen-binding protein of Sertoli cell origin. Bound testosterone is present also in high concentration in the sperm-containing tubular fluid and is transported with the tubular fluid to the excurrent duct system, which itself is androgen dependent for its full functional and morphologic development.

EXCURRENT DUCT SYSTEM

Intratesticular Ducts

The seminiferous tubules may be considered coiled tubular holocrine (cytocrine) glands by the conventions of classification outlined in Chapter 2. Their duct system, however, is unique. The seminiferous tubular loops secrete via tubuli recti (straight tubules) into the rete testis, contained within the mediastinum of each testis.

The straight portions of the seminiferous tubules represent the short terminal segments of the seminiferous tubule, which narrow abruptly and are lined with a simple cuboidal to columnar epithelium bearing microvilli; the epithelium is thought not to be secretory and is considered to be derived from the Sertoli cell population of the germinal epithelium. The labyrinthine, anastomosing channels of the rete testis are lined by a similar cuboidal epithelium that is underlaid by the connective tissue of the mediastinum, the posterior invagination into the testis of the testicular capsule (tunica albuginea). A centrally placed, single motile flagellum projects from these cells; its functional role in moving spermatozoa is difficult to visualize.

Draining these spaces are 10 to 20 tubules termed the *ductuli efferentes,* or efferent ducts. These cross the tunica albuginea and emerge on the posterosuperior aspect of the testis, where they enter the overlying epididymis. The ductuli constitute a major portion of the initial portion (head) of the epididymis in humans, where they are present as highly coiled lobuli or coni. The wall of the efferent ducts is thin, consisting of an epithelium, its tunica propria, and a thin, circularly disposed layer of smooth muscle. The simple epithelium exhibits a unique arrangement of groups of tall columnar, ciliated cells that are broader at their apices than at their bases and that alternate with populations of cuboidal, nonciliated cells. This arrangement of tall and short cells imparts a distinctive puckered appearance to the luminal profiles of efferent ducts in cross-section (Fig. 17–12). The ciliary beat within the efferent ducts facilitates fluid and sperm transport. This is the only site in the human male excurrent duct system exhibiting such ciliary transport of sperm. The cuboidal nests of cells bear numerous apical microvilli and surface invaginations, features consistent with experimental studies implicating this system of ducts in fluid resorption and endocytosis.

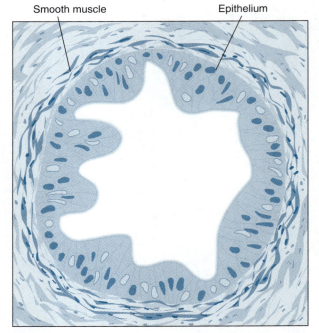

FIGURE 17–12. *Histologic structure of an efferent duct. The presence within the epithelium of populations of columnar and cuboidal cells gives rise to the undulating appearance of the lining epithelium. A thin layer of smooth muscle encircles the duct.*

Extratesticular Ducts

Epididymis

The very name of the organ, *epididymis* (from the Greek epi, upon, and *didymus*, testicle) denotes its placement on the posterolateral surfaces of each testis. The organ consists of three anatomic regions, an apically placed caput (head), a corpus (body), and a cauda (tail) situated at the inferior pole of the testis (see Fig. 17–2). The head of the epididymis consists of cone-shaped, highly contorted collections of the ductuli efferentes, identical in histology to that just described.

The efferent ducts join within the head of the epididymis to form a single duct that constitutes the body and tail. The epididymal duct is tortuously coiled upon itself; were it unraveled, it would measure some 6 m in length. The duct consists of a thin-walled tube lined with a tall, pseudostratified columnar epithelium with conspicuous stereocilia (Fig. 17–13). The epithelium rests on a thin tunica propria, which is surrounded by a scanty layer of circularly arranged smooth muscle with occasional longitudinal fibers. The size of the duct, the diameter of the lumen, and the thickness of the smooth muscle investment all increase as the cauda is reached. The epithelial height of the tail correspondingly is decreased to about half that of the head. Finer subdivisions of the duct may be made on the basis of histologic characteristics too detailed for inclusion here.

A mass of sperm is usually present within the lumen; it is moved distally by weak peristaltic action of the tubular wall. It is well established that the epididymis fosters the functional maturation of sperm and plays

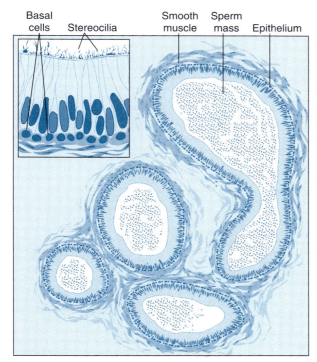

FIGURE 17-13. Histologic section of the human epididymal duct in its midsection. Note the tall pseudostratified columnar epithelium bearing long stereocilia and enclosing a luminal sperm mass. Inset, showing epithelial detail.

important roles in absorption, secretion, and sperm storage. In the ductuli efferentes and the epididymal duct, 90% of the testicular fluid is resorbed. During the 3 to 5 days' sojourn within the head and body of the epididymis, the sperm become capable of directional motility and are capable of fertilizing ova. Glycoprotein moieties are secreted by the epididymal epithelial cells into the lumen, are adsorbed onto the sperm cell surface, and possibly are incorporated into the plasma membrane during transit through the epididymis. Other secretions of the epididymis are glycerylphosphorylcholine, sialic acid, carnitine, glycoproteins, and possibly steroids, but their significance is currently not defined.

Vas (Ductus) Deferens

The tail of the epididymis is directly continuous at the lower pole of the testis with the scrotal portion of the vas deferens (see Fig. 17–1). This large duct, the most muscular of any of the excurrent ducts, is readily palpable within the scrotal *spermatic cord* (muscular and connective tissue bundle transmitting the ductus deferens, testicular artery, and testicular venous plexus and nerves from the abdomen to the scrotal testis). The scrotal vas is the site of *vasectomy*, the surgical section and ligation of the vas for the purpose of sterilization. The vas passes from the scrotum into the pelvic cavity through the inguinal canal and terminates in a dilated ampulla, which lies in relation to the posterior surface of the bladder, adjacent to the seminal vesicles (see Fig. 17–1). The wall of the vas deferens consists of a mucosa, robust muscularis, and adventitia (Fig. 17–14). The epithelium is similar in many respects to that of the tail of the epididymis; it is pseudostratified columnar and exhibits many apical stereocilia. The muscularis, which measures in the order of 1 to 1.5 mm in diameter, consists of well-developed layers of smooth muscle arranged as inner longitudinal, middle circular, and outer longitudinal layers. An adventitia of loose connective tissue surrounds the organ. The dilated ampullary portion has numerous glandular outpocketings that contain low columnar secretory cells.

Ejaculatory Duct

The ejaculatory duct is formed by the confluence of the vas deferens distal to the ampulla with the duct of the seminal vesicle. These paired ducts are approximately 2 cm in length and run a straight course through the substance of the prostate gland. The ducts empty within the prostatic urethra, in relation to the prostatic utricle (see Chapter 12). The ducts are thin-walled, lacking a smooth muscle layer; the epithelium may be pseudostratified or simple columnar.

ACCESSORY GLANDS

Like the excurrent ducts, the accessory glands depend for their full structural and functional development upon testosterone. The three major male accessory glands in the human are the seminal vesicle, the prostate gland, and the bulbourethral glands (Cowper's glands).

Seminal Vesicle

The paired seminal vesicles lie on the posterior surface of the urinary bladder, just lateral to the ampullae of the vasa deferentia (see Fig. 17–1). As their name implies, these organs earlier were thought to be reservoirs of sperm. Although sperm may be found within the folds of the gland, this likely represents a postmortem artifact. The vesicles are, in fact, an important secretory organ; the thick, viscid, yellowish fluid represents on the order of three fourths of the volume of human semen. An important component of the fluid is fructose, the principal carbohydrate in semen, which is considered nutritive to sperm, aiding motility. Flavins are responsible for the yellow cast of the secretion and can themselves assume a measure of importance in forensic medicine studies; semen and seminal stains fluoresce in ultraviolet light, owing to their flavin content. Prostaglandins (biologically active lipids), found in high concentration in the seminal fluid, are of seminal vesicle origin.

Developmentally, the seminal vesicles arise as outgrowths of the ductus (vas) deferens. They are hollow, sacculated organs, some 5 to 10 cm in length, that are bounded by an unremarkable connective tissue capsule. Underlying the capsule is a layer of smooth muscle thinner than that of the vas deferens and ar-

316 CHAPTER SEVENTEEN MALE REPRODUCTIVE SYSTEM

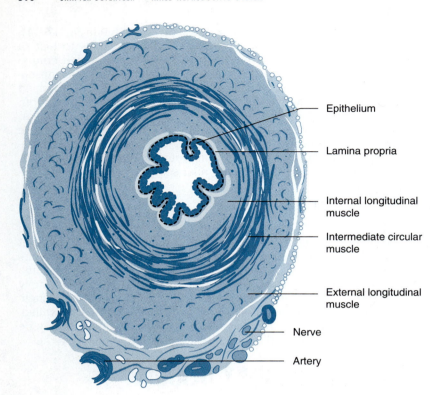

FIGURE 17–14. *Human ductus (vas) deferens in cross-section. Note the characteristic puckered appearance of the mucosa and the robust musculature arranged in three layers.*

FIGURE 17–15. *Cross-section through the human prostatic urethra in the region of the prostatic utricle. A, Note the raised posterior portion of the urethra, the colliculus seminalis. The prostatic ducts from various portions of the gland empty into the urethra, according to the diagram presented in B.*

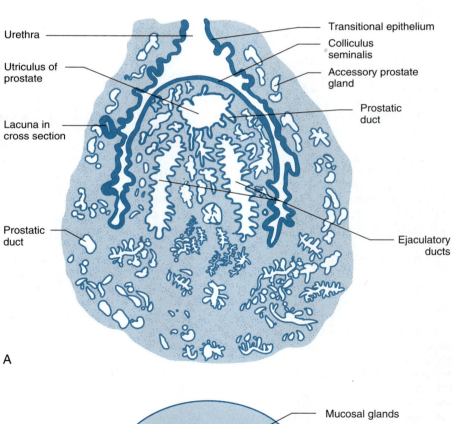

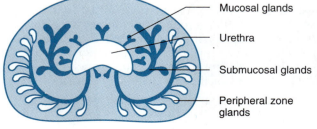

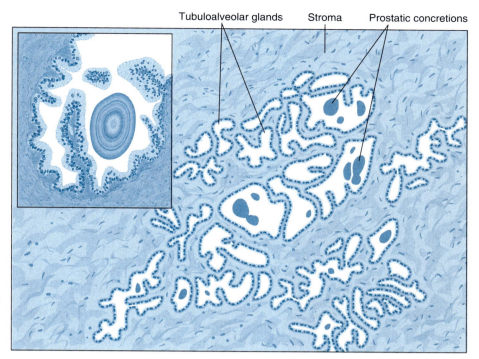

FIGURE 17-16. Histologic features of the prostate gland. Tubuloalveolar secretory units and numerous ducts lie within a fibromuscular stroma. Inset shows detail of an acinus containing a lamellated prostatic concretion (corpus amylaceum). These unique structures become more numerous with advancing age.

ranged in indistinct inner circular and outer longitudinal layers. The mucosa consists of a tall columnar or pseudostratified columnar epithelium, underlaid by a tunica propria. In histologic section, the mucosa appears honeycombed with basal pockets, an appearance derived from the many diverticula that arise from the wall of the vesicle, and the deep primary, secondary, and branching tertiary folds within the mucosa itself (see Fig. 17-17). The diverticula communicate with the central lumen of the vesicle, and a slender duct joins that of the terminal vas deferens, as noted previously, to form the ejaculatory duct. Rough endoplasmic reticulum and abundant secretory granules characterize the fine structure of the secretory cells of the epithelium, substantiating their role in active protein secretion.

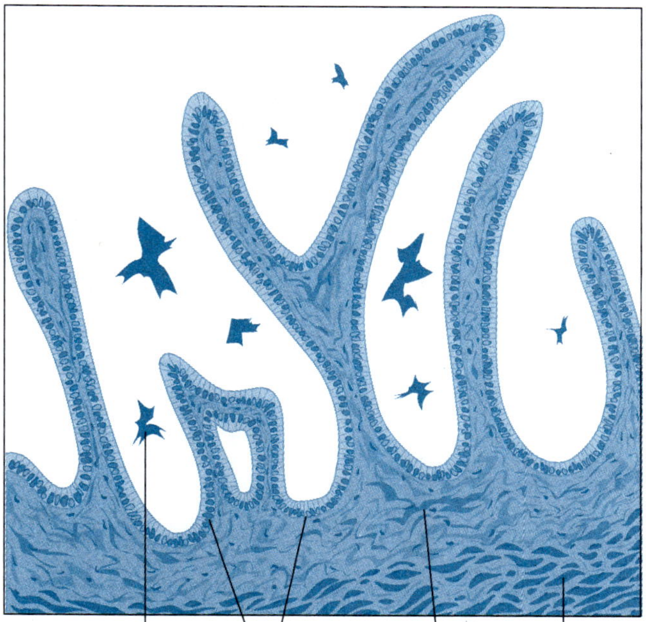

Prostate Gland

The prostate (from the Latin, meaning to stand before) lies immediately before the neck of the bladder and completely encloses the first portion of the urethra, which courses inferiorly through the substance of the gland as the prostatic urethra. The largest of the male accessory sex glands, the prostate is covered by a thin capsule of connective tissue interspersed with smooth muscle. Smooth muscle is present, as well, within the stromal connective tissue supporting the numerous branched, tubuloalveolar glands that compose the secretory portion of the gland. Septa from the capsule divide the prostate into indistinct lobes. The secretory units bud from the ductal system, forming units that exhibit a variable shape and epithelial lining.

Within the ducts and alveoli, particularly in older men, spheroidal concretions are commonly observed. These bodies, the *corpora amylacea* (Fig. 17-16, *inset*), are composed of glycoprotein that may become secondarily calcified. The concretions may block secretion, causing swelling of the gland. Commonly, smaller

FIGURE 17-17. Histologic features of the seminal vesicle. Note the branching and anastomosing mucosal folds that project into the lumen of the seminal vessel. The folds are lined by a columnar or pseudostratified columnar epithelium.

concretions are expelled by the prostate into the semen at the time of ejaculation. This results from the forceful contraction of the fibromuscular stroma and the expression of the stored secretion product into the prostatic urethra.

Typically, under androgen stimulation, the epithelium is simple to pseudostratified columnar. Abundant rough endoplasmic reticulum, a well-developed Golgi apparatus, and associated secretory granules characterize the cytoplasm of the secretory epithelial cells. Components of the slightly acidic prostatic secretion are acid phosphatase, citric acid, amylase, zinc, and the proteolytic enzyme fibrinolysin, which is imputed to cause liquefaction of the semen following ejaculation.

The glands of the prostate are collected into three major groups, arranged concentrically. They are designated the *mucosal glands,* the *submucosal glands,* and the *main glands,* each of which is drained by a discrete ductal system. The mucosal group consists of those short glands disposed immediately adjacent to the prostatic urethra (see Fig. 17–15B). This portion of the prostate develops from a primordium separate from the remainder of the gland and is partitioned from the outer portions of the adult prostate gland by smooth muscle. Some 30 to 40 in number, the mucosal glands drain by individual ducts into the urethra. The more peripherally situated submucosal group drains through fewer, larger ducts. The main (peripheral zone) glands constitute the greater proportion of the secretory tissue of the prostate and contribute the bulk of the organ's secretory product. The main glands discharge their secretion via long ducts emptying into the lateral recesses of the urethra, on either side of the colliculus (verumontanum).

Two common, threatening clinical conditions of the prostate gland that affect older men are benign nodular prostatic hyperplasia (BPH) and prostatic adenocarcinoma. Benign enlargement is typically confined to the mucosal group of glands, whereas the submucosal and peripheral zone components are the usual sites of adenocarcinoma. BPH can lead to devastating urinary tract and renal sequelae owing to obstruction of the prostatic urethra and urinary retention. Cancer of the prostate is second only to lung cancer as a cause of cancer-related deaths in men in the United States. Acid phosphatase secreted by the normal prostate is also secreted by tumors, both in situ and in metastatic tumors distant from the gland—commonly, of the pelvic bone or abdominal viscera. In clinical practice, an elevated serum acid phosphatase level is commonly indicative of prostatic adenocarcinoma, as is elevation over time of a more recently validated serum antigen marker, prostate-specific antigen (PSA).

Bulbourethral Glands

Also known as Cowper's glands, the paired bulbourethral glands are small, the size of a pea, and located within the musculature of the pelvic diaphragm that surrounds the membranous portion of the urethra. The glands are characterized as compound tubuloalveolar; their mucous secretory epithelium is variable, ranging from cuboidal to columnar. Their secretion consists of a clear, mucus-like material that contains sialic acid, galactose, galactosamine, galacturonic acid, and a methylpentose. Under erotic stimulation, the gland secretes through ducts ending in the penile urethra; its clear, viscous fluid is considered to act as a urethral lubricant. These secretions augment the lubricating mucus formed in the mucosal glands of Littre (see Chapter 12), found in the epithelial lining of the penile urethra.

PENIS

The pendulous copulatory organ, the *penis* (from Latin, meaning a tail), consists of three bodies of cylindrically arranged erectile tissue, bound together by dense white connective tissue, termed the *tunica albuginea,* and covered by a loosely adherent fascia and integument. The erectile bodies are arranged as paired dorsal structures, the corpora cavernosa penis, and a single ventral body, the corpus cavernosum urethrae, or corpus spongiosum, which transmits the penile portion of the urethra (Figs. 17–1 and 17–18). The dilated terminal end of the corpus spongiosum is termed the glans (Latin, acorn), which bears the opening of the external urethral meatus (orifice). The epithelial lining of the dilated terminal portion of the penile urethra, the fossa navicularis, is stratified squamous, mucosal variety, which is continuous with the nonkeratinized

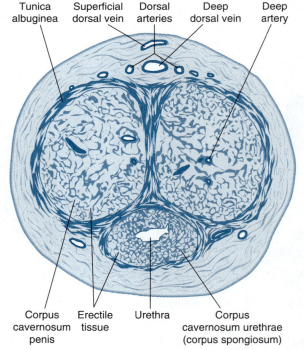

FIGURE 17–18. *Cross-section of the human penis. The ventrally placed urethra is surrounded by the corpus cavernosum urethrae (corpus spongiosum). Two additional, dorsally situated erectile bodies, the corpora cavernosa penis, are enclosed by a strong sleeve of dense irregular tissue, the tunica albuginea. Note the presence of the numerous cavernous spaces within the erectile bodies.*

epithelium of the glans. The glans is well endowed with sebaceous glands and is exquisitely innervated with numerous varieties of sensory receptors, including specialized genital papillae.

Erectile or cavernous tissue consists of endothelially lined vascular spaces, separated by trabeculae containing fibroelastic tissue and smooth muscle. Filling of the spaces under conditions of sustained arterial pressure and reduced venous outflow causes engorgement of the erectile bodies, limited by the indistensible surrounding connective tissue tunics. Consequent hemodynamic elongation and swelling of the organ occurs, a condition termed *erection* or *tumescence*. The degree of rigidity attained by the erectile bodies is in part a function of the degree of elastic distensibility of the surrounding tunica albuginea. This layer surrounding the corpus spongiosum is much less robust and is more pliable and distensible than that surrounding the paired dorsal bodies. Consequently, less rigidity is achieved within the spongiosum, fortuitously preventing occlusion of the penile urethra during erection and ejaculation.

Filling of the cavernous spaces is under complex autonomic control, involving, it is currently thought, both the arterial and venous sides of the penile vascular bed. Two systems of vessels supply the cavernous spaces, the trabecular capillaries and highly coiled small arteries (capable of elongation upon tumescence) that empty directly into the spaces. Relaxation of the muscular tone of the walls of these coiled helicine arteries under parasympathetic stimulation increases the blood flow to the cavernous spaces, filling them to a degree and compressing venous outflow channels against the inner aspect of the tunica albuginea. (The significance to erection of this latter aspect has been the subject of continuing debate among investigators.) Equally controversial is the possible role played in reducing venous outflow by the raised cushions of smooth muscle (termed *polsters*) present within the intima of these effuent veins. Contraction of the smooth muscle component of the trabeculae may also abet the increase of hemodynamic pressure within the cavernous spaces. *Detumescence* or flaccidity of the penis is restored following ejaculation (orgasm) as a result of sympathetic outflow, which restores vascular smooth muscle tone of the helicine arteries, with consequent reduction of blood inflow to the cavernous spaces and release of venous outflow compression.

SEMEN

Semen (*ejaculum*) refers to the complex melange of sperm, exfoliated cells of the ductal system, and fluid and secretions from the testis, epididymis, vas deferens, and the accessory sex glands. Less than 10% of semen consists of spermatozoa (some 60×10^6 per ml, on average). Semen is forcefully ejaculated (L., *jacere*, to throw) from the penile urethra at orgasm. Contributions to semen from the various components of the male reproductive tract have been cited in previous sections. It should be noted here that the process of ejaculation is a *sequential* one. The release upon erotic stimulation of the secretions of the bulbourethral glands and the glands of Littre has been previously noted. At orgasm, the prostate gland delivers its secretion to the prostatic urethra by constriction of its capsule and fibromuscular stroma, concomitantly with the addition, through the ejaculatory ducts, of sperm and fluid from the rhythmic contractions of the musculature of the epididymis and vas deferens. The contraction of the seminal vesicles and the addition of its contribution to semen is accomplished last in this process. In human semen, significant numbers of structurally abnormal sperm (e.g., doubling of heads or tails) are commonly recorded; too high a proportion of such sperm disposes to infertility.

BIBLIOGRAPHY

GENERAL REFERENCES: CELL, TISSUE, AND ORGAN BIOLOGY

Alberts, B., et al. Molecular Biology of the Cell, 3rd ed. New York: Garland, 1994.

Austen, B. M., Westwood, O. M. R. Protein Targeting and Secretion. Oxford: IRL Press at Oxford University Press, 1991.

Avery, J. K., and Steele, P. F., eds. Oral Development and Histology. Section V, Structure of the Soft Tissues. New York: Thieme Medical Publishers, 1994.

Bergman, R. A., Afifi, A. K., and Heidger, P. M. Atlas of Microscopic Anatomy—A Functional Approach: Companion to Histology and Neuroanatomy, 2nd ed. Philadelphia: W.B. Saunders, 1989.

Bock, G., and Clark, S., eds. Junctional Complexes of Epithelial Cells. New York: Wiley, 1987.

Bourne, G. H., ed. Cytology and Cell Physiology, 4th ed. International Review of Cytology Suppl. 17. San Diego: Academic Press, 1987.

Case, R. M., Lingard, J. A., and Young, J. A., eds. Secretion: Mechanisms and Control. Manchester, UK: University of Manchester Press, 1984.

Cotran, R. S., Kumar, V., and Robbins, S. L. Robbins' Pathologic Basis of Disease, 5th ed. Philadelphia: W.B. Saunders, 1994.

Darnell, J., Lodish, H., and Baltimore, D. Molecular Cell Biology, 2nd ed. New York: Scientific American Books, 1990.

Fawcett, D. W. Bloom and Fawcett, A Textbook of Histology, 12th ed. New York: Chapman & Hall, 1994.

Fawcett, D. W. The Cell. Philadelphia: W.B. Saunders, 1981.

Guyton, A. C. Human Physiology and Mechanisms of Disease, 5th ed. Philadelphia: W.B. Saunders, 1992.

Guyton, A. C. Textbook of Medical Physiology, 8th ed. Philadelphia: W.B. Saunders, 1991.

Junqueira, L. C., Carneiro, J., and Kelley, R. O. Basic Histology, 7th ed. Norwalk: Appleton & Lang, 1992.

Kessel, R. G., and Kardon, R. H. Tissues and Organs: A Text-Atlas of Scanning Electron Microscopy. San Francisco: W. H. Freeman, 1979.

Leeson, C. R., Leeson, T. S., and Paparo, A. A. Atlas of Histology, 2nd ed. Philadelphia: W.B. Saunders, 1985.

Muggleton-Harris, A. L., ed. Membrane Research: Classic Origins and Current Concepts. New York: Academic Press, 1981.

Murakami, M., et al., eds. Epithelial Transport: Energetics, Mechanisms, and Control, 11th Seiriken Conference on Epithelial Transport. Tokyo: Biomedical Research Foundation, 1986.

Roberts, R. L., Kessel, R. G., and Tung, H.-N. Freeze Fracture Images of Cells and Tissues. Oxford: Oxford University Press, 1991.

Sawyer, R., and Fallon, J., eds. Epithelial-Mesenchymal Interactions in Development. New York: Praeger, 1983.

Shih, G., and Kessel, R. G. Living Images: Biological Microstructures Revealed by Scanning Electron Microscopy. Boston: Science Books, 1982.

Stevens, A., and Lowe, J. Histology. London: Gower Medical Publishing, 1992.

Weiss, L., ed. Cell and Tissue Biology: A Textbook of Histology, 6th ed. Baltimore: Urban & Schwarzenberg, 1988.

Wight, N. A., and Alison, M. The Biology of Epithelial Cell Populations. New York: Oxford University Press, 1984.

Williams, P. L., Warwick, R., Dyson, M., and Bannister, L. H., eds. Gray's Anatomy, 37th ed. Edinburgh: Churchill Livingstone, 1989.

CONNECTIVE TISSUES

Avery, J. K., and Steele, P. F., eds. Oral Development and Histology. Section IV, Structure of the Teeth: New York: Thieme Medical Publishers, 1994.

Bourne, G. H., ed. The Biochemistry and Physiology of Bone, 2nd ed., Vols. 1–4. New York: Academic Press, 1971–1976.

Creyer, A., and Van, R. L. R., eds. New Perspectives in Adipose Tissue: Structure, Function, and Development. Boston: Butterworths, 1985.

Diggs, L. W., Strum, D., and Bell, A. The Morphology of Human Blood Cells, 5th ed. Chicago: Abbott Laboratories, 1985

Noda, M., ed. Cellular and Molecular Biology of Bone. San Diego: Academic Press, 1993.

Stockwell, R. A. Biology of Cartilage Cells. New York: Cambridge University Press, 1979.

Zucker-Franklin, D., et al., eds. Atlas of Blood Cells: Function and Pathology, Vols. 1 and 2. Philadelphia: Lea & Febiger, 1981.

NEUROMUSCULAR TISSUE

Afifi, A. K., and Bergman, R. A. Basic Neuroscience: A Structural and Functional Approach, 2nd ed. Baltimore: Urban & Schwarzenberg, 1986.

Barr, M. L., and Kiernan, J. A. The Human Nervous System: An Anatomical Viewpoint, 6th ed. Philadelphia: J.B. Lippincott, 1993.

Bergman, R. A. Ultrastructural configuration of sarcomeres in passive and contracted frog sartorius muscle. Am. J. Anat. 166:209–222, 1983.

Bourne, G. H., ed. The Structure and Function of Muscle. New York: Academic Press, 1972.

Gluhbegovic, N., and Williams, T. H. The Human Brain—A Photographic Guide. Philadelphia: Harper & Row, 1980.

Junge, D. Nerve and Muscle Excitation, 3rd ed. Sunderland, MA: Sinauer Associates, 1992.

Matthews, G. G. Cellular Physiology of Nerve and Muscle, 2nd ed. Boston: Blackwell Scientific Publications, 1991.
Meredith, G. E., and Arbuthnott, G. W., eds. Morphological Investigations of Single Neurons in Vitro. New York: Wiley, 1993.
Peters, A., Palay, S. L., and Webster, H. deF. The Fine Structure of the Nervous System: Neurons and Their Supporting Cells, 3rd ed. New York: Oxford University Press, 1991.
Terzis, J. K., and Smith, K. L. The Peripheral Nerve: Structure, Function, and Reconstruction. New York: Raven Press, 1990.

CARDIOVASCULAR SYSTEM

DeBakey, M. E., and Gotto, A. The Living Heart. New York: D. McKay Co., 1977.
Fozzard, H. A., et al., eds. The Heart and Cardiovascular System: Scientific Foundations. New York: Raven Press, 1991.
Schlant, R. C., and Alexander, R. W., eds. The Heart, Arteries, and Veins, 8th ed. New York: McGraw-Hill, Health Professions Division, 1994.
Smith, J. J., and Kampine, J. P. Circulatory Physiology: The Essentials, 2nd ed. Baltimore: Williams & Wilkins, 1984.

LYMPHOID TISSUE AND IMMUNITY

Alberts, B., et al. The Immune System. In: Molecular Biology of the Cell, 3rd ed. New York: Garland, 1994.
Bowdler, A. J., ed. The Spleen: Structure, Function, and Clinical Significance. London: Chapman & Hall, 1990.
Henry, K., and Symmers, W. St. C., eds. Thymus, Lymph Nodes, Spleen and Lymphatics, 3rd ed. New York: Churchill Livingstone, 1992.
Lockey, R. L., and Bukantz, S. C. Fundamentals of Immunology and Allergy. Philadelphia: W.B. Saunders, 1987.
Stites, D. P., and Terr, A. I., eds. Basic and Clinical Immunology, 7th ed. Norwalk, CT: Appleton & Lange, 1991.

INTEGUMENT

Montagna, W. The Structure and Function of Skin, 3rd ed. New York: Academic Press, 1974.
Montagna, W., Kligman, A. M., and Carlisle, K. S. Atlas of Normal Human Skin. New York: Springer-Verlag, 1992.
Montagna, W., Prota, G., and Kenney, J. A. Jr. Black Skin: Structure and Function. San Diego: Academic Press, 1993.

DIGESTIVE SYSTEM

Avery, J. K., and Steele, P. F., eds. Oral Development and Histology, 2nd ed. New York: Thieme Medical Publishers, 1994.
Becker, F. F., ed. The Liver, Normal and Abnormal Functions, Vols. 1 and 2. New York: Dekker, 1974–1975.
Bolt, R. J., et al., eds. The Digestive System. New York: Wiley, 1983.
Mason, D. K., and Chisholm, D. M. Salivary Glands in Health and Disease. Philadelphia: W.B. Saunders, 1975.
Molta, P. M., Fujita, H., and Correr, S., eds. Ultrastructure of the Digestive Tract. Boston: Nijhoff (distributed by Kluwer Academic Publishers), 1988.
Rouiller, C., ed. The Liver: Morphology, Biochemistry, and Physiology, Vols. 1 and 2. New York: Academic Press, 1963–1964.
Toner, P. G., Carr, K. E., and Wyburn, G. M. The Digestive System—An Ultrastructural Atlas and Review. New York: Appleton-Century-Crofts, 1971.
Wight, D. G. D., ed. Liver, Biliary Tract and Exocrine Pancreas, 3rd ed. New York: Churchill Livingstone, 1994.
Young, J. A., and Van Lennep, E. W. The Morphology of Salivary Glands. New York: Academic Press, 1978.

URINARY SYSTEM

Bergman, H., ed. The Ureter, 2nd ed. New York: Springer-Verlag, 1981.
Brenner, B. M., and Rector, F. C. Jr., eds. The Kidney, 4th ed. Philadelphia: W.B. Saunders, 1991.
Bulger, R. E., and Dobyan, D. C. Recent advances in renal morphology. Annu. Rev. Physiol. 44:147–179, 1982.
Jones, T. C., Mohr, U., and Hunt, R. D., eds. The Urinary System. New York: Springer-Verlag, 1986.
Rouillier, C., and Muller, A. F., eds. The Kidney: Morphology, Biochemistry, and Physiology, Vols. 1–4. New York: Academic Press, 1969–1971.
Walsh, P. C., et al., eds. Campbell's Urology, 6th ed. Philadelphia: W.B. Saunders, 1992.

RESPIRATORY SYSTEM

Farmer, S. G., and Hay, D. W. P., eds. The Airway Epithelium: Physiology, Pathophysiology and Pharmacology. New York: Dekker, 1991.
Gil, J. Organization of the microcirculation of the lung. Annu. Rev. Physiol. 42:177–186, 1980.
Gil, J., ed. Models of Lung Disease: Microscopy and Structural Methods. New York: Dekker, 1990.
Kuhn C., III. The cells of the lung and their organelles. In: Crystal, R. G., ed. The Biochemical Basis of Pulmonary Function. New York: Dekker, 1976.
Massaro, D., ed. Lung Cell Biology. New York: Dekker, 1989.
Thurlbeck, W. M., and Abell, R. M., eds. The Lung: Structure, Function and Disease. Baltimore: Williams & Wilkins, 1978.

EYE AND EAR

Hogan, J. J., et al. Histology of the Human Eye. Philadelphia: W.B. Saunders, 1971.
Hudspeth, A. J. The hair cells of the inner ear. Sci. Am. 248:54–64, 1983.
Lim, D. J. Functional structure of the organ of Corti: A review. Hear. Res. 22:117–146, 1986.
McDevitt, D., ed. Cell Biology of the Eye. New York: Academic Press, 1982.

ENDOCRINE SYSTEM

Baulieu, E.-E., and Kelly, P. A., eds. Hormones: From Molecules to Disease. New York: Chapman & Hall, 1990.
Bhatnagar, A. S., ed. The Anterior Pituitary Gland. New York: Raven Press, 1983.
DeGroot, L. J., et al., eds. Endocrinology, 3rd ed. Philadelphia: W.B. Saunders, 1995.
Greer, M. A., ed. The Thyroid Gland. New York: Raven Press, 1990.
Hazelwood, R. L. The Endocrine Pancreas. Englewood-Cliffs, NJ: Prentice-Hall, 1989.
Hess, M., Heidger, P. M., Dyer, R. F., and Ruby, J. R., eds. Electron Microscopic Concepts of Secretion. Ultrastructure of Endocrine and Reproductive Organs. New York: Wiley, 1975.
James, V. H. T., ed. The Adrenal Gland, 2nd ed. New York: Raven Press, 1992.
Motta, P. M., ed. Ultrastructure of Endocrine Cells and Tissues. Boston: Nijhoff (distributed by Kluwer, Boston), 1984.
Nussdorfer, G. Cytophysiology of the adrenal cortex. In: Bourne, G., and Danielli, J., eds. International Review of Cytology, Vol. 98. Orlando: Academic Press, 1986.

FEMALE REPRODUCTIVE SYSTEM

Adashi, E. Y., and Leung, P. C. K., eds. The Ovary. New York: Raven Press, 1993.
Austin, C. R., and Short, R. V., eds. Reproduction in Mammals, Vols. 1–6. London: Cambridge University Press, 1972–1976.
Familiari, G., Makabe, S., and Motta, P., eds. Ultrastructure of the Ovary. Boston: Kluwer Academic Publishers, 1991.
Greep, R. O., ed. Handbook of Physiology: Endocrinology. Vol. 11, Section 7, Female Reproductive System. Washington: American Physiological Society, 1975.
Mossman, H., and Duke, K. L. Comparative Morphology of the Human Ovary. Madison: University of Wisconsin Press, 1973.
Neville, M. C., and Daniel, C. W., eds. The Mammary Gland: Development, Regulation, and Function. New York: Plenum Press, 1987.
Peters, H., and McNatty, K. P. The Ovary: A Correlation of Structure and Function in Mammals. Berkeley: University of California Press, 1980.
Wynn, R. M. Obstetrics and Gynecology: The Clinical Core, 5th ed. Philadelphia: Lea & Febiger, 1992.

Wynn, R. M., ed. Biology of the Uterus. New York: Plenum Press, 1977.
Zuckerman, S., and Weir, B. J., eds. The Ovary, 2nd ed. Vol. 1, General Aspects. New York: Academic Press, 1977.

MALE REPRODUCTIVE SYSTEM

Burger, H., de Kretser, D. M., eds. The Testis, 2nd ed. New York: Raven Press, 1989.

de Kretser, D. M., and Kerr, J. F. The cytology of the testis. In: Knobil, E., et al., eds. Physiology of Reproduction. New York: Raven Press, 1988, p. 121.

Fawcett, D. W. The mammalian spermatozoon. Dev. Biol. 44:394–436, 1975.

Fawcett, D. W., Leak, L. V., and Heidger, P. M., Jr. Electron microscopic observations on the structural components of the blood-testis barrier. J. Reprod. Fertil. Suppl. 2, 10:105–122, 1970.

Fitzpatrick, J. M., and Krane, R. J., eds. The Prostate. New York: Churchill Livingstone, 1989.

Hafez, E. S. E., and Spring-Mills, E., eds. Accessory Glands of the Male Reproductive Tract. Ann Arbor, MI: Ann Arbor Science, 1979.

Hafez, E. S. E., and Spring-Mills, E., eds. Prostatic Carcinoma: Biology and Diagnosis. Boston: Nijhoff (distributed by Kluwer, Boston), 1981.

Hamilton, D. W., and Greep, R. O., eds. Handbook of Physiology: Endocrinology, Vol. 5, Section 7, Male Reproductive System. Washington: American Physiological Society, 1975.

Kline, T. S. Prostate. New York: Igaku-Shoin, 1985.

Tindall, D., et al. Structure and biochemistry of the Sertoli cell. Int. Rev. Cytol. 94:127–149, 1985.

INDEX

Note: Page numbers in *italics* refer to illustrations; numbers followed by t indicate tables.

A

A bands, 81, 83
  in skeletal muscle, 78, 79–82, *80–82*
A-alpha (α) axon, 120, 120t
A-beta (β) axon, 120, 120t
ABO blood group, 97
Absorbing cell, in columnar epithelium of digestive tract, 27
Accessory glands, male, 315–318, *317*
Accessory prostate gland, *316*
Accessory thyroid gland, 268
Acetabular fossa, *74*
Acetabular labrum, *74*
Acetabular ligament, transverse, *74*
Acetabular notch, *74*
Acetabulum, *74*
Acetic acid, as fixative, 3
Achilles tendon, *80*
Achromatic, defined, 249
Acid maltase deficiency, 16
Acid vesicle system, 16, *17*
Acidophils, 105
  of adenohypophysis, 261–262, *262–263*
Acinus(i), 36–37, *36*
  hepatic, as unit of hepatic function, 208, *209*
    zones of, *209*
  of exocrine gland, *38*
  of exocrine pancreas, *207*
  of lacrimal gland, 251
  of salivary gland, *206*
  of sebaceous gland, 173
Acrosomal cap, *311*
  maturation of, *310*
Acrosomal phase of spermiogenesis, 309, *310*
ACTH (adrenocorticotropic hormone), 262t, *263*
Actin, composition of, *84–85*, 85
  filaments of, 18
ADCC (antibody-dependent cell-mediated cytotoxicity), 152
A-delta (δ) axon, 120, 120t

Adenohypophysis, 260–265, *262–264*, 262t.
  See also specific cell type.
  composition of, 261–264, *262–264*
  hormones of, 262t
  secretion mechanisms of, 265
Adenoids, 143
Adenosine triphosphate (ATP), in muscle contraction, 86–88, *87*
Adhesion belt, *131*
  of intestinal epithelial cells, *32*, 198
Adipocytes. See *Fat cells.*
Adipose tissue, *48*, 57–58, *157*. See also *Fat cells.*
  of breast, 299
  of lymph node, 145
Adluminal compartment, of seminiferous epithelium, *306*
Adrenal glands. See *Suprarenal glands.*
Adrenocorticotropic hormone (ACTH), 262t, *263*
Adventitia, 178
  of colon, 201
  of ureter, *224*
  of vagina, 298, *298*
A-gamma (γ) axon, 120, 120t
Age pigment, 16
Agranulocytes, 99–100, *99–100*
Airway, 228–229, *228–229*, 228t
  epithelium of, 228–229, *229*
Albumin, in blood plasma, 103
α cells, of islets of Langerhans, 276–278, *278*
Alpha granules, in platelet, 102
Alveolar bone, of mandible, *187*
Alveolar capillaries, 235–236
Alveolar cells, *34*
  free, *236*, 237–238
  types I and II, 235, *235*
Alveolar connective tissue, 42, *42*
Alveolar ducts, 233–234, *234*
  epithelium in, 228t
Alveolar epithelium, 228t
  types I and II, 233–234, 236, *236–237*
Alveolar glands, 36–37, *36*, 36t
Alveolar macrophages, *236*

Alveolar macrophages *(Continued)*
  interleukin–8 produced by, 150
Alveolar process, gingival, *183*
Alveoli, 234–238, *234–235*
  in alveolar wall, 235–236
  in bronchial wall, *232*
  in interalveolar septa, 236–238, *236–237*
  in respiratory tissue surrounding bronchiole, *233–234*
  interface with capillaries, 236–237, *237*
Amacrine association cells, in retina, 247–248, *247*
Ameloblasts, in developing tooth, *188*
Amine precursor uptake and decarboxylation (APUD) cells, sites of, 279t
Amines, 259, 260t
Amino acid radicals, *271*
Amphiarthroses, 74–75, *74*
Amphipathic, defined, 6, *9*
Ampulla, Henle's, *304*
  of oviduct, *283*, 287
Anagen, 172
Anamnestic immune response, 153
Anaphase, *22*, 23
Androgen-binding protein, 307
Androstenediol, secreted by ovarian follicle, 285
Anemia, 98
Anisocytosis, 98
Anisotrophy, 79–81, *81*
Ankyrin, 18
Annulospiral nerve fiber endings, 128, *128*
Annulus, of mitochondrial sheath of spermatozoon, 311
Anterior horn, of spinal cord, cell of, *113*
Antibody(ies), humoral immunologic response and, 151
  labeling of, 5, *5*
Antibody-dependent cell-mediated cytotoxicity (ADCC), 152
Antidiuretic hormone, action and regulation of, 265t
Antigen-presenting cell (APC), in immune response, 150–151

Antigen-presenting cell (APC) *(Continued)*
  in lymph node, 144
  in spleen, 148
Antrum, of secondary ovarian follicle, *284–285*, 285
Anulus fibrosus, 74–75
Anus, 201–202, *202*
Aorta, *135*, 137, *137*
APC (antigen-presenting cell). See *Antigen-presenting cell (APC).*
Apical compartment, of seminiferous epithelium, 307
Apocrine glands, 37, *37*, *175–176*, 176
Aponeurotic structure of scalp, *170*
Appendix, 201, *201*
APUD cells, sites of, 279t
Aqueous humor, 246
Arcuate vessels, of kidney, *214–215*
  in fetus, *273*
Areola, *299*, 300
Areolar connective tissue, 42, 57
Argentaffin cells, of gastric glands, 193–194, *193–194*
  of intestine, 196, *199*
Aromatase, 290
Arrector pili muscle, *93*, *170*, 172–173, *173*
Arteries, 137–139, *137–139*. See also *Arterioles; Capillaries;* specific artery.
  large elastic, 137, *137*
  of intestine, *198*
  of kidney and ureter, 215–216, *216–217*, *220*, 223–224
  of penis, *318*
  of uterine lining, during menstrual cycle, *293*
  of vas deferens, *316*
Arterioles, 138, *138–139*
  central, of spleen, *147–148*, 148–149
  of intestinal villus, *198*
  of liver, *210*
  of renal corpuscle, *216*
  of suprarenal gland, *277*
Articular capsule, *74*
Articular cartilage, *74*
Artifacts, in light microscopy, 2
Astrocyte, 117–118, *118–119*
Atomic force microscopy, 2
ATP (adenosine triphosphate), in muscle contraction, 86–88, *87*
Atresia, follicular, 283, *286*
Atrioventricular bundle, *136*, 136
Atrioventricular (AV) node, 91, *91*, *136*, 136
Atrium of heart, *135*
  polypeptide hormones in, 90–91
Atrophy, defined, 77
Attachment proteins, 17
Audition, mechanics of, 252
Auditory canal, external, 251
Auditory end organ, 253–254, *253–254*
Auditory physiology, 254–255
Auerbach's plexus, 190
  ganglion of, *197*
  intestinal tract and, *178*
Auricle, 251
Auricle of heart, *135*
Autonomic ganglion, 119
  cells of, *116*
Autophagolysosomes, 16, *17*
Autoradiography, 5–6, *6*
AV (atrioventricular) node, 91, *91*, *136*, 136
Axillary sweat gland, 175
Axoaxonic synapse, *123*, 124, *124*
Axodendritic synapse, *123*, 124, *124*
Axon, *113*, 114–117, *116–117*, *121*, *123*, 125
  degeneration of after injury, 129–130, *130*
  myelinated, of tactile corpuscle, *166*

Axon *(Continued)*
  olfactory, *241*
  sprouting and regeneration of, 129–130, *130*
Axon hillock, *123*
  of neuron, *113*, 114, *116*
Axon terminal, 125
Axonal process, of rods, 247, *247*
Axonal transport, 122, *123*
Axonotmesis, 131
Axoplasm, neurofilaments in, 115
Axosomatic synapse, *123*, 124, *124*

B

B lymphocytes, 45, 99, 107, *109*, 152–153, 153t
  clusters of differentiation (CD) of, 152
  in primary cortical follicles of lymph node, 144
  memory, 99
  T lymphocytes and, 153–154
  transformed. See *Plasma cells.*
B lymphocyte–stimulating factor, 150
B nerve fibers, 120, 120t
Band patterns, in relaxed and contracted skeletal muscle, 81–82, *82*
Banded cells, 107
Bands, basophilic, *107*
  eosinophilic, *106*
  in immature neutrophils, 100
  neutrophilic, *106–107*
Bands of Büngner, 130, *130*
Barr body, 100, *101*
Basal cells, in olfactory epithelium, 241, *241*
  in respiratory epithelium, 228–229
  in taste buds, *242*, 243
  invaginations in, in specialized epithelia, *33*
  of epidermis, *30*
Basal compartment, of seminiferous epithelium, *306*, 307
Basal lamina, 56, *56*, 159
  alveolar, *237*
  of epidermis, *30*
  of glomerular endothelium, 218, *218*
  of mammary gland, *34*
  of primary ovarian follicle, *284*
  of seminiferous tubule, *306*
  of small intestine, *32*
  of specialized epithelia, *33*
  of vestibulary sensory receptor, *256*
Basal striations, in ducts of parotid gland, *205*
  in kidney tubules, *33*
  in specialized epithelia, 27–28, *33*
Basement membrane, 28, *33*, 55–57, *56–57*
  of eccrine sweat gland, *175*
  of epidermis, *159*, 164–165
  of intestinal epithelium, 27, *197*
  of respiratory epithelium, 28, *229*
  of specialized epithelial cells, *33*
  of thyroid follicle, *270*
  of uroepithelium, *31*
Basilar membrane, of cochlea, 253, *253*
  of organ of Corti, *253*
  vibrations of, 254–255, *254*
Basket cells. See *Myoepithelial cells.*
Basophilic bands, *107*
Basophilic erythroblasts, 103
Basophilic metamyelocytes, *107*
Basophilic normoblasts, 103
Basophils, 102, *102–103*, 105
  in normal adult human blood, 98t
Basophils (β cells) of hypophysis cerebri, 262–264, *262–264*

Bell stage of tooth development, *185*
Benign nodular prostatic hyperplasia (BPH), 318
Bertin, renal column of, *214*, 215
β cells, of islets of Langerhans, 276–278, *278*
BFU-E (burst-forming unit–erythroid), *109*
Bicuspid valve, 134
Bile canaliculi, at surfaces of hepatocytes, *208–209*
Bile ducts, 209–210, *210*
Bile ductule, *210*
Billroth's cords, in red pulp of spleen, 147–148, *148*
Biostructure, size dimensions in, 2
Bipolar cells, of retina, 247, *247–248*
Bipolar neuron, defined, 117
Bitemporal hemianopia, 251, *251*
Bladder, 225, *225*, 282, 304
  epithelium of, *31*
Blastocyst, 295
Blindness, 251
  color, 250
  night, 250
Blood, 97–110. See also specific cell.
  description of, 97
  growth factors, 108–110
  normal adult human, numbers and types of leukocytes in, 98, 98t
Blood cells, development of. See *Hematopoiesis.*
  in arteriole, *138*
  in red pulp of spleen, *148*
Blood clot, 102
Blood group antigens, 97
Blood plasma, 97, 103
Blood pressure regulation, renin-angiotensin-aldosterone mechanism of, 222
Blood space, placental, *296*
Blood supply, of bronchus, 232
  of digestive tract, *198*, 202–203
  of hair root, *172*
  of hypophysis cerebri, 265
  of intestine, *198*
  of lung, 238
  of pancreas, 278
  of peripheral nerve, 121, *121*
  of retina, 248, *248*
  of skin, 168, *168*
  of stomach wall, *198*
  of striated skeletal muscle, 78
Blood vessels. See also specific vessel type.
  in developing bone, *70*
  in primary ovarian follicle, *284*
Blood-testis barrier, 307
Blood-thymus barrier, 145–147
Boettcher, cells of, 253, *254*
Bone, 64–73
  cartilaginous, development of, 62, 65–66, *68–70*, 69–70
  cell types in, 64–66, *64–66*
  collagen of, 73
  compact, 67, *70–71*, 73
  ground substance of, 73
  Haversian systems of, 70–72, *71–72*
  histogenesis of, 66–70, *67–70*
  in embryonic mesenchyme, *60*
  matrix of, 72–73
  membranous, development of, 66–69, *67*
  methods of studying, 64–65
  ossification of connective tissue, 73
  woven, 67
Bone marrow, blood cell development in, *104*
  fatty, in cartilaginous bone, *72*
  granulocyte types produced in, 100, 100t
  interleukin-7 produced by, 150

Bone marrow *(Continued)*
  megakaryocytes and platelets in, 102, *103*
  primitive, *69*
  smears of, *105, 107–108*
Bone marrow cavity, of long bone, *68, 71*
Bony collar, of long bone, *69*
Booster immune response, 151, 153
Border cells, of organ of Corti, *253*
Bouin's fluid, as fixative, 3
Bowel. See *Colon; Small intestine.*
Bowman's capsule, *216*
Bowman's gland, 241–242, *241*
Bowman's membrane, *244,* 245
BPH (benign nodular prostatic hyperplasia), 318
"Brain sand," 267
Branching fibers, in cardiac muscle, 88, *88, 136*
Bridges, intercellular. See *Desmosomes.*
Broad ligament, of uterus, *283*
Bronchial tree, *228,* 231–236, *231–236.* See also specific structure.
  arteries of, 238
  epithelium of, 228t
  veins of, 238
Bronchioles, 232–233
  contracted and relaxed, *233–234*
  epithelium of, 228t
Brown fat, 48, *48,* 58
Bruch's membrane, 246
von Brücke, Ernst Wilhelm, 79
Brunner's glands, in duodenum, *197,* 200
  intestinal tract and, *178*
Brush border. See *Microvilli; Villi.*
Buccal smear, sex chromatin in, *101*
Bud stage of tooth development, *185*
Buffy coat, 97
Bulbar conjunctiva, 244
Bulbourethral glands, 318
Bundle of His, 136, *136*
Büngner, bands of, 130, *130*
Bursa, infrapatellar, *74*
Burst-forming unit–erythroid (BFU-E), *109*
Button, terminal, *123*

C

C nerve fibers, 120, 120t
Cachectin (TNF-α), 150
Calcification, endochondral, 62, 65–66, 68–70, 69–70
Calcitonin, action and regulation of, 269t
Call-Exner body, in ovarian follicle, *284*
Calyces, of kidney, 214–215, *214*
Canaliculi, bile, *209*
Cancellous bone, of skull, *73*
Cap phase, of spermiogenesis, 309
Cap stage, of tooth development, *185*
Capacitation, of spermatozoa, 289
Capillaries, 138–139, *139*
  alveolar, *235–237*
  continuous, 139, *139*
  fenestrated, *217, 270*
  in muscle, *81*
  in small intestine, *199*
  lymphatic, 168
  of seminiferous tubule, *306*
  of spleen, 149
  of suprarenal gland, *277*
  of sweat gland, *176*
  pineal, *267*
Capillary bed, airway alveolus and, *235*
Capillary/alveolar interface, 236–237, *237*
Capsular artery, of suprarenal gland, *277*
Capsular matrix, 62

Capsule, articular, *74*
  in lymphatic organs, 150t
  of corpus luteum, *287*
  of kidney, *215*
  of lymph node, 143–145, *144–145*
  of suprarenal gland, *273, 277*
  of thymus, 145, *146*
Capsule cells, surrounding autonomic ganglion cells, *116*
Carbohydrates, in plasma membrane, 10
Cardia, of stomach, *191*
Cardiac glands, 190, *190,* 194
Cardiac muscle, 88–89, *89*
  electron microscopy of, *90*
  excitation-contraction coupling in, 89–90
  fibers of, 89–91, *90–92, 136, 137*
  intercalated disks in, *88–91,* 90, *91*
  pacemaking and stimulus conduction in, 91, *91–92*
Cardiac skeleton, 134
Cardiodilatin, 90–91, 136
Cardionatrin, 90–91, 136
Cardiovascular system, 134–154
  arteries in, 137–139, *137–139.* See also specific artery.
  heart in, 134–137, *134–137*
  veins in, 139–141, *140.* See also specific vein.
Carina, of trachea, *231*
Carotid body, APUD cells of, 279t
Cartilage, 60–64, *60–63.* See also specific type.
  calcified, remodeling of, *65*
  of airway, 230, *231–232,* 232
Cartilaginous bone, development of, 68–70, 69–70
Catagen, 172
CD (clusters of differentiation), 152
Cell cycle, 22, *22*
Cell division, 21–23, *22*
Cell membrane. See *Plasma membrane.*
Cells, 2–23
  activation of, by protein hormones, *261*
  communication between, plasma membrane in, 11
  fractionation of, 6, *7*
  of connective tissue, 42–48, *42–48*
  of nervous system, 112–119
  structure and function of, 6–23
  types of, in cerebellum, *112*
  "typical" eukaryotic, 6, *8*
Cellular immune response, 99, 151–152
Cementum, *183,* 184
  deposition of, 188, *189*
Central arteries, of spleen, 149, *149*
Central veins, of liver, 207, *209*
Centrifugation, differential, *7*
Centriole, structure of, 17, *18*
Centroacinar cells, in exocrine pancreas, *207*
Ceruminous glands, 176
  of external auditory canal, 251
Cervical glands, 297
Cervix uteri, *282–283,* 292, 297–298, *297*
CFU (colony-forming unit), *109*
Characteristic frequency, of nerve fiber, 255
Cheeks, 178–179, *179*
Chief cells, of gastric gland, *192–194,* 193
  of parathyroid gland, *272*
Cholesterol, in plasma membrane, 9
Choline, in plasma membrane, 9
Chondroblasts, 60
  division of, 61, *61*
Chondrocytes, 60, *60,* 61
  in mature elastic cartilage, *62*
Chondrogenesis, 60–61, *61*

Chondroitin sulfate, tissue distribution of, 50t
Chondronectin, 55
Chorionic gonadotropin, 286
  maintenance of corpus luteum and, *294,* 295
Chorionic plate, *296*
Chorionic villi, *296,* 297
Choroid, 246
  of eye, 243
Chromaffin cells, of suprarenal gland, *276*
Chromaffin reaction, 275
Chromatin, 19–21, *21, 101*
Chromatolysis, of Nissl bodies, 129, *129*
Chromatophore, dermal, 48, *162*
Chromophil substance. See *Nissl bodies.*
Chromophobe cells, of adenohypophysis, *262, 264*
  of islets of Langerhans, 276–278, *278*
Chromosomes, 19–21, *21, 101.* See also *Meiosis.*
  metaphase, *21–22,* 23
Chylomicrons, moving across intestinal epithelial cell membrane, *198*
Cilia, *28.* See also *Microvilli; Villi.*
  motile, of respiratory tract, 27, *28, 229*
  nonmotile (stereocilia), of epididymis, 27, 32
  of vestibulary receptor, 256–257, *256*
  structure of, 17, *18*
Ciliary body, 245–246
Ciliary processes, 246
Ciliary zonules, 246
Ciliated epithelium, columnar, *26*
  columnar pseudostratified, *57*
  of airway, 228–229, *229,* 232, *232–233*
  of respiratory bronchiole, *235*
  structure and function of, 31, *32*
Circular furrow, of tongue, *181*
Circular muscle bundles, of ureter, *224*
Circular muscle layer, of appendix, *201*
  of bladder wall, *225*
  of duodenum, *197*
  of small intestine, *197–198*
  of stomach wall, *198*
  of vas deferens, *316*
Circulation, in spleen, closed vs. open, 149, *149*
Circumferential lamellae, in cartilaginous bone, *71,* 72
Circumvallate papillae, 180, *180–181*
Cis face, of Golgi complex, 15–16, *15, 114*
Cisternae, of endoplasmic reticulum, 13–14
  perinuclear, 19, *20*
Cisternal membrane, of endoplasmic reticulum, *13*
Clara's cells, in terminal bronchioles, 232
Clathrin, 10, *11*
Claudius, cells of, 253, *254*
Clavicular notch, *73*
Clear cells, 175, *175*
Clear receptor cells, in taste buds, 242
Clear terminal, of vestibulary sensory receptor, 256, *256*
Clitoris, 300
Closed circulation, in spleen, open circulation vs., 149, *149*
Clotting, of blood, 97, 102
Clubbing, of nails, 170
Clusters of differentiation (CD), of B lymphocytes, 152
Coated pits, in cell surface, 10, *11*
Coated protein, in cell surface, *11*
Coated vesicle, at cell surface, *11*
Cochlea, 252, *253*
  duct of, *254*

Cochlea *(Continued)*
  microphonic potential of, 255
  nerve of, *254*
Collagen, *159*
  banded, molecular structure of, 52
  fibers of, *42*, 49, *49–50*, 49t
    in mesentery, *43*
  in cartilage matrix, 62
  in human dermis, *49*
  of arteriole, *138*
  of axillary sweat gland, *175*
  of bone, 73
  structure of, *50*
  synthesis of, 50, *51*
  types of, 49, 49t, 50–51, 50t
Collagenous connective tissue, of lymph node, *145*
  of tongue, *180*
Collecting ducts, of kidney, 219–220, 221–222
  countercurrent multiplier and exchange mechanisms and, *224*
Collecting tubules, of kidney, *27*, 215, 219–220, 221–222, 223
Collecting veins, in spleen, 149, *149*
Colliculus seminalis, *316*
Colloid, of adenohypophysis, *262*
  of thyroid follicle, *270*
Coloboma, 246
Colon, *191*, 199–201, *200–201*
Colony-forming unit (CFU), *109*
Colony-stimulating factor (CSF), 108, 150
Color blindness, 250
Color vision, 250
Colostrum, 301–302
Columnar cells, in stratified columnar epithelium of gland, *31*
Columnar epithelium, 26, 28
  cuboidal epithelium vs., *27–28*, 31–32
  defined, 25
  locations in body, 26t
  of gallbladder wall, *210*
  of seminal vesicle, *317*
  of uterus, during menstrual cycle, *293*
  pseudostratified, in airway, 228–229, *229*, 232, *232–233*
  simple, in bronchiole, *233–234*
    in digestive tract, *27*
    lining stomach, 190–191, *190*
    of oviduct, *288*
  pseudostratified, 32–33, *32*
  stratified, 26
    and cuboidal epithelium, *31*, 35
    defined, 25
    glandular, *31*
    locations in body, 26t
Compact bone, 67
Compound glands, 36–37, *36*, 36t
  exocrine, 37
Conduction, of nerve impulses, 122
  saltatory, defined, 122
Conduction block, 131
Conductive deafness, 255
Cones, *48*, 246–247, *247–248*
Conjunctiva, 244
Connecting piece, of spermatozoon, 311
Connective tissue, 42–58
  cells of, 42–48, *42–48*
    collagenous, forming capsule of lymph node, *145*
    in dermis, *175*
    of tongue, *180*
  dense, 57, *57*
  fetal, 58, *58*
  forming capsule and septa of thymus, 145, *146*

Connective tissue *(Continued)*
  in dermis, *166*
  in hypodermis, *169*
  irregular, *42*, 57–58, *57*
  loose, *42*, *42*, 57
    of corpus luteum, *287*
  matrix of, 48–57, *49–51*, 53–57
  microscopic appearance of, *42*, 57–58, *57–58*
  mucoid, 58, *58*
  of duodenum, *197*
  of gallbladder wall, *210*
  of hair follicle, *173*
  of lymphatic organ capsules, 150t
  of tongue, *181*
  pigmented, 58, *58*
  regular, *43*, 58
  renal interstitial, 222–223
  uterine, during menstrual cycle, *293*
Contact dermatitis, T lymphocytes in, 152
Continuous capillaries, 139, *139*
Contraception, oral, 291
Contraction, of muscle, cardiac, 93–94
  molecular basis of, 86–88, *86–88*
  smooth, 93, *94*
  striated skeletal, 79
Convoluted tubules, of kidney, *216*, 218–220, *219*
Cooperativity, of immune system elements, 151
Corium. See *Dermis*.
Cornea, 244–245, *244*
Corneocytes. See *Stratum corneum*.
Corona radiata, of mature ovarian follicle, *284–285*, 285
Coronoid process, *74*
Corpora amylacea, of prostate gland, 317–318, *317*
Corpora arenacea, 267
Corpora cavernosa penis, 318, *318*
Corpus albicans, 283, 286
Corpus cavernosum urethrae, 318, *318*
Corpus luteum, 283, *283*, 286, *287*
Cortex, of cell, 18
  of hair shaft, 171, *171–172*,
  of lymph node, 144, *144*, 145
  of thymus, 145, *146–147*
  organized, in tissue from lymphatic organs, 150t
  renal, *224*
Corti, organ of, 252–254, *253–254*
Cortical nephrons, *220*, 223
Cortical reaction, in ooplasm, 289
Cortical sinus, of lymph node, *144–145*
Corticotrophs, of adenohypophysis, 262, *263*
Costal cartilage, *73*
Costal notches, *73*
Cough, smoker's, 232
Countercurrent exchange mechanism, renal/vascular, *223*, 224
Cowper's gland, *304*
Craniospinal ganglia, 119
Creases, in skin, *166*
Cricoid cartilage, 230, *231*
Crista ampullaris, 252, *256*
Cristae, of mitochondrion, 12, *12*
Cross-bridges, of myosin filaments, 84–85
Cross-linking, of collagen, 49, *50*
Crown, of tooth, *182*, *183*
Cryostat, 5
Crypt of Lieberkühn, *28*
  at rectoanal junction, *202*
  in appendix, *201*
  in colon, *191*, 200
  in duodenum, *197*
  in small intestine, 196–197, *197–200*

Crypt of Lieberkühn *(Continued)*
  tonsillar, 143
CSF (colony-stimulating factor), 108, 150
Cuboidal epithelium, 26, 27
  columnar epithelium vs., *27–28*, 31–32
  defined, 25
  in respiratory bronchiole, *235*
  locations in body, 26t
  simple, in kidney tubules, *27*
  stratified, 26
    and columnar epithelium, *31*, 35
    defined, 25
    follicular cells surrounding ovum, *30*
    locations in body, 26t
Cumulus oophorus, 285, *285*
  free surface of, *30*
  of mature ovarian follicle, *284*
Cutaneous area, of lips, 178–179, *179*
Cuticle, of hair shaft, 171, *171–172*
  of inner root sheath of hair, *171–172*, 172
  of nail, 169
Cutis. See *Skin*.
Cycle, menstrual. See *Menstrual cycle*.
  of seminiferous epithelium, 311–312, *313*
Cysts, Nabothian, *297*, 298
Cytochemistry, 4–5
Cytocrines, secretion of, 163
Cytokines, 108, 150–151. See also specific cytokine.
Cytokinesis, 23
Cytology, defined, 2
Cytomatrix, 11
Cytoplasm, 6, 11, *11*
Cytoplasmic body, residual, development of, *310*
Cytoskeleton, 11, 16
  intermediate filaments, 19, 19t
  microfilaments, 18
  microtubules, 16–18, *18*
Cytosol. See *Cytoplasm*.
Cytotoxic T (Tc) lymphocytes, 152
Cytotoxicity, antibody-dependent cell-mediated (ADCC), 152
Cytotrophoblast, 295, *296*

D

Dark adaptation, 249–250
Dark cells, of eccrine sweat gland, 175
Deafness, 255
Decidua, 295–297, *296*
Degranulation, of mast cells, *45*
Delayed-type hypersensitivity T (Tdh) lymphocytes, 152
δ basophils, of adenohypophysis, 264, *264*
δ cells, of islets of Langerhans, 276–278, *278*
Delta granules, in granulomere region of platelet, 102
Demilunes, serous cells in, in salivary glands, *205*
Demyelination, defined, 122
Dendrites, *113*, 115–116, 117, *123*
  retrograde changes in after nerve cell injury, 129
Dendritic cells. See *Melanocytes*.
  epidermal. See *Langerhans' cells*.
Dendrodendritic synapse, 124
Denervation atrophy, 77
Dense bodies, in smooth muscle, 93
Dense core terminal, of vestibulary sensory receptor, 256, *256*
Dense receptor cells, in taste buds, 242
Dental follicle, 185, *187–188*
Dental lamina, 185–186, *188*
  permanent, *187*

Dental papilla, *185–186*
   in developing tooth, *188*
Dental pulp, *187*
Dental sac, 185, *188*
Dentin, 182–184, *183*
   formation of, 186–187, *187–188*
Dermal papillae, *127, 166, 181*
Dermal sheath, of hair follicle, *171, 172*
Dermatan sulfate, tissue distribution of, 50t
Dermatitis, contact, T lymphocytes in, 152
Dermis, *30, 49,* 156t, *162,* 165, *165–166, 175*
   lymphatic capillaries of, 168
   of foot, shoulder, and scalp, *157*
   of nail bed, *169*
   papillary layer of, 165, *166*
   reticular layer of, 165, *165*
Descemet's membrane, 245
Desmin, 19t, 86
Desmosomes, formed by epithelial cells of small intestine, *32*
   formed by stratified squamous epithelium, 27, *32*
   in cardiac muscle, 90
   in epithelial cells of skin, *32*
   in stratified columnar epithelial cells, *131*
   in stratified squamous epithelium, 34
   in stratum spinosum, *159, 160*
Desquamation, in stratified squamous epithelium, *161*
Diads, in striated cardiac muscle, 90
Diaphysis, of long bone, *68,* 69
   penetration of vessels into, *69*
Diarthroses, *74, 75*
Diastole, 137
Differential interference microscopy, 4
Diffuse neuroendocrine system, 279, 279t
Digestive tract, 178–211. See also specific organ.
   blood supply to, *198,* 202–203
   cells of, 194, 195t
   description and functions of, *178, 178*
   lymphatics of, 203
Digestive tube, 188–203. See also specific organ.
   blood supply to, *198,* 202–203
   description of, *178,* 188–189
   lymphatics of, 203
   smooth muscle of, *95*
Dioptric system, of eye, 243–244
Diploë, 67
Diplotene, mixing of parental genomes in, 307–308
Discontinuous capillaries, *139, 139*
Disks, intervertebral, *74*
Distal convoluted tubule, countercurrent multiplier and exchange mechanisms and, *224*
   macula densa of, 222
Distributing arteries, 138, *138*
Disulfide bonds, *51*
Disuse atrophy, 77
DNA, nuclear organizer, 21
Dorsal root ganglia, 119
Duct cells, striated, of salivary gland, *206*
Duct glands, 36t
Ductless glands, 36t
Ducts, collecting, of kidney, 219–220, 221–222
   countercurrent multiplier and exchange mechanisms and, *224*
   ejaculatory, 315
   excurrent system of, 314–315, *314–316*
   extratesticular, 314–315, *315–316*
   in exocrine gland, *38*
   intratesticular, 304–305, *304, 314, 314*
   of intestinal tract, *178*

Ducts *(Continued)*
   of salivary glands, 205–206, *205–206*
   of sweat glands, *175*
   prostatic, *316*
Ductules, bile, *210*
   efferent, *57*
   of testis, 304, *304,* 314
Ductus deferens, *304*
Duodenum, *191*
Dynein, 17
   in cilia, 17–18, *18*
   in fast retrograde axonal transport, 122

E

Ear, 251–252
von Ebner, serous glands of, *181*
Eccrine sweat glands, *170,* 174–176, *174–175*
Ectopic ossification, 73
Ectopic pregnancy, 288
Effector phase, in life of cytotoxic T lymphocyte, 152
   of cellular immune response, 152
Effector T lymphocytes, types of, 151–152
Efferent arteriole, of renal corpuscle, 216
Efferent ducts, *57*
   of testis, 304, *304,* 314
Efferent lymphatic vessels, of lymph node, *144*
Efferent nerve fiber endings, 128, *128*
Egg, capture and transport of, 288–289
Ehlers-Danlos syndromes, 52
Ejaculatory ducts, 315, *316*
Elastic arteries, 137, *137*
   near lymph node, *145*
Elastic cartilage, 62–63, *62*
Elastic lamina, internal, in arteriole, *138*
Elastica interna, in vena cava, *140*
Elastin fibers, in connective tissue, *42,* 52–53, *54*
   in dermis, *49*
   in elastic cartilage, *62,* 63
   in mesentery, *43*
   in vena cava, *140*
Elaunin, 53
Elbow joint, *74*
Electrical synapse, 124
Electromagnetic spectrum, microscopy and, *3*
Electron cytochemistry, 5
Electron microscopy, limit of resolution in, 2, *3*
   preparation of tissues for, 3–4
Eleiden, in stratum lucidum, 160
Embedment, for microscopy, 3
Embryo, implantation of, *294,* 295
Embryonic connective tissue, *58, 58*
E-mega (erythrocyte/megakaryocyte progenitor cell), *109*
Enamel, 182, *183*
   cervical loop of, *188*
Enamel cap, *187*
Enamel epithelium, *187–188*
   reduced, 187–188
Enamel organ, *186*
   enamel deposition and, *185,* 187–188, *188*
   primordium of, *186, 188*
End bulbs of Krause, *127,* 128
End piece, of spermatozoon tail, 311, *311*
Endocardium, *92, 134, 136*
Endochondral ossification, 62, 65–66, *68–70,* 69–70
Endocrine glands, 25, 38–39, *38,* 259, 259t
Endocrine system, 259–279. See also specific gland or system.

Endocrine system *(Continued)*
   description and function of, 259–260, *259–261,* 259t, 260t
Endocytosis, 10–11, *11*
Endocytosis vesicle, 10, *11*
Endolymph, 252
Endolysosomes, 16, *17*
Endometrial stroma, 292
Endometrium, *283,* 292
   during menstrual cycle, *293*
   of pregnancy, 295–296, *296*
Endomysium, *78,* 79
Endoneurium, 116–117, 120–121, *120–121*
Endoplasmic reticulum (ER), 13–15, *13–15*. See also *Rough endoplasmic reticulum (RER); Smooth endoplasmic reticulum (SER)*.
   granular, 114, *114*
   in hepatocyte, *208*
   in "typical" cell, *8*
   isolation of, *7*
Endosome, 10, *11*
Endosteum, 64
Endothelium, 25
   cardiac, *136*
   corneal, 245
   fenestrated, 218, *218*
   in mesentery, *43*
   interleukin-8 produced by, 150
   vimentin filaments in, 28
Enzymatic cleavage, *51*
Enzyme histochemistry, 5
Eosin, 3, 44
Eosinopenia, 101
Eosinophilia, 98, 101
Eosinophilic bands, *106*
Eosinophilic metamyelocytes, *106*
Eosinophilic myelocytes, *106*
Eosinophiloblasts, *109*
Eosinophils, 46, 101–102, *101*
   in jejunum, *48*
   in lamina propria, *46*
   in normal adult human blood, 98t
   mature, *109*
   segmented, *106*
Ependymal cells, 118, *119*
Epicardium, 134, *134*
Epidermal dendritic cells. See *Langerhans' cells.*
Epidermal pegs, *166*
   in Meissner's corpuscle, *127*
   of tongue, *181*
Epidermis, 156–165, *163*
   basement membrane of, *159,* 164–165
   description of, 156, *158*
   epithelial cells of, 156–162, 156t, *157–161*
   keratinization of, 161–162, *161*
   nonepithelial cells of, 162–165, *162–163*
   of lip, *186*
Epididymis, 304, *304,* 314–315, *315*
Epiglottis, *180,* 228, *230*
   epithelium of, 228t
Epimysium, 79, *81*
Epinephrine, norepinephrine vs., 275t
   secreted by medulla of suprarenal gland, 274–275
Epineurium, 117, 120, *120–121*
Epiphyseal cartilage, 69
Epiphyseal cavity, *68*
Epiphyseal line, *71*
Epiphyseal plate, 69
Epiphysis, *68,* 69
Episclera, 244
Epithelial pearls, *187*
Epithelial reticular cells, in thymus, 145–147, *146–147*

Epithelial sheet, basal lamina and, *56*
Epithelium, 25–39. See also specific type or site.
  classification of, 25–28, *26*, 26t
  defined, 25
  glandular, classification of, *36*, 36t
    compound, 36–37, *36*
    endocrine, 38–39, *38*
    exocrine, 27–28, *33*, 37–38, *37–38*
    simple, 36, *36*
  of airway, 228–229, 228t, *229*
  of lymphatic organs, 150t
  of small intestine, 195–196, *198–199*
  simple, cuboidal/columnar, 27–28, 31–34, *33*, *34*
    pigmented, *29*, 34
    pseudostratified, 32–33, *32*
    squamous, *27*, 28–31
    specialized, 31, *33*
    stratified, keratinized, *30*, *32*, 34–35
      nonkeratinized, *30*, 35
      squamous, *30*, *32*, 34–35
    transitional, *26*, 26t, *31*, 35, 223–224
      of lower urinary tract, *224–225*
      of male reproductive system, *316–317*
Eponychium, 169
ER. See *Endoplasmic reticulum (ER)*.
Erectile bodies, of penis, 318, *318*
Erythroblasts, 44
  acidophilic, 105
  basophilic, 103
  early, 103
  intermediate, 105
  late, 105
  normochromatic, 105
  orthochromatic, 105
  polychromatophilic, *97*, 105
Erythrocyte/megakaryocyte progenitor cells (E-mega), *109*
Erythrocytes, 44, 97–98, *97*, *99*, 105
  destroyed in spleen, 149
  development of, *104*
  diffusely basophilic, 105
  in alveolar capillary, *236*
  in liver sinusoid, *210*
  mature, 105, *106*, *108*, *108–109*
  phagocytosis of, *43*
  polychromatic, 105
  polychromatophilic, 105
Erythropoiesis, 103–105, *104–105*
Erythropoietin, 105
  as growth factor in hematopoiesis, 108
Esophagus, 189–190, *189–191*, 228
  epithelium of, *30*
  gastric junction with, glands in, 190, *190*
Estradiol, 285–286
Estrogen, mammary gland development and, 301
  uterine changes and, *290*
Estrus cycle, 286
Euchromatin, 19, *20*
Eumelanin, 163
Eustachian tube, 251
Excitation-contraction coupling, in striated cardiac muscle, 89–90
Excretory ducts, of salivary glands, 205–206, *205*
Excurrent duct system, 314–315, *314–316*
Exocrine glands, 37–38, *37–38*
  duct system in, 38, *38*
Exocrine pancreas, 206–207, *207*
Exocytosis, 10–11, *11*, *15*, 265
External ear, 251
Extracellular hydrated gel. See *Ground substance*.
Extracellular leaflets, of plasma membrane, *9*

Extrafusal muscle fibers, 79
Extratesticular ducts, 314–315, *315–316*
Extrinsic coat, 10
Eye, conjunctiva of, 244
  cornea of, 244–245, *244*
  eyelid of, 251
  lacrimal gland of, 251
  lens of, 246
  pigment-containing cells of, *48*
  retina of, 246–250, *247–248*
  sclera of, 244
  uvea of, 245
  visual pathways of, 250–251, *251*
  vitreous body of, 246
Eyelid, 251

F

F-actin filament, *80*
Fallopian tube. See *Oviduct*.
False ribs, 73
Fascia, superficial, 168, *169–170*, 174
Fascia adherens, in cardiac muscle, 90
Fascicles in muscles, 77–79, *80*
Fascin, 18
Fat cells, 46–48, *48*. See also *Adipose tissue*.
  brown, 48, *48*, 58
  in dermis, *169*
  in salivary gland, *204*
  in tongue, *180*
  in ureter, *224*
  in wall of colon, *200*
  subpatellar, *74*
  surrounding external anal sphincter, *202*
Fatty acids, in plasma membrane, *9*
  metabolism of, *12*
Female reproductive system. See also specific structure or process.
  description and functions of, 282, *282–283*
Femur, *74*
Fenestrae, endothelial, 218, *218*
Fenestrated capillaries, 139, *139*, *270*
Fertility, sperm production and, 312
Fertilization, *288*, 289, *294*
Fetal chorionic villi, maternal blood space and, *296*
Fetal connective tissue, 58, *58*
Fetal mesenchyme, *296*
Fetal/placental circulation, *296*, 297
Feulgen reaction, 4–5
Fibers, elastic. See *Elastin fibers*.
Fibrinogen, 103
Fibroblasts, 43
  in connective tissue, *42–43*
  in dermis, *49*, *162*
  synthesis of, 52
Fibrocartilage, 63–64, *63*
  collagen types in, 51
Fibrocytes, *42–43*, 43
Fibronectin, 55, *56*
Fibrosa, of esophagus, *189*, 190
Fibrous sheath, of spermatid flagellum, *310*
  of spermatozoon tail, 311, *311*
Filaggrin, in stratum corneum, 161
Filiform papillae, *180–181*
Filopodia, of growth cones, 130, *130*
Filtration slits, of renal capillary endothelium, 218, *218*
Fimbriae, of oviduct, *283*, *288*
Fimbrin, 18
Fine structure, defined, 2
Fingernails, 169, *169*
Fingerprints, 166
Fixatives, 3

Flagellum, contraction of, 309
  development of, *310*
Flexure lines, of skin, 166
Floating ribs, 73
Flower-spray nerve fiber endings, 128, *128*
Fluid-mosaic model of membrane structure, 9, *9*
Fluorescence labeling, *5*
Foliate papillae, *180–181*
Follicles, 38
  dental, 185, *187–188*
  hair, 171–172, *171–172*
  lymph node, 144
  ovarian. See *Ovarian follicle*.
  thyroid, 30, 38, 268, 270
Follicle-stimulating hormone (FSH), action and regulation of, 262t
  ovarian follicle and, 290, *290–291*
  secreted by adenohypophysis, *264*
Follicular phase, of ovarian cycle, uterine changes and, *290*
Follicular regulatory protein, 286
Fontanelle, 67
Foot, skin of, *157*
Foramen caecum, *180*
Formaldehyde, 3
Formalin, 3
Forming face *(cis)*, of Golgi complex, 15–16, *15*, *114*
Fornix, vaginal, *282–283*, 292, 297
Fovea centralis, *247–248*
Fractionation, of cells, 6, *7*
Freeze-fracture microscopy, 3–4
FSH. See *Follicle-stimulating hormone (FSH)*.
Fundus, gastric, *191*
  uterine, *283*, 291–292
Fungiform papillae, of tongue, 180, *180*, 242
Fuzzy coat, 10

G

G_0 phase, 22
G_1 phase, 22, *22*
G_2 phase, 22, *22*
G-actin molecules, *80*
GAG-proteins. See *Glycosaminoglycans*.
Galea aponeurotica, *170*
Gallbladder, *210*, 211
Gametogenesis, 304
Gamma efferent nerve fiber endings, 128, *128*
Gamma globulins, in blood plasma, 103
Ganglion(a), *113*, *116*, 119
  of Auerbach's plexus, *197*
  of retina, *247*, 248
  sympathetic, APUD cells of, 279t
GAP (growth-associated proteins), 123
Gap junctions, in bone, 64
  in neural tissue, 124
  in small intestine, 32
  in smooth muscle, 93
  in striated cardiac muscle, 90, *91*
  plasma membrane and, 11
Gastric glands, 191–194, *193–194*, 195t, *196*
Gastric pits, *191*
Gastrocnemius muscle, *80*
Gastroenteropancreatic endocrine (GEP) system, 278
Gastrula, *294*
G-CSF (granulocyte colony-stimulating factor), 150
  as growth factor in hematopoiesis, 108
Gelsolin, 18
Gemmules, on dendrite, 117
Geniculate nucleus, lateral, 251, *251*

Geniculocalcarine tract, *251*
Genitalia, female, *282,* 300
 male, 304, *304*
GEP (gastroenteropancreatic endocrine) system, 278
Germ cells, female, 283
 male, 304, 307–309, *308, 310*
Germinal center, in lymph nodule, 143, *143, 145*
 secondary, *144*
Germinal epithelium, of ovary, 283
Germinal matrix, 169, *169*
Germinal vesicle, of primary ovarian follicle, 285
GFAP (glial fibrillary acidic protein), in astrocytes, 117
GH (growth hormone), 262t, *263*
Gingiva, *183,* 184
Glands, 35–39, *36–38,* 36t. See also specific gland or site.
 classification of, 36t
 compound, 36–37, *36*
 description and functions of, 35, *36*
 endocrine, 38–39, *38*
 exocrine, 37–38, *37–38*
 large, emptying into intestinal tract, *178*
 mixed tracheal, *231*
 of Moll, 176
 of Montgomery, 173–174
 simple, 36, *36*
 stratified columnar epithelium of, *31*
 unicellular, 26, 31–32, *33*
 locations in body, 26t
 uterine, during menstrual cycle, *293*
Glans clitoridis, *282,* 300
Glans penis, *304*
Glassy membrane, of hair follicle, *171–172,* 172
 of ovarian follicle, 286
Glial cells, function of, 118–119
Glial fibrillary acidic protein (GFAP), in astrocytes, 117
Glial filaments, 19t
Globular units, mitochondrial, 12
Glomerular filtration barrier, *217, 218,* 218
Glomeruli, *215*
Glottis, *231*
Glucagon, action and regulation of, 277t
Glucocorticoids, action and regulation of, 275t
Glutaraldehyde, 3
Glycerol, in plasma membrane, *9*
Glycocalyx, 10
Glycogen granules, in cardiac muscle, 89, *90*
 in hepatocyte, *208*
Glycolipids, in plasma membrane, 9–10, *9*
Glycoproteins, in plasma membrane, *9*
 structural, 54–55, *54,* 56
Glycosaminoglycans, 55
 in cartilage matrix, 62
 tissue distribution of, 50, 50t
GM-CSF (granulocyte-macrophage colony-stimulating factor), 150
 as growth factor in hematopoiesis, 108
GnRH (gonadotropin-releasing hormone), FSH and LH and, 290, *291*
Goblet cells, 37
 in bronchial epithelium, 232
 in colon, *200*
 in columnar epithelium, *57*
 in duodenal lining, *196*
 in intestinal epithelium, *198–199*
 in intestinal villus, *197*
 in respiratory epithelium, 228, *229*
 secretions of, 238t

Goblet cells *(Continued)*
 structure and function of, 27–28, 31–32, *33*
Gold/protein A labeling, 5
Golgi complex, *14,* 15–16, *15–16,* 114, *114*
 in Brunner's gland, *200*
 in digestive tract epithelium, *27,* 198
 in fibroblast, *51*
 in hepatocyte, *208*
 in myoepithelial cell, *34*
 in nerve cell, *123*
 in neuron, *116*
 in pancreatic acinar cell, *207*
 in respiratory epithelial cell, *28*
 in salivary gland cells, *204, 206*
 in secretory cell, *32*
 in seminiferous epithelial cells, *306*
 in "typical" cell, *8*
Golgi hydrolase vesicle, 16, *17*
Golgi phase, of spermiogenesis, 309
Golgi tendon organ, *77,* 79, 128–129, *128*
Golgi-Mazzoni corpuscle, 127
Gonadocorticoids, action and regulation of, 275t
Gonadotrophs (δ basophils), of adenohypophysis, 264, *264*
Gonadotropin, chorionic, 286
 pituitary, uterine changes and, *290*
Gonadotropin-releasing hormone (GnRH), FSH and LH and, 290, *291*
Goose bumps, of scalp, 173, *173*
Graafian follicle, *284,* 286
Graft-vs.-host reaction, T lymphocytes in, 152
Granular cell layer, of esophageal epithelium, *30*
Granular layer, of Tomes, *183*
Granular membrane, of mature ovarian follicle, *284*
Granule cells, small, in respiratory epithelium, 229
Granules, in mast cells, *42–43,* 44, *45*
 in neutrophils, 101
Granulocyte colony-stimulating factor (G-CSF), 150
 as growth factor in hematopoiesis, 108
Granulocyte-macrophage colony-stimulating factor (GM-CSF), 150
 as growth factor in hematopoiesis, 108
Granulocytes, 44. See also specific type.
 description of, 100, 100t
 development of, 105–107, *106–107*
Granulomere, of platelet, 102
Granulosa, of developing ovarian follicle, *284,* 285
Granulosa lutein cells, *101,* 286, *287*
Ground substance, in connective tissue cells, 49, 54–55, *54–56*
 of bone matrix, 73
Growth cone, of regenerating nerve fiber, 129–130, *130*
Growth factors, in hematopoiesis, 108–110, *109–110.* See also specific growth factor.
 T-cell (interleukin-2), 150
Growth hormone (GH), 262t, *263*
Growth-associated proteins (GAP), *123*
Gums, 179, *187*
Gustatory neuroepithelium, *26,* 29

H

H zone, in skeletal muscle, *78,* 80–82, *81–82, 84*
Hair bulb, 171–172, *171*
Hair cells, of inner ear, 253, *253–254,* 256–257, *256*

Hairs, *93,* 170–173, *170–173*
Hard palate, 179
Hassall's corpuscles, in thymus, 145–146, *146–147,* 150t
Haversian canals, in cartilaginous bone, *71*–72
 in membranous bone, 67
Haversian lamellae, in cartilaginous bone, *71*
Haversian systems, 70–72, *71–72*
H&E (hematoxylin and eosin) stain, 3
Head, of spermatozoon, *311*
Hearing, assessment of, 255
 cochlea in, 252, *253*
 ear, general description of, 251–252
 impairment of, 255
 mechanics of, 252
 organ of Corti in, 253–254, *253–254*
 physiology of, 254–255
Heart, 134–136, *135*
 APUD cells of, 279t
 atrial fibers of, polypeptide hormones in, 90–91
Heavy chains, in myosin molecule, 84, *84*
Helicotrema, *253*
Helly's fluid, 3
Helper T lymphocytes, 99
Hematocrit, 98
Hematopoiesis. See also specific cell or process.
 description of, 103, *104*
 erythropoiesis and, 103–105, *105*
 granulopoiesis and, 105–107, *106–107*
 growth factors and, 108–110, *109–110*
 lymphocytopoiesis and, 107
 megakaryocytopoiesis and, 108, *108*
 monocytopoiesis and, 107–108, *108*
 spleen and, 149
Hematoxylin, 4–5, 44
Hematoxylin stain, 3
 Verhoeff's, for elastin, 51–52
Hemianopia, *251, 251*
Hemidesmosomes, 35
 attaching stratum basale to basal lamina, 156, *159*
 formed by epithelial cells of small intestine, *32*
Hemochorial placenta, 297
Hemocytoblasts, *105*
Hemoglobin, 98
Henle, loops of, *27,* 218–221, *219*
 countercurrent multiplier and exchange mechanisms and, *224*
 vasa recta and, 223, *223*
Henle's layer, of inner root sheath of hair shaft, *171,* 172
Hensen, cells of, 253–254, *253–254*
Heparin, tissue distribution of, 50t
Hepatic acinus, 208, *209*
Hepatic arteriole, *210*
Hepatic artery, *209*
Hepatic cord, *209*
Hepatic lobule, as unit of hepatic function, 208, *209*
Hepatocytes, *207–210*
Herring body, *266*
Heterochromatic staining, of lymphocytic nuclei, 45
Heterochromatin, 19, *20*
Hilum, of kidney, *214*
 of lung, 231
 of lymph node, 144–145, *144*
Hinges, of myosin cross-bridges, 84–85
Hip, *74,* 75
Histiocytes, phagocytic, *108*
 in diarthroses, 75

Histochemistry, 4–5
  enzyme, 5
Histocompatibility complex, major (MHC), 151
  restriction of cytotoxic T cells by, 152
Histology, defined, 2, *2*
HLA (human leukocyte antigens), 151
  cytotoxic T cell restriction and, 152
Holocrine glands, 37, *37*
Holocrine secretion, 174
  of apocrine glands, 176
Homonymous hemianopia, 251, *251*
Horizontal association cells, of retina, 247, *247*
Hormones, 259–260, *260–261*, 260t
  adenohypophysial, 262t
    secretion mechanisms of, 165
  feedback mechanisms and, *291*
  of adrenal cortex, 274, 275t
  of adrenal medulla, 275t
  polypeptide, in atrial fibers of heart, 90–91
  types of, 260t
Horny cells. See *Stratum corneum*.
Howship's lacunae, 66
Humerus, *74*
Humoral immunologic responses, 151
Huxley's layer, of inner root sheath of hair shaft, *171*, 172
Hyaline cartilage, 60–62, *60–61*
  of airway, 231, *231–233*
Hyaline membrane disease, 236
Hyalomere, of platelet, 102
Hyaluronic acid, in proteoglycans, 55
  tissue distribution of, 50t
Hybridization, in situ, 6
Hydroxylysine, 50
Hydroxyproline, 50
Hyperimmune response, modulated by T suppressor lymphocytes, 152
Hypochromic anemia, 98
Hypodermis, 168, *169–170*, *174*
Hypophysis cerebri, adenohypophysis of, 260–265, *262–264*, 262t
  blood supply of, 265
  description and function of, 260, *261*
  endocrine functions of, 259t
  neurohypophysis of, 265, 265t, *266*
Hypothalamus, APUD cells of, 279t
  control of neurohypophysis and, *266*
  endocrine functions of, 259t

I

I band(s), in skeletal muscle, *78*, 79–81, *80–81*, *83*, *85*
  in contraction, 81–82, *82*, *86*, *86*
ICSH (interstitial cell–stimulating hormone), action and regulation of, 262t
Ig (immunoglobulin), 153, 153t
  surface (sIg), 151
IL. See *Interleukins (IL)*.
Immune interferon, 150
Immune response, primary vs. secondary, 153
Immune system, 149–154
  cellular response of, 99, 151–152
  cytokines in, 150–151. See also specific cytokine.
  description and functions of, 143, 149–150
  humoral response in, 151
  lymphocytes in, 151–154, 153t. See also specific cell.
  major histocompatibility complex in, 151
Immunization, booster, 151

Immunoblasts, 107, 143, 145
Immunocompetence, defined, 143
Immunocytochemistry, 5, *5*
Immunoglobulins, 153, 153t
  surface (sIg), 151
Immunologic memory, 151
Implantation, of embryo, *294*, *295*
Impulse conduction, in heart, sequence of, *136*
Incisura angularis gastris, *191*
Inclusions, cytoplasmic, 11
Incremental lines of Retzius, 182, *183*
Induction phase, of cellular immune response, 152
Infrapatellar bursa, *74*
Infundibulum, of hair follicle, 172
  of hypophysis cerebri, *261*
  of oviduct, *283*, 287–288, *288*
Inhibin, 307
Inhibitory postsynaptic potential (IPSP), 249
Initial segment, of neuron, 114
Inner ear, 252
Insulin, action and regulation of, 277t
Integral membrane protein, 10
Integument. See *Skin*.
Interalveolar septa, cells of, 236–238, *236–237*
Intercalated disks, in cardiac muscle, 88–91, *90*, 136, *136*
Intercalated ducts, of salivary glands, 205–206, *205–206*
Intercapsular matrix, 62
Intercellular bridges, *32*, 306
Intercisternal vesicles, in Golgi complex, 15
Intercostal spaces, 73
Interferon, 150
Interleukins (IL), 150
  as growth factors in hematopoiesis, 108
Interlobular artery and vein, of kidney, *214–215*, *220*, *223*
Intermediate filaments, 16, 19, 19t
  in skeletal muscle, *78*, 83, *83*
  in smooth muscle, 93–94, *94*
Intermediate normoblasts, 105
Intermediate sinus, of lymph node, *144*
Intermembranous space, of mitochondrion, 12, *12*
Interphase, 22, *22*
Interrod substance, of tooth enamel, 182
Interstitial cell–stimulating hormone (ICSH), action and regulation of, 262t
Interstitial connective tissue, of interalveolar septum, 237
  of kidney, 222–223
  of oocyte, *284*
  of testis, 304, *305*
  of uterus, during menstrual cycle, *293*
"Interstitial growth," 61
Interstitial lamellae, in cartilaginous bone, *71*, 72, *72*
Interstitial space, in interalveolar septa, 237
Interterritorial matrix, 62
Interventricular septum, *135*
Intervertebral disks, *74*
Intestine. See *Colon; Small intestine*.
Intracellular space, in plasma membrane, *9*
Intracristal space, of mitochondrion, 12, *12*
Intraepithelial glands, 37, *37*
Intrafusal muscle fibers, *79*
  nuclear bag and nuclear chain, 128, *128*
Intramembranous ossification, 66–69, *67*
Intramural ganglion, 119
Intratesticular ducts. See also specific structure.
  description and functions of, 304–305, *304*, 314, *314*

Iodide, thyroid cell and, *271*
Iodopsin, 247
IPSP (inhibitory postsynaptic potential), 249
Iris, 245
  epithelium of, 58, *58*
Iron deficiency, 98
Ischium, *74*
Islets of Langerhans, 276–278, 277t, *278*
  endocrine functions of, 259t
Isometric contraction, 86–88, *88*
Isotonic contraction, *86–88*, 88
Isotrophy, 79–81, *81*
Isthmus, of oviduct, *283*, 287, *288*
  of thyroid gland, 267

J

Jejunum. See also *Small intestine*.
  epithelium of, *198*
  plasma cells in, *48*
JG (juxtaglomerular apparatus), 222
Joints, 73–75, *73–74*
Junctional complexes, in seminiferous epithelium, 306
  in small intestinal epithelium, *32*
Junctional folds, in postsynaptic membrane of muscle, 125
Juxtaglomerular apparatus (JG), 222
Juxtaglomerular cells, *216*, 222
Juxtaglomerular nephron, 220, *220*
Juxtamedullary nephron, 223

K

Kartagener's immotile cilia syndrome, 18
Karyotype, 20, *21*
Keith-Flack node, 91, 136
Keratan sulfate, in proteoglycan aggregates, 55
  tissue distribution of, 50t
Keratin filaments, 19, 19t, *159*
  in small intestinal epithelium, *32*
Keratinization, 161–162, *161*
Keratinized skin, cross section of, *157*, *158*
Keratinocytes, *163*
Keratohyalin, 35
Keratohyalin granules, in stratified squamous epithelium, *161*
Kidney, 214–223. See also specific structure.
  description and function of, 214–215, *214–215*
  fetal, *273*
  interstitial tissue of, 222–223
  juxtaglomerular apparatus of, 222
  regulation of urine concentration by, histopathology of, 223, *223–224*
  tubular system of, 217–222, *217–220*
  urine production in, 215–216
  vascular system of, 215–216, *216–217*, *220*, *223*, *223–224*
Killer cells, 99, 152
Kinesin, 17
  in fast anterograde axonal transport, 122
Kinocilium, in vestibulary sensory receptor, 256, *256*
Knee joint, *74*
Korff's fibers, 186
Krause's corpuscles, *127*, 128
Kupffer's cells, immune response and, 151
  lining liver sinusoids, *210*

L

Labeling, fluorescence, *15*

Labia, *282*, 300
Labiogingival groove, *186*
Labiogingival lamina, *185*
Labyrinth, of inner ear, 252
Lacrimal caruncle, 244
Lacrimal gland, 251
Lactation, 301–302, *301*
Lacteal, central, in intestinal villus, *198*
Lactiferous ducts, *299*, 300–301
Lactiferous sinuses, *299*, 300
Lacunae, endometrial, 295
　in cartilage, 60–61, *62*
　in cartilaginous bone, *71*
LAF (lymphocyte-activating factor), 150
LAK (lymphokine-activated killer) cell, 152
Lambda granules, in granulomere region of platelet, 102
Lamellae, in cartilaginous bone, 71–72, *71*
　in membranous bone, 67
Lamellar bodies, 160
Lamellipodia, of growth cones, 130, *130*
Lamina densa, *33*, 56, *56*
Lamina lucida, 56
Lamina propria, 28–29, *31*, *57*
　at rectoanal junction, *202*
　cells in, *46*
　of cervix, 297
　of colon, *200*
　of digestive tract, 27, *178*
　of esophagus, 189–190
　of gallbladder, *210*
　of larynx, 230, *231*
　of seminal vesicle, *317*
　of small intestine, 197, *197–198*
　of stomach, 190–192
　of tongue, *180*
　of trachea, *229*
　of ureter, *224*
　of uterine lining, during menstrual cycle, *293*
　of vaginal wall, *298*
　of vas deferens, *316*
Lamina rara, *33*, 56
Lamina reticularis, 56
　of basement membrane, *33*
Laminin, 55, *56*
Langerhans, islets of, 276–278, 277t, *278*
　endocrine functions of, 259t
Langerhans' cells, *163*, 164
　immune response and, 151
Lanugo, 173
Large intestine, *191*, 199–202, *200–202*. See also specific segment.
Larynx, *228*, 230, *231*
　epithelium of, 228t
Lens, 246
Leptotene spermatocyte (L), *313*
Leukoblasts, 105, 107
Leukocytes, agranulocytic, 99–100, *99–100*. See also specific type.
　description and functions of, 98–99, 98t
　destruction of, 149
　development of, *104*
　granulocytic, 100–102, *100–102*, 100t. See also specific type.
　polymorphonuclear. See Neutrophils.
Leukocytosis, 98
Leukopenia, 98
Levator ani muscle, *202*
Leydig cells, 304, *305–306*, 312–314
LH. See Luteinizing hormone (LH).
Lieberkühn, crypts of, *178*
　at rectoanal junction, *202*
　in appendix, *201*
　in colon, *200*
　in small intestine, *197–198*

Ligament, broad, of uterus, *283*
　ovarian, *282*
　round, of uterus, *282*
　spiral, 253, *254*
　suspensory, of lens, 246
　transverse acetabular, *74*
Ligamentum teres, *74*
Light adaptation, 250
Light chains, in myosin molecule, 84, *84*
Light microscopy (LM), limit of resolution in, 2, *3*
　preparation of tissues for, 2–3
Limiting membranes, of cornea, anterior, 244, 245
　posterior, 245
　of retina, 247
Lingual papillae, 180, *180*
Lingual tonsil, 143
　crypt of, *181*
Lining cells, in red pulp of spleen, *148*
Lipid bilayer, in plasma membrane, 9, *11*
Lipid droplets, in red muscle fibers, 83
　in seminiferous epithelium, 306
　in "typical" cell, *8*
Lipids, in plasma membranes, classes of, 9
　intestinal absorption of, *198*
　synthesis of, *12*
Lipochrome pigment, in nerve cells, 114, *115*
Lipocytes. See Adipose tissue; Fat cells.
Lipofuscin, 16
Lips, 178–179, *179*, 185–186
Liquor folliculi, *284*, 285
Liver, 207–211, *207–210*
　bile ducts of, *209–210*, 210
　blood supply to, 208–210, *209–210*
　cells of, *207–210*
　description of, 207
　function of, 210–211
　parenchyma of, 207–208, *207–209*
　sinusoids of, Kupffer's cells and, *210*
LM. See Light microscopy (LM).
Lobule, hepatic vs. portal, as unit of hepatic function, 208, *209*
　of breast, *299*, 301
Long bone, cartilage "model" of, 68
Longitudinal folds, of esophagus, *189*
　of stomach, *191*
Longitudinal muscle bundles, of ureter, *224*
Longitudinal muscle layer, of appendix, *201*
　of bladder wall, *225*
　of duodenum, *197*
　of small intestine, *197–198*
　of stomach wall, *198*
　of vas deferens, *316*
Longitudinal striations, in skeletal muscle, 77, *77*
Loops of Henle, 218–221, *219*
　countercurrent multiplier and exchange mechanisms and, *224*
　vasa recta and, 223, *223*
Loose connective tissue, 42, *42*, 57
　of corpus luteum, *287*
Lumbar vertebra, first, *73*
Lung, *228*. See also specific structure
　APUD cells of, 279t
　blood supply of, 238
　innervation of, 239
　lymphatic vessels of, 238–239
　protective mechanisms of, 238, 238t
　section of, *234*
Lunule, of nail, 169
Luteal phase, of ovarian cycle, uterine changes and, *290*
Lutein cells, 286, *287*
Luteinizing hormone (LH), action and regulation of, 262t

Luteinizing hormone (LH) *(Continued)*
　corpus luteum and, 286, 290, *290–291*
　secreted by adenohypophysis, 264
Lymph, lymphocytes in, 99
Lymph nodes, 143–145, *144–145*
　tissue from, cytologic characteristics of, 150t
Lymph nodules, 143
　of anal canal, *202*
　of appendix, *201*
　of colon, *200*
　of lingual tonsil, *181*
　of small intestine, *197*
　of stomach, *191*
　tissue from, cytologic characteristics of, 150t
Lymphatic capillaries, 168
　in thyroid gland, 270
Lymphatic organs, tissue from, characteristics of, 150t
Lymphatic system, description and functions of, 143
Lymphatic vessels, afferent, *144–145*
　of digestive tract, 203
　of liver, *210*
　of lung, 238–239
　of stomach wall, *198*
　plexus of, in small intestine, *198*
Lymphoblasts, 107
　in lymph nodules, 143
　in thymus, 145
Lymphocyte-activating factor, 150
Lymphocytes, 44, 45–46, *46–47*, 99–100, *99*. See also specific type.
　B. See B lymphocytes.
　classes of, 151
　development of, 107
　immune system and, 151–154, 153t
　in alveolar tissue, *42*
　in blood, 98t
　in dermis, *49*
　in jejunum, *48*
　in small intestine, *199*
　in spleen, *148*
　in thymus, 145
　mature, *108*
　pre-B, *109*
　pre-T, *109*
　T. See T lymphocytes.
Lymphocytic infiltrate, in esophagus, *190*
　in tongue, *181*
Lymphocytopoiesis, 107
Lymphoid stem cell(s), *109*
Lymphoid tissue, 143–149, *143–149*, 150t
　cytologic characteristics of, 150t
　diffuse, 143
　of lymph nodes, 143–145, *144–145*
　of lymph nodules, 143
　of spleen, 147–149, *147–149*
　　accessory, 149
　　cytologic characteristics of, 150t
　of thymus, 145–147, *146*
　of tonsils, 143, *143*
Lymphokine, defined, 150
Lymphokine-activated killer (LAK) cell, 152
Lymphotoxin (TNF-β), 150
Lysosomal glycogen storage disease, 16
Lysosomes, 16, *16–17*
　fusion of, in thyroid cell, 271
　in axons, 116
　in hepatocyte, *208*
　in jejunal epithelium, *198*
　in Paneth's cell, *200*
　in pseudostratified epithelium, *28*
　in "typical" cell, *8*
　primary, *15*

Lysosomes (Continued)
  synthesis of, in thyroid cell, 271
Lysozyme, in mucus of endocervix, 297, 298

M

M–1 (first meiotic division), 313
M line, 84
  in skeletal muscle, 78, 80
Macrocytes, 98
Macrophage colony-stimulating factor (M-CSF), 108
Macrophage-like cells, 163, 164
  immune response and, 151
Macrophages, 43–44, 43, 43–44
  alveolar, interleukin-8 produced by, 150
  in lumen of bronchiole, 234
  in thymus, 146
Macula adherens. See Desmosomes.
Macula densa, of distal convoluted tubule, 222
Macula pellucida, of ovarian follicle, 287
Macula sacculi, 252
Macula utriculi, 252
Major histocompatibility complex (MHC), 151
  restriction of cytotoxic T cells by, 152
Male reproductive system. See also specific structure or process.
  description and functions of, 304, 304
Malleus, 252
Mallory's connective tissue stains, 49
Mallory's hyaline, 19
Malpighian corpuscles, 147, 147, 148. See also Stratum malpighi.
Malpighian layer, of nail bed, 169
Mammalian cell, "typical," 8
Mammary glands, description and function of, 299, 300–301
  inactive, 299–300, 301
  lactating, 301–302, 301
  of pregnancy, 300, 301
Mammillary body, 261
Mammotrophs, of adenohypophysis, 261–262, 263
Manchette, 310
Mandible, 186, 188
Mantle zone, in cortex of lymph node, 145
Manubrium, 73
Marginal (subcapsular) sinus, in tissue from thymus, 150t
  of lymph node, 144, 145
Marginal zone, in spleen, 148
Marrow. See Bone marrow.
Mast cells, 44–45, 45, 270
  in alveolar tissue, 42
  in mesentery, 43
Maternal blood lake, placental, 296, 297
Matrix, germinal, 169, 169
  in mature elastic cartilage, 62
  of hyaline cartilage, 61–62
Matrix space, of mitochondrion, 12, 12
Matrix-forming precursor (MFP), 131
Maturation phase, of spermiogenesis, 309, 310
Maturing face (trans), of Golgi complex, 15–16, 15, 114
Maxilla, 186
M-CSF (macrophage colony-stimulating factor), 108
M-CSF (monocyte colony-stimulating factor), 150
Meckel's cartilage, 60
Median sulcus, of tongue, 180
Mediastinum testis, 304

Medulla, of hair shaft, 171, 171
  of lymph node, 144, 144
  of suprarenal gland, 276–277
  of thymus, 145–147, 146–147
  organized, in tissue from lymph node and thymus, 150t
  renal, 224
Medullary cavity, 68, 71
Medullary cords, in lymph node, 145
Medullary rays, of kidney, 214, 215
Medullary sinus, of lymph node, 144
Megakaryoblast, 108, 109
Megakaryocytes, 44, 102, 102–103, 108
  destruction of, 149
  mature, 109
Megakaryocytopoiesis, 108, 108
Megaloblast, 44, 103, 105
Meibomian glands, 174, 251
Meiosis, in oocyte, 287
  in oogonium, 283
  in seminiferous tubule, 306
  in spermatocyte, 307–308
Meissner's plexus, ganglion cells of, 95
  intestinal tract and, 178
Meissner's tactile corpuscles, 126–127, 127, 165, 166, 167
Melanin granules, in nerve cells, 114, 116
Melanization, 163–164
Melanocytes, 162–163, 162–163
  of iris, 58
  of retina, 29, 48, 246, 247
Melanocyte-stimulating hormone (MSH), 163
  action and regulation of, 262t
  origin of, 264
Melanocytic nevi, 164
Melanomas, 164
Melanophores, 48
Melanosomes, 162–163, 162–163
Membrana granulosa, of mature ovarian follicle, 284
Membrana preformativa, in developing tooth, 186
Membrane, Bruch's, 246
  Nasmyth's, 187
Membrane pore, of rough endoplasmic reticulum, 13
Membrane protein, inner, in plasma membrane, 9
Membrane structure, fluid-mosaic model of, 9, 9
Membrane trafficking, defined, 11
Membrane transport, 10–11, 11
Membrane-coating granules, 160
Membranous bone, formation of, 66–69, 67
Membranous labyrinth, 252
Membranous ossification, 66–69, 67
Memory, positive and negative, in immunologic response, 151
Memory B cells, 99
  in lymph node, 144
Memory phase, in life of cytotoxic T lymphocyte, 152
  of cellular immune response, 152
Menarche, 292
Meniscus, articular, 74
  tactile, 164
Menopause, 292
Menstrual cycle, 290, 292
  menstrual phase of, 290, 293–294, 294–295
  proliferative phase of, 290, 292–294, 293
  secretory phase of, 290, 293–294, 294
Mercuric chloride, as fixative, 3
Merkel's cells, 164
Merocine secretion, of apocrine glands, 176
Merocrine glands, 37, 37

Mesangial cells, in renal corpuscle, 218
Mesenchymal cells, undifferentiated, 109
Mesenchymal tissue, 58, 58
  of tooth, 185
Mesenchyme, cartilage and bone developing in, 60
  fetal, 296
Mesentery, 43, 178
Mesoappendix, 201
Mesoderm, 42
Mesothelial cells, nuclei of, 43
  vimentin filaments in, 28
Mesothelium, 25
  intestinal tract and, 178
  of duodenal serosa, 197
Messenger RNA (mRNA), 13, 13
Metachromatic staining, 60
  of fibrocartilage, 63
  of mast cells, 44, 45
Metamyelocytes, 106–107, 107
  eosinophilic, 106
Metaphase, 21–22, 23
Metaphysis, of long bone, 68
Metarubricyte, 44, 103, 105, 105
MFP (matrix-forming precursor), 131
MHC (major histocompatibility complex), 151
  restriction of cytotoxic T cells by, 152
Microbodies, 16
Microcyte, 98
Microfibrils, 50, 52
Microfilaments, 16, 18
  in axoplasm, 115
  in myofibrils, 80, 84
Microglia, 118, 118
Microlobule, in gland, 38
Micrometer, defined, 2
Microphonic potential, cochlear, 255
Microscopy, freeze-fracture, 3–4
  limits of resolution in, 2, 3
Microtome, 3
Microtrabecular lattice, 11
Microtubules, 16–18, 18
  in axoplasm, 115
  in seminiferous epithelium, 306
Microvilli. See also Villi.
  in uriniferous tubules, 216, 219
  of columnar epithelium of digestive tract, 27
  of simple gustatory neuroepithelium, 29
  of small intestinal epithelium, 32, 198
  of specialized epithelia, 33
  of stratified columnar epithelium of gland, 31
  of thyroid follicle, 270
  structure and function of, 31, 33
Micturition, 214
Middle ear, 251–252
Middle piece, of spermatozoon tail, 311, 311
Midget bipolar cells, 248
Midget ganglion cells, of retina, 248, 248
Milk secretion, 301–302, 301
Mineralocorticoids, action and regulation of, 275t
Minimyosin, 18
Mitochondria, 12, 12, 83, 114, 123, 125
  in axons, 116, 116
  in cardiac muscle, 89, 91
  in columnar epithelium of digestive tract, 27
  in exocrine pancreas, 207
  in hepatocyte, 208
  in ovarian follicle, 284
  in perikaryon of neuron, 116
  in pseudostratified epithelium, 28
  in salivary gland, 204, 206

Mitochondria *(Continued)*
  in "typical" cell, *8*
Mitochondrial sheath, of fibrous sheath of spermatid, *310*
  of middle piece of spermatozoon tail, 311, *311*
Mitosis, 21–23, *22*
Mitotic division figure, *22*
  in cartilage, 61, *61*
  in intestinal epithelium, *199*
  in late primary ovarian follicle, *284*
Mitral valve, 134
Mixed nerve, 119–120, *120–121*, 120t
Mixed serous and mucous glands, 37–38
MN blood group, 97
Mobility, of immune system elements, 151
Modiolus, of cochlea, *253*
Moles, 164
Moll, glands of, 176
Monoblast, 44, *109*
Monocyte colony-stimulating factor (M-CSF), 150
Monocyte-macrophage, mature, *109*
Monocytes, 43, *44*, 100, *100, 108*
  development of, 107–108, *108*
  in normal adult human blood, 98t
  interleukins produced by, 150
Monocytopoiesis, 107–108, *108*
Monokine, defined, 150
Mononuclear cells, 44, *44*
Monosynaptic stretch reflex, 128
Montgomery, glands of, 173–174
Morula, *294*, 295
Motor end-plate, 124–125, *125, 179*
Motor nerve, defined, 120
Motor unit, defined, 125
Mouth, 178–182, *179–181, 185–187*
mRNA (messenger RNA), 13, *13*
MSH. See *Melanocyte-stimulating hormone (MSH).*
Mucoid connective tissue, 58, *58*
Mucosa, of anal canal, *202*
  of bladder, *225*
  of colon, *191*, 200, *200*
  of digestive tract, *178*
  of esophagus, 189, *189–190*
  of mouth, 178–179, *179*
  of small intestine, 195, *197–198*
  of stomach, *198*
  of trachea, *231*
  of vagina, 298, *298*
Mucosal glands, of prostate, *316*, 318
Mucous cells, in crypt of Lieberkühn, *199*
  in salivary glands, *33*, 203, *204–205*
Mucous epithelium, of pylorus, *196*
Mucous glands, 38, *38*
  of cervix, *297*, 298
  of respiratory tract, secretions of, 238t
  of tongue, 181, *181*
Mucous granules, in salivary gland cell, *204*
Mucous membrane. See *Mucosa.*
Mucous neck cells, of gastric glands, *192*, 193–194, *196*
Mucous surface cells, of gastric glands, *196*
Mucus, composition and function of, 32, *33*
  endocervical, lysozyme in, *297*, 298
  in goblet cell, *28, 198*
  produced by respiratory epithelium, *229*
Multilocular fat cells, 48, *48, 58*
Multipolar neuron, defined, 117
Muscle, bundles of, of ureter, *224*
  contraction of, isometric, *86*
    molecular basis of, 86–88, *86–88*
  fibers of, cardiac, *136, 137*
    heterogeneity of, 83, *83*
    nuclear bag, 128, *128*

Muscle *(Continued)*
  nuclear chain, 128, *128*
  layers of, of duodenum, *197*
    of small intestine, *197–198*
    of stomach wall, *198*
  motor end-plate of, 79, 124–125, *125*
  sensory receptors of, 79
Muscle cells, plasma membrane of, *56*
Muscular (distributing) arteries, 138, *138*
Muscular tissue, 77–95. See also specific muscle type.
  cardiac, 88–91, *88–92*
  myoepithelial, 95, *95*
  skeletal. See *Skeletal muscle.*
  smooth. See *Smooth muscle.*
Muscularis, of bladder, *225*
  of vagina, 298, *298*
Muscularis externa, layers of, of digestive tract, 178, *178*
  of appendix, *201*
  of esophagus, *189*
  of stomach, *191*
Muscularis mucosae, 28
  of colon, *200*, 201
  of esophagus, 189, *189–190*
  of intestinal tract, *178*
  of rectoanal junction, *202*
  of small intestine, *197–198*, 198
  of stomach, *191, 198*
  smooth muscle of, 95
Myasthenia gravis, neuromuscular junction and, 125
Myelin sheath, 116–117, *117, 121,* 125
  degeneration of, *129*
Myelinated nerve fibers, 121–122, *121*
Myeloblasts, *105–106,* 108, *109*
Myelocytes, 44, *106,* 107
Myenteric plexus of Auerbach. See *Auerbach's plexus.*
Myocardial pacemakers, 91, *91–92, 136*
Myocardium, 134, *134*
  ventricular, *92, 136*
Myoepithelial cells, 26, 33–34, *34,* 95, *95*
  of sweat glands, 175, *175–176*
Myoepitheliocytes, *26*
Myoepithelium, 95, *95*
Myofibrils, 79, *80, 83,* 125
  in skeletal muscle, *82*
  thick and thin microfilaments in, *80, 84*
Myofilaments, 80
  in myoepithelial cell, *34*
  in skeletal muscle, *82*
Myoglobin, in red muscle fibers, 83
Myoid cells, of seminiferous tubule, *306*
Myometrium, *283,* 292, *296*
Myoneural junction, 124–125, *125, 179*
Myosin, 18
  molecule of, *80,* 84–85, *84*
Mucous granules, in salivary gland cell, *204*
Myxedema, 55

N

Nabothian cysts, *297,* 298
Nail bed, 169, *169*
Nails, 168–170, *169*
Naris, anterior, *228*
Nasal cavity, *228,* 229–230, *230*
Nasal conchae, 229–230
Nasal fossae, 229, *229*
Nasal sinuses, 230
Nasal vestibule, *228*
Nasmyth's membrane, 187
Nasopharynx, 230
  epithelium in, 228t
Natural killer (NK) cells, 152

Neck, of spermatozoon, 311, *311*
  of tooth, 182
Negative feedback, hormonal, *261*
Negative immunologic memory, 151
Nephron, cortical, *223*
  description and function of, 217, *217–218*
  distal tubule of, *216,* 221
  juxtamedullary, *223*
  loop of Henle of, *219–220,* 220–221
  proximal convoluted tubule of, *216,* 218–220, *219*
Nerve cells, *123*
  body of, retrograde changes in, 129, *129*
  in dermis, *169*
Nerve fascicle(s), *120*
Nerve growth factor (NGF), 130–131
Nerve impulses, conduction of, 122
Nerve supply, to mouth and tongue, 181–182
  to pancreas, 278
Nerves, endings of, encapsulated, 126–129, *127–128*
  free, 126, *126*
  fibers of, axonal transport by, 122, *123*
    characteristic frequency of, 255
    description and functions of, 119–121, *120–121,* 120t
    efferent and afferent endings of, 128, *128*
    impulse conduction by, 122
    in skeletal muscle, 79, *81*
    in taste buds, *242,* 243
    in tongue, *180–181*
    myelinated, 121–122
    unmyelinated, 122
  of lung, 239
  of pineal gland, 267
  of skin, 167
  of vas deferens, 316
  reactions to injury to, 129–132, *129–131,* 131t
Neural tissue, 112–132. See also specific structure.
Neurapraxia, 131
Neurite-promoting factor (NPF), 131
  advance of growth cone and, *130*
Neuroendocrine system. See also *Hypophysis cerebri.*
  diffuse, 279, 279t
Neuroepithelium, *26,* 33, *34*
  locations in body, 26t
  simple gustatory, 29
Neurofibrils, *123*
  in neuron, 114, *115*
Neurofilaments, 19, 19t, 114
  in axoplasm, 115
  in neuron, *116*
Neuroglia, 117–119, *118–119.* See also specific cell.
  of pineal gland, 267, *267*
Neurohypophysis, 260, 265, 265t, *266*
Neurolemma, 121, *121,* 125
Neuroma, 130
Neuromuscular junction, 124–125, *125, 179*
Neuromuscular spindles, in skeletal muscle, 128, *128*
Neuromuscular synapse, 124
Neuronotropic factor (NTF), *123,* 130–131
  advance of growth cone and, *130*
Neurons. See also specific type.
  axon of, 114–117, *117*
  dendrites of, *113,* 117
  description and functions of, 112, *112–113*
  perikaryon of, 112–114, *113–116*
  plasticity of, 132

Neurons (Continued)
  reactions to injury to, 129–132, 129–131, 131t
  sensory, receptor organs of, encapsulated endings of, 126–129, 127–128
    free nerve endings of, 126, 126
Neuropil, 116, 118
Neurosecretory cells, 266
Neurotmesis, 131
Neurotubules, 116
Neutrophilic bands, 106–107
Neutrophilic metamyelocytes, 106
Neutrophilic myelocytes, 106
Neutrophils, 100–101, 100–101, 106–107, 107
  in normal adult human blood, 98t
  mature, 109
Nevi, melanocytic, 164
Nexins, in cilia, 18, 18
Night blindness, 250
Nipple, 299, 300
Nissl bodies, 113–114, 114, 123
  chromatolysis of, 129, 129
NK (natural killer) cells, 152
Nodal fibers, in heart muscle, 91, 91
Node of Ranvier, 116, 121
Nodule, in cortex of lymph node, 144
Nomarski microscopy, 4
Nonfenestrated capillaries, 139, 139
Norepinephrine, epinephrine vs., 275t
  secreted by suprarenal gland, 274–275
Normoblasts, 44, 103, 105, 105
Normochromatic erythroblasts, 105
Nose. See also Nasal entries.
  vestibule of, 228
    epithelium in, 228t
NPF (neurite-promoting factor), 131
  advance of growth cone and, 130
NTF (neuronotropic factor), 123
  advance of growth cone and, 130
Nuclear bag muscle fibers, 128, 128
Nuclear chain muscle fibers, 128, 128
Nuclear envelope, 19, 20
  in "typical" cell, 8
Nuclear lamins, 19, 19t
Nuclear layers, of retina, 247
Nuclear membranes, 19, 20
Nuclear organizer DNA, 21
Nuclear pores, 19, 20
Nucleolus, 20–21, 21
  of epithelial cells of skin, 32
  of epithelium of kidney tubules, 33
  of fibroblast/fibrocyte, 42
  of goblet cell, 198
  of nerve cell, 123
  of neuron, 113, 116
  of oocyte, 284
  of stratified squamous epithelial cells, 160
  of "typical" cell, 8
Nucleolus-associated chromatin, 21
Nucleosome, 20, 21
Nucleotide phosphorylation, in mitochondrion, 12, 12
Nucleus, chromatin of, 19–20, 21
  description of, 19
  envelope of, 19, 20
  geniculate lateral, 251, 251
  in cardiac muscle cells, 88, 89, 92
  in eosinophils, 101
  in epithelial cells, of bladder, 31
    of digestive tract, 27
    of esophagus, 30
    of kidney tubules, 33
    of skin, 32, 160
    specialized, 33
    with stereocilia, 32

Nucleus (Continued)
  in erythroblasts, 97
  in fibroblasts/fibrocytes, 42
  in goblet cells, 198
  in hepatocytes, 208
  in lymphocytes, 99, 99
  in mixed glandular cells of exocrine pancreas, 207
  in monocytes, 100
  in mucous cells of Brunner's gland, 200
  in neurons, 113, 116, 123
    after nerve injury, 129, 129
    multipolar, 115
  in neutrophils, 100, 100–101
  in oocytes, 284
  in ova, 30
  in salivary gland cells, 204
  in Schwann cells, 121
  in secondary ovarian follicle, 285
  in skeletal muscle cells, 81–82, 125
  in smooth muscle cells, 92
  in spermatids, 310
  in taste receptor cells, 29
  in thyroid follicle cells, 268
  isolation of, 7
  phagocytized, 108
Nucleus pulposus, 74–75
Null cells, 99
Nyctalopia, 250

O

Odland bodies, 160
Odontoblasts, 183, 187–188
Oil red O dye, 46
Olecranon bursa, 74
Olecranon process, 74
Olfaction, 241–242, 241
Olfactory epithelium, 26
Oligodendroglia, 116, 118, 118
Olivocochlear bundle of Rasmussen, 254
Oocyte, 284
  capture and transport of, 288–289
  entering oviduct, 294
  nucleus of, 30
  primary, 283
  secondary, 287
Oogonium, 283
Open circulation, in spleen, closed circulation vs., 149, 149
Optic chiasm, 250, 251, 261
Optic nerve, 247, 250–251, 251
Optical microscopy. See Light microscopy (LM).
Ora serrata, 248
Oral cavity, 178–182, 179–181, 185–187
Oral epithelium, 185–186
Oral mucosa, 178–179, 179
Orcein stain, for elastin, 52
Oropharynx, 230
  epithelium of, 228t
Os, external, of cervix, 297
Osmium tetroxide, 46
Osseous labyrinth, 252
Ossification, centers of, primary, 67
  ectopic, 73
  intramembranous, 66–69, 67
  of bones, age at completion of, 69, 70t
  of cartilage, 62, 65–66, 68–70, 69–70
Osteoarthritis, 75
Osteoblasts, 64, 64, 65–66, 65–66, 72
  in developing bone, 70
  in embryonic mesenchyme, 60
Osteoclasts, 64, 64–66, 66, 72
  in developing bone, 70

Osteocytes, 65–66
Osteoid, 65, 65–66
Osteonectin, 55
Osteoprogenitor cells, 65, 69
Ostium, of oviduct, 289
Otolithic membrane, 256
Outer basic lamellae, in cartilaginous bone, 71, 72
Outer membrane, of mitochondrion, 12, 12
Outer nuclear membrane, 20
  rough endoplasmic reticulum and, 14
Oval window, 252, 253
Ovarian cycle, endocrine regulation of, 289–291, 290–291
Ovarian follicle, atretic, 286
  development of, 283, 284
    uterine changes and, 290–291
  primary, 284, 285
  primordial, 283–285, 284
  secondary, 284–285, 285–286
  tertiary, 284, 286
Ovarian ligament, 282
Ovaries, corpus luteum of, 283, 283, 286, 287
  description and functions of, 282–283, 282–283
  follicles of. See Ovarian follicle.
  ovulation and first meiotic division, 286–287
  zona vasculosa of, 138
Oviduct, 282–283, 294
  description and functions of, 287–288, 288
  egg capture and transport in, 288–289
  embryo transport in, 289, 294
  fertilization in, 288, 289
Ovulation, 286–287
  uterine changes and, 290
Ovum, 30, 289
  fertilized, transit of through oviduct, 294, 294
  follicular cells surrounding, 30
Oxyphil cells, of parathyroid gland, 272
Oxytalan, 53
Oxytocin, action and regulation of, 265t
  myometrium and, 292

P

P (protoplasmic) leaflets, of plasma membrane, 9, 9
Pacemakers, myocardial, 91, 91–92, 136
Pachytene spermatocyte (P), 313
Pacinian (Vater-Pacini) corpuscles, 127, 127, 157, 169
Palate, 179, 228
Palatine tonsil, 143, 143, 180
Palpebral conjunctiva, 244
Pancreas, APUD cells of, 279t
  blood and nerve supply of, 278
  exocrine, 206–207, 207
  hormones of, action and regulation of, 277t
  islets of Langerhans of, 276–278, 277t, 278
  endocrine functions of, 259t
Paneth's cell, 200
  in crypt of Lieberkühn of intestine, 196, 199
Papillae, dental, 185–186
  foliate, 180–181
  in dermis of foot, 157–158
  lingual, 180, 180, 181
  of hair, 93, 170
  of renal pyramid, 215
Papillary blood supply to skin, 168
Papillary ducts, of kidney, 215, 220, 223

Papillary ducts *(Continued)*
  countercurrent multiplier and exchange mechanisms and, *224*
Papillary layer, of dermis, 156t, *158*, 165, *165*
Papillary muscles, ventricular, 134, *135*
Papillary plexus, 168
Papillary ridges, 166
Paracrine chemical mediators, 11
Parafollicular cells, 270, *270–271*
Parathyroid glands, 270–272, *272*
  APUD cells of, 279t
  endocrine functions of, 259t
Parathyroid hormone (PTH), 271–272
Parietal cells, of gastric glands, *192–194*, 193
Parietal layer, of renal corpuscle, *216*
Parotid gland, 203–204, *205*
PAS (periodic acid–Schiff) stain. See *Periodic acid-Schiff (PAS) stain.*
Patella, *74*
Pedicels, *217*, 218
Pelvis, of kidney, *214*
Penicillus, of spleen, 149
Penis, *304*, 318–319, *318*
  polsters in, 140–141, *140*
Peptides, in chemical transmission, 124
  synthesis of, on rough endoplasmic reticulum, *13*
Pericardium, 134
Perichondrium, *61*, 69
  hyaline cartilage developing in, *60*
Pericytes, of capillaries, 138
Perikaryon, of a neuron, 112–114, *113–116*
Perilymph, 252
Perimetrium, *283*, 292
Perimysium, 79, *81*
Perineurium, 117, 120, *120–121*
Perinuclear cisterna, 19, *20*
Perinuclear space, rough endoplasmic reticulum and, *14*
Periodic acid–Schiff (PAS) stain, 4
  for cartilage matrix, 62
  for reticular fibers, 52
Periodontal membrane, *183*, 184
Periosteal bud, 69
Periosteal circumferential lamellae, in cartilaginous bone, *71*
Periosteum, 64, *64*, *72*
  formation of, 67
  gingival, *183*
Peripheral blood, cells in, *100–102*
  smear of, 98–99
Peripheral nerve, 119–120, *120–121*, 120t
Peripheral nuclei, in cross section of skeletal muscle, *82*
Peripheral membrane proteins, 10
Peripheral zone glands, of prostate, *316*, 318
Peritoneal cavity, *282*
Peritoneum, 202, *304*
Perivascular cells, in dermis, *49*
Perivascular limiting membrane, 118
Peroxidase labeling, 5
Peroxisomes, 16
Peyer's patches, 154, 197–198
Phaeomelanin, in red hair, 163
Phaeomelanosomes, 163
Phagocytes, wandering, *108*
Phagocytosis, 10–11
  by Sertoli cells, 307
  in spleen, 149
Phagolysosomes, 16, *17*
Phalangeal cells, of organ of Corti, 253, *253–254*
Pharyngeal tonsil, 143
Pharynx, 182, *228*, 230
Phase microscopy, 4

Phospholipids, in plasma membranes, 9, *9*
Phosphorylation, in myoepithelial cells, 95
  in skeletal muscle, 86–88, *86–88*
  in smooth muscle, 93–94
  oxidative, in Golgi complex, *16*
  in mitochondria, 12, *12*
Photosensitive process, 247, *247*
Picric acid, as fixative, 3
Pigment, of hair shaft, *171*
Pigment cells, 48, *48*. See also *Melanization; Melanocytes; Melanosomes.*
Pigment epithelium, 26t, 34
  of iris, *58*, 245
  of retina, *29*, 48, 246, *247*
Pigmented basal cells, *162*, *162*
Pigmented connective tissue, 58, *58*
Pili. See *Hairs.*
Pillar cells, of organ of Corti, 253, *253–254*
Pineal gland, 267, *267*
  APUD cells of, 279t
  endocrine functions of, 259t
Pinealocytes, 267, *267*
Pinocytosis, 103
  defined, 10
Pits, coated, in cell surface, 10, *11*
  gastric, *191*
Pituicyte, of neurohypophysis, 265, *266*
Pituitary gland. See *Hypophysis cerebri.*
Placenta, APUD cells of, 279t
  implantation and formation of, 295–297, *296*
Placental villi, formation of, 297
Plasma, 97, 103
Plasma cells, 44, 46, *47*
  immunoglobulins produced by, 152–153
  in jejunum, *48*
  in lamina propria, *46*
  in lymph node, 144
  mature, *109*
Plasma membrane, 6–11, *8–11*, *14*
  as viewed with electron microscopy, 10, *10*
  carbohydrates of, 10
  description and functions of, 6–9, *9*
  in cell-to-cell communication, 11
  of microvillus, *31*
  of specialized epithelial cells, *33*
  of stratified epithelial cells, *27*, *31*
  transport across, 10–11, *11*
Plasmablasts, *109*
Plasmalemma. See *Plasma membrane.*
Plasmin, 287
Plasminogen, 287
Plasminogen activator, 287
Platelets. See *Megakaryocytes.*
Pleura, visceral, *234*
Plexiform layers of retina, *247*
  synapses in, 248–249
Plica circularis, of small intestine, *197*
Plicae palmatae, of cervix, 297
Pluripotent colony-stimulating factors, 108
PMNs (polymorphonuclear neutrophils). See *Neutrophils.*
Pneumocytes, 233–234, 236, *236–237*
Podocytes, 217–218, *217–218*
Polar body, first, 287
  second, 289
Polsters, in penis, 140–141, *140*
Polychromatic erythroblasts, 105
Polychromatic normoblasts, 105
Polychromatophilic erythroblasts, 105, *105*
Polychromatophilic normoblasts, 105
Polycythemia, 98
Polymorphonuclear neutrophils (PMNs). See *Neutrophils.*

Polyribosomes, 13
Polyspermy, 289
Polysynaptic ganglion cells, of retina, 248, *248*
Pores, in plasma membrane, 9
Portal lobule, triangular, as unit of hepatic function, 208, *209*
Portal vein, *209*
Portal venule, *210*
Positive immunologic memory, 151
Postacrosomal region, of spermatozoon, *311*
Posterior chamber, of eye, 246
Postsynaptic membrane, 125
Postsynthesis phase (G_2), 22, *22*
Potassium bichromate, as fixative, 3
Power stroke, in muscle contraction, 86
Pre-B lymphocytes, *109*
Precapillary sphincter, 138
Precursor cell, single-lineage, *110*
Precursor phase, in life of cytotoxic T lymphocyte, 152
Pre-DNA synthesis phase (G_1), 22, *22*
Prepatellar bursa, *74*
Preprophase, 22
Pre-T lymphocytes, *109*
Prickle cell layer of epidermis. See *Stratum spinosum.*
Prickle cells, *127*, 166
Primary immune response, 153
Primary nodule, in cortex of lymph node, 144, *145*
Primordial follicle, 283
Principal piece, of spermatozoon tail, 311, *311*
Proacrosomal granules, 309
Procollagen, 49–50, *51*
Proerythroblasts, 103, *109*
Proerythrocytes, 105
Profilaggrin, 160
Progenitor osteoblastic cells, 65, 69
Progesterone, implantation and, 292
  mammary gland development and, 301
  secreted by corpus luteum, 286
  uterine changes and, *290*
Progranulocytes, *106*, 107
Prohormones, 266
Prolactin, action and regulation of, 262t
  secreted by adenohypophysis, 263
Proliferative phase, of menstrual cycle, *290*, 292–294, *293*
Promegakaryocytes, 108
Promelanosomes, 163
Promyelocytes, *106*, 107
Pronormoblasts, 103
Pronuclei, *294*
Prophase, 22–23, *22*
  meiotic, in oogonia, 283
Prorubricytes, 103, *105*
Prostaglandins, uterine contractions and, 292
Prostate gland, *304*, 316–317, *317*–318
Prostatic utricle, *304*
Protein envelope, of stratum corneum, 160
Protein hormones, 259, 260t
Proteins, attachment, 17
  follicular regulatory, 286
  in plasma membranes, *9*, 10
  synthesis of, 15, *15*
    hormone-induced, 260
    in thyroid cell, *271*
    on rough endoplasmic reticulum, *13*
Proteoglycan heparan sulfate, 218
Proteoglycans, 54–55, *54–55*
  in cartilage matrix, 62
Protoplasmic astrocytes, 118, *118*
Protoplasmic (P) leaflets, of plasma membrane, *9*

Proximal convoluted tubule, *216*, 218–220, *219*
Pseudopodia, of megakaryocyte, *108*
　of phagocytic histiocyte, *108*
Pseudostratified epithelium, 25, *26*
　simple, of respiratory system, *28*
　sites of, 26t
Pseudo-unipolar neuron, 112
　defined, 117
Pseudoxanthoma elasticum, 52
PTH (parathyroid hormone), 271–272
Pubis, female, *282*
　male, *304*
Pulmonary arteries, 137, *137*
Pulmonary capillary endothelial cells, 236–237, *237*
Pulmonary innervation, 239
Pulmonary surfactant, 235–236
Pulmonary veins, *135*, 238
Pulp, of spleen, 147–149, *147–148*
　of tooth, *183*, 184
　　primordium of, *188*
　white, in tissue from lymphatic organs, 150t
Pulp arterioles, of spleen, 149
Pulp cavity, of tooth, *183*, 184
Pulp veins, of spleen, 149, *149*
Pupil, 245
Purkinje fibers, 91, *92*, 136, *136*
Pyloric antrum, *191*
Pyloric canal, *191*
Pyloric glands, 194, *196*
Pyloric sphincter, *191*
Pylorus, *191*
　mucous epithelium of, *196*
Pyramid, of kidney, *214*, 215

Q

Quadriceps tendon, *74*

R

Radius, *74*
Ranvier, node of, 116, 121, *121*
Rasmussen, olivocochlear bundle of, 254
Receptor cells, of olfactory epithelium, 241, *241*
　of taste buds, 242, *242*
Receptor organs of sensory neurons, description and functions of, 126
　encapsulated endings of, 126–129, *127–128*
　free nerve endings of, 126, *126*
Receptor-mediated endocytosis, 10
Rectoanal junction, *202*
Rectum, 201–202, *202*, *282*
Red area, of lips, 178–179, *179*
Red blood cells. See *Erythrocytes.*
Red muscle fibers, 78, *81*, 83, *83*
Red pulp, of spleen, 147–149, *147–148*
Reflex, monosynaptic stretch, 128
Regulator T lymphocytes, 152
Regulatory phase, of cellular immune response, 152
Reissner's membrane, 252, *253*
Rejection of graft, chronic, cytotoxic T lymphocytes and, 152
Relaxin, corpus luteum and, 286
　uterine cervix and, 292
Renal artery, *214*
Renal column of Bertin, *214*, 215
Renal corpuscle, *216*
Renal filtration barrier, *217*, 218, *218*

Renal vasculature, uriniferous tubules and, 223, *223*
Renal vein, *214*
Renewing cell populations, defined, 22
Renin, 222
Renin-angiotensin-aldosterone mechanism, of blood pressure regulation, 222
Replicability, of cellular immune system components, 151
Reproductive system, female. See also specific structure or process.
　description and functions of, 282, *282–283*
　male. See also specific structure or process.
　description and functions of, 304, *304*
RER. See *Rough endoplasmic reticulum (RER).*
Residual bodies, 16, *17*, 308
　of Regnaud (RB), *313*
　　development of, *310*
　phagocytized by Sertoli cells, 307
Resolving power, of human retina, 2
Resorcin-fuchsin stain, 52–53
Respiratory bronchioles, 233, *234–235*
Respiratory chain ATP production, in mitochondrion, 12, *12*
Respiratory distress syndrome, 236
Respiratory epithelium, 228–229, *229*
　in bronchiole, 233–234
　in bronchus, 232, *232–233*
Respiratory system. See also specific structure.
　description of, 228, *228*
Rete cutaneum, 168
Rete mirabile, *223*
Rete testis, *57*, 304, *304*
Reticular blood supply to skin, 168
Reticular cells, in lymph node, 53
　in thymus, 145–147, *146*
Reticular lamina, 56
Reticular layer of dermis, 156t, 165, *165*, 168
　of foot, *158*
　of scalp, *173*
Reticular plexus, 168
Reticulin, 51
Reticulocytes, 97, *97*, 105
Retina, color vision and, 250
　dark and light adaptation of, 249–250
　layers of, 246–248, *247*
　　ganglion cell, 248
　　limiting membranes, 247–248
　　nuclear, 247–248
　　optic nerve, 248
　　pigment epithelium, *29*, *48*, 246, *247*
　　plexiform, 247–248
　　rods and cones, 246–247, *247–248*
　photochemistry and physiology of, 249
　resolving power of, 2
　structure and blood supply of, 248
　synaptic organization of, 248–249, *248*
Retinal, 247
Retinal epithelium, *29*, *48*, 246, *247*
Retrograde axonal transport, 122, *123*
Retrograde nerve cell changes, 129, *129*
Retzius, incremental lines of, 182, *183*
Rhodopsin, 247
Ribonucleic acid (RNA), 13, *13*
Ribosomal ribonucleic acid (rRNA), 13
Ribosomes, 13, *13*
　in perikaryon of neuron, *116*
　isolation of, *7*
　on rough endoplasmic reticulum, *14*
Ribs, 73
Rigor mortis, 86, *87*
RNA (ribonucleic acid), 13, *13*

Rod bipolar cell, 248
Rods, of retina, *48*, 246–247, *247*, 248
　of tooth enamel, 182
Root, of hair, sheaths of, *171–173*, 172
　of tooth, 182
Rough endoplasmic reticulum (RER), 13–15, *13–14*
　in fibroblast, *51*
　in germ cell, *306*
　in goblet cell, *28*
　in hepatocyte, *208*
　in jejunal epithelial cell, *198*
　in pancreatic acinar cell, *207*
　in Paneth's cell, *200*
　in perikaryon of neuron, *116*
　in salivary gland cell, *204*
　in Sertoli cell, 305
　in "typical" cell, *8*
　melanosome synthesis in, 163
　synthesis of prohormones in, 266
Round ligament, of uterus, *282*
Round window, 252, *253*
rRNA (ribosomal ribonucleic acid), 13
Rubriblasts, 103, *105*
Rubricytes, 105, *105*
Ruffini's corpuscles, 127, *127*
Ruffled border, of osteoclasts, 66
Rugae, of stomach, *191*

S

SA (sinoatrial) node, 91, 136
Saccular glands, 36–37, *36*, 36t
Saccule, of vestibular end organ, 252, *256*
Saliva, 203
Salivary glands, description and functions of, 203, *204*
　ductal system of, 205–206, *206*
　parotid, 203–204, *205*
　striated ducts in, *33*
　sublingual, 205, *205*
　submandibular, 204–205, *205*
Saltatory conduction, 116
Sarcolemma, *83*, *87*, 125, *125*
Sarcomere, *80–81*
　defined, 81
　in rigor mortis, *87*
　in skeletal muscle, 81–82, *82*
　molecular composition of, *84*
Sarcoplasm, 125
Sarcoplasmic reticulum, 15, *83*. See also *Smooth endoplasmic reticulum (SER).*
　in cardiac muscle, 89–90
Scala media, 252–253, *253–254*
Scala tympani, 252, *253–254*
Scala vestibuli, 252, *254*
Scalp, dermis of, *157*
　goose bumps of, *173*
　hypodermis of, *170*
　section through hair follicles, *170*
Scanning electron microscopy (SEM), 3
Scarring, fibrous astrocytes in, 118
Schmidt-Lanterman cleft, *121*, 122
Schwann, sheath of, 121, *121*, 125
Schwann cell (SC), 116, *117*, 121, *121*
　formation of band of Büngner and, 130, *130*
Sclera, *29*, 243–244
Scleral foramen, 244
Scrotum, *304*
Scurvy, 52
Sebaceous glands, of scalp, 93, *170*, 173–174, *173*
Sebum, 173–174
Secondary (flower-spray) afferent nerve fiber endings, 128, *128*

Secondary cortical follicles, of lymph node, 144
Secondary cortical nodules, in cortex of lymph node, *145*
Secondary (wallerian) degeneration, of severed axon, 130, 131t
Secondary immune response, 153
Secretory cells, myoepithelium and, 95, *95*
　of salivary glands, 203, *204*
　of sweat glands, *175*
Secretory ducts, of salivary glands, *133*, 205–206, *206*
Secretory epithelium, of sweat glands, *175–176*
Secretory granules, in Paneth's cell, *200*
Secretory phase, of menstrual cycle, *299*, 293–294, *294*
Secretory vesicles, in axons, 116
　in Golgi apparatus, *15–16*, *114*
　in "typical" cell, *8*
Seddon classification of nerve injury, 131
Segmented granulocytes, *106*, 107
SEM (scanning electron microscopy), 3
Semen, 319
Semicircular canals, *256*
Semilunar fold, of conjunctiva, 244
Semilunar valves, 134, *135*
Seminal vesicle, *304*, 315–317, *317*
Seminiferous epithelium, 305–309, *305–306*, *308*, *310*. See also specific cells.
　cycle and wave of, 311–312, *313*
　description and functions of, 305, *306*
　stages of, *313*
Seminiferous tubules, *57*
　description and functions of, 304–305, *304*
　sperm production in, *306*
　fertility and, 312
Senses, general, description of, 241
　special, 240–257. See also specific sense or structure.
Sensorineural deafness, 255
Sensory cells. See *Neuroepithelium*.
Sensory nerve, defined, 120
　receptor organs of, 126–129, *126–128*
SER. See *Smooth endoplasmic reticulum (SER)*.
Seromucinous gland, bronchial, *232*
Seromucous acini, in submandibular gland, 204, *205*
Seromucous gland, in bronchiole, *233*
Serosa, of appendix, *201*
　of colon, 201
　of intestinal tract, 178, *178*
　of small intestine, *197*, 199
　of stomach, *191*, 195
Serous acini, of lacrimal gland, 251
　of parotid gland, *205*
　of submandibular gland, *205*
　of tongue, *180*
Serous cells, of salivary glands, *33*, 203, *204–205*
Serous demilune, of sublingual gland, *205*
Serous glands, 37, *38*
　of respiratory tract, secretions of, 238t
　of von Ebner, 81, *81*
Sertoli cell, 305–307, *305–306*, *310*, *313*
Serum, 97
　blood, 103
Sex chromatin, 20, 100, *101*
Sharlach R dye, 46
Sheath of Schwann, 121, *121*, 125
Sheathed arterioles, of spleen, 149
Shoulder, skin of, *130*, *157*
Siderosomes, 103
sIg (surface immunoglobulin), 151
Signal sequence, in peptide, 15

Signaling molecules, in tissue fluids, 11
Silver salts, for staining of reticular fibers, 52
Simple epithelium. See under *Epithelium*; specific type.
Simple glands. See also specific gland.
　defined, 37
Single-lineage precursor cell, *110*
Sinoatrial (SA) node, 91, 136
Sinuses, of lymph node, *144*
　of nose, 230
　of spleen, 147–148, *148*
Sinusoidal capillaries, 139, *139*
Sinusoids, hepatic cords and, *209*
　in suprarenal gland, 273–275, *277*
　liver, Kupffer's cells and, *210*
Skeletal muscle, band patterns of, in contraction, 81–82, *82*
　molecular basis of, 79–81, *80–81*
　description and function of, 77, *77–78*
　early observation of, 77
　fibers of, contraction of, molecular basis of, 86–88, *86–88*
　molecular basis of, 84–86, *84–85*
　orientation of, *78*, 81–83, *82–83*
　types of, *78*, 81, 83, *83*
　histologic organizaiton of, 77–79, *78–81*
　of palatine tonsil, *143*
　of tongue, *181*
　striations in, 81–82, *82*
　as seen in modern microscopes, *78*
　in cardiac muscle, 88, *88*
　longitudinal, 77, *77*
　molecular basis of, 79–81, *80–81*
　ultrastructure of, 83–84
Skin. See also *Dermis; Epidermis*.
　aging of, 167
　appendages of, gland, *170*, 173–176, *173–176*. See also specific gland.
　hair, 170–173, *170–173*
　nail, 168–170, *169*
　APUD cells of, 279t
　blood supply to, 168, *168*
　color of, 163, 167
　creases in, 166
　cross section of, *30*
　description and functions of, 156, 156t, *157*
　hypodermis of, 168, *169–170*, *174*
　lines in, 166–167
　lymphatic capillaries of, 168
　nerves of, *157*, 167
　thickness of, 156, *157*
Small intestine, APUD cells of, 279t
　crypts of Lieberkühn of, 196–197, *199–200*
　description of, 195, *197*
　endocrine functions of, 259t
　epithelium of, 195–196, *198–199*
　lamina propria of, 197, *197–198*
　mucosa of, description of, 195, *197–198*
　muscularis mucosae of, *197–198*, 198
　muscularis of, *197–198*, 199
　Peyer's patches of, 197–198
　serosa of, *197*, 199
　submucosa of, *197*, 198–199, *200*
Smell, sense of, 241–242, *241*
Smoker's cough, 232
Smooth endoplasmic reticulum (SER), 13–15, *13–15*
　in axon, *116*
　in germ cells, *306*
　in hepatocyte, *208*
　in intestinal epithelial cells, *198*
　in muscle. See *Sarcoplasmic reticulum*.
　in pigment epithelial cell of eye, *29*
　in Sertoli cells, 305
　in "typical" cell, *8*

Smooth muscle, 92–95
　description and function of, 92–94, *92–94*
　molecular basis of function of, 94
　nerve supply of, 94–95
　of arteriole, *138*
　of artery, 137
　of bronchiole, 233–235
　of bronchus, 232, *232–233*
　of gallbladder wall, *210*
　of lamina propria, *46*
　of large vein, *140*
　of seminal vesicle, *317*
　of small intestine, *199*
　of ureter, 224–225, *224*
Soft palate, 179, *228*
Solenoid, 20
Soleus muscle, *80*
Somatic capillaries, 139, *139*
Somatotrophs, of adenohypophysis, 261, *263*
Specific recognition system, 149
Specificity, of immune system cells, 151
Spectrin, 18
Spermatic cord, 315
Spermatids, *308*, *308*, 309
　in seminiferous tubule, 305–306
　release of as spermatozoa, *310*
　stages of differentiation of, *313*
Spermatocytes, in seminiferous tubule, 306
　primary and secondary, 305, *308*, 309
Spermatogenesis, *306*, *307*, *308*
Spermatogonia, 305–306, *307*, *308*
　types A and B, 308
　types of, *313*
Spermatozoa, 309–311, *311*
　capacitation of, 289
　development of, *308*
　in testis, 305
　production of, fertility and, 312
　receptors for, in zona pellucida of oocyte, 289
Spermiation, 307
Spermiogenesis, 308–309, *308*, *310*
Spiral lamina, osseous, of cochlea, *253*
Spiral ligament, 253, *254*
Spiral prominence, *254*
Spleen, 147–149, *147–149*
　tissue of, cytologic characteristics of, 150t
Spongiosa, 67, *70–72*
Spot desmosomes. See *Desmosomes*.
Squames, epithelial, *30*
　in stratum corneum, 161
　of inner root sheath of hairs, 172
　of nails, 169
Squamous epithelium, 26–27, 28–31, *30*
　defined, 25
　of distal alveolar duct, 233–234
　stratified, *30*, *32*, 34–35
　keratinization of, *161*
　keratinized, *166*
　melanocytes in, *162*
　of esophagus, *189–190*
　of lip, *187*
　of palatine tonsil, 143, *143*
　of tongue, *181*
　prickle cell, *160*
Stable cell population, defined, 21–22
Stains, eosin, 3
　for elastin, 52–53
　for light microscopy, 3
　for peripheral blood smears, 99
　hematoxylin, 3
　Verhoeff's, 52–53
　hematoxylin and eosin, 3
　Mallory's, 49
　orcein, 52
　osmium tetroxide, 46

Stains *(Continued)*
　PAS, 52, 62, 216
　resorcin-fuchsin, Wright's, 52–53
　silver salts, 52
　Sudan black, 4, 46
　Sudan III, 46
　toluidine blue, 4–5, 44, 52–53
Stapedius muscle, 252
Stapes, 252
Static cell population, defined, 21–22
Stato-acoustic epithelium, *26*
Stellate reticular cell, in thymus, 145, *146*
Stellate reticulum, *186*
　in developing tooth, *188*
Stellate vein, of kidney, 215
Stem cells, development of, 108–110, *109–110*
　of thymus, 145
　pluripotent, 44
Stereocilia, of epididymis, 27, *32*
　of vestibular receptor, 256–257, *256*
Sterile matrix, 169
Sternum, *73*
Steroid hormones, 259, 260t
Stomach, 190–195, *190–194*, 195t
　APUD cells of, 279t
　description of, 190, *191*
　glands of, *178*, 192–194, *192–196*. See also specific gland.
　junction of, with esophagus, 190, *190*
　lamina propria of, 191, *191*
　mucosa of, 190–191, *191*
　muscularis mucosae of, 191–192, *192*
　muscularis of, *178*, 194
　serosa of, 195
　submucosa of, 194
　wall of, *198*
Stratified epithelium, *30–32*, 34–35. See also specific type.
Stratum basale, *32*, 34–35, 156–159, 156t, *158–160*
　of endometrium, during menstrual cycle, *293*
Stratum compactum, of placenta, *296*
Stratum corneum, 35, 156, 156t, 160–161, *162*, 165
　basic protein of, 160
　of foot, shoulder, and scalp, *157*
　of scalp, *173*
　of skin of foot, *158*
Stratum disjunctum, of skin of foot, *158*
Stratum germinativum. See *Stratum malpighi.*
Stratum granulosum, 35, 156, 156t, 159–160, *165–166*
　of skin of foot, *158*
　of skin of scalp and foot, *157*
Stratum intermedium, of developing tooth, *187–188*
Stratum lucidum, 156, 156t, 160
　of skin of foot, *157–158*
Stratum malpighi, *165*
　of scalp, *173*
　of skin of foot, *157–158*
Stratum spinosum, *30, 32*, 35, 156, 156t, 159, *159–160*
Stratum spongiosum, of placenta, *296*
Stretch marks, 166–167
Stretch reflex, monosynaptic, 128
Stria vascularis, of cochlea, 253, *254*
Striae, of skin, 166–167
Striated ducts, of salivary glands, *33*, 205–206, *205–206*
Striated muscle. See *Cardiac muscle; Skeletal muscle.*
Striations, basal, in ducts of parotid gland, *205*

Striations *(Continued)*
　in cardiac muscle, 88, *88, 136*
Stroma, endometrial, 292
　of iris, 245
Stromal cell, *284*
Subcapsular epithelium, of eye, 246
Subcapsular sinus, of lymph node, *144, 145*
Subcutaneous tissue, 168, *169–170, 174*
Subendocardium, 134
Subepicardial space, 134, *134*
Sublingual gland, 205, *205*
Submandibular gland, 204–205, *205*
Submucosa, 28
　of appendix, *201*
　of bladder wall, *225*
　of bronchus, *232*
　of colon, *200,* 201
　of digestive tract, 178, *178*
　of duodenum, *197*
　of esophagus, 189, *189–190*
　of small intestine, *197–198,* 198–199
　of stomach, *191,* 194, *198*
Submucosal glands, of prostate, *316,* 318
Subneural sarcolemma, 125
Subpapillary blood supply, to skin, 168
Subpapillary rete, 168
Subpatellar fat, *74*
Substantia propria, of cornea, 245
Sudan black dye, 4, 46
Sudan III dye, 46
Sunderland classification, of nerve injury, 131, 131t
Superficial dorsal vein, of penis, *318*
Superficial plexus, 168
Supporting cells, in olfactory epithelium, 241, *241*
　in taste buds, 242–243, *242*
Suppressor T lymphocytes, 99
Suprarenal glands, blood supply of, 275–276, *277*
　cortex of, 273–274, *273–275*
　　endocrine functions of, 259t
　　hormones of, 274, 275t
　description of, 272
　fetal, *273*
　histologic features of, 272–273, *273, 277*
　medulla of, 274–275, 275t, *276*
　　APUD cells of, 279t
　　endocrine functions of, 259t, 275t
Surface epithelium, of colon, *200*
　of intestine, *198*
Surface immunoglobulin (sIg), 151
Surface membrane protein, in plasma membrane, *9*
Surface mucous cells, of pylorus, *196*
Surfactant, pulmonary, 235–236, *237*
Suspensory ligament, of lens, 246
Sustentacular cells, of tongue, *181*
　Sertoli cells as, 305–306
Suture, of skull, *73*
Sweat glands, 37, *37,* 93
　and duct, *166*
　apocrine, 175–176, *176*
　description of, *163,* 174, *175*
　eccrine, *170,* 174–176, *174–175*
　of scalp, *170*
　of skin of foot, *157–158*
Sympathetic ganglia, APUD cells of, 279t
Symphysis pubis, *74*
Synapses, degeneration of, after nerve injury, 129, *129*
　description and function of, 122–124, *123–124*
　in retina, 248–249, *248*
　neuromuscular junction, 124–125, *125*
Synapsins, 124

Synaptic vessel, 125
Synaptobrevin, 124
Synaptophysin, 124
Synarthroses, 73–74, *73*
Synchondroses, 73
Syncytiotrophoblast layer, of chorionic villus, *296*
Syncytiotrophoblasts, 295
Syndesmoses, 73, *73*
Syngamy, 289
Synostoses, 73–74
Synovial fluid, 75
Synovial fold, *74*
Synovial membrane, *74,* 75
Synthesis phase, 22, *22*
Systole, 137

T

T_3 (triiodothyronine), 269, 269t, *271*
T_4 (thyroxine), 269, 269t, *271*
T helper (Th) lymphocytes, 152
T lymphocytes, 45, *47,* 99, 107, *109,* 151–152
　B lymphocytes and, 153–154
　interleukins produced by, 150
　mature, 146–147
　phases of action of, in immune response, 152
T suppressor (Ts) lymphocytes, 152
T system, in striated cardiac muscle, 89–90
Tactile corpuscles, Meissner's, 126–127, *127*
Tail, of spermatozoon, *311*
Target organ, defined, 259
Tarsal glands, 174, 251
Taste, 242–243, *242*
Taste buds, 180, *180–181,* 242–243, *242*
　in stratified squamous epithelium, *29*
Taste cell, *181*
Taste pore, *29, 181*
Tattooing, 165
Tawara, node of, 91, *91, 136, 136*
Tay-Sachs disease, 16
Tc (cytotoxic T) lymphocytes, 152
TCA cycle, in mitochondrion, *12*
T-cell growth factor (interleukin-2), 150
T-cell receptor (TCR), 151
Tdh (delayed-type hypersensitivity) T lymphocytes, 152
Tear film, 245
Tectorial membrane of cochlear duct, 253–254, *253–254*
Teeth, attachment of gingiva to, *183,* 184
　cementum of, *183,* 184
　　deposition of, 188, *189*
　dentin in, 182–184, *183*
　　formation of, 186–187, *187–188*
　description of, 182, *183*
　development of, 184–186, *185–188*
　enamel of, 182
　enamel organ of, enamel deposition and, 187–188, *188*
　periodontal membrane and, *183,* 184
　pulp and pulp cavity of, *183,* 184
Tela subcutanea, 168, *169–170,* 174
Telodendria, of axons, 116
Telogen, 172
Telophase, *22,* 23
TEM (transmission electron microscopy), 3
Tendon organs of Golgi, 128–129, *128*
Tension receptor organ, *79*
Tensor tympani muscle, 252
Terminal bar. See *Adhesion belt.*
Terminal bronchioles, Clara's cells in, 232
Terminal button, *123*
Terminal capillaries, of spleen, 149

Terminal web. See *Adhesion belt.*
Territorial matrix, 62
Testis, 304, *304*
Tetanic contraction, 77
Tetraiodothyronine (T$_4$), 269, 269t, *271*
TGF-α (transforming growth factor-α), 151
TGF-β (transforming growth factor-β), 151
Th (T helper) lymphocytes, 152
Theca folliculi, *30*, *284–285*, 285
Theca lutein cells, 286, *287*
Thiamine pyrophosphatase activity, in Golgi apparatus, *114*
Thick filaments, 84–86, *84*
Thin filaments, 84–85, *85–86*
Thoracic vertebra, first, *73*
Thrombus, 102
Thymus, *135*, 145–147, *146*
  interleukin–7 produced by, 150
  tissue from, cytologic characteristics of, 150t
Thyrocalcitonin, action and regulation of, 269t
Thyroglobulin, *38*
  colloidal iodinated, *268*, *271*
Thyroid cartilage, 230, *231*
Thyroid cell function, 269, *271*
Thyroid gland, 267–270, *268*, 269t, *270–271*
  APUD cells of, 279t
  endocrine functions of, 259t
  follicular cells of, *38*, 269–270, *271–272*
  hormones of, 269t
  parafollicular cells of, 270, *271*
Thyroid-stimulating hormone (TSH), 262t, *263*
Thyrotrophs, of adenohypophysis, 262–263, *263*
Thyroxine (T$_4$), 269, 269t, *271*
Tibia, *74*
Tight junctions. See *Gap junctions.*
Tissue, preparation of, for electron microscopy, 3–4
  for light microscopy, 2–3
TNFs (tumor necrosis factors), 150
Toenails. See *Nails.*
Tolerance, acquired, 151
Toluidine blue stain, 4–5, 44
  for elastin, 52–53
Tomes' fibers, 184, 186
Tomes' granular layer, *183*
Tongue, 85–86, 180–182, *180–181*
Tonofibrils, 35
Tonofilaments, *159*
Tonsils, lingual, *180–181*
  palatine, 143, *143*, *180*
  tissue from, cytologic characteristics of, 150t
Tooth. See *Teeth.*
Touch receptors, 126–127, 165, *166*, 167
Toxic granules, of neutrophils, 101
Trabeculae, in bone, *71*
  development of, *65*
  in lymph node, *144*
  in penile tissue, *140*
  in red pulp of spleen, *147*
Trabecular veins, in red pulp of spleen, *147*
Trachea, *228*, 231, *231*
  epithelium of, 228t
Trans face, of Golgi complex, 15–16, *15*, *114*
Transfer RNA (tRNA), 13
Transforming growth factors (TGFs), 150–151
Transitional epithelium, 26, 26t, *31*, 35, 223–224
  of bladder, *225*
  of ureter, *224*
Transmembrane protein, in plasma membrane, *9*, 10

Transmission electron microscopy (TEM), 3
Transmitter substances, in chemical synapses, 124
Transneural degeneration, 130
Transverse acetabular ligament, *74*
Transverse tubules, *83*
Tricuspid valve, 134
Triiodothyronine (T$_3$), 269, 269t, *271*
tRNA (transfer RNA), 13
Trochanter, greater, *71*
Trochlea, *74*
Trophoblasts, 295
Tropocollagen, 49–50, *50–51*
  molecular structure of, 52, 61
Tropoelastin, 53, *54*
Tropomyosin, *84*, 85
Troponin, *84*, 85
Ts (T suppressor) lymphocytes, 152
TSH (thyroid-stimulating hormone), 262t, *263*
Tubal pregnancy, 288
Tuber cinereum, *261*
Tubular glands, 36, *36*, 36t
Tubules, of kidneys, *216–220*, 217–222, *224*
  straight, of testis, 304, *304*
Tubulin, 16, *18*
Tubuloalveolar glands, 36t
Tumescence, of penis, 319
Tumor necrosis factors (TNFs), 150
Tunica adventitia, of artery, *137*, *137*
  of large vein, *140*, *140*
Tunica albuginea, of ovary, 283
  of penis, 318, *318*
  of testis, *57*, 304, *304*
Tunica intima, of artery, *137*, *137*
  of large vein, *140*, *140*
Tunica media, of artery, *137*, *137*
  of large vein, *140*, *140*
Tunica muscularis, of colon, *200–201*, 201
  of small intestine, *197–198*, 199
  of stomach, *178*, 194
Tunica serosa, of colon, *200*
Tunica vaginalis testis, *304*
Tunnel, of cochlear duct, *254*
Twitch contraction, 77
Tympanic membrane, 251
Tympanic reflex, 252
Tyson, glands of, 174

U

Ulna, *74*
Ultimobranchial body, APUD cells of, 279t
Ultramicrotome, 3
Ultraviolet light, melanization and, 164
Unilocular fat cells, 46–48, *48*
Unipolar neuron, 112
Unit membrane, 10, *10*
Unmyelinated nerve fibers, 122
Ureter, *214*, *224*, *304*
  fetal, *273*
Urethra, 225–226
  female, *282*
  male, *140*, *304*
    cross section of, *316*, *318*
Urinary bladder, female, 225, *225*, *282*
  epithelium of, *31*
  male, *304*
Urinary space, of renal corpuscle, *216*, 217
Urinary tract. See also specific structure.
  lower, clinical considerations for, 226
  description and function of, 223
  epithelium of. See *Transitional epithelium.*
  urethra in. See *Urethra.*

Urinary tract *(Continued)*
  wall of, 224–225, *224*
Urine, concentration of, 223, *223–224*
  production of, 215–216
Uriniferous tubules, *219*, 221–222
  description and function of, 217, *219*
  nephron and, *216–220*, 217–221
  renal vasculature and, 223, *223*
Uroepithelium. See *Transitional epithelium.*
Urogenital tract, APUD cells of, 279t
Uterine cervix, *282–283*, 292, *297*, 297–298
Uterus, *283*, 291–292, *293*
  changes in, during menstrual cycle, *290*, *293*
Utricle, of inner ear, 252, *256*
  of prostate, *304*
Uvea, 245–246

V

Vagina, *282–283*, 298, *298*
Vallate papillae of tongue, 242
Valves, in afferent lymphatic vessels, *145*
  in small and medium-sized veins, 140
  mitral, 134
  tricuspid, 134
Vas deferens, 315, *316*
Vasa recta, 215, 216, 220
  countercurrent multiplier and exchange mechanisms and, *224*
  loops of Henle and, *223*
Vasa vasorum, 137
  of large veins, *140*, *140*
Vascular channels, in endocrine glands, *38*
Vascular smooth muscle fibers, 94–95
Vasectomy, 315
Vater-Pacini corpuscles, 127, *127*, *157*, *169*
Veins, 139–141, *140*
  central, of liver lobule, *207*
  collecting, of spleen, *149*
  of intestinal villus, *198*
  of kidney, 215–216, *216–217*, 220, *223*
  of rectoanal junction, *202*
  of ureter, *224*
  trabecular, of spleen, *147*
Vellus hairs, 173
Vena cava, 140
Venous sinuses, in penile tissue, *140*
  in red pulp of spleen, 147–148, *148*
Ventricles of heart, *135*
Venules, 140
  portal, *210*
Verhoeff's hematoxylin stain, for elastin, 52–53
Vermiform appendix, 201, *201*
Vertebra(e), *73*
  body of, *74*
Vestibular end organ, *256*
Vestibular folds, 230, *231*
Vestibular membrane, *254*
Vestibular sensation, system for, 252, 255–257, *256*
Vestibule, nasal, *228*, *229*
Villi. See also *Cilia; Microvilli.*
  of duodenum, *191*, *197*
  of placenta, *296*
  formation of, *297*
  of small intestine, *197*
Vimentin filaments, in mesothelia and endothelia, 28
  tissue distribution of, 19t
Visceral capillaries, 139, *139*, *270*
Visceral pleura, *234*
Visceral smooth muscle, 94–95

Visceral striated muscle, 77
Vision, 243–244. See also *Eye;* specific structure.
Visual cortex, *251*
Visual pathways, 250–251, *251*
Vitamin B_{12} deficiency, 98
Vitreous body, 246
Vitreous membrane, of hair follicle, *171–172*, 172
Vocal apparatus, 230–231, *231*
Volkmann's canal, *71*
Vulva, 300

W

Wallerian degeneration, 130, 131t
Wandering cell, in respiratory epithelium, *229*
Wave, of seminiferous epithelium, 311–312, *313*
Wharton's jelly, 58
White blood cells. See *Leukocytes.*
White muscle fibers, *78, 81,* 83, *83*
White pulp, of lymphatic organs, 150t
of spleen, 147–149, *147–148*
Windows, of cochlea, 252, *253*
Woven bone, 67
Wright's resorcin-fuchsin stain, 52–53

X

X chromosome, *101*
Xyphoid process, *73*

Z

Z lines, in cardiac muscle, *91*
in skeletal muscle, *78, 80–84,* 81–82
Zenker-formol fixative, 3
Zona adherens, *31*
Zona fasciculata, of suprarenal cortex, 273, *274,* 276, *277*
Zona glomerulosa, of suprarenal cortex, 273, *273,* 276, *277*
Zona occludens, of plasma membrane, *31*
Zona pellucida, *30*
of oocyte, *284,* 285, 289
Zona reticularis, of suprarenal cortex, 274, *275,* 276, *277*
Zona vasculosa, of ovary, *138*
Zonula adherens. See *Desmosomes.*
Zonula ciliaris, 246
Zygote, 289
Zygotene spermatocyte, *313*
Zymogen granules, in exocrine pancreas, *207*
in serous secretory cell of salivary gland, *204*

Illustration Credits

The authors gratefully acknowledge the sources listed below for allowing us to modify and redraw the following figures:

Figures 1–2, 1–5, and 12–7, kind courtesy of Don W. Fawcett, M.D.

Figures 1–4 and 16–12 from Ham, A.W.: Histology, 6th edition. Philadelphia, J. B. Lippincott Company, 1969.

Figures 1–6, 12–8, 16–4, 16–8, 17–6, and 17–10 from Fawcett, D. W.: Bloom and Fawcett, A Textbook of Histology, 12th edition. New York, Chapman & Hall, 1994.

Figure 1–21 from Alberts et al: Molecular Biology of the Cell, 2nd edition. New York, Garland Publishing, Inc., 1989.

Figure 1–24 from Young, R. W.: Cell proliferation and specialization during endochondral osteogenesis in young rats. J. Cell Biol. 14:357–370, 1962.

Figures 12–1A and 12–1C from Gray's Anatomy, 27th edition. Malvern, PA, Lea & Febiger, 1959.

Figures 12–2 and 12–11 from Hammersen, F.: Sobotta/Hammersen, Histology—A Colour Atlas of Cytology, Histology and Microscopic Anatomy. Malvern, PA, Lea & Febiger, 1976.

Insets for Figures 12–3, 12–4, 12–6, and 12–11 from Lentz, T. L.: Cell Fine Structure. Philadelphia, W. B. Saunders Company, 1971.

Figure 12–5 from Kanwar, Y. S., and Farquhar, M. G.: Anionic sites in the glomerular basement membrane. J. Cell Biol. 81:137–153, 1979.

Figure 12–6 from Bevelander, G., and Ramaley, J. R.: Essentials of Histology, 8th edition. St. Louis, Mosby–Year Book, Inc., 1979.

Figures 16–9 and 16–16 from Van de Graaff, K.: Human Anatomy, 2nd edition. Dubuque, IA, William C. Brown Publishing Co., 1988.

Figure 16–10 from Martini, F.: Fundamentals of Anatomy and Physiology. Englewood Cliffs, NJ, Prentice-Hall, Inc., 1992.

Figures 16–11, 16–14, 16–15, and 16–18 from di Fiori, M.: Atlas of Normal Histology, 6th edition. Malvern, PA, Lea & Febiger, 1989.

Figure 16–13 from Duplessis, G. D. T., and Haegel, P.: Embryologie. New York, Springer-Verlag, 1972.

Figures 16–13, insets A to C, 17–16, and 17–17 from Bergman, R. A., Afifi, A. K., and Heidger, P. M. Atlas of Microscopic Anatomy: A Companion to Histology and Neuroanatomy, 2nd edition. Philadelphia, W. B. Saunders Company, 1989.

Figure 16–19 from Neville, M. C., et al.: *In* Lactation: Physiology, Metabolism and Breast-feeding. New York, Plenum Press, 1983.

Figure 17–7 from Fawcett, D. W., Anderson, W. A., and Phillips, D. M.: Dev. Biol. 26:220, 1971.

Figure 17–8 from Fawcett, D. W. *In* Segal, S. J., et al., eds.: The Regulation of Mammalian Reproduction. Springfield, IL, Charles C Thomas, 1973.